Feature Boxes

"Neuropsychological Celebrity"

Rather than focus on important researchers in the field, these boxes highlight famous **case studies relevant to the material.** They provide fascinating and valuable insights into the functioning of the human brain and add a more engaging and personal approach.

Neuropsychological Celebrity

Anosognosic Woman Examined by P. H. Sandifer

In July 1945, a 66-year-old woman was admitted to

Examiner: "Now give me your left hand."
(Patient presented the right hand again.)
The right hand was then held. (by the examiner)
Examiner: "Give me your left hand."
(Patient looked puzzled and moved neither arm.)
Examiner: "Is anything wrong with your left hand?"
Patient: "No doctor."

"Current Controversy"

Found throughout the text, these features highlight **more general questions in neuropsychology,** such as ethical issues, general philosophical issues, and issues of current debate in the field. "Current Controversy" features allow the reader to apply the concepts as well as use critical thinking skills.

Current Controversy

Are you really born with all the neurons that you will ever have?

The regeneration of damaged cells is something that we take for granted. A small cut on the hand typically heals quickly and without incident, leav-

is one site in the adult human brain, the hippocampus, that appears to generate new neurons regularly (Eriksson et al., 1998). As you learned earlier in this chapter, the hippocampus appears to play an important role in memory, although it is not the storage site for memories. The hippocampus is also extremely vulnerable to damage from a stroke, so its

---

"Real World"

Students can put the material into context with these thought-provoking boxes. Each one addresses a **question drawn from real-life experiences** that will be familiar to many students, drawing the information out of the text and into an approachable framework.

---

the **Real** world

Mad Cow Disease

Bovine spongiform encephalopathy (BSE), widely known as "mad cow disease" was first noticed in the United Kingdom in 1986 and has affected over 200,000 cattle worldwide. BSE is a degenerative prion-based neuropathy that affects the central nervous systems of cattle. There are a number of prion diseases, including

Neuropsychology

Neuropsychology
Clinical and Experimental Foundations

Lorin J. Elias
University of Saskatchewan

Deborah M. Saucier
University of Saskatchewan

PEARSON

Boston • New York • San Francisco
Mexico City • Montreal • Toronto • London • Madrid • Munich • Paris
Hong Kong • Singapore • Tokyo • Cape Town • Sydney

Executive Editor: Karon Bowers
Editorial Assistant: Deb Hanlon
Executive Marketing Manager: Pamela Laskey
Editorial Production Service: Omegatype Typography, Inc.
Composition Buyer: Linda Cox
Manufacturing Buyer: JoAnne Sweeney
Electronic Composition: Omegatype Typography, Inc.
Interior Design: Carol Somberg
Cover Administrator: Linda Knowles

For related titles and support materials, visit our online catalog at
www.ablongman.com.

Between the time website information is gathered and then published, it is not unusual
for some sites to have closed. Also, the transcription of URLs can result in typographi-
cal errors. The publisher would appreciate notification where these errors occur so that
they may be corrected in subsequent editions.

Library of Congress Cataloging-in-Publication Data

Elias, Lorin J.
  Neuropsychology : clinical and experimental foundations / Lorin J. Elias, Deborah M.
Saucier.— 1st ed.
      p.   cm.
  Includes bibliographical references and index.
  ISBN 0-205-34361-9
    1. Neuropsychology. 2. Clinical neuropsychology. 3. Brain damage. I. Saucier, Deborah
M. (Deborah Michelle). II. Title
QP360.E435 2006
612.8'2—dc22
                                                            2005051341

Printed in the United States of America

10 9 8 7 6 5 4 3 2 1   10 09 08 07 06 05

To Phil and Doreen

Brief Contents

Contents

ix

Unit
II

Functional Systems and Associated Disorders

5 | **The Sensorimotor System**   139

6 | **Sensation and Perception: Vision**   **177**

11 | Attention and Consciousness   345

16 | Recovery of Function   468

Preface

Like so many textbooks, this one was born out of frustration rather than a deep desire to spend years working on a project of this scale. Both of us were teaching neuroscience courses with the available textbooks, and we found that our course outlines read like a puzzle: Read Chapter 1, then Chapter 13, then Chapters 8, 9, 11, and 18–22, but read pages 453–459 of Chapter 26 with Chapter 18, pages 459–463 of Chapter 26 with Chapter 19, and so on. Most neuroscience textbooks separate discussions of structure and function, often by hundreds of pages. Even worse, most discuss intact functional systems in one chapter but detail what happens when the system is broken in a different chapter. This type of organization makes the material more difficult to learn and more difficult to teach.

A second frustration that we shared was that the available neuropsychology textbooks generally fell into two groups: those that emphasized clinical neuropsychology and those that emphasized experimental neuropsychology. Neither one of these perspectives is more important than the other, and ideally, the two perspectives should be balanced within the same book.

We were fond of many of the features that are commonly included with current introductory psychology textbooks, such as interim summaries, self-tests, and sections that related the material to the student's daily life. We wished that a neuroscience textbook was available with these same beneficial features. Eventually, we chose to try to create a book that was well organized, balanced, and easy to read and relate to. The product of our efforts is now in your hands.

Organization of This Book

We took a primarily functional approach when organizing this book, grouping most of the chapters by functions such as visual perception, language, and memory. Within each chapter, we discuss both intact and lesioned/dysfunctional systems (e.g., discussing the visual perceptual system and visual agnosias within the same chapter). Further, each chapter is organized into two or three related, self-contained modules. Each module opens with a brief description of what is to come in the module, and each module ends with a summary of the significant concepts contained within the subunit. Although this approach is not unique in psychology textbooks, these features do not appear within the currently available neuropsychology textbooks. In terms of balance, we sought to incorporate representative clinical and experimental content. Even the title of our book, *Neuropsychology: Clinical and Experimental Foundations,* was meant to reflect this balance.

Pedagogical Aids

There are a number of features that appear throughout the book. These are meant to engage, to inform, and, in some cases, to help students study as they read the book.

Neuropsychological Celebrity: Some neuroscience textbooks feature interviews with "neuroscience celebrities," namely, researchers who have made major contributions to their field of study. However, we believe that neuropsychology is unique in that the real celebrities are not the researchers, but the remarkable people whom neuropsychologists study. So much of neuropsychology has been founded on famous case studies (see the two volumes of Code et al.'s *Classic Cases in Neuropsychology* for more examples). We have provided descriptions of topical case studies in most chapters to engage the student and put a human face on the conditions (abilities and disabilities) being described.

The Real World: These feature boxes focus on questions drawn from real-life and familiar experiences. Each feature box is directly related to the material in the chapter in which it appears and is meant to make the material relevant to the student's own life. For an example, see the "Real World" section in Chapter 10 about how people give directions to others.

Current Controversy: These feature boxes highlight more general questions in neuropsychology. The questions include ethical issues, more general philosophical issues, and issues of current debate in neuropsychology. They are meant to enhance critical thinking with respect to issues in neuropsychology, to integrate the material among the chapters and modules, to place the study of neuropsychology within society, and to help the student develop a larger perspective of brain and brain function. For an example, see the discussion of nutriceuticals in Chapter 7.

Self-Tests: These short quizzes are designed to help gauge mastery of the material, encourage independent learning, and enhance critical thinking skills. Two to four quizzes appear in most chapters, and answers to the questions can be found in the instructor's manual.

We hope that you find this book both useful and enjoyable. Your feedback is more than welcome; we can be contacted via e-mail at: Lorin.Elias@Usask.ca or Deb.Saucier@Usask.ca.

Acknowledgments

This project was dependent on the efforts of many, and the names of only two of these people appear on the cover. In this section, we attempt to thank all of those who helped this project from concept to completion.

Students motivated this project, and they also contributed to its development. Among these were Alastair MacFadden, Kate Goodall, Karen Gilleta, Laurie Sykes Tottenham, Brent Robinson, Marla Pender, Marianne Hrabok, Josh Gitlin, Kelly Suschinsky, Nicole Thomas, Crystal Ehresman, Jennifer Burkitt, Avril Keller, and numerous sections of Psychology 246.3 at the University of Saskatchewan.

Our colleagues here and around the world also made very valuable contributions, including Barbara Bulman-Fleming, Mike Dixon, Tom Wishart, Margaret Crossley, William Calvin, and Mel Feany. The following reviewers provided helpful comments on the manuscript: Mark S. Aloia, Brown University; Ruth Ann Atchley, University of Kansas; Stephen C. Chamberlain, Syracuse University; Paul J. Currie, Barnard College, Columbia University; Dr. Rosemary Fama, SRI International; Deborah Fein, University of Connecticut; Lisa Goehler, University of Virginia; Ken Green, California State University, Long Beach; Dr. Thomas Guilmette, Providence College; Dr. Kaira Hayes, Fort Hayes State University; Charles Long, University of Memphis; Vedran Lovic, University of Toronto at Mississauga; J. V. Lupo, Creighton University; Antoinette Miller, Clayton College and State University; Lisa Partlo, University of Calgary; Patricia A. Rueter-Lorenz, University of Michigan; Bonnie Sherman, St. Olaf College; Patti Simone, Santa Clara University; Jim Tanaka, University of Victoria, British Columbia; Alexander Troster, University of Washington; Christine Wagner, University of Albany; and Anastasia Yasik, Pace University. Many talented artists are featured in this book, including Paul Janzen. Duncan Mackinnon at Pearson Canada got the ball rolling for us, and an excellent team at Allyn and Bacon picked it up and did a most efficient and wonderful job, including Karon Bowers, Deb Hanlon, Carolyn Merrill, Lara Torsky, Susan Hartman, Kelly May, Adam Whitehurst, Marlana Voerster, Lara Zeises, and Jonathan Bender.

Perhaps most of all, we should thank our families. Living with someone who is writing a book is like taking in a new family member, and this new member is quite needy, impolite, resource intensive, and generally unrewarding. We thank our families for tolerating us through this process and welcoming this manuscript into their lives. We think it was worth it, and we hope you do too.

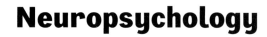

Neuropsychology

1

Introduction to Neuropsychology

I used to think that the brain was the most wonderful organ in my body.
Then I realized who was telling me this.

—EMO PHILLIPS

MODULE **1.1**

Introduction to Neuropsychology

The 10% Myth

Have you ever heard the claim that humans use only 10% of their brain? When people find out that I study the brain, I am often asked this question, and I usually reply, "There is no evidence to suggest that there is any part of your brain that you do not use." Admittedly, this answer is somewhat of a cop-out. After all, there is a big difference between claiming that humans use their brains to their fullest potential and claiming that all parts of the brain are used for at least some functions.

The mythical claim that humans use only 10% of their brain has unknown origins, although both Marie-Jean-Pierre Flourens (1794–1867) and Karl Lashley (1890–1958) performed experiments that involved damaging or removing large portions of brain of animals. Following these procedures, the animals were observed, and often the animals could still perform basic functions—even when they had sustained injury to as much as 90% of their brain. These results apparently led others to the overinterpretation (and exaggeration) that the animals used only 10% of their brains, a finding that was then generalized to humans. Throughout the years, a number of prominent individuals, including William James (1842–1910), Albert Einstein (1879–1955), and Margaret Mead (1901–1978), have been quoted as stating that humans use only a very small portion of their brains, which no doubt increased the popularity of the 10% myth.

Of course, this is only a myth, and throughout this book, we will be documenting the role that the brain plays in producing human behavior. Although not every morsel of the brain will be discussed in exhaustive detail, we will pass the 10% mark early in Chapter 2!

WHERE WE ARE GOING ➤ The following sections describe the domain and goals of neuropsychology. Although the brain is currently regarded as the source of thought and behavior, early investigators attributed these functions to other organs of the body. In addition to describing these attributions and their impact on popular culture, we will introduce the mind–body problem that still plagues philosophers and psychologists today.

What Is Neuropsychology?

Broadly defined, **psychology** is the study of behavior. More specifically, psychology is an attempt to describe, explain, and predict behavior. In some cases, psychology is also the study of how to change behavior. **Neuropsychology** is a speciality within the larger field of psychology. Neuropsychology is also the study of behavior; neuropsychologists attempt to describe, explain, predict, and change behavior. However, neuropsychology is the study of the relation between behavior and the activity of the brain. Implicit within this definition is the assumption that an individual's behavior is at least in part the result of the activity in the brain. As you will discover in detail in Chapter

15, there are two main types of neuropsychologists. **Clinical neuropsychology** is "the branch of neuropsychology concerned with psychological assessment, management, and rehabilitation of neurological disease and injury" (Beaumont, 1996, p. 525). This is qualitatively different from **experimental neuropsychology** in that this branch focuses on how human behavior arises from brain activity, which includes explaining how patterns of behavioral impairments can be explained in terms of disruptions to the damaged neural components. Experimental neuropsychology is also referred to as **cognitive neuropsychology** or more commonly as **cognitive neuroscience**.

Heart, Mind, and Brain: The Early History of Neuropsychology

Before I get too far in this module, I might address the larger question "Why study history?" Alternately, you might ask, "Why not just study what is known to be true now rather than wasting some of my brain learning what we know isn't true?" There are two simple answers to these questions. First, it is important to study the history of any discipline because it provides important insights into the development of the science and because it gives us information about what is left to discover. In a sense, any time we read a research report, we are studying what is known, which is, in essence, history. Second, studying the history of neuropsychology is also important because it illustrates the many instances within the discipline in which researchers were wrong about the nature of brain–behavior relationships. As you will learn in the following chapters, there are many unexpected features of the nervous system, and often many of the most firmly held views are now known to be false (e.g., you are born with all the neurons you will ever have). When teaching, I often tell my class that if I were to design the brain, I would do it in a much more organized way (although anyone who has seen my office should doubt that statement). When we want to apply common sense to understanding the brain, we should remember that the brain is not common, nor on a superficial level does it make much obvious sense (although we hope that this text will help with the making sense part).

There are many ways to organize a unit on the history of neuropsychology—for example, starting with the earliest dates and moving forward through time. However, we have decided to discuss the history of neuropsychology by dividing our discussion into sections on early history and recent history, employing a systems approach to the organization of each module. In other words, we have organized the module into sections that reflect the functional unit that was studied. In our opinion, a systems approach makes it easier to integrate the information and more truly reflects the means by which the research was done. However, within each module, there is still the standard chronological progression of events.

The assumption that the brain plays a central role in behavior is not particularly contentious today (e.g., it is presumed in the quote that starts this chapter). However, human thoughts and behaviors were not always attributed to the brain. Empedocles (495–435 B.C.) was a philosopher (best known for his position that all matter was composed of four elements: fire, air, water, and earth) who believed that the heart was the source of human behavior, a position that became known as the **cardiac** or **cardiocentric hypothesis.** Aristotle (384–322 B.C.) came to the same conclusion, although for different reasons. Because the heart is normally very active and warm, Aristotle concluded that the heart was the source of thought and sensation. Knowing that heat rises and that the brain is covered with a network of vasculature, Aristotle argued that the brain served as a radiator, cooling the blood. Aristotle was incorrect on both counts. The brain does not cool blood; in fact, blood helps to cool the brain. Furthermore, the heart is not the source of human behavior. As argued by Hippocrates (430–350 B.C.) and Galen (A.D. 129–199), the brain is responsible for these functions, a view that is referred to as the **cephalocentric hypothesis** or the **brain hypothesis.** Both Hippocrates and Galen were incorrect about many of the details (e.g., Galen thought that the brain's ventricles and the cerebrospinal fluid within them play a central role in cognition), but these errors were corrected by later investigators such as Albertus Magnus in the thirteenth century and Vesalius in the sixteenth century. (See Table 1.1 for a chronological listing of some important milestones in the history of neuroscience.)

Although the cardiac hypothesis might seem hopelessly out of date now, the symbols of this perspective are common throughout our culture. For instance, have you ever seen a Valentine's Day card with a picture of a brain on it? I have not. If you ask someone which organ of the body they associate with the emotion "love," they will most likely indicate the heart, not the brain. What about the expression "It makes my blood boil"? How many songs have you heard about having a broken heart? How about a broken brain? These are all remnants of the cardiac hypothesis that live on in popular culture.

Surgically Opened (and Healed) Skull That Has Been Subjected to Trephination, a Procedure That Was Probably Performed over 7000 Years Ago

Figure 1.1

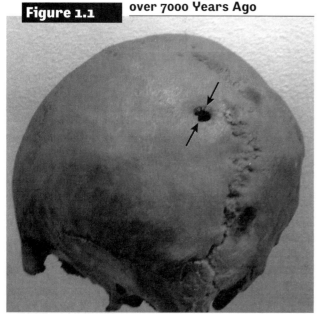

Source: Image courtesy of Murray Stokely.

Despite ancient claims of the role of the heart in human emotion and intellect, there is good evidence that other people were tinkering with brain function long before that. On the basis of observations of fossilized skull fractures in early hominids (and the prey of early hominids), Finger (1994) suggests that there was recognition that damaging the brain (or at least the head) would result in the death or disabling of an individual. However, there are also ancient skulls that have been surgically excised or cut open, presumably for its therapeutic value. For instance, the skull in Figure 1.1 is over 7000 years old, and the arrows indicate the points at which the skull was surgically opened (two times!!). Importantly, the individual survived these operations (as demonstrated by the bone regrowth). It is unknown what the ancient surgeon was trying to achieve with the **trephination,** although it seems safe to conclude that this operation was designed to cure something (if the "doctor" had wanted to kill the

Table 1.1

Neuroscience History Timeline

ca. 5000 B.C.	The first "functional neurosurgeries" are performed.
ca. 1700 B.C.	Edwin Smith surgical papyrus is written.
460–379 B.C.	Hippocrates claims that the brain is the seat of intelligence.
ca. 445 B.C.	Empedocles claims that the heart is the seat of mental process.
335 B.C.	Aristotle also claims that the heart is the seat of mental process.
A.D. 177	Galen claims that sensation is produced in the cortex and movement in the cerebellum.
1543	Vesalius publishes *On the Workings of the Human Body*.
1649	Descartes claims that the pineal gland is the interface between the mind and body.
1808	Gall publishes work on phrenology.
1811	Legallois claims that the medulla controls respiration.
1811	Bell describes the functional differences between the dorsal and ventral roots of the spinal cord.
1821	Magendie also describes the functional differences between the dorsal and ventral roots of the spinal cord.
1824	Flourens uses experimental lesions to study brain–behavior relationships.
1825	Bouillaud claims that loss of speech results after frontal lesions.
1836	Marc Dax claims that left hemisphere damage impairs speech.
1861	Aubertin also claims that loss of speech results after frontal lesions.
1861	Paul Broca presents the case of "Tan."
1864	Hughlings-Jackson writes about speech impairment following brain injury.
1870	Hitzig and Fritsch use electrical stimulation to map the motor area of the dog.
1873	Golgi publishes his first description of the silver nitrate method.
1874	Wernicke publishes *Der Aphasische Symptomencomplex* on aphasias.
1875	Ferrier uses electrical stimulation to map the motor cortex of several species.
1889	Cajal claims that neurons are independent elements.
1892	Goltz caries out lesion experiments on three dogs and argues against localization of function.
1906	Golgi and Cajal share the Nobel Prize.
1909	Brodmann describes fifty-two cytoarchitectonically discrete cortical areas.

"patient," it would have been fairly easy to do so). There are also writings from ancient Egypt dating back 5000 years that document the symptoms of brain damage, although the ancient Egyptians did not consider the brain important enough to mummify. These observations suggest that ancient peoples appreciated the importance of the brain in behavior and perhaps in some disease states.

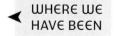 **WHERE WE HAVE BEEN**   Early theories of brain function did not typically recognize the importance of the brain in higher cognitive functions. Instead, the brain was viewed as a passive interpreter of signals, whereas the mind was often characterized as a separate entity from the brain.

The Mind–Body Problem

Identifying the brain as the primary organ responsible for thought and behavior is a good start, but other daunting philosophical questions remain. Physically, how does the brain control behavior? What is the relationship between the inner "mental life" that we experience and the body? Does the mind or soul have physical form? If not, how can it interact with the body? Perhaps the most influential arguments on this topic were first advanced by René Descartes (1596–1650). He presented a "reflexive" theory of the control of behavior in which he described the flow of "animal spirits" through "valvules" within nervous tissue filaments. This theory accounted for reflexive behaviors by describing how external stimuli would move the skin, in turn moving the filaments, releasing the animal spirits and innervating the muscles. Although this theory appeared to account for some involuntary behaviors (such as withdrawing one's hand from a hot stimulus), it could not account for voluntary behavior.

Descartes believed that voluntary behaviors depended on the interface of the mechanistic body with a rational, decision-making soul. The location that Descartes identified for this interaction was the pineal gland. Many descriptions of this position state that he chose the pineal gland on the basis of its unitary nature. Most structures in the brain are paired; there are often two very similar copies of a structure, one on the left and one on the right side of the brain. This is not the case with the pineal gland. It is composed of a single structure along the midline of the brain. Although this anatomical feature probably played a significant role in Descartes' selecting the pineal gland, the fact that it is surrounded by **cerebrospinal fluid** (a clear fluid that supports and cleanses the brain) was also important. Descartes believed that cavities of cerebrospinal fluid were reservoirs for the animal spirits necessary for action. Therefore, voluntary action would produce small movements of the pineal gland, resulting in the release of animal spirits throughout the body and producing movement of the body.

At the time, new hydraulic machines and mechanical dolls were on exhibit in Paris and the parts, movements, and complexity of "behaviors" influenced Descartes' theory. Descartes' theory relied heavily on what was modern technology at the time: hydraulics. As you will see later in this chapter, numerous other theories of brain function also rely heavily on technological metaphors. For instance, in the 1940s and 1950s, the brain was thought to operate much like a switchboard, forging new connections when learning. Later analogies relied heavily on computer technology to describe the ways in which the brain encodes and stores information. Current analogies of brain function resemble current technologies. Instead of describing the brain as a single computer, some analogies refer to networks of relatively independent computers, processing information in parallel as well as in series, much like today's supercomputers.

Of course, one of the problems with all of these mechanical accounts of mental life is their relative inability to account for variability in behavior. When any living organism is placed in an identical situation multiple times, its behavior in the situations is often variable. The same is not usually true of most machines. Provided that it is maintained in proper working order, a hydraulic press crushes ten similar apples on ten different occasions in a virtually identical fashion. Similarly, when a connection is made on a switchboard, then this connection is disconnected, and then it is connected again, the connection functions virtually identically the second time as it did the first time. Even computers exhibit very little variability (though still more than we would like). Given the same command under the same conditions, the computer should produce the same response. Complex biological systems are considerably less predictable. According to the Harvard Law of Animal Behavior, "under carefully controlled experimental circumstances, an animal will behave as it damned well pleases."

The account of mind–body interaction provided by Descartes has a much more daunting problem than accounting for variability in behavior. Descartes proposed that the mind and body are separate but interacting entities, a position that is referred to as **dualism.** However, dualists must then explain how the mind and body can interact, if at all. Some have argued that the mind and body do interact in a causal fashion without specifying how. Other dualists propose that the mind and body function in parallel without interacting. Still others claim that the mind can affect the body but the body cannot affect the mind.

The opposing position, called **monism,** posits that the mind and body are unitary. Gilbert Ryle paraphrases the monist position nicely with his statement "There is no ghost in the machine." Although most neuropsychologists are monists, the material in this book is consistent with either position. Both positions assume that the brain is, at the very least, involved in behavior and thought. Remember that neuropsychology is the study of the relationship between behavior and brain activity, and whether the brain is influenced by a nonmaterial entity is not a central question for this field of study.

The following module outlines the development of neuropsychology, beginning with the discovery that the brain played a central role in human thoughts, feelings, and actions. In contrast to some of the material that was reviewed in the previous section, wherein opinions from hundreds of years ago were described, much of the material in this section focuses on research that has been performed in the last 100 years.

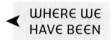

We have explored the history and accuracy of the myth that humans only use 10% of their brain capacity, we have introduced the field of neuropsychology, and we have reviewed the early history of neuropsychology.

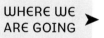

The following sections provide an overview of the early scientists who catalogued the effects of damage to the brain. Some of the scientists discussed include Broca, Bell, Magendie, and Gall.

MODULE **1.2**
The Recent History of Neuropsychology

The year 1990 began with a declaration that the 1990s would be the decade of the brain, and given the advances that have been made, some people suggest that we have acquired more knowledge about the brain since 1990 than was acquired during all the time previous. Indeed, much of the research that you will read about in this book has been performed since 1990. However, all research relies on the works of others, and the focus of this module is the discovery of the pioneers in neuropsychology and their breakthroughs. Although the field of neuropsychology is rather young, neuropsychology draws from a number of very established disciplines, including anthropology, biology, physiology, and neurology. This module is designed to give you an appreciation of how these fields contributed to the development of neuropsychology and an idea of how neuropsychology relies on a breadth of information to provide insight into brain–behavior relations.

Cataloging the Effects of Lesions

Serious critiques of the passive role for the brain in the production of behavior proposed by Descartes began with the observations of Jean-Cesar Legallois (1770–1840), Charles Bell (1774–1842), and Francois Magendie (1783–1840). Legallois was a French physiologist who discovered that **lesioning** (destroying tissue in) the medulla resulted in the immediate cessation of breathing. The discovery of the respiratory center within the medulla was the first widely accepted function to be localized within the brain (Finger, 1994). Bell, a Scottish physiologist, and Magendie, a French physiologist, studied the nerves that exited the spinal cord. They observed that the dorsal roots (the nerves that leave the spinal cord on the back of the spinal cord) had sensory functions, whereas the ventral roots (the nerves that leave the spinal cord on the front) were responsible for motor functions. Thus, even at the level of the spinal cord, function was segregated. This view of functional segregation of the spinal cord set the stage for others to examine whether or not the brain was also organized into separate sensory and motor components (Finger, 1994). In 1811, Bell suggested that the entire nervous system should be investigated for functional and anatomical segregation (Finger, 1994).

Franz Joseph Gall (1758–1828) and his colleague Johann Spurzheim (1776–1832) undertook the challenge, suggesting that the cortex was functionally localized. Gall, who was a respected anatomist and physician, stated that there were twenty-seven distinct cognitive abilities (which he called *faculties*) that could be localized on the cortex of the human brain (nonhuman animals had only nineteen of these faculties). These faculties included such poorly defined cognitive abilities as love of friends, wisdom, acquisitiveness, and destructiveness. To his credit, Gall also suggested that cognitive skills, such as mathematical ability, memory for words, and spoken language, were mediated by separate areas of the brain (which is true). However, Gall also believed that the cortex behaved like muscles, in that increased size of an area was associated with increased function. Simply put, if a person was exceptionally wise, then the corresponding area of the brain also should be large. The increase in size of the cortical area would result in a deformation of the skull, or a bump, which then could be empirically measured by using a technique called cranioscopy. Measurements of the skull and pronouncements on personality became known as **phrenology**, which was exceptionally popular in the early nineteenth century.

The reaction against phrenology was strong, and one of the strongest critics of phrenology was Marie-Jean-Pierre Flourens (1794–1867), the French anatomist. One of Flourens's firmest beliefs was that phrenology was at best subjective and that all the analyses were performed post hoc. That is, if a person was supposed to be a musical genius, then a phrenologist would look for a large bump on the skull and pronounce that this was the music center. If another musical genius did not have a corresponding center, no worries for the phrenologist. Obviously, the person was a genius in a different aspect of music and therefore would have a large bump in a different area. Flourens was a firm believer in the empirical method, and he performed numerous studies with nonhuman animals using lesioning techniques to study corresponding effects on behavior (recall our earlier mention of Flourens in discussing the 10% myth). Some of his contributions were the observations that the cerebellum was responsible for coordinated movement and that the medulla performed vital functions for the organism.

In an observation that will become more important in Chapter 16, Flourens also observed that sometimes following lesions, function may be restored. However, Flourens believed that once one function recovered, all functions had recovered, which he used as support for the concept of cortical equipotentiality. Flourens was firmly opposed to the localization of cognitive function, instead proposing that the cortex functioned as a whole and that there was no functional specialization within the cortex (a position that was later termed **equipotentiality**). This viewpoint was also held by German physiologist Friedrich Goltz (1834–1902). Goltz performed a number of experiments involving the removal of the cortex in dogs and cats and observed that only the size of the lesion, not the location of the lesion, affected the behavior of the nonhuman animal. On the basis of these observations, he concluded that the cortex could not be specialized for specific cognitive functions.

Although many scientists of the early nineteenth century believed in cortical equipotentiality, this position was not universally held. Using the same preparations as Goltz, the English physiologist David Ferrier (1843–1928) suggested that the behavioral observations of decorticate dogs and monkeys were inconsistent with the position of cortical equipotentiality. Ferrier suggested that the results of the lesion experiments were consistent with the localization of sensory and motor functions within discrete portions of the cortex. Furthermore, research by Gustav Fritsch (1838–1927), an anatomist, and Eduard Hitzig (1838–1907), a psychiatrist, demonstrated quite convincingly that the frontal cortex of the dog was essential for the production of normal movement. Together, they successfully demonstrated that careful use of the techniques of Goltz and others (e.g., lesioning portions of the frontal cortex) resulted in abnormal motor movements and intact sensation. Finger (1994) states that the work of Fritsch and Hitzig successfully overturned the theory of cortical equipotentiality. As it turns out, then, Gall was right, but for the wrong reasons, whereas Goltz and Flourens used the right techniques but came to the wrong conclusions. History has been unkind to Gall, largely because the focus has been on his work in phrenology rather than recognizing his truly innovative ideas about the localization of language (Selnes, 2001).

Although many basic functions had been successfully localized within the brain (e.g., movement and respiration), the first higher cognitive function that was successfully localized was language. Paul Broca (1824–1880), a French anthropologist, was

Neuropsychological Celebrity

Monsieur Leborgne

Monsieur Leborgne, better known as "Tan" acquired a deficit in speech production, but not speech comprehension. A meeting of the Societe d'Anthropologie early in 1861 set the stage for Broca's discoveries. At the meeting, Aubertin stated that it would take only one patient with a cognitive deficit and a localized lesion to nullify the leading belief of cortical equipotentiality. Furthermore, Aubertin suggested that speech loss would always be associated with large anterior lesions of the brain. On April 12, 1861, Broca came upon such a person, a Monsieur Leborgne, a fifty-one-year-old epileptic who had recently been transferred to Broca's care. Monsieur Leborgne was incapable of speech, with the exception of the ability to utter a few obscenities and the sound "tan." In fact, Monsieur Leborgne was referred to by Broca's other clients as *"Tan,"* a name that is used to describe the case today. In reviewing Tan's medical history, it became apparent that he had lost the ability to speak in 1840. On April 18, 1861, Tan died, and Broca examined his brain. There was a large lesion of the anterior left hemisphere, within what we now call the frontal lobes. Broca recognized that Tan's deficit was related to articulate speech and not to comprehension of language or other types of cognitive deficits.

It took Broca two more years to propose that the left hemisphere was special for speech in most people. It took Broca much longer to recognize that comprehension of speech was also affected when individuals had damage to Broca's area. Thus, the contributions of Broca to understanding the neural mechanisms of speech were tremendous. Furthermore, the general acceptance of Broca's observations led to widespread emulation of Broca's techniques. Indeed, one could state that Broca led others to look for and examine individuals with discrete brain damage in an attempt to localize other cognitive functions.

the first to gain widespread acceptance for the role of the frontal cortex in the production of speech. Broca based his conclusions on the observations of an individual with left frontal damage. In 1861, Broca presented a case study (of a man he referred to as "Tan") in which a circumscribed lesion of the left frontal lobe (now called *Broca's area*) resulted in an individual who was incapable of productive speech. Broca suggested that Tan had lost the capacity for speech but retained the ability to understand language. Originally, Broca referred to this phenomenon as **aphemia;** it later came to be known as *aphasia* or **Broca's aphasia.** It is interesting to note that Broca did not initially prescribe a special role for the left hemisphere in the production of speech, waiting until 1865 to suggest a role for the left hemisphere in speech for right-handed individuals.

Although researchers such as Jean-Baptiste Bouillaud (1796–1881), his son-in-law Simon Aubertin (1825–1865), and the father-and-son team of Marc Dax (1770–1837) and Gustave Dax (1815–1893) suggested that the left hemisphere was important for speech, they did not receive the recognition that Broca did. One reason for this was that Dax did not publish his findings until after Broca's were published. Another reason was the detailed description of the speech deficits in the paper by Broca; for instance, Broca suggested that only articulate speech had been affected, not other aspects of speech. Finally, at the time at which Broca was publishing his results, the scientific climate had changed (Finger, 1994; Selnes, 2001; Young, 1990), and individuals, especially individuals who were as well respected as Broca, who suggested that function could be lateralized, were no longer immediately categorized as phrenologists.

Two major components of speech that Broca did not study directly were the emotional tone of speech (**prosody**) and the loss of comprehension of language associated with the preservation of speech. The British neurologist John Hughlings-Jackson (1835–1911) first articulated that the content and emotional tone of speech were separable. Among Hughlings-Jackson's many contributions to the field of neuropsychology is his observation that speech is a complex process that involves linguistic ability as well as complex motor skills. Furthermore, on the basis of his clinical observations

Current Controversy

Historical Methods Revisited

There are some people who suggest that some historical methods have their place alongside modern techniques. Although techniques that were developed in times past are not necessarily abandoned for new techniques (e.g., sterile surgery), there are a number of dubious techniques that appear to be enthusiastically promoted on the Internet. Two examples of this are trephination and phrenology.

As you recall from Module 1.1, *trephination* is the production of a hole in the skull, which was practiced widely throughout the ancient world. (Figure 1.1 is an example of a 7000-year-old-skull that underwent trephination.) It is unclear what the purpose of trephinations in ancient cultures was, although it is possible that they were early attempts to treat mental illness, brain disease, or skull fractures. However, advocates for modern trephination (e.g., Amanda Fielding, Bart Holding) suggest that trephination is a technique for expanding consciousness as well as an effective technique for relieving depression, addiction, and neuroses. Advocates for trephination suggest that trephination works by increasing the flow of blood and oxygen to the brain, which is reduced by our upright posture and rigid skull. They cite research that suggests that trephination was performed on high priests in the ancient world to enhance their spirituality. However, there is no evidence that trephination produces any change in cognitive function, oxygen ratios, or blood flow. Furthermore, there are a number of anthropologists who firmly suggest that trephination took place only as a medical treatment and not as

a religious experience. Finally, although advocates of trephination indicate that there are highly qualified neurosurgeons who will perform this surgery for you, it must be recognized that your intact skull is one of your brain's best defenses and that tampering with the integrity of the skull to "enhance consciousness" is something that no reputable neurosurgeon would engage in.

Phrenology is the study of the skull as a means of understanding an individual's cognitive strengths and weaknesses, personality traits, and other character traits. Phrenology was proposed by Franz Joseph Gall, who suggested that there were twenty-seven traits (e.g., wisdom, love of children) that could be reliably localized on the skull. When a specific trait was strong in an individual, the skull would protrude in the spot over the area of the brain responsible for the trait; when the trait was weak in an individual, the skull would have a depression in it. Thus, the phrenologists suggested that "reading" the skull was a good method by which to detect traits such as criminality and intellect. Although there is no scientific basis for phrenology, it still has followers. For instance, in 1983, Peter Cooper founded the London Phrenology Company to rekindle interest in the "science" of phrenology. Advocates of phrenology suggest that knowledge of phrenology can help those in law enforcement (distinguishing criminals from noncriminals), as well as providing personal opportunities for self-knowledge and spiritual growth. Modern phrenological maps attempt to localize such poorly defined terms as *eventuality* and *human nature*. Like readings in astrology, a phrenological reading is based on vague statements that are difficult to either prove or disprove.

of clients who were unable to verbally name objects but could swear aloud when they were upset, he suggested that there could be dissociations between the semantic content of language (the meaning) and the emotional tone.

Carl Wernicke (1848–1904) was a German neurologist who made significant contributions to neuropsychology in a number of areas. Perhaps his best-known research was in a paper that he wrote in 1874 (when he was only twenty-six years old). In this paper, he suggested that there was an auditory center (now known as *Wernicke's area*) in the temporal lobes that, when damaged, would result in an individual who could still produce speech but would be incapable of using words correctly and be unable to understand the speech of others. Today, this type of aphasia is still called **Wernicke's aphasia.** Wernicke also suggested that there should be a number of different aphasias that would produce different symptoms based on the site and extent of the lesions. Wernicke suggested that total or global aphasia (a complete inability to understand or produce language) would result from lesions of both Wernicke's and Broca's areas. This will be discussed in more depth in Chapter 8.

◄ **WHERE WE HAVE BEEN** The late seventeenth and early eighteenth centuries were times of great progress in understanding brain function. Much of the research that was performed at this time went far to overthrow the ideas of cortical equipotentiality, instead establishing that the brain is functionally segregated. One of the first higher cognitive functions to be localized was speech, which individuals such as Broca localized to the left frontal lobe. Other researchers, such as Hughlings-Jackson and Wernicke, realized that speech was a complex ability and investigated facets of speech other than simple production.

WHERE WE ARE GOING ► The remainder of this module will investigate those who examined the cellular components of the brain and those who mapped the cortex of the brain. Within this module will also be a brief examination of early methods of treating organic brain disease.

Focus on the Neuron

The working unit of the brain is the neuron. This section will describe the pioneers who researched the neuron and their major discoveries.

ANATOMICAL STUDIES. There were three main hurdles that had to be overcome to study the cellular constituents of the brain: the size of the cells, the texture of the brain, and the lack of pigmentation in much of the brain. Each of these problems had to be solved for the study of the fine structures of the brain to progress.

Cells in the body range from 0.01 to 0.05 millimeter in diameter, although most neurons are approximately 0.02 millimeter in diameter. Because your eyes can see two points only if they are separated by at least 0.1 millimeter (otherwise they appear as one point), some type of magnification must be used to observe neurons. In the early 1800s, the development of the compound microscope allowed individuals to observe animal tissue at high levels of magnification. By 1839, Theodore Schwann (a German zoologist) proposed that all living tissue was composed of microscopic units called *cells* (now referred to as the *cell doctrine*), and other researchers began to study neurons.

To study neurons, very thin slices of brain must be made (often not much thicker than the neurons themselves). Early histologists developed the microtome to produce these slices. However, because the brain has a consistency somewhat like that of toothpaste, it must be hardened before it can be sliced. Many researchers fix the brain (i.e., harden it) by soaking it in formaldehyde for an extended period of time (days to weeks). Unlike other tissues in the body, thinly sliced fixed brain has no obvious color and must be treated with a type of stain to make the cells visible. The study of thinly sliced, fixed, and stained tissues is called **histology.** Histology is still a very powerful technique for studying the brain, and the development of new stains and staining techniques continues to lead to new insights into the brain.

The histological study of the brain has had many pioneers, and many of the early researchers in the field were those who developed the tissue stains. In fact, many of the stains that were developed during this period are still widely used today. One such is the **Nissl stain,** developed in the nineteenth century by Franz Nissl (a German neurologist). The Nissl stain distinguishes neurons from other cells in the brain, staining the central portions of neurons (also called the cell body) wherever it is applied.

Another example is the **Golgi stain** (also referred to as the Golgi-Cox stain), which was developed in 1873 by Camillo Golgi (1843–1926), an Italian histologist. Golgi discovered that when tissue was soaked in a silver solution (often silver chromate), some of the neurons became darkly stained, revealing their structure. As a result of his staining, Golgi was able to determine that the neuron had three distinct parts: the cell body and two parts that radiate away from the cell body—the axon and the dendrites. (Chapter 2 gives details about these components.) Golgi staining provided evidence that the axons travel great distances from the cell body and that these processes must be involved in carrying the output of the activity of the neuron.

Although Golgi invented the stain, the Spanish histologist and artist Santiago Ramon y Cajal (1843–1926) used the stain to trace the connections of the brain. Over a period of twenty-five years, Cajal traced the circuitry of much of the brain. Furthermore, Cajal was instrumental in defining the features of the neuron, including the observation that dendrites are covered in spines, something that had previously been dismissed as an artifact of staining. Throughout their careers, Golgi and Cajal were great rivals. Golgi was a proponent of the view that neurons fuse together with each other to form a continuous circuit, whereas Cajal proposed that neurons are not continuous and that they must communicate by contact (now known as the **neuron doctrinc**). Research done in the 1950s demonstrated that Cajal was correct. Neurons do not form continuous circuits. In an interesting twist of fate, Golgi and Cajal shared the Nobel Prize for Medicine in 1906 in recognition for their advances in understanding neurons. Golgi was recognized for developing the stain that allowed Cajal to receive the prize for developing the neuron doctrine.

ELECTRICAL PROPERTIES OF THE NEURON. We now know that neurons conduct electrical impulses throughout their entire length. As we will see in Chapter 2, the electrical impulses in the axon are called action potentials, which are different from the electrical impulses in the dendrites. However, research on the electrical properties of the neuron began with research into electricity. For instance, Finger (1994) suggests that studies of the electrical properties of neurons began with the work of Luigi Galvani (1737–1798). In 1780, Galvani constructed what would today be considered a crude battery and discovered that muscle and nerve cells produce electricity. (Contemporaries of Galvani included Benjamin Franklin, who in 1751 published his research on electricity). In 1848–1849, the German physiologist—Emil du Bois-Reymond (1818–1896) used the newly developed galvanometer to measure the movement of the current in muscle and tied the internal production of current to movement. Taken together, the discoveries of Galvani and du Bois-Reymond finally dismissed the notion of fluid-based neural communication (Finger, 1994).

The team of Fritsch and Hitzig, along with Ferrier and Charles Sherrington (1857–1952), were scientists who studied the relationship between brain, movements, and electricity. Fritsch and Hitzig observed that discrete electrical stimulations of parts of the cortex of a dog could result in movements (Finger, 1994). Among Ferrier's many contributions was to extend Fritsch and Hitzig's work to monkeys, rats, and cats. Another distinguished researcher was Sherrington, a British physiologist who studied the control of reflex movements in mammals. Among his many contributions are the naming of the gap between neurons (**synapse**) that Cajal had hypothesized to be there, the observation of reciprocal innervation of muscles (e.g., when your bicep is contracted, your tricep must be relaxed), and the neural control of reflexes. Sherrington received the Nobel Prize in 1932 for his research on the neural control of behavior.

Despite understanding that neurons could be excited by electricity and that electrical impulses in neurons were responsible for movement, there was no clear idea of how a neuron could produce and/or conduct electricity. Julius Bernstein (1839–1917), a German physiologist, was one of the first researchers to measure the speed of an electrical signal in the axon (called an *action potential*) and to determine that the membrane that covered the axon had a specific charge when it was at rest (called the *resting membrane potential*). Bernstein also proposed that the neuron could conduct electricity by changing the concentrations of ions that were concentrated in its intracellular fluid. However, much of the progress in the understanding of the role of ions in producing an electrical charge across the membrane came from the work of British physiologists Alan Hodgkin (1914–1998) and Andrew Huxley (1917–). They initially began their work by studying the electrical propagation of neural impulses in the sciatic nerve in the frog. However, John (known as J.Z., pronounced "Jay-Zed") Young (1907–1997), a British neurobiologist, suggested that the giant axon of the squid was a better preparation for these types of studies, because the giant axon of the squid is approximately 1000 times larger than mammalian axons (it is roughly the length and width of a pencil lead) and can be studied for about six hours after dissection. In 1952, Hodgkin and Huxley published a series of papers that demonstrated that the electrical impulse or action potential that occurs in such axons was due to changes in the relative concentrations of ions. They discovered that the movement of the ions into and out of the membrane was facilitated by changes in the ability of these ions to enter and exit the neuron (also referred to as permeability) and that this change in permeability was an active process of the axon. In recognition of their work in understanding how a neuron could produce electrical charge and how this charge was conducted over the length of the axon, Hodgkin and Huxley received the Nobel Prize in Physiology or Medicine in 1963.

CHEMICAL PROPERTIES OF THE NEURON. We now know that neurons communicate with each other by releasing chemicals, called *neurotransmitters*. As you will see in Chapter 2, there are a variety of neurotransmitters that are distributed throughout the brain. However, the existence of neurotransmitters had to be demonstrated via a number of very clever experiments by numerous brilliant scientists.

One of the early pioneers in the field was the American/German physiologist, Otto Loewi (1873–1961). At the time of his experiments, it was well known that a frog's heart could be dissected and placed in a solution, and it would remain beating. It was also known that if the dissection was done carefully, one can stimulate the vagus nerve (a nerve that enervates the heart) and observe a reduction in heart rate. Loewi performed a unique series of experiments that he collectively attributed to an idea he had in a dream. He demonstrated that the vagus must release a substance (which he termed *vagusstoff*) that produces a change in heart rate. In one experiment, Loewi stimulated one heart and collected the fluid immediately after the stimulation and placed a second heart into the solution. The second heart exhibited a slowing of heart rate, despite the fact that Loewi had not stimulated the vagus. In a series of experiments, he demonstrated that the slowing of the heart was a result of the release of *vagusstoff* by the vagus.

Subsequent experiments by Loewi (and others) demonstrated that *vagusstoff* was the neurotransmitter now known as acetylcholine. One of Loewi's lifelong friends, Henry Dale (1875–1968), an English physiologist, was responsible for identifying and characterizing acetylcholine and for determining that mammalian nervous systems behave similarly to those of amphibians. An American scientist, Julius Axelrod (1912–2004), was responsible for determining how neurons store, release, and deactivate neurotransmitters. All three of these scientists received Nobel Prizes in Physiology or Medicine for their work—Loewi and Dale jointly in 1936, and Axelrod in 1970. (As an aside, when the Nazis invaded Austria, they arrested Loewi and forced him to give them his Nobel Prize money before he could leave the country. In 1940, Loewi emigrated to the United States, where he remained until his death.)

Table 1.2 lists the accomplishments of a few of the pioneers in neuroscience.

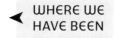

WHERE WE HAVE BEEN We have examined the pioneers in the fields of histology, electrophysiology, and neurochemistry or pharmacology. What is interesting to note is that much of this research was dependent on the development of new technologies. This is still the case, as many of the exciting new discoveries that have been made in these fields are a direct result of technology. Another interesting point is that many of the discoveries associated with the electrical and chemical properties of the central nervous system were made by studying the peripheral nervous system, not by studying the central nervous system.

Table 1.2	Pioneers in Histology, Electrophysiology, Neurochemistry, and Pharmacology
1780	Galvani discovers that muscle and nerve cells produce electricity.
1839	Schwann proposes that all living tissue is made of microscopic units (cells).
1848–1849	Galvani and du Bois-Reymond refute fluid-based neural communication theory.
1873	Golgi publishes the first description of the silver nitrate method.
1894	Nissl stain is developed to distinguish neurons from other brain cells.
1906	Cajal shares the Nobel Prize for Medicine with Golgi in recognition of the importance of Golgi's stain in making possible Cajal's drawings of brain circuitry.
1932	Sherrington receives the Nobel Prize for Research on neural control of behavior.
1902, 1912	Bernstein's membrane hypothesis—discovered the resting potential and action potential in nerves, proposed that neurons could conduct electricity.
1936	Loewi and Dale share the Nobel Prize for Physiology for the discovery of the neurotransmitter acetylcholine.
1952	Hodgkin and Huxley discover that an axon's action potential is due to changes in relative concentrations of ions and receive the Nobel Prize in 1963.
1970	Axelrod wins the Nobel Prize for discovering how neurons store, release, and deactivate neurotransmitters.

WHERE WE ARE GOING ➤ We are going to describe some early attempts at making functional maps of the brain. Earlier investigations focused on the microscopic differences in structure between brain regions, presuming that regions of different structure would also have different function. Later studies tested this position experimentally in animals, and even later work tested this position using electrical stimulation during human brain surgery.

The Brain Mappers

KORBINIAN BRODMANN. The Nobel Prize–winning work of Golgi and Cajal laid the foundation for the subsequent work of German neuroanatomist Korbinian Brodmann (1868–1918). As Golgi and Cajal noted, neurons come in a variety of shapes and sizes, and neurons of similar shape and size tend to be grouped together. Therefore, different regions of the brain can be described in terms of the typical physical features, or **cytoarchitecture,** of the neurons that are found there. At the beginning of the twentieth century, Brodmann divided the cortex into regions of similar cytoarchitecture, forming a cytoarchitectural map (see Figure 1.2). His work was published in 1909, and Brodmann's book *Vergleichende Lokalisationslehre der Grosshirnrinde in ihren Prinzipien dargestellt auf Grund des Zellenbaues*, is one of the major classics of the neuroscience literature. Although relatively few people have read the book (for those with rusty German, there is an English translation), the maps that are contained within it are among the most reproduced figures in neuroscience.

Figure 1.2	**Sample of Brodmann's Cytoarchitectural Map**

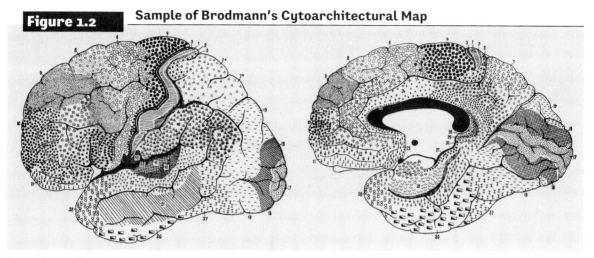

Source: Figure 85 from *Brodmann's Localisation in the Cerebral Cortex,* translated and edited by Laurence J. Garey, p. 110. Copyright © 1999, World Scientific Publishing. Reprinted by permission.

According to Brodmann's maps, each cortical region of different cytoarchitecture is denoted by a different number. The numbering system does not appear to be particularly logical in its ordering. One might expect the numbers to increase as one moved from the front of the brain to the back or from the top to the bottom. Some of the lower-numbered Brodmann areas *are* located at the top of the brain (areas 1, 2, and 3, corresponding to primary somatosensory areas, and area 4, corresponding to primary motor cortex), but beyond this trend, the guiding principles that govern the numbering system are lost on us. Rather than attempting to extract a rule to help predict which number corresponds to which reason, we suggest that you simply memorize the Brodmann numbers for some relatively famous brain regions (see Table 1.3).

Brodmann was of the opinion that regions of different cytoarchitecture would have different functions, although he had very little evidence to support this claim. Over the past 100

Table 1.3	**Brodmann Numbers Corresponding to Several Primary and Secondary Motor and Sensory Areas of the Cortex**

Function	Brodmann Number
Vision	
Primary	17
Secondary	18, 19, 20, 21, 37
Audition	
Primary	41
Secondary	22, 42
Somesthesis	
Primary	1, 2, 3
Secondary	5, 7
Movement	
Primary	4
Secondary	6
Eye movement	8
Mouth movement (speech)	44, 45
Olfaction	
Primary	34

years, much of the evidence has supported this view. However, even neighboring regions of different cytoarchitecture can have vastly different functional properties despite their physical proximity. For example, Brodmann areas 37 and 22 border on one another. Area 37 is specialized for visual object recognition and naming, whereas area 22 (particularly the part toward the back of the brain) is specialized for perceiving spoken words.

Brodmann's approach to the brain was not unique; others have come up with differing systems. For instance, Cecile Vogt (1875–1962) and Oscar Vogt (1870–1950) claimed that there are over 200 unique cortical cytoarchitectonic areas. More recent (and more accurate) cytoarchitectonic maps have also been published, but none have caught on as have Brodmann's. Despite these other systems, Brodmann's numbering system is still standard today, and as you will see, it is commonly used to describe the results of functional neuroimaging experiments.

KARL LASHLEY AND SHEPHARD IVORY FRANZ. After receiving his Ph.D. from Johns Hopkins University, Karl Lashley (1890–1958) started his collaboration with Shephard Ivory Franz (1874–1933) in Washington. Starting in 1916, the two investigated memory functions in rodents. More specifically, they trained rats to make relatively simple sensory discriminations (such as judging brightness) and to navigate mazes, after which Lashley and Franz studied the effects of relatively large cortical lesions on the rats' ability to continue performing the tasks. As we discussed in the section on the 10% myth, Lashley and Franz found that most of these abilities remained intact following cortical lesions. Most of their experiments appeared to have been motivated by Lashley's desire to discover the location of the **engram,** a hypothetical change in the brain that is responsible for storing memories (Pinel, 2003). When impairments were evident, they were related more to the size of the lesion than to the location of the lesion, which seemed to contradict the idea that the engram had a specific location.

These findings led Lashley to formulate two interdependent "laws." The first he called the **Law of Equipotentiality,** first used by Lashley and Franz in 1917 (Lashley & Franz, 1917) and defined later in 1929:

> The term "equipotentiality" I have used to designate the apparent capacity of any intact part of a functional area to carry out, with or without reduction in efficiency, the functions which are lost by destruction of the whole. This capacity varies from one area to another and with the character of the functions involved. It probably holds only for the association areas and for functions more complex than simple sensory or motor co-ordination. (Lashley, 1929 [1963 reprinting], p. 24)

Lashley's second law, the **Law of Mass Action,** was defined in the following paragraph:

> I have already given evidence, which is augmented in the present study, that the equipotentiality is not absolute but is subject to a law of mass action whereby the efficiency of performance of an entire complex function may be reduced in proportion to the extent of brain injury within an area whose parts are not more specialized for one component of function than for another. (Lashley, 1929 [1963 reprinting], p. 24)

Although most accounts of Lashley's work describe it in terms of his opposition to opinion about cortical specialization, he was clearly willing to accept that there was some form of cortical specialization for primary sensory and motor functions. However, Lashley strongly argued that the cortex was not specialized in the same manner for functions such as memory and intelligence (an argument that was also advanced by Flourens). This position is still held by many. As you will discover in the following section and later chapters, the human cerebral cortex is clearly specialized for many sensory and motor tasks, but attempts to localize more broadly defined functions such as "consciousness" or "intelligence" (as the phrenologists attempted to do) have not been very successful.

WILDER PENFIELD. Wilder Penfield (1891–1976) was born in Spokane, Washington, but after winning one of the newly established Rhodes scholarships, he trained in England, Germany, and Spain before moving to Canada to become Montreal's first neurosurgeon. After ten years of fundraising and campaigning in Montreal, he established the now famous Montreal Neurological Institute in 1934. Penfield is perhaps best known for the clinical and experimental work that he completed between the 1930s and 1950s. In an effort to treat intractable epilepsy (uncontrollable seizures), neurosurgeons of that time were starting to remove the brain tissue that they suspected caused the seizures. For the most part, these surgeries were proving to be successful, although the challenge was to remove as little of the healthy tissue as possible. Thus, successful surgeries were those that reduced seizures and spared as much structure and function as possible.

In an attempt to minimize the amount of tissue that was removed in these surgeries, Penfield sought to identify the diseased areas in a very direct fashion. He relied on the earlier experimental work of Ferrier and Fitsch and Hitzig and devised a technique for stimulating the cortex of his awake epileptic patients during their brain surgery. Knowing that many epileptics experience **auras** (a perceptual experience that occurs without sensory stimulation, such as smelling burnt toast when there is no such smell in the room) before the onset of seizures, Penfield reasoned that when low levels of electrical stimulation were applied to the regions within or surrounding the brain areas most involved in starting a seizure, the person should experience the same aura. To determine whether he was stimulating the correct spot, Penfield operated on his patients while they were awake and able to communicate, using a local anaesthetic. Because the brain itself has no somatosensory receptors, Penfield's stimulation of the surface of the brain was not painful to the patient. Instead, following stimulation of a particular area, the patient could report what (if anything) he or she perceived. When areas in the center of the auditory cortex in the temporal lobe were stimulated, patients would report hearing sounds such as "a bell ringing" or a "buzzing noise." When Penfield stimulated the areas that surrounded the primary auditory cortex, patients described the sounds with greater specificity. Instead of giving generic labels for the sounds, such as "ringing" or "buzzing," the patients described the sounds with more specific terms, such as "a cricket chirping." Penfield's suspicion that he could localize the source of seizure activity by stimulating the areas that produce auras in epileptics proved to be correct. These auras could often be provoked by stimulating areas in the temporal lobe, and when the aura-producing areas were removed, seizures were much less common (Penfield & Rasmussen, 1950).

As a clinical technique, this strategy was very effective, and it is still used for the treatment of intractable epilepsy. Penfield was able to remove the source of seizure activity while leaving much of the surrounding healthy cortex intact. However, together with his colleague Herbert Jasper, Penfield's most famous contribution to neuroscience was his mapping of somatosensory and motor cortex (Penfield & Boldrey, 1937; Penfield & Jasper, 1954). When areas just behind the frontal lobe of the brain (the **postcentral gyrus of the parietal lobe**) were stimulated, Penfield's patients reported feeling tactile sensations in various parts of their body. When the stimulation was right at the top of the brain, they reported sensations in their legs or trunk. Stimulation farther down the side of the brain produced sensations in the face or mouth. This discovery, that the human cortex is organized according to a map of the surface of the body (called *somatropic*) led to his development of a sensory and motor map called a **somatosensory homunculus** (*homunculus* means "little man"). These drawings (see Figure 1.3) illustrate the parts of the body in different sizes, depending on how much cortical area is devoted to sensation from that area. Note that some relatively large body parts (e.g., trunk, leg) have little cortical representation, whereas other, smaller body parts (e.g., hand, mouth) have extensive cortical representation. As you might guess from Figure 1.3, people are extremely sensitive to stimulation of the areas with

Figure 1.3   **A Drawing of a Somatosensory Homunculus**

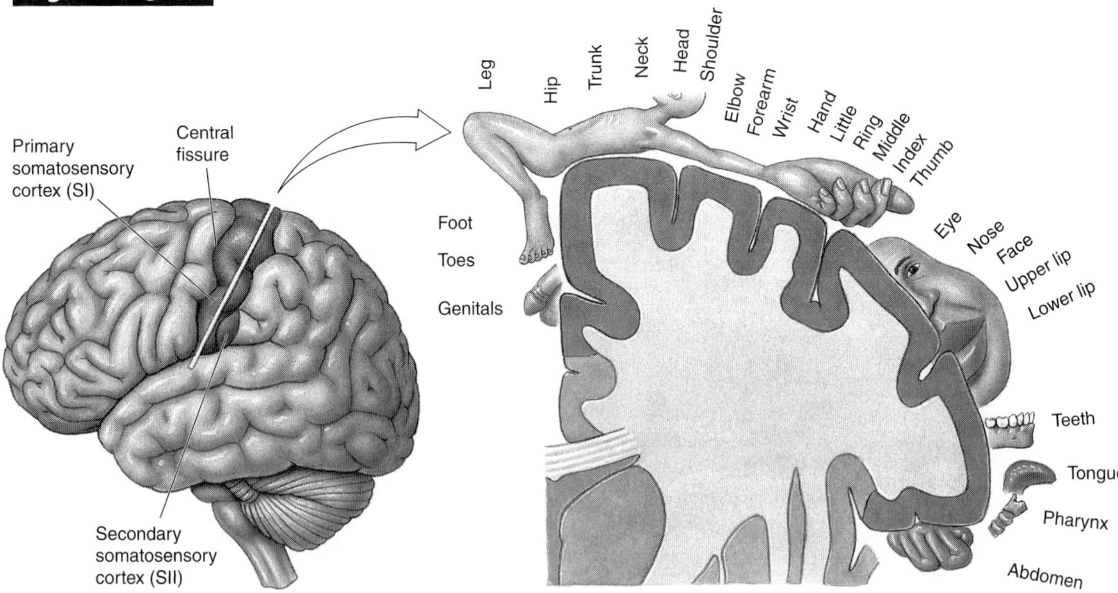

Source: John P. J. Pinel, *Biopsychology,* 5e. Published by Allyn and Bacon, Boston, MA. Copyright © 2003 by Pearson Education. Reprinted by permission of the publisher.

Table 1.4	Brain Mapping Pioneers
1909	Brodmann publishes his book on cytoarchitecture (physical features of neurons that are found in certain areas of the cerebral cortex).
1917	Lashley and Frantz investigate memory function in rodents and develop the Law of Equipotentiality and the Law of Mass Action.
1934	Penfield becomes Montreal's first neurosurgeon; best known for his clinical and experimental work related to epilepsy during the 1930s–1950s.
1954	Penfield and Jasper map the somatosensory and motor cortex.

extensive representation. In Chapter 5, we discuss this homunculus further (including criticism that part of it is incorrect) along with the homunculus that describes the cortical representation of movement. Adaptations of Penfield's drawings appear in textbooks almost as commonly as Brodmann's maps. Like Descartes, Penfield spent considerable time (particularly late in his life) pondering the scientific basis of the human soul. As was the case with Descartes, he did not find one.

Table 1.4 lists the accomplishments of some of the pioneers of brain mapping.

Functional Neurosurgery

With the knowledge that particular parts of the brain have specific functions came the temptation to alter the brain's anatomy to alter its functioning. The work of Goltz, Fritsch and Hitzig, and Ferrier laid some of the foundation for the neurosurgery that became so popular in the nineteenth century. More specifically, Goltz's observation that dogs with temporal lobe damage were more tame than unlesioned dogs inspired Swiss physician Gottlieb Burkhardt to perform operations in 1892 on six of the schizophrenic patients in the "insane asylum" that he supervised. Before the surgery, all six patients experienced hallucinations and were easily agitated. After the surgeries, some of the patients appeared to be calmer—although two died. Understandably, the medical authorities at the time opposed this type of experimental treatment, and very few functional neurosurgeries were performed over the next forty years.

Goltz's early work on docility in dogs following cortical lesions was followed up by a number of experiments in the United States in the early nineteenth century. Testing primates instead of dogs, investigators such as Carlyle Jacobson discovered that frontal cortical lesions (damaging frontal and/or prefrontal cortex) reduced aggressive behavior. These reductions appeared to emerge without other major changes or losses in functions such as object recognition or memory. Providing converging evidence that the frontal lobes were involved in neurosis, John Fulton attempted to induce an experimental neurosis in chimpanzees with large frontal lesions. Despite being able to successfully induce neuroticlike behavior in chimpanzees with intact frontal lobes, Fulton could not produce the same changes in the lesioned chimpanzees.

The first physician to attempt to apply the findings to people was Portuguese neuropsychiatrist Antônio Egas Moniz. Together with his colleague Almeida Lima, Moniz developed a technique called a **leucotomy** (meaning "white matter cutting"), wherein the tracts between the thalamus and the frontal lobe were severed by using a specially developed knife called a leukotome. The surgery was first performed in 1935. First, two small holes were created in the sides of the skull by trepanning (similar to the trephination method described in Module 1.1). Then the leukotome was inserted and moved side to side, severing the white matter connections to the frontal lobes. The procedure seemed to be more effective than any other treatment that was available at the time (antipsychotic drugs had not yet been developed), and the global medical community quickly adopted the procedure. Moniz was awarded the Nobel Prize in Physiology or Medicine in 1949 "for his discovery of the therapeutic value of leucotomy in certain psychoses."

As a modern reader who knows that frontal leucotomies are no longer performed, you might think that Moniz does not sound like a particularly cautious physician. Actually, Moniz was conservative in comparison to other advocates of psychosurgery. In fact, Moniz argued that psychosurgery should be performed only as a last resort; psychosurgery was recommended only if no other forms of treatment produced satisfactory results and only for patients who remained a danger to themselves or others. (As an aside—Moniz retired after being shot in the spine and rendered paraplegic by one of his former patients. It is perhaps ironic that he would suffer nervous system damage at the hand of his patient.)

Despite Moniz's cautions, others were considerably more enthusiastic about his procedure, and the leucotomy was quickly adopted and adapted by American neurologist Walter Freeman. After hearing of the results of Moniz's first procedures performed in 1935, Freeman teamed up with neurosurgeon James Watts, and they first attempted the procedure in September 1936. Pleased with the results, Freeman and Watts (particularly Freeman) went on to promote the procedure through the press, referring to it as a **prefrontal lobotomy.** After performing many of the procedures with Watts, Freeman became dissatisfied with the trephining that was required during the procedure. After hearing about an alternative method, in which the leukotome was inserted through an eye orbit, Freeman and Watts developed a simpler technique in 1945. Substituting a common icepick for a leukotome similar to that designed by Moniz, Freeman could insert the pick through a tear duct and use a small hammer to perforate the skull; then the pick could be used to destroy the connections to the prefrontal cortex. The same procedure would then be performed through the other eye orbit. Unlike Moniz's procedure, this adaptation could be performed quickly, under local anaesthetic. This procedure greatly increased Freeman's capacity to perform the operations. His production line approach to neurosurgery horrified even the most seasoned neurosurgeons of the time, especially because he had no licence to perform surgery. Even his partner, James Watts, became uncomfortable with this approach, eventually distancing himself from Freeman. According to Freeman's records, he performed 3439 lobotomies. It is estimated that between 1936 and 1960, physicians (including Freeman) completed 40,000–50,000 lobotomies in the United States.

Table 1.5	Pioneers in Functional Neurosurgery
1892	Burkhardt is inspired by Goltz's work and performs neurosurgeries on patients with schizophrenia.
Early 1930s	Jacobson discovers that cortical lesions reduce aggressive behavior in chimpanzees.
	Fulton induces neurosis in chimpanzees with intact cortex but cannot with lesioned chimpanzees.
1935	Lima and Moniz develop the leucotomy to treat patients with brain disorders; Moniz wins the Nobel Prize for Physiology in 1949 for his contribution to the treatment of psychoses.
1936	Neurologist Freeman teams up with neurosurgeon Watts, and they conduct their first leucotomy, a procedure later renamed lobotomy.
1945	Freeman and Watts develop a slightly different procedure, and the popularity of the procedure continues to increase until the development of psychiatric drugs in the 1950s.

New drug therapies for psychoses, anxiety disorders, and depression were developed starting in the 1950s. These developments, combined with mounting criticism about the efficacy of the lobotomy, led to its demise in North America. Although very few controlled studies were performed, on the basis of the available evidence, retrospective analyses suggest that lobotomies do not appear to be particularly effective in treating psychotic symptoms. At best, one third of patients who received lobotomies appeared to improve following the surgery. Considering that 25–30% of individuals suffering from these conditions will improve spontaneously (with no treatment), this success rate is not impressive and perhaps no different than chance.

Table 1.5 lists the accomplishments of some of the pioneers of functional neurosurgery.

The Paradigm Shift in Neuropsychology

The goal of neuropsychology is to study the relationship between brain activity and behavior. Given this goal, what if there were a way to tell exactly what brain areas were active (and how much) during any given task? Would that make neuropsychology's goal easy to reach? Of course it would—wouldn't it? Newly developed techniques for providing three-dimensional representations of brain metabolism (such as oxygen or glucose use) have been developed, and collectively, these methods are referred to as **functional neuroimaging.** Initially, when these methods were just starting to become popular, some people predicted that they would rapidly put an end to experimental neuropsychology. After all, given a tool that could map out what parts of the brain are required for a given task, how long would it take to map out the entire brain? Although the task of human brain mapping has certainly been revolutionized by neuroimaging, the job is far from complete. Furthermore, current imaging

Neuropsychological Celebrity

Frances Farmer

According to Leonard Maltin's *Movie Encyclopedia* (1994), Frances Farmer was a "beautiful, intelligent, talented leading lady of the 1930s and 1940s whose unfortunate life story has become the preeminent cautionary fable describing the bleak underside of Hollywood success." Frances studied drama at the University of Washington and then moved to Hollywood in 1936. Shortly thereafter, she signed a seven-year contract with Paramount Studios and starred in films such as *Too Many Parents* and *Border Flights*.

She was a popular box office draw, but she developed a reputation among filmmakers for being contemptuous and rebellious. She refused to "play the Hollywood game," both professionally and socially. Paramount Studios dropped her contract, and she started performing in supporting actress roles in lesser-quality films. One night in 1942, she received a traffic ticket for drunk driving. According to some accounts, she was very verbally abusive to the arresting officer, and the event degenerated to a shoving match for which she was eventually sentenced to 180 days in jail. She became hysterical during the subsequent court appearance, was jailed, and behaved even less appropriately within the confines of the prison. She was later declared mentally incompetent by her own mother and spent the subsequent years in various institutions.

According to biographer William Arnold (1978), Farmer met the famous lobotomist Walter Freeman in the late 1940s at Western State Hospital in Steilacoom, Washington. There, Freeman reportedly performed what has become the most infamous lobotomy of all time. According to most sources (but not Farmer's own family), Freeman performed a lobotomy on Frances Farmer in front of a gallery of observers. According to Walter Freeman's son Frank, Walter verified that he had operated on Farmer and identified her in a photograph. Although the picture clearly depicts Freeman performing a lobotomy, the identity of the patient is not clear. Interviews with Farmer after this date depicted a detached woman with very flat affect. This is certainly consistent with the outcome of a lobotomy, but it is also consistent with an individual who is on any number of a variety of medications. Did Frances Farmer have a lobotomy? Is she the patient depicted in the most famous photograph of functional neurosurgery? According to most of the popular press and her biographer, yes. According to her family, no.

methods can have very serious technical and methodological limitations (more on this in Chapter 3).

One problem that plagues all of the imaging tools is individual variation. It might sound like a cliché, but everyone's brain is different. Just as people are different on the outside, each person looks different on the inside too. This creates a serious challenge for researchers who wish to use neuroimaging, because there is no "average" brain. What, then, does one do with functional neuroimaging from a group of ten people? Morph them together into one image? Discuss them separately? Although both techniques are used, there is no consensus about which is more appropriate.

Before functional neuroimaging had its impact on experimental neuropsychology, structural imaging (generating an image of the brain's physical structure, regardless of its structure, such as a computed tomography scan or magnetic resonance imaging) had already revolutionized clinical neuropsychology. Before the advent of these techniques, the neuropsychological assessment was concerned primarily with determining whether brain damage was present (sometimes called *organicity*), and if there was evidence of damage, the neuropsychologist attempted to localize it. Now these scanners are available in most major urban centers in the developed world. Whereas we used to rely on the results of hours of behavioral testing to determine the nature and extent of brain damage, now the person being assessed need not even be conscious. After a brief scan, the examining physician knows both the location and the extent of the injury, if any.

Does this mean that clinical neuropsychologists are now obsolete? Certainly not. In fact, clinical neuropsychologists are in great demand, and the size and number of training programs keep growing to try to meet this demand. A number of reasons can account for this increase. One is that the average age of the population in the Western world is increasing, and along with this increase comes increased prevalence in diseases of older age such as Alzheimer's disease and Parkinson's disease. Clinical neuropsychologists are also in demand because the nature and goals of neuropsychological assessments have changed dramatically since the advent of neuroimaging. Instead of seeking to determine and localize damage, the neuropsychological assessment seeks to diagnose conditions that are not readily detectable by using neuroimaging (e.g., early stages of Alzheimer's disease), to assess the client's quality of life, and to evaluate the client's capacity to succeed in his or her present environment (e.g., assessing whether the person will be able to return to work or whether the person should move from home to a managed care facility). Most recently, the clinical neuropsychologist has become more involved in rehabilitation following brain injury (see Chapter 16).

◄ **WHERE WE HAVE BEEN** Brodmann's cytoarchitectonic mapping and Penfield's sensory and motor mapping continue to be used to this day. Lashley's views on the equipotentiality of the cortex with regards to memory and intellect are also held in high regard today. These early investigations of which behaviors are localized helped to inform the psychosurgical practices that were adopted later in the twentieth century to try to treat mental illness. Although these procedures were very popular for a short while, they quickly fell into disrepute and were replaced by psychoactive medications. Other advancements, such as the development of structural and functional neuroimaging, had dramatic impact on the goals and means of both experimental and clinical neuropsychology.

Glossary

Aphemia (Broca's aphasia)—The deficit suffered by individuals who, as a result of a left hemisphere frontal lobe lesion, are incapable of productive speech. Broca suggested that these individuals had lost the capacity for speech but retained the ability to understand language.

Auras—A perceptual experience that many epileptics experience, which occurs without sensory stimulation before the onset of seizures. Smelling burnt toast is one such aura that is commonly experienced by epileptics.

Cardiocentric hypothesis (also referred to as the cardiac hypothesis)—The hypothesis that the heart was the center for cognitive and emotional function.

Cephalocentric hypothesis (also referred to as the brain hypothesis)—The hypothesis that the brain is the center for behavior.

Cerebrospinal fluid—Fluid in the brain that supports, nourishes, and cleans the brain.

Clinical neuropsychology—A specialty area of neuropsychology that is concerned with the diagnosis, treatment, and rehabilitation of individuals with neurological disorders.

Cytoarchitecture—Typical physical features of the neurons that reside in different regions of the brain.

Dualism—Originally proposed by Descartes, the idea that the mind and body are separate but interacting entities.

Engram—A hypothetical change in the brain that is responsible for storing memories that was posited by Karl Lashley.

Equipotentiality (Law of Equipotentiality)—Proposal that the cortex functions as a whole, with no functional specialization within the cortex.

Experimental neuropsychology (also referred to as cognitive neuropsychology or cognitive neuroscience)—A specialty area of neuropsychology that is concerned with understanding how the brain produces behavior in both neurological intact and damaged individuals.

Functional neuroimaging—Techniques that provide three-dimensional representations of brain metabolism (such as oxygen or glucose use) while the person is performing various mental tasks. Functional magnetic resonance imaging (fMRI) and positron emission tomography (PET) are two such functional imaging techniques.

Golgi stain—A stain developed by Italian histologist Camillo Golgi that stains only some neurons and stains the entire neuron, revealing parts other than the cell body. This is done through soaking tissue in a silver solution (often silver chromate), making stained neurons appear a dark color.

Histology—Examination of thin, fixed sections of brain that have been stained with different techniques (e.g., Golgi stain).

Law of Mass Action—The proposal that the degree of deficit is directly related to the proportion of brain that has been lesioned.

Lesioning—The process by which brain tissue is experimentally damaged or removed.

Leucotomy—The procedure pioneered by Moniz in which the thalamus is disconnected from the frontal lobe with a special knife, called a leukotome.

Monism—The idea that the mind and body are the same thing, a position that most neuropsychologists take.

Neuron doctrine—A proposal by Spanish histologist and artist Santiago Ramon y Cajal that neurons were not continuous and that they must communicate by contact.

Neuropsychology—The study of the relationship between behavior and activity of the brain.

Nissl stain—A stain developed by German neurologist Franz Nissl that distinguishes neurons from other cells in the brain by staining the central portions of neurons (cell body) wherever it is applied.

Phrenology—The pseudo-scientific practice of inferring personality and other traits from bumps on the skull.

Postcentral gyrus of the parietal lobe—Somatosensory cortex; an area of the brain that, when stimulated electrically, results in sensations being touched.

Prefrontal lobotomy—A technique, practiced starting in the 1930s by Walter Freeman, which involved inserting a sharp instrument through the eye orbit or tear duct, perforating the skull, and destroying the connections to the prefrontal cortex.

Prosody—The emotional tone of speech.

Psychology—The study of the attempt to describe, explain, predict, and, in some cases, change behavior.

Somatosensory humunculus—A sensory and motor map of the surface of the human brain.

Synapse—The term coined by Sherrington to describe the gap between neurons.

Trephination—Surgically opening the skull as a means of treatment. Although this form of treatment was practiced in ancient times, it still has somewhat of a following today.

Wernicke's aphasia—Aphasia caused by lesions in the left temporal lobes that results in the ability to produce speech but not to use words correctly or to understand the speech of others.

2

Neuroanatomy

If the human brain were so simple that we could understand it, we would be so simple that we couldn't.
—EMERSON M. PUGH

MODULE **2.1**

Cells of the Nervous System

We must start somewhere, so let's start small. Every living thing is made up of cells. What makes the human a higher-functioning organism is the fact that humans have aggregates of specialized cells that perform specialized functions. Although the brain is composed of many parts, all of which have multiple functions, the larger components of the brain are made up of individual cells, which are the focus of this unit. **Neurons** and **glia** are the specialized cells of the nervous system, and they are specialized in both structure and function. As you will see in this unit, glia provide support functions, and neurons are the communicators. Neurons react and respond to stimuli, and they are the basis of behavior. Neurons also learn and store information about their external environment. Before we can investigate higher functions, it is important to consider what a neuron is and what a neuron does to achieve all of this.

WHERE WE ARE GOING ➤ We are going to begin this module with a discussion of the types of cells (neurons and glia) that make up the nervous system. We will discuss the means by which information is transmitted within the neuron and how neurons communicate with each other. The second module will focus on the major divisions of the nervous system and the structures and systems within these divisions. Finally, we will discuss how the brain is protected from damage.

Neurons and Glia: Structure and Function

GROSS ANATOMY OF THE NEURON. Although there are many types of neurons, most are similar to the one depicted in Figure 2.1. Perhaps the most distinctive structural feature of a neuron is its shape. As you will see, the neuron's shape is closely related to its function: to receive, conduct, and transmit signals—to collect information and send it on (or not). The neuron consists of three main components: (1) the **dendrites,** which receive incoming information from other neurons; (2) the **soma,** or cell body, which contains the genetic machinery and most of the metabolic machinery needed for common cellular functions; and (3) the **axon,** which sends neural information to other neurons. Information is passed from the axon to the dendrite across a gap (about 20–50 nanometers wide), which is called a **synapse.** On the basis of their positions relative to the synapse, you will often see events that occur in the axon referred to as **presynaptic** and events that happen in the dendrite referred to as **postsynaptic.**

Dendrites essentially increase the surface area available for the reception of signals from the axons of other neurons. The extent of branching of the dendrites gives an indication of the number of connections or synapses it makes with incoming axons. In some cases, dendrites from one neuron can receive as many as 100,000 inputs. All of this information is sent to the rest of the neuron in the form of an electrical charge, or action potential. Dendrites are often covered with tiny spines, which grow and retract in response to experience. The spines themselves can form synapses with other neurons.

The axon is commonly thought of as an information sender. The neuron has only one axon, although an axon can divide at its far end into many branches (thereby

Figure 2.1   **Major Features of the Neuron**

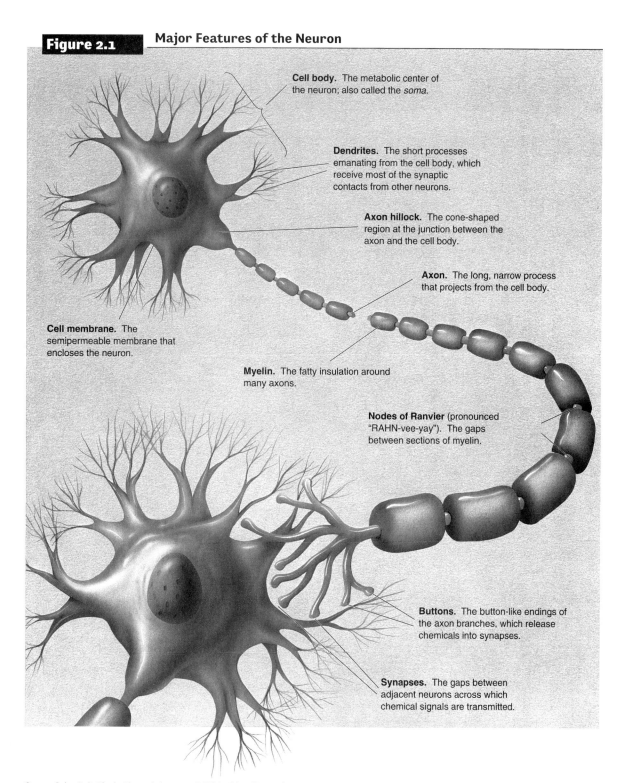

Cell body. The metabolic center of the neuron; also called the *soma*.

Dendrites. The short processes emanating from the cell body, which receive most of the synaptic contacts from other neurons.

Axon hillock. The cone-shaped region at the junction between the axon and the cell body.

Axon. The long, narrow process that projects from the cell body.

Cell membrane. The semipermeable membrane that encloses the neuron.

Myelin. The fatty insulation around many axons.

Nodes of Ranvier (pronounced "RAHN-vee-yay"). The gaps between sections of myelin.

Buttons. The button-like endings of the axon branches, which release chemicals into synapses.

Synapses. The gaps between adjacent neurons across which chemical signals are transmitted.

increasing the number of synapses it can form). The axon is essentially a long thin fiber or wire that can pass its message along to many different cells simultaneously. Consistent with the wire analogy, many axons in the mammalian nervous system are covered with insulation, called **myelin**. Myelin helps to speed the rate of information transfer and to ensure that the message gets to the end of the axon. The end of an axon is called the **terminal button**. Information is sent from the terminal button across the synapse to the dendrite. Information that passes from the axon across the synapse is in the form of a neurochemical message (by substances referred to as **neurotransmitters**), which may be transformed into an electrical message within the dendrite.

INTERNAL ANATOMY OF THE NEURON. Like all animal cells, the neuron is covered with a membrane. There is nothing obvious that sets neural cell membranes apart from other animal cell membranes. The **plasma membrane** consists of a bilayer of continuous sheets of phospholipids that separate two fluid (H_2O) environments—one inside the cell (cytoplasm) and the other outside the cell. Within this membrane are proteins and channels that allow the passage of materials into and out of the neuron. Inside the main cell body, small components of the cell, called organelles, form a complex environment in which organelles perform the various genetic (**nucleus**), synthetic (**ribosomes, endoplasmic reticulum**), and metabolic (**mitochondria**) processes that keep the neuron functioning.

The cell nucleus is probably the most recognizable organelle under the microscope. Functionally, the nucleus packages and controls the genetic information contained in DNA (deoxyribonucleic acid). In two very crucial steps, the nucleus processes the genetic information needed to complete a series of events that form a path from the recipe that the genetic information provides to form proteins that the neuron needs. The nucleus also contains all of the genetic information needed to code proteins such as those for eye or hair color, as well as those that are thought to underlie complex processes such as linguistic ability.

STRUCTURE AND FUNCTION OF NEURONS. Neurons can be classified according to structure and function. The variety of patterns of branching in both axons and dendrites aids in our classification of neurons into different functional and structural classes. In the nervous system, structure and function are often related. Structurally, some common neurons are labelled as **unipolar, bipolar,** and **multipolar** (the most common). Unipolar neurons have only one process emanating from the cell body; bipolar neurons have two processes; and multipolar have numerous processes extending from the cell body. Neurons with no axons or only very short axons are called interneurons, and they tend to integrate information within a structure rather than sending information between structures.

Functionally, neurons can be classified by the type of signals that they process. For instance, the signals that motor neurons convey may represent muscle contraction. Sensory neurons process information elicited from sensory-type stimuli, whereas interneurons make connections between cells, enabling a sort of convergence and combination of behavioral responses. Thus, the type of information that is represented by neural activity relates to the function of the neuron. Neurons can also be classed as being **afferent** (bringing information to the central nervous system or structure) or **efferent** (sending information from the brain or away from a structure). Nonetheless, it is important that you appreciate that neurons do vary in size, shape, and function and that a neuron can change shape as a result of experience.

GLIA. As was mentioned in the introduction to this module, neurons are not the only type of cell in the nervous system; there are also glia, which perform an essential role in the functioning of the central nervous system. Generally, glia perform support functions, different types of glia providing different types of support. (Support cells outside of the brain and spinal cord are called **satellite cells.**) There are at least three different types of glia: astrocytes, oligodendrocytes, and microglia.

Astrocytes are the largest glia and are named *astrocytes* because they tend to be star-shaped. Astrocytes fill the space between neurons, resulting in close contact between neurons and astrocytes. (There is often as little as 20 nanometers between neurons and astrocytes.) It is thought that this close contact between astrocytes and neurons can affect the growth of neurons (Sheppard, 1994). As you will see in the next module, astrocytes are involved in the blood–brain barrier, a protective system that keeps the brain separate from the rest of the body. Astrocytes also perform nutritive and metabolic functions for neurons. Astrocytes are also essential for the regulation of the chemical content of the extracellular space; that is, because they envelop the synapse, they can regulate how far neurotransmitters and other substances released by the terminal button can spread. Similarly, astrocytes are important in the storage of neurotransmitters. It is clear that we do not know all of the functions of the astrocyte, as recent evidence suggests that astrocytes may even play a role in the transmission of information in the nervous system.

Oligodendrocytes, however, have one very clear function: to make myelin (Peters, Palay, & Webster, 1991). Oligodendrocytes wrap their processes around most axons in the brain and spinal cord (Figure 2.2). These processes are made of myelin, which is a fatty substance that acts to insulate the axon. Axons outside of the brain and spinal cord are also frequently myelinated, with the myelin provided by **Schwann cells.** Beyond their location in the nervous system, one major difference between Schwann cells and oligodendrocytes is that Schwann cells provide only one segment of myelin to an axon, whereas oligodendrocytes can contribute many segments to many axons.

Microglia are named with reference to their size—they are the smallest of the glia. Microglia are **phagocytes** that remove debris from the nervous system. Debris can accumulate in the brain as a result of injury, disease, infection, or aging. Microglia are very different from the other cells of the nervous system: They are made outside of the brain and spinal cord by macrophages. Excessive activation of microglia has been implicated in neurodegenerative diseases such as multiple sclerosis and Alzheimer's disease.

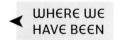
WHERE WE HAVE BEEN

We have discussed the structure and functions of neurons and glia. Neurons are the communicators of the nervous system, whereas glia tend to perform support functions. Neurons and glia can be categorized by structure or by function.

| **Figure 2.2** | **Myelination of Peripheral and Central Nervous System Axons** |

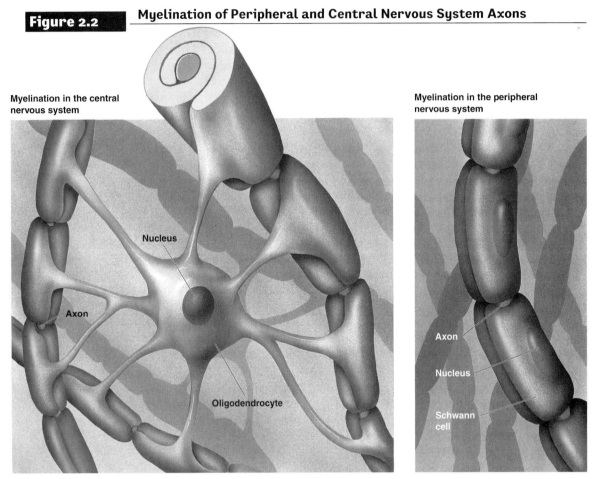

Source: John P. J. Pinel, *Biopsychology,* 5e. Published by Allyn and Bacon, Boston, MA. Copyright © 2003 by Pearson Education. Reprinted by permission of the publisher.

WHERE WE ARE GOING ▶ We will now discuss the means by which information is transmitted within the neuron and how neurons communicate with each other. The second module will focus on the major divisions of the nervous system and the structures and systems within these divisions. Finally, we will discuss how the brain is protected from damage.

Communication within the Neuron: The Action Potential

When a neurotransmitter diffuses across the synapse to interact with the postsynaptic site, a series of electrical events can occur, some of which act to send information to other neurons and some of which inhibit sending information to other neurons.

The electrical events that underlie the transmission (or inhibition) of information rely on the balance of ions between the inside of the neuron (intracellular) and the outside of the neuron (extracellular). When the neuron is at rest, it maintains an electrical charge of about −70 millivolts (mV), which means that the electrical charge on the inside of the neuron is 70 mV less than the charge on the outside. This initial state of the neuron is called the **resting potential.**

The resting potential of the neuron depends on the difference between the concentrations of ions across the neuron membrane. Neurons contain a variety of ions, although the ones that are important for understanding the electrical properties of the neuron are sodium ions (Na^+) and potassium ions (K^+). At rest, the extracellular fluid contains high concentrations of Na^+, and the intracellular fluid contains high concentrations of K^+. In simple solutions, ions are distributed homogeneously, that is, they are found in equal amounts throughout the solution. However, in the brain, ions are concentrated in either the extracellular or intracellular fluid.

The neuron has two properties that promote the uneven distribution of ions. The first property relates to the permeability of the cell membrane that covers the neuron. The membrane is not permeable to all types of ions. Ions cross the membrane through proteins embedded in the membrane, which are known as **ion channels.** At rest, K^+ readily crosses the membrane, whereas Na^+ cannot easily enter the neuron. However, given enough time, enough Na^+ would sneak into the cell and enough K^+ would leak out of the neuron that there would be homogeneous distribution of the ions. Thus, the second property of the neuron that promotes uneven distribution of ions is the neuron active transport of ions by the neuron. Neurons actively import K^+ and actively export Na^+ through a transport mechanism known as a **sodium–potassium pump.** The sodium–potassium pump requires the neuron to use energy, thereby ensuring that the uneven distribution of ions is maintained. The sodium–potassium pump exchanges three Na^+ ions inside the cell for two K^+ ions that are outside the cell.

When a neurotransmitter diffuses across the synapse, it can open ion channels that allow the rapid influx (inflow) of Na^+ into the neuron and the rapid efflux (outflow) of K^+ from the neuron. The opening of the sodium channels allows Na^+ to rapidly enter the neuron, which makes the intracellular space more positive. When the change in the membrane potential moves from its resting state of about −70 mV to about +50 mV (this change in the membrane potential is called **depolarization**), an **action potential** occurs. When an action potential occurs, neurotransmitters are released from the terminal buttons. Thus, although action potentials occur entirely within one neuron, they result in neurotransmitter release that results in communication between neurons.

However, Na^+ entering the neuron is not the entire story. As the neuron becomes depolarized, K^+ channels open, and K^+ ions rapidly leave the neuron. The efflux of K^+ triggers the closing of the sodium channels, and eventually, the neuron returns to its resting state of −70 mV, also called repolarization (Figure 2.3). Because the K^+ channels take longer than necessary to close, some additional K^+ leaks out, which results in a temporary change in the membrane beyond −70 mV (called **hyperpolarization**).

There are several features of an action potential that must be considered. The first is that there are times when an action potential cannot be triggered. For instance, when

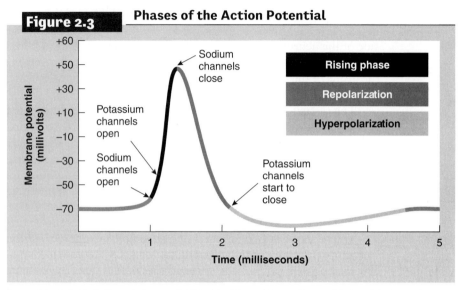

Source: John P. J. Pinel, *Biopsychology,* 5e. Published by Allyn and Bacon, Boston, MA. Copyright © 2003 by Pearson Education. Reprinted by permission of the publisher.

the neuron is strongly depolarized, sodium channels close and cannot be reopened. Because action potentials require the movement of Na⁺, the inability to open sodium channels results in a period of time during which an action potential cannot be triggered (known as the **absolute refractory period**). The second feature of action potentials is that they are "all or none." That is, once the neuron becomes sufficiently depolarized, sodium channels open and an action potential occurs. The features of the sodium channels also result in similar levels of depolarization, which ensures that all action potentials are the same size.

Another feature of action potentials relates to the myelination of axons. Myelin is not uniformly located on the axon; there are a number of small gaps in the myelin, known as **nodes of Ranvier.** In myelinated neurons, ion channels and sodium–potassium pumps occur only at the nodes of Ranvier. Thus, in myelinated axons, ions can cross the membrane only at the nodes of Ranvier.

When an action potential first reaches the axon, it is passively propagated to the first node of Ranvier. This initial depolarization results in the production of a new action potential at the node of Ranvier. This depolarization jumps to the next node of Ranvier, and the sequence of events occurs again. The jumping of the action potential from one node of Ranvier to another is called **saltatory conduction,** and this series of events occurs down the entire length of the axon. Each node of Ranvier actively generates a new action potential, resulting in an action potential that is of uniform size. Furthermore, because the action potential is actively propagated, neural transmission in myelinated neurons is faster than transmission in neurons without myelination.

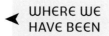

We have discussed the structure and functions of neurons and glia. Neurons use electrical signals to send information internally. These electrical signals are called action potentials, and action potentials tend to be all or none, tend to be equivalent in size, and are actively propagated by neurons. Myelin is the insulation on the neuron that speeds up neurotransmission.

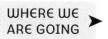

The next section will focus on communication between neurons and the chemicals (or neurotransmitters) that are used to send messages across the synapse. The second module will focus on the major divisions of the nervous system and the structures and systems within these divisions. Finally, we will discuss how the brain is protected from damage.

Communication between Neurons: The Synapse

Within the neuron, communication is largely electrical, relying on the action potential to transmit information. However, between neurons, communication is largely chemical. This section will focus on the details of how neurons communicate with each other across the synapse. Although most synapses are **axodendritic** (see Figure 2.4), that is, they consist of axons that form synapses with dendritic spines, there are other types of synapses. Axosomatic synapses are made up of axons forming synapses with the soma of the neurons, and they are also very common. There are also dendrodendritic synapses (dendrites forming synapses with other dendrites) and axoaxonic synapses (axons forming synapses with other axons). For the purposes of this chapter, we will consider axodendritic synapses, beginning with the presynaptic events and ending with the postsynaptic events that result in an action potential.

The terminal button of an axon contains dozens of small packages (vesicles) that contain neurotransmitters (Figure 2.4). Often the neurotransmitters are located next to active zones, which are areas of protein accumulation on the membrane that allow the vesicle to deposit its contents into the synapse. Neurotransmitter release is triggered by the arrival of an action potential at the terminal button of the axon. The action potential causes calcium (Ca^{2+}) channels to open, and Ca^{2+} rushes into the neuron. The increase in concentration of Ca^{2+} causes the neurotransmitter to be released into the synapse by a process known as **exocytosis**. During exocytosis, the membrane of the vesicle fuses with the axonal membrane (at the active zone), which results in an opening in the vesicle (or pore), allowing the neurotransmitter to flow into the synapse.

Once the neurotransmitter has been released, it diffuses across the synapse to produce postsynaptic effects. Postsynaptic effects occur when the neurotransmitter binds to a protein embedded in the postsynaptic membrane known as a receptor. For the most part, receptors are specific; that is, only one type of neurotransmitter can bind to a given receptor (although there are many subtypes of receptors for the same neurotransmitter). Commonly, this specificity is described by using the analogy of a lock and key. That is, you may have many keys to many locks, but only one key opens a given lock (hopefully!). Two types of receptors are located on the postsynaptic membrane: transmitter-gated ion channels and G-protein-coupled receptors. Often

Figure 2.4 | The Synapse

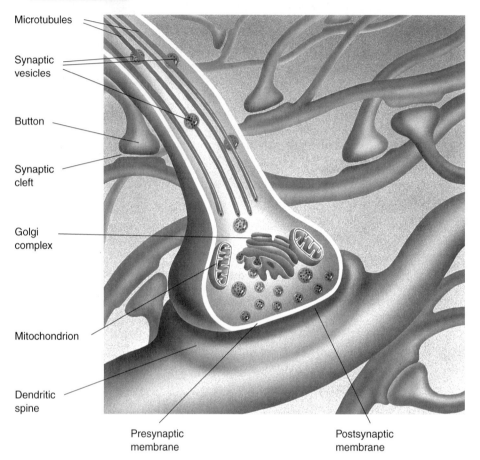

Microtubules

Synaptic vesicles

Button

Synaptic cleft

Golgi complex

Mitochondrion

Dendritic spine

Presynaptic membrane

Postsynaptic membrane

Source: John P. J. Pinel, *Biopsychology,* 5e. Published by Allyn and Bacon, Boston, MA. Copyright © 2003 by Pearson Education. Reprinted by permission of the publisher.

dendrites will have a mixture of the two types of receptors located in their membranes. Additionally, these different receptors (located on the same cell membrane) frequently bind different neurotransmitters.

Transmitter-gated ion channels (Figure 2.5) or **ionotropic** receptors are proteins that control an ion channel. When a neurotransmitter binds to a transmitter-gated ion channel, the channel changes conformation (either opening or closing). Ionotropic receptors result in quick changes in ionic concentrations and often appear in situations in which a fast response is required.

The functional consequence of receptor binding often depends on the ion that is controlled by the receptor. For instance, if the receptor controls a channel that is permeable to Na+, the net effect will be to depolarize the dendrite (often resulting in

Figure 2.5   Neurotransmitter Receptors

An ionotropic receptor

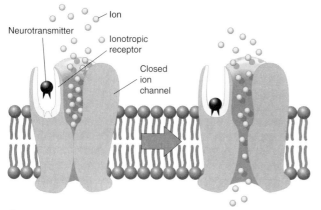

Some neurotransmitter molecules bind to receptors on ion channels. When a neurotransmitter molecule binds to an ionotropic receptor, the channel opens (as in this case) or closes, thereby altering the flow of ions into or out of the neuron.

A metabotropic receptor

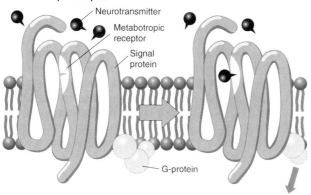

Some neurotransmitter molecules bind to receptors on membrane signal proteins, which are linked to G-proteins. When a neurotransmitter molecule binds to a metabotropic receptor, a subunit of the G-protein breaks off into the neuron and either binds to an ion channel or stimulates the synthesis of a second messenger.

Source: John P. J. Pinel, *Biopsychology,* 5e. Published by Allyn and Bacon, Boston, MA. Copyright © 2003 by Pearson Education. Reprinted by permission of the publisher.

an action potential). If the receptor controls a channel that is permeable to chloride (Cl–), which is highly concentrated in the extracellular fluid, the net effect will be to hyperpolarize the dendrite. When a dendrite is depolarized (moved toward producing an action potential) by the release of a neurotransmitter from the presynaptic site, we call the electrical event an excitatory postsynaptic potential (**EPSP**). Conversely, when a dendrite is hyperpolarized (moved away from producing an action potential) by the release of a neurotransmitter from the presynaptic site, we call the electrical event an inhibitory postsynaptic potential (**IPSP**). Unlike action potentials, postsynaptic potentials are not actively propagated; they get smaller the farther they travel, and they can differ in the degree to which they depolarize or hyperpolarize the neuron.

G-protein-coupled receptors or **metabotropic** receptors (Figure 2.5) produce slower, more diverse, and more sustained responses than transmitter-gated ion channel receptors do. Metabotropic receptors also occur more frequently in the nervous system than do transmitter-gated ion channel receptors. Metabotropic receptors use a multistep process to produce their responses, which begins with the neurotransmitter binding to the receptor. Once the neurotransmitter is bound, a subunit of the G-protein breaks away and can either move along the inside of the membrane and bind to an ion channel or trigger the synthesis of other chemicals. Thus, binding of G-protein receptors can result in IPSPs or EPSPs, or they can result in changes in gene expression. Thus, G-protein receptors can have more diverse effects than ionotropic receptors.

As a final note, there are also neurotransmitter receptors on the presynaptic membrane (**autoreceptors**). Autoreceptors are metabotropic receptors that are located on the presynaptic cell membrane and bind the neurotransmitter released by the presynaptic axon. It is thought that their primary function is to regulate and monitor the amount of neurotransmitter in the synapse.

There must be some mechanism to terminate the action of a neurotransmitter binding to a receptor; otherwise, once neurons were activated, they would remain active. Once the neurotransmitter is bound to the receptor, it will break away from the receptor and diffuse back into the synapse. However, the neurotransmitter must be removed from the synaptic cleft, or it will rebind with the receptor. Two mechanisms are responsible for terminating the activity of neurotransmitters: reuptake and enzymatic degradation. Reuptake is more common and involves the presynaptic neuron reabsorbing the neurotransmitter from the synapse and repackaging it in vesicles to be used again. Enzymatic degradation is when a neurotransmitter is broken down into an inactive form by an enzyme present in the synapse. Often the inactive forms are absorbed into the presynaptic neuron to be resynthesized into the neurotransmitter.

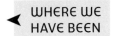 We have discussed how neurons communicate between themselves. When neurotransmitters bind to ionotropic receptors, postsynaptic potentials (either EPSPs or IPSPs) are generated. Unlike action potentials, postsynaptic potentials are not propagated and can vary in size. Metabotropic receptors can also produce EPSPs or IPSPs, although they also produce a variety of more general responses in the neuron.

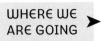 The next section will examine a number of common neurotransmitters in the nervous system. The second module will focus on the major divisions of the nervous system and the structures and systems within these divisions. Finally, we will discuss how the brain is protected from damage.

Neurotransmitters

There are a variety of neurotransmitters, which often are observed in specific types of neurons and are associated with specific behaviors. Commonly, neurotransmitters are divided into small and large molecule neurotransmitters. Within the small-molecule neurotransmitter group are four classes of neurotransmitters: acetylcholine, monoamines, soluble gases, and amino acids. Within the large-molecule group, there is only one class of neurotransmitter: neuropeptides. Most neurotransmitters are either excitatory or inhibitory (although there are some exceptions that depend on receptors). Small-molecule neurotransmitters tend to be released in a directed fashion, activating either ionotropic or metabotropic receptors that act directly on ion channels. Large-molecule neurotransmitters tend to be released diffusely, activating metabotropic receptors, and produce either metabolic or genetic alterations within the neuron. Thus, small-molecule neurotransmitters are associated with fast responses (either excitatory or inhibitory), whereas large-molecule neurotransmitters are associated with slower, longer-lasting responses.

ACETYLCHOLINE. Acetylcholine (ACh) was the first neurotransmitter to be identified, and neurons that release this neurotransmitter are called **cholinergic**. ACh is the neurotransmitter that is used by all motor neurons in the brain and spinal cord (although other neurons in the nervous system also use ACh). ACh is synthesized by enzymatic conversion from choline, which is commonly found in vegetables and egg yolks. ACh is deactivated into choline and acetic acid by acetylcholinesterase (AChE). The rate of degradation is very fast (among the fastest in the nervous system), and choline is reabsorbed presynaptically. Drugs that inhibit AChE prevent the breakdown of ACh and are often used as insecticides and as nerve gases in chemical warfare. Effects of these drugs include decreases in heart rate, blood pressure, and respiration and death.

There are two types of receptors for ACh: muscarinic and nicotinic receptors (named for the exogenous ligands, muscarine and nicotine, that bind to them). The most common receptor subtype is **muscarinic,** which is a metabotropic receptor. Muscarinic receptors are commonly found throughout the brain and in cardiac and smooth muscle (e.g., stomach). Conversely, **nicotinic receptors** are ionotropic and excitatory, and their activity can be blocked by the poison curare. Although nicotinic receptors are found in all striated muscles, they occur in only a few locations within the brain (Feldman, Meyer, & Quenzer, 1997).

MONOAMINES. The **monoamine** class of neurotransmitters is derived from a single amino acid, of which there are two groups: those derived from tryptophan (**indoleamines**) and those derived from tyrosine (**catecholamines**). Both tryptophan and tyrosine are readily available in the diet. (Common sources include meat and dairy products.)

Serotonin (abbreviated as 5-HT) is the only indoleamine neurotransmitter, and it is relatively rare in the nervous system. 5-HT-containing neurons tend to be involved in brain systems that regulate eating, sleep, and emotional behavior. 5-HT is removed from the synapse by reuptake into the presynaptic neuron. Drugs that affect the rate at which 5-HT is reabsorbed are potent antidepressants (e.g., Prozac). Almost all 5-HT receptors are metabotropic, and many different subtypes of receptors are currently known (labeled as 5-HT_{1A}, $5\text{-HT}2_{1B,}$ 5-HT_2, etc.).

There are three catecholaminergic neurotransmitters: dopamine (DA), norepinephrine (NE), and epinephrine (E). Catecholamine-containing neurons are numerous in the nervous system and tend to be involved in brain systems that regulate movement, mood, motivation, and attention. Catecholamines are converted by using different enzymes from the original amino acid tyrosine to a compound called dopa, which is then converted into DA. DA can be converted into NE (also known as noradrenaline, or NA), and NE can be converted into E (also known as adrenaline, or A).

Dopaminergic neurons are located in the areas of the brain involved with movement and reward, and all known DA receptor subtypes are metabotropic. Depletion of DA in the brain occurs in individuals with the movement disorder Parkinson's disease. (For more discussion of Parkinson's disease, see Chapter 7.) Replacement of DA (by using the drug L-dopa) often results in an improvement of the symptoms of Parkinson's disease. Drugs that stimulate the release of DA (e.g., amphetamines) are very addictive, suggesting that DA also plays a role in the neural systems underlying addiction.

Adrenergic neurons (neurons that use either NE or E) are located throughout the brain, although many originate in the locus coeruleus. In addition to acting as a neurotransmitter in the brain, E also acts as a hormone that is released by the adrenal glands.

All known adrenergic receptors are metabotropic and appear to play a broad role in mediating the hormonal effects of catecholamines (mainly E). Drugs that are used to treat the acute symptoms of asthma affect adrenergic neurons and act by causing the stimulation of adrenergic receptors, which results in the relaxation of the bronchial muscles (widening airways) and the contraction of the smooth muscles in the bronchi (reducing inflammation).

SOLUBLE GASES. The soluble gases are the most recently discovered group of neurotransmitters. These neurotransmitters are actually the gaseous molecules nitric oxide (NO) and carbon monoxide (CO). Both NO and CO are rapidly synthesized within the nervous system and undergo very rapid degeneration. Because NO is small, it can easily cross the neural membrane and does not need a receptor to produce effects. The functions of NO are better known than those of CO. (In fact, some researchers are not sure whether or not CO is a neurotransmitter.) NO is thought to play a role as a retrograde messenger, as NO is released from the postsynaptic site and acts on the presynaptic site (Feldman et al., 1997). The most famous drug that affects NO is Viagra™, although in the brain, NO plays an important role in the brain's ability to learn.

AMINO ACIDS. There are at least four amino acids that act as neurotransmitters: aspartate, glutamate, glycine, and gamma-aminobutyric acid (GABA). For the most part, the receptors for the amino acids are all ionotropic, which suggests that amino acid neurotransmitters are involved in all fast responses within the nervous system. Indeed, receptors for the amino acid neurotransmitters are located throughout the brain and are thought to be involved in a variety of neural activity, including learning and memory. The most prevalent excitatory amino acid neurotransmitter is **glutamate,** and the most prevalent inhibitory amino acid neurotransmitter is **GABA.**

NEUROPEPTIDES. Over fifty peptides qualify as neurotransmitters, including endorphins, substance P, cholycystokinin, and insulin (Feldman et al., 1997). Endorphins are known to play a role in pain mediation. Drugs such as codeine and heroin act on endorphin receptors, providing potent relief from pain (among other things). Substance P is a neurotransmitter that plays a significant role in sensory transmission, especially related to the transmission of touch, temperature, and pain. Capsaicin (a compound that is found in chili peppers) produces a strong "hot" feeling in the mouth when it is ingested, which is due to the stimulation of cells in the mouth that release substance P. Cholycystokinin and insulin are examples of peptide neurotransmitters that are involved in the regulation of hunger and ingestion.

Neuropeptides are different from standard neurotransmitters not only because they are large molecules. For the most part, peptides are made, stored, and transported differently from the small-molecule neurotransmitters. However, more important, peptide neurotransmitters tend to modulate the responses of neurons. That is, they tend not to induce action potentials in neurons by themselves; rather, they adjust the sensitivity of neurons. Thus, the primary function of a neuropeptide appears to be related to its ability to modulate the effects of other neurotransmitters.

1. Name three differences between EPSPs and action potentials.

2. Complete this chart with the following words: fewer, greater, less, longer, more, shorter (some words may be used twice).

Ionotropic Receptors		Metabotropic Receptors	
_____ response latency		_____ response latency	
_____ common		_____ common	
_____ response duration		_____ response duration	
_____ range of actions		_____ range of actions	

3. What three actions can a metabotropic receptor produce when it is bound to a neurotransmitter?

4. Compare the actions and functions of small-molecule and peptide neurotransmitters.

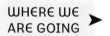

◄ WHERE WE HAVE BEEN   The means by which the cells of the nervous system communicate within themselves and among themselves have been discussed. Within the neuron, the primary form of communication is electric (either action potentials or postsynaptic potentials). Between neurons, neurotransmitters are used to communicate (by diffusing across the synapse and binding to receptors). There are a variety of neurotransmitters, and the type of receptor that they bind to often affects their impact in the nervous system.

WHERE WE ARE GOING ►   The second module in this chapter will focus on the major divisions of the nervous system and the structures and systems within these divisions. Finally, we will discuss how the brain is protected from damage.

MODULE **2.2**
The Nervous System

The human brain has been called the most complicated object in the known universe. These are not exactly encouraging words for the student who is sitting down to explore its anatomy for the first time! It can be similarly discouraging for the textbook writer who aspires to summarize the most critical elements of neuroanatomy in a few short pages. When lecturing to my introductory neuropsychology class, I find this topic particularly frustrating. Why? There are two main reasons, listed next. Providing them might appear as though I am complaining (probably because I *am* complaining), but my primary goal in listing them is to help you learn neuroanatomy. If you are aware of some of the pitfalls of learning this content, you might be able to avoid them. My top two frustrations with teaching neuroanatomy are as follows:

1. *Its Complexity.* The brain is not a particularly heavy object (approximately 1300 grams, or 3 pounds), but it contains 50 to 100 billion neurons. These cells are interconnected, and some people estimate that there are over 1 quadrillion connections within an average brain. The brain's complexity is not simply the product of the number of its parts. It is also a result of how the brain evolved. As we will discuss in more detail in Chapter 12, the brain's structure and function were shaped by evolution, a slow and clumsy process based on random mutations in genes. Therefore, the brain is not organized as if it were engineered. If it were, your visual cortex would be behind your eyes, not at the back of the head. (A large amount of space and energy is wasted transmitting visual information to the very back of your head, only to have it start heading toward the eyes again as it is processed in more and more complex ways.) Similarly, the primary motor and somatosensory areas would not be at the very top of your head, as far away as possible from your spinal cord! The nervous system is extremely complex in its design, and its layout often does not appear to make much sense.

2. *Its Inconsistencies.* There is considerable variability between human brains (presumably reflecting differences in genetics and environment between people); but in addition to the brain's own variability, there are inconsistencies in how it has been described. Some names for brain structures refer to what an object looks like. For example, the convoluted outer surface of the brain is called **cortex,** which means "bark." A small, almond-shaped object in the temporal lobe is called the **amygdala,** which, surprisingly enough, means "almond-shaped object." A nearby structure is called the **hippocampus,** which means "sea horse," but it does not look much like a sea horse to me! Other structures are named according to *where* they are. The superior temporal gyrus is not named *superior* because it is better than the other gyri of the temporal lobe; instead, the term *superior* refers to the gyrus closest to the top. Other structures are named after the investigators who described them. For example, the nucleus basalis of Meynert was named after Theodore Meynert, an Austrian neurologist in the 1800s. Structures are also named according to their *function.* The **sensory cortices** (*cortices* is the plural of *cortex*) are often referred to by function, such as the **primary visual cortex.**

In addition to the many different types of names, some structures have more than one name. To make matters worse, it isn't just the small, obscure nuclei buried deep in the recesses of your brain that have multiple names; even the major landmarks have multiple aliases. For example, the large fissure that runs between the temporal lobe and frontal/parietal lobes can be called the Sylvian fissure, Sylvian sulcus, lateral fissure, lateral sulcus, fissure of Sylvius—you get the idea. In addition to the anatomical terms used to describe brain areas, they can also be referred to by their location relative to other structures, corresponding Brodmann area, or even function. As you will discover in Chapter 8, the terms primary auditory cortex, the posterior portion of the superior temporal gyrus, Heschl's gyrus, and Brodmann's area 41 all refer to the same structure! There are also different systems of grouping neuroanatomical structures together. For example, in this chapter, we discuss the **hypothalamus** as part of the **diencephalon,** whereas other sources often discuss it as part of the **telencephalon** (the limbic system, to be more exact—more on that later). Some say that the brain has four lobes, whereas others claim that there are five!

When I first encountered these inconsistencies as a student, I wondered which name was correct or which system of classification was correct. I quickly discovered that although there were no "correct" answers, there certainly are incorrect answers (to my knowledge, there is no system that classifies the amygdala as a hindbrain structure). Instead, there are a variety of systems of nomenclature, each of which has its own merits. After all, the brain is an extremely interconnected structure, and defining borders between regions is often an arbitrary exercise rather than an exact science. Where does the parietal lobe end and the occipital lobe begin? It depends on whom you ask!

These inconsistencies plague both the student and instructor of neuroanatomy. To simplify matters somewhat, we have chosen to provide what we consider the most common name for each structure (not listing all possible names but occasionally listing popular synonyms), and we have provided an account of the most commonly taught system of subdivisions for these structures. However, depending on when and where they were taught, your instructor(s) might prefer different terms (such as fissure of Rolando instead of central fissure) or a different system for dividing the structures into a hierarchy. The best advice we can offer is to ask your instructor when you encounter inconsistent information.

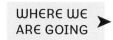 We are going to begin this module with a description about how locations in the nervous system are described. Then we will examine the major divisions of the nervous system and the structures and systems within these divisions. Finally, we will discuss how the brain is protected from damage.

Positional Terms

Learning the terms to describe the relative position of parts of the nervous system serves two functions. First, it allows you to describe a location quite precisely. For example, if someone suffers a lesion to part of his or her temporal lobe, the part running along the bottom surface that curls up underneath toward the midline of the brain, these terms allow you to describe the location precisely and economically (using few words). The location of the temporal lesion described above can also be referred to as medial inferior temporal (using three words instead of sixteen). There is a second advantage to learning these terms: As was previously mentioned, many parts of the nervous system are named after where they are. Therefore, the names sometimes are directions to the location of these objects.

Neuroanatomical directions are always given in relation to the spinal cord. This system is particularly convenient when describing structures in four-legged animals (quadrupeds), such as the crocodile in Figure 2.6. In such animals, the spinal cord is connected to the most rearward portion of the brain. If you could draw an imaginary line that extended through the spinal cord and up through the front of brain, this line would be relatively straight. This imaginary line is called the **neuraxis**. Straight neuraxes are the rule for quadrupeds, but for us bipeds, our neuraxis has a large

| **Figure 2.6** | **Terms Used to Describe Anatomical Directions** |

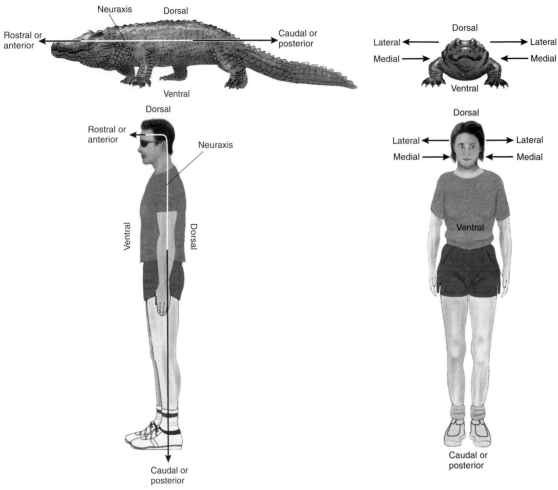

Source: Neil R. Carlson, *Physiology of Behavior,* 8e. Published by Allyn and Bacon, Boston, MA. Copyright © 2004 by Pearson Education. Reprinted by permission of the publisher.

(almost 90 degree) bend in it. This has major implications for some (but not all) of the directional terms used to describe the human brain versus the human spinal cord.

The part of your spinal cord closest to your back is referred to as **dorsal** (if you speak some French, the easy way to remember this is to remind yourself that *dos* means "back"). Conversely, the part of the spinal cord closest to your front is referred to as **ventral.** However, because of the bend in the human neuraxis, the part of your head closest to your back is *not* the dorsal portion. Instead, the dorsal portion of the brain runs along the top of your head. (See Figure 2.6 to clarify this, and remember that all positional terms are given relative to the spinal cord, not the brain.) Similarly, the part of your brain closest to your front is *not* the ventral portion. Instead, ventral refers to the part of the brain running along the bottom surface and the part of the spinal cord closest to your belly. The term **anterior** refers to objects located toward the head. Therefore, in the human nervous system, objects in the brain that are closest to one's nose are relatively anterior, and parts of the spinal cord that are closest to the brain are also anterior. Conversely, the term **posterior** refers to objects toward one's behind. Therefore, in the human brain, the back of the head is the most posterior, as is the lower portion of the spinal cord. Other sources might refer to anterior objects as **rostral** and posterior objects as **caudal.** Two other commonly used positional terms are **superior** (above or topmost) and **inferior** (below or bottommost).

For all the terms described in the preceding paragraphs, the differences between the directions relevant to the spinal cord and those referring to the human brain are easier to remember if you imagine a human in a position in which the person does *not* have a 90 degree bend in the neuraxis. What is this position? When teaching my students, I illustrate this by getting up on all fours on a table at the front of the classroom and tilting my head back as if I were a quadruped (see Figure 2.6). In this position, the dorsal portion of my spinal cord and the dorsal portion of my brain are now parallel to one another.

Other directional terms refer to the relative distance of objects from the neuraxis. The term **medial** refers to objects that are located close to the neuraxis (midline), whereas the term **lateral** refers to objects that are relatively farther from the midline. There are two other convenient words for describing location relative to the midline, but instead of describing whether objects are close to the midline, they refer to different sides of the midline. The term **ipsilateral** refers to two objects, lesions, or behaviors that are located on the same side (right or left) of the body. Conversely, the term **contralateral** refers to two objects, lesions, or behaviors that are localized to opposite sides of the body.

Relative to the human brain, here is a summary of the positional terms in plain English:

> *neuraxis:* an imaginary line running along the length of the nervous system, extending from the bottom of the spinal cord to the most frontward portion of the brain
> *dorsal:* toward the back (top of the brain, back of the spinal cord)
> *ventral:* toward the front (bottom of the brain, front of the spinal cord)
> *anterior:* toward the head (front of the brain, top of the spinal cord)
> *posterior:* toward the tail (back of the brain, bottom of the spinal cord)
> *superior:* above or topmost
> *inferior:* below or bottommost
> *medial:* toward the middle
> *lateral:* away from the middle (toward the outside)
> *ipsilateral:* on the same side
> *contralateral:* on opposite sides

In addition to these terms, it is useful to describe three planes into which the central nervous system is usually "cut" (see Figure 2.7). Of course, there are almost an infinite number of planes in which any object can be cut. (If you have every tried to cut up a mango efficiently, you know this firsthand.) However, the standard approach to slicing the brain is to use one of three planes. These terms are useful not only for describing dissected nervous systems. Medical procedures such as **magnetic resonance**

Figure 2.7   **Planes of the Nervous System**

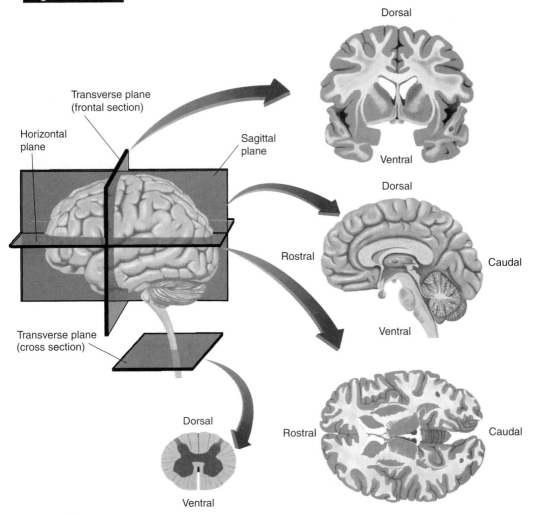

Source: Neil R. Carlson, *Physiology of Behavior,* 8e. Published by Allyn and Bacon, Boston, MA. Copyright © 2004 by Pearson Education. Reprinted by permission of the publisher.

imaging allow the visualization of the brain and spinal cord in these three planes as well. Further, many of the drawings and scans that you see of brains and spinal cords will show the nervous system cut into one of these three planes. **Horizontal** sections are slices through the neuraxis taken in the plane parallel to the horizon. **Sagittal** sections are those taken parallel to a line cut down the center of the brain, between the two hemispheres (the line right down the center is called **midsagittal**). Sagittal sections that are not midsagittal do not cross the neuraxis. Sections taken across the neuraxis running parallel to one's face (perpendicular to the ground, such as a section cut between both ears from above) are **coronal** (sometimes called **frontal** or **transverse**).

Relative to the human brain, here is a summary of the three planes:

Horizontal section: a brain slice taken parallel to the ground
Sagittal section: a brain slice taken parallel to the side of the brain
Coronal section: a brain slice taken parallel to the face; also known as *frontal* or *transverse*

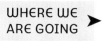

◀ **WHERE WE HAVE BEEN**

We have described the manner in which locations in the nervous system are described and the planes in which slices of the nervous system are examined.

WHERE WE ARE GOING ▶

We are going to examine the major divisions of the nervous system and the structures that are located within these divisions. We will mention the function of these structures only briefly; their functions will be described in much more detail in the following chapters.

Divisions of the Nervous System

The following sections detail the major divisions of the nervous system and the systems and structures within the divisions. Within the nervous system, structures or systems within the same division have similar locations and functions. For example, structures within the **basal ganglia** are more similar in function and location than are, for example, the **tectum** (a **midbrain** structure) and the **cerebellum** (a hindbrain structure). Thus, knowing the division(s) in which a nervous system structure or system falls provides information about its location and function.

There are two major divisions in the nervous system of the human (and other vertebrates). The **central nervous system (CNS)** is the part of your nervous system that is encased by bone. This includes your brain (protected by your skull) and spinal cord (protected by the spinal column). Because humans are **endoskeletal** (i.e., we wear our skeleton on the inside), some of our nervous system exists outside of protection from bone. This part is called the **peripheral nervous system (PNS)**.

The PNS itself has two major divisions. The **autonomic nervous system (ANS)** is primarily responsible for regulating internal states, such as temperature. Therefore, it contains nerves that convey information to the CNS

Match the following definitions with the appropriate terms.

neuraxis	away from the middle (toward the outside)
dorsal	below or bottommost
ventral	on the same side
anterior	on opposite sides
posterior	toward the back (top of the brain, back of the spinal cord)
superior	toward the front (bottom of the brain, front of the spinal cord)
inferior	toward the tail (back of the brain, bottom of the spinal cord)
medial	toward the head (front of the brain, top of the spinal cord)
lateral	above or topmost
ipsilateral	toward the middle
contralateral	an imaginary line running along the length of the nervous system, extending from the bottom of the spinal cord to the most frontward portion of the brain

from internal organs. Nerves that convey information to the CNS are called afferent nerves. The ANS also contain nerves from the CNS, projecting motor information. These projections are called efferent nerves. Therefore afferent nerves go toward the CNS, whereas efferent nerves carry information from the CNS (an easy way to remember the distinction is to think "e" is for "exit" and "a" is for "approach"). The efferent nerves of the ANS are of two types. **Sympathetic nerves** form a network that serves to prepare the body for vigorous activity (e.g., in response to a threatening or exciting situation) whereas **parasympathetic nerves** form a network that sustains nonemergency behaviors. More specifically, sympathetic and parasympathetic projections tend to oppose one another, helping to maintain a balance. When environmental circumstances warrant a shift in this balance, one of the two systems becomes relatively more active.

The second division of the PNS is primarily responsible for interacting with the external environment. This division is called the **somatic nervous system (SNS).** It perhaps comes as no surprise to you that this system is composed largely of afferent projections. After all, to interact with the external environment, one must receive sensory signals from organs such as the eyes, ears, nose, skin, muscles, and joints. The ANS also projects efferents that convey motor signals from the CNS. Figure 2.8 summarizes the components of the CNS and PNS.

| Figure 2.8 | Summary of the Components of the Nervous System |

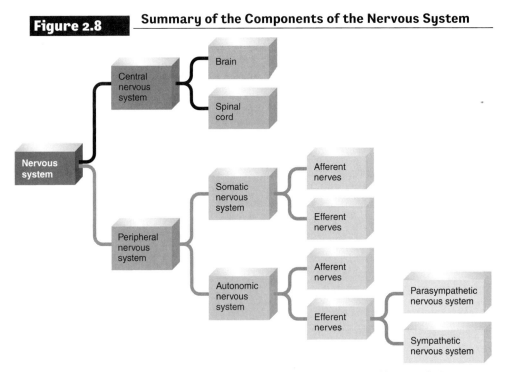

Source: John P. J. Pinel, *Biopsychology,* 5e. Published by Allyn and Bacon, Boston, MA. Copyright © 2003 by Pearson Education. Reprinted by permission of the publisher.

The Spinal Cord

The CNS (all of which is encased by bone) has two major divisions: the brain and the spinal cord. Superficially, these two divisions look very different. One is very long and skinny, weighing about 35 grams; the other is a larger, roundish structure, weighing 40 times as much. Furthermore, the brain is a grayish color on the outside with more white on the inside, whereas the spinal cord is gray on the inside and white on the outside. The **gray matter** is mostly composed of cell bodies (including somas) and some blood vessels; **white matter** is mostly composed of myelinated axons. As you learned in the previous module, myelin is a fatty substance, which is also why white matter has a white and glossy appearance. In cross section, the spinal cord appears to have a gray H-shape in the middle.

The spinal cord has thirty-one segments, and each of these segments has a pair of spinal nerves (one on the left and one on the right) attached to it. According to the **Bell-Magendie law,** the dorsal projections entering the spinal cord (efferents) carry sensory information, whereas the ventral projections from the spinal cord (afferents) carry motor information to muscles and glands. The thirty-one segments are divided into five groups. The eight most anterior segments are **cervical segments,** followed by twelve **thoracic segments,** five **lumbar segments,** five **sacral segments,** and one **coccygeal segment.** If the spinal cord is damaged at a given segment, the brain loses both sensation and control from that segment downward.

Divisions of the Brain

The other division of the CNS, the brain, has three major divisions within it. These three divisions are the **forebrain** (prosencephalon), the midbrain (mesencephalon), and the **hindbrain** (rhombencephalon).

THE HINDBRAIN. The hindbrain is the interface between the brain and the spinal cord and is divided into the **metencephalon** and **myelencephalon.** The myelencephalon is a heavily myelinated region that houses tracts conveying signals between the brain and the rest of the body. The lowest portion of the hindbrain is the **medulla oblongata,** which helps to regulate basic or "vegetative" functions such as one's breathing and heartbeat. Therefore, damage to the medulla oblongata is often fatal.

Just superior to the myelencephalon is the metecephalon. This division contains two major structures: the **pons** and the cerebellum. The pons (which means "bridge") looks like a bulge above the medulla, and its function is relaying sensory information from the spinal cord to the cerebellum and other brain structures, mostly via the **thalamus.** Posterior to the pons is the cerebellum (which means "little brain"). It looks like a miniature version of the rest of the brain, with very small ridges called **gyri** and grooves called **sulci.** Traditionally, the cerebellum has been regarded as a structure that is responsible for coordinating and initiating movement. However, recent evidence has implicated it in a wide variety of other behaviors, such as language processing.

THE MIDBRAIN. The midbrain (or mesencephalon) also has two subdivisions: the tectum and **tegmentum** (Figure 2.9). The tectum (which means "roof") is primarily

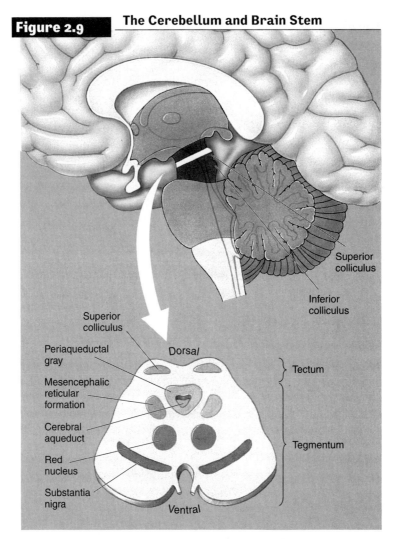

Figure 2.9   **The Cerebellum and Brain Stem**

Source: Neil R. Carlson, *Physiology of Behavior,* 8e. Published by Allyn and Bacon, Boston, MA.
Copyright © 2004 by Pearson Education. Reprinted by permission of the publisher.

involved with relaying visual and auditory sensory information. It looks like four small bumps on the dorsal surface of the midbrain. The bottom two bumps are the **inferior colliculi,** and they relay auditory information and help to control auditory reflexes (such as orienting oneself to a loud sound). The top two bumps are the **superior colliculi,** and they relay visual information and control simple visual reflexes (such as blinking).

The tegmentum (meaning "covering") is located ventral to the tectum. The tegmentum is a very vigorously studied portion of the brain because of the **nuclei** (groups of cells of similar shape and function) located within it. The substantia nigra (meaning "black substance") and **red nucleus** are motor nuclei, and **Parkinson's disease** is associated with the degeneration of the substantia nigra (see Chapter 7). The other nucleus of interest in the tegmentum is the **periaqueductal gray,** which is the gray matter surrounding the central canal. The periaqueductal gray appears to play a role in pain perception. Electrical stimulation of this area can relieve even severe pain in some cases. The periaqueductal gray contains large numbers of opioid and cannabinoid receptors, which might help to explain the analgesic (pain-relieving) characteristics of drugs that affect these neurotransmitter systems.

THE FOREBRAIN. The forebrain (prosencephalon) makes up the bulk of the human brain. It has two major divisions: the diencephalon and the telencephalon. The diencephalon is a relatively small portion of the forebrain containing the thalamus and hypothalamus. The thalamus is an egg-shaped structure that is located right over the top of the midbrain (*thalamus* means "inner chamber"). It serves as the main sensory and motor relay station in the brain. More specifically, most afferents to or efferents from the rest of the forebrain pass through the thalamus. It contains quite a number of nuclei, which are specialized for relaying specific types of sensory or motor information. For example, the **lateral geniculate nucleus,** located on the lateral posterior surface of the thalamus, is the primary relay for visual information. Just posterior and toward the midline, the **medial geniculate nucleus** relays auditory sensory information. Somatosensory information is relayed via the **ventral posterior nucleus, pulvinar nucleus,** and **lateral posterior nucleus.** Olfactory information is relayed via the **dorsal medial nucleus.** Motor information is relayed via the **ventrolateral nucleus.** The two lobes of the thalamus are connected through a structure called the **massa intermedia.**

The other, smaller component of the diencephalon within the forebrain is the hypothalamus. Although the hypothalamus is often referred to as a unitary structure, it is, like the thalamus, composed of a number (about twenty-two, in this case) of smaller nuclei (see Figure 2.10). The hypothalamus is more of a cluster of these small nuclei rather than the more homogeneous-looking egg-shaped thalamus, with its clearly defined borders. As is implied by its name, the hypothalamus is located underneath (hence "hypo") the thalamus. The nuclei of the hypothalamus are relatively small in comparison to the rest of the brain (they make up 0.3% of the brain, according to Hoffman and Swaab, 1994), but their influence on a wide variety of behaviors is considerable.

The hypothalamus is a very famous structure, and you probably recall learning about it in your introductory psychology class. One of the functions of the hypothalamus that makes it so famous is its role in **satiety**—the feeling of being full after eating. If the **lateral nuclei** of the hypothalamus are damaged, an animal will eat much more than it normally would. (Most introductory psychology students are presented with a picture of a very fat rat with a lateral hypothalamus lesion sitting beside a normal-looking rat of the same age and strain to emphasize this point.) In addition to its role in satiety, the hypothalamus has a much broader role: It controls both the autonomic and endocrine systems. Its control of the endocrine system is accomplished through hormones and its control of the **pituitary gland,** the so-called master gland of the body, which hangs below the hypothalamus. The hypothalamus also regulates

Figure 2.10   The Hypothalamus

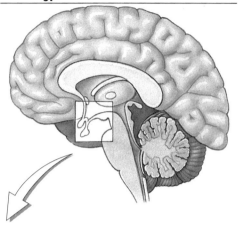

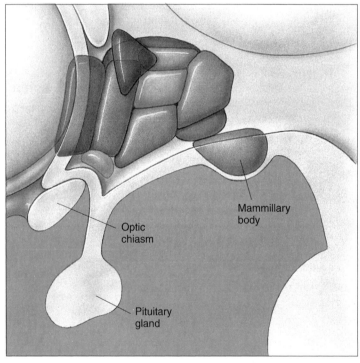

Optic chiasm

Mammillary body

Pituitary gland

Source: John P. J. Pinel, *Biopsychology,* 5e. Published by Allyn and Bacon, Boston, MA. Copyright © 2003 by Pearson Education. Reprinted by permission of the publisher.

behaviors that appear to be critical to all mammals, the so-called four Fs: fighting, fleeing, feeding, and, um, well, fornicating! (Every instructor of neuropsychology makes this same joke.)

The other main division of the forebrain is the telencephalon. It contains the **cerebral cortex,** the **limbic system,** and the basal ganglia. The cerebral cortex is the largest part of the brain (filling most of the skull), and it covers most of the other parts of the brain, including the other parts of the telencephalon. It is usually simply called the cortex (meaning "bark"). Its crumpled appearance allows it to have a relatively large surface area (2500 square centimeters, 2.5 square feet) in a small space, much as crumpling a piece of paper allows one to fit it into a space that is smaller than its original dimensions. The folds in the cortical surface produce ridges called gyri (the singular of which is gyrus) and sulci (the singular of which is sulcus). Depending on the depth of the sulcus, it may also be referred to as a **fissure.** Fissures are sulci that reach so far into the cortex that they touch one of the **ventricles** (more about ventricles later in this module). Not all sulci are this deep; therefore, although all fissures are sulci, not all sulci are fissures. There are three fissures that you should be able to locate and name: the **lateral fissure, central fissure,** and **longitudinal fissure** (see Figure 2.11). Two of these fissures serve as borders between different **lobes** of the brain, whereas the other divides the brain into right and left halves called **hemispheres.**

There are four (reasonably) anatomically and functionally distinct regions of the brain called lobes. Some of the borders between these regions can be easily identified;

Figure 2.11	**Lobes and Fissures of the Brain**

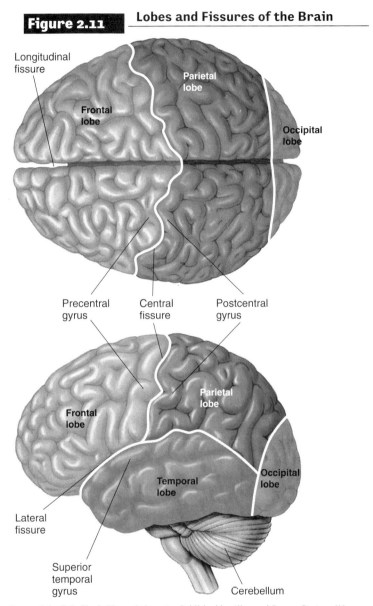

Longitudinal fissure

Parietal lobe

Frontal lobe

Occipital lobe

Precentral gyrus

Central fissure

Postcentral gyrus

Parietal lobe

Frontal lobe

Occipital lobe

Temporal lobe

Lateral fissure

Superior temporal gyrus

Cerebellum

Source: John P. J. Pinel, *Biopsychology,* 5e. Published by Allyn and Bacon, Boston, MA. Copyright © 2003 by Pearson Education. Reprinted by permission of the publisher.

others are somewhat arbitrary. The **frontal lobe** is bordered by the central fissure and lateral fissure. The major gyri and sulci of the frontal lobe can be seen in Figure 2.12. The major gyri are the superior frontal gyrus, middle frontal gyrus, inferior frontal gyrus, orbital gyrus, and precentral gyrus. The major sulci are the superior frontal sulcus, middle frontal sulcus, inferior frontal sulcus, and precentral sulcus. Functionally, the frontal lobe performs a wide variety of functions, including the panning and control of movement, memory, inhibition, regulating complex social behavior, and influencing (if not subserving) personality. The functions of the frontal lobes are discussed in detail in Chapter 7 (sensorimotor system), Chapter 8 (language), Chapter 9 (memory), Chapter 10 (emotion), and Chapter 12 (attention and consciousness), which should give you an idea how broad their functions are.

The lateral fissure and an imaginary line called the parieto-occipital sulcus border the **temporal lobe.** In most people, this is not really a sulcus at all, but rather an imaginary line that extends between the preoccipital notch and the transverse occipital sulcus (see Figure 2.13). Within the temporal lobe, the major gyri are the superior temporal gyrus, middle temporal gyrus, and inferior temporal gyrus (see Figure 2.13). The most anterior section of the temporal lobe is called the temporal pole. The major sulci of the temporal lobe are the superior temporal sulcus, middle temporal sulcus, and inferior temporal sulcus. The temporal lobe is mostly involved in language processing and memory, but it also plays a role in complex object recognition and emotion.

Figure 2.12 — Major Gyri of the Brain

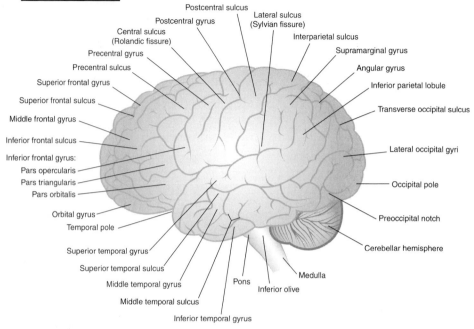

Postcentral sulcus
Postcentral gyrus
Central sulcus (Rolandic fissure)
Lateral sulcus (Sylvian fissure)
Interparietal sulcus
Precentral gyrus
Supramarginal gyrus
Precentral sulcus
Angular gyrus
Superior frontal gyrus
Inferior parietal lobule
Superior frontal sulcus
Transverse occipital sulcus
Middle frontal gyrus
Inferior frontal sulcus
Lateral occipital gyri
Inferior frontal gyrus:
Pars opercularis
Pars triangularis
Occipital pole
Pars orbitalis
Orbital gyrus
Preoccipital notch
Temporal pole
Cerebellar hemisphere
Superior temporal gyrus
Superior temporal sulcus
Medulla
Middle temporal gyrus
Pons
Middle temporal sulcus
Inferior olive
Inferior temporal gyrus

Source: Martin (1998) p. 89. Copyright © 1998 Prentice Hall. Reprinted with permission.

Figure 2.13 — The Basal Ganglia

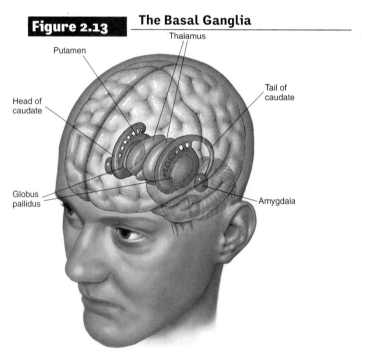

Thalamus
Putamen
Head of caudate
Tail of caudate
Globus pallidus
Amygdala

Source: John P. J. Pinel, *Biopsychology,* 5e. Published by Allyn and Bacon, Boston, MA. Copyright © 2003 by Pearson Education. Reprinted by permission of the publisher.

The **parietal lobe** is bordered by the central fissure, lateral fissure, and parieto-occipital sulcus. Its major gyri include the postcentral gyrus, angular gyrus, and supramarginal gyrus. The major sulci of the parietal lobe include the postcentral sulcus, interparietal sulcus, and transverse occipital sulcus. Two other anatomical regions of interest within the parietal lobe include the superior parietal lobule and inferior parietal lobule. Functionally, the parietal lobe plays many sensory functions, including primary somatosensory functions (discussed in Chapter 7), sensory integration, and spatial cognition (discussed in Chapter 11).

The **occipital lobe** is bordered by the parieto-occipital sulcus and contains one major fissure: the calcarine fissure. The cortex surrounding this fissure is called primary visual cortex; it is discussed in detail in Chapter 6 (vision). The most posterior portion of the occipital lobe is called the occipital pole.

The second major division of the telencephalon is the basal ganglia (Figure 2.13). The basal ganglia are composed of three structures: the **caudate nucleus,** the **putamen** (which together are called the **striatum,** meaning "striped structure"), and the **globus pallidus.** Although the globus pallidus and putamen can be collectively called the **lentiform nucleus,** to my knowledge, there is no special name for the caudate nucleus and globus pallidus. The globus pallidus looks similar in shape and size to the thalamus—just lateral to the egg-shaped thalami (plural for thalamus) are the two globus pallidi. These egg-shaped structures are encased in the putamen, and the caudate extends from the putamen in a C-shaped curling taillike structure. All three structures are named after their appearance (*globus pallidus* means "globe," *putamen* means "shell," and *caudate* means "nucleus with a tail").

The basal ganglia are critically important for initiating movements and maintaining muscle tone. The basal ganglia receive projections from the part of the midbrain that is most famous for its degeneration in Parkinson's disease: the substantia nigra. However, another common motor disorder also involves the basal ganglia. Huntington's disease results from damage to the striatum—both the caudate nucleus and the putamen.

The third division of the telencephalon is the limbic system (summarized in Figure 2.14). The limbic system (sometimes referred to as the limbic lobe) is essentially a circuit of structures that surround both the basal ganglia and the thalamus. Located at the anterior end of the base of the

Figure 2.14	**The Limbic System**

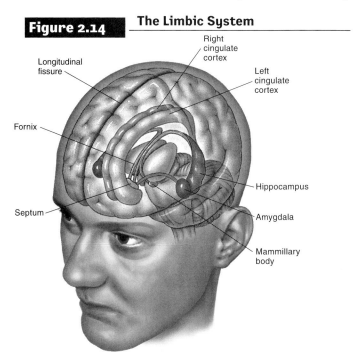

Longitudinal fissure

Right cingulate cortex

Left cingulate cortex

Fornix

Hippocampus

Septum

Amygdala

Mammillary body

Source: John P. J. Pinel, *Biopsychology,* 5e. Published by Allyn and Bacon, Boston, MA. Copyright © 2003 by Pearson Education. Reprinted by permission of the publisher.

temporal lobe, the almond-shaped amygdala plays a central role in the expression of emotions such as anger and fear. The amygdala also appears to play a central role in learning, particularly when the material being learned provokes emotional responses. Just posterior to the amygdala lies the hippocampus, so named because of its apparent resemblance to a sea horse in shape. Similar to the amygdala, the hippocampus (and the cortex that surrounds it) appears to play a very important role in memory. The most posterior portion of the tail of the hippocampus curls forward, superior to the thalamus, eventually forming an arcing bundle of axons called the **fornix** (*fornix* means "arc"). Among other things, the fornix connects the hippocampus with the **mamillary bodies,** small protrusions along the ventral surface of the brain that also appear to play a role in memory. At the anterior base of the fornix, the **cingulate cortex** curls superior to the other structures of the basal ganglia and limbic system, encircling the thalamus (*cingulate* means "encircling"). The functions that are subserved by the cingulate have yet to be clearly defined, but the anterior portion of the structure appears to have a role in response selection, particularly when two conflicting pieces of information are provided (such as in the Stroop task, wherein color names are presented in colors that are not congruent with the word, such as the word red being presented in green). Therefore, the limbic system is not a unified circuit of structures serving similar (and exclusively emotive) functions. Instead, the limbic system contains a variety of structures with roles in functions such as emotion, sexual behavior, response selection, and memory.

Some neuroanatomical classifications include the hypothalamus as part of the limbic system. Functionally, this classification makes a lot of sense. Just as the limbic system is involved in regulating emotion, motivation, and the four Fs, so too does the hypothalamus. However, most consider the hypothalamus to be part of the diencephalon, as we have here. A summary of the major divisions of the nervous system and the components associated with each division can be found in Figure 2.15.

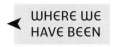

WHERE WE HAVE BEEN

We have described the major divisions of the nervous system and the structures that are located within these divisions.

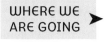

WHERE WE ARE GOING

We are going to examine how these structures are connected between the two halves of the brain, how they are provided with blood, and how they are protected from damage.

Connections between the Two Halves of the Brain

There are a number of structures that link the two halves of the brain; these are often called **commissures.** The link between the two hippocampi is called the **hippocampal commissure.** There are three structures that connect cortical areas between the two hemispheres: the **anterior commissure,** the **posterior commissure,** and the

Figure 2.15   Summary of the Divisions of the Central Nervous System

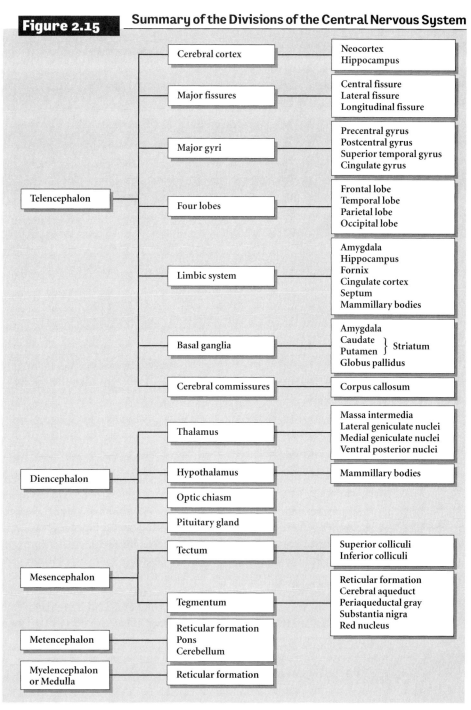

| Figure 2.16 | **The Commissures** |

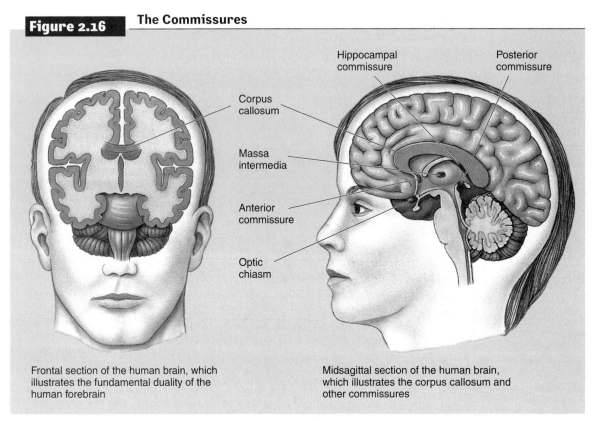

Frontal section of the human brain, which illustrates the fundamental duality of the human forebrain

Midsagittal section of the human brain, which illustrates the corpus callosum and other commissures

Source: John P. J. Pinel, *Biopsychology,* 5e. Published by Allyn and Bacon, Boston, MA. Copyright © 2003 by Pearson Education. Reprinted by permission of the publisher.

corpus callosum. The largest (by far) of all these structures is the corpus callosum (see Figure 2.16). It is a large white matter structure consisting of approximately 200 million fibers connecting cortical centers in similar locations between the two hemispheres (e.g., connecting areas along the superior temporal gyrus of the left hemisphere to the same area on the right hemisphere).These types of connections are called **homotopic,** but the corpus callosum also contains some **heterotopic** connections between dissimilar cortical areas. Anatomically, there are four main regions of the corpus callosum. The most posterior area is called the splenium. Anterior to the splenium lies the body of the corpus callosum, and the bend at the anterior tip of the corpus callosum is called the genu (meaning "knee"). The portion of the corpus callosum inferior to the body, at the end of the bend of the genu is called the rostrum.

Cranial Nerves

The cranial nerves are twelve pairs of nerves that are visible along the ventral surface of the brain. Many of these nerves are attached to the brain at the level of the medulla

Neuropsychological Celebrity

A Family with Three Acallosal Girls

So far in this chapter, we have discussed components of the brain that are normally present. However, we have not discussed the possibility of an individual missing one of these components. In one such condition, called **callosal agenesis** (also called *acallosal*), an individual is born without a corpus callosum (see Figure 2.17). This rare condition runs in families, and on the basis of the pattern on inheritance (it is much more common in males), it is probably an autosomal-recessive, or an X-linked recessive, trait. Most individuals who are born without a corpus callosum also display other neurological pathologies, including epilepsy. However, approximately 15% of acallosal people exhibit normal intelligence (Fischer, Ryan, & Dobyns, 1992), and many have no obvious neurological symptoms. This could be because other parts of the brain compensate for the missing corpus callosum. For example, the anterior commissure is often relatively larger in cases of callosal agenesis. Finlay and colleagues (2000) reported a family with five young girls, three of whom were acallosal. Relative to their siblings, the acallosal girls had borderline to low-average intelligence, and neuropsychological testing indicated that they had difficulties with transferring tactile information between the hemispheres and difficulties in some areas of memory.

Figure 2.17 — **An Acallosal Brain**

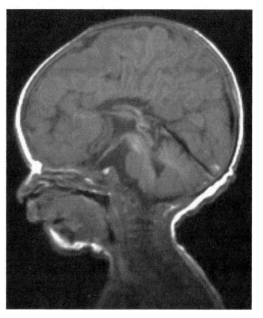

Source: Copyright protected material used with permission of Jeff Goree and the University of Iowa's Virtual Hospital, www.vh.org.

oblongata and pons, but two of them, numbers II and III (cranial nerves are usually referred to by number using Roman numerals), are at the level of the midbrain (see Figure 2.18). Some of these nerves are efferents, carrying motor information; others are afferents, conveying sensory information to the brain. Some are both afferent and efferent. Most of the nerves serve sensory and motor functions for the head, but one of the nerves, the vagus nerve (number X), extends to the viscera, including the intestines, heart, and liver. This long and convoluted route probably earned the nerve its peculiar name (*vagus* means "wandering"). The cranial nerves and their respective functions are summarized in Table 2.1.

There are a number of mnemonics (some of which are off-color) that can help one to remember the names and numbers of the cranial nerves. The most common (and G-rated) one is "On Old Olympus Towering Tops, A Finn And German Vault, Skip, And Hop." A variant of this, wherein nerve XI is called *accessory* instead of *spinal accessory*, is "On Old Olympus Towering Tops, A Foolish Austrian Grew Vines

Figure 2.18 — Cranial Nerves

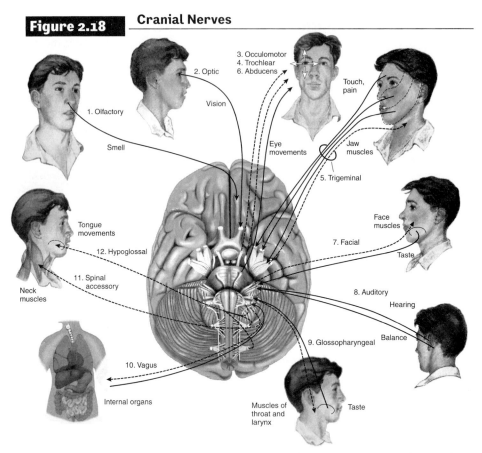

Source: Neil R. Carlson, *Physiology of Behavior,* 8e. Published by Allyn and Bacon, Boston, MA. Copyright © 2004 by Pearson Education. Reprinted by permission of the publisher.

And Hops." To help you remember whether the nerves are motor (M), sensory (S), or both (B), try "Some Say 'Mary May.' But My Brother Says, 'Better Beware Mary's Mother!'" or "Some Say Marry Money, But My Brother Says, 'Bad Business Marry Money.'"

Blood Supply

The brain is a bit of a hog when one considers blood and energy supply. It makes up only about 2% of a human's body weight, but it receives 20% of the blood flow from the heart and consumes approximately 25% of the body's available energy. Because the brain cannot store excess energy, it is extremely sensitive to interruptions in energy supply. An interruption in blood flow as short as 6 seconds can result in a loss of consciousness. An interruption in blood flow as short as 10 minutes can cause all cells in the affected region to die.

Table 2.1

The Cranial Nerves

Number	Name	Function
I	Olfactory nerve	Smell
II	Optic nerve	Vision
III	Oculomotor nerve	Eye movements and pupil dilation
IV	Trochlear nerve	Eye movements
V	Trigeminal nerve	Somatosensory information from the face
VI	Abducens nerve	Eye movement
VII	Facial nerve	Taste (anterior tongue) and tongue control
VIII	Acoustic (vestibulocochlear) nerve	Hearing and balance
IX	Glossopharyngeal nerve	Taste (posterior tongue), tongue control, swallowing
X	Vagus nerve	Sensory and motor control of viscera
XI	Spinal accessory nerve	Head movement
XII	Hypoglossal nerve	Controls muscles of tongue

The blood flow into the brain comes from two groups of arteries (see Figure 2.19). The more posterior parts of the brain are irrigated by the two **vertebral arteries** (one on each side of the neuraxis); the two internal **carotid arteries** serve anterior areas.

Figure 2.19

Cerebral Arteries

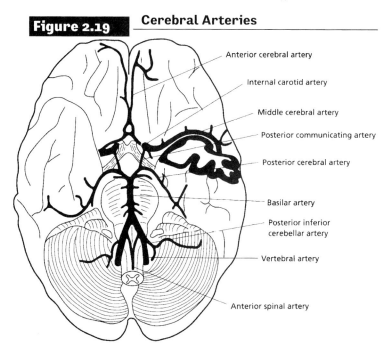

Anterior cerebral artery

Internal carotid artery

Middle cerebral artery

Posterior communicating artery

Posterior cerebral artery

Basilar artery

Posterior inferior cerebellar artery

Vertebral artery

Anterior spinal artery

Source: Martin (1998) p. 101. Copyright © 1998 Prentice Hall. Reprinted by permission.

The vertebral arteries supply the posterior inferior cerebellar arteries (which irrigate the posterior portion of the cerebellum) and the anterior inferior cerebellar arteries (which irrigate the anterior portion of the cerebellum) before joining to form the **basilar artery.** The basilar artery then gives rise to several other arteries, including the posterior cerebral arteries (which irrigate the occipital lobe). The internal carotid arteries give rise to the **anterior cerebral arteries** (irrigating the medial frontal and parietal lobes), the **middle cerebral artery** (irrigating the lateral frontal, temporal, and parietal lobes), and several smaller arteries.

The blood supply from the vertebral and internal carotid arteries are joined together in a link between the middle cerebral artery and posterior cerebral artery, a link called the **posterior communicating artery.** The **anterior communicating artery** joins the two internal carotid arteries, and these two communicating arteries complete a vascular circle called the **circle of Willis.** This vascular arrangement is odd and somewhat redundant, but it might help to compensate for local interruptions in blood flow as well as to allow for an equalization of blood pressure in the brain.

Blood exits the brain through external or internal cerebral and cerebellar veins. Most of the internal veins feed into the great cerebral vein before emptying into the heart. The external veins take a more indirect route to the heart. Many of the veins first drain into the dural sinuses.

Protection

As you will discover in Chapter 13, there are many different ways to damage one's nervous system, and it is very sensitive to this damage. Fortunately, the nervous system is protected in a variety of ways.

BONE. Perhaps the most obvious protection of the CNS is also the most familiar: bone. The bone that encases the CNS (skull and spinal column) normally provides excellent protection to the CNS. However, in the event of serious injury, these structures (or fragments of them) can actually inflict serious damage on the CNS. It is relatively rare for a foreign object (such as a knife or bullet) to pierce the bones surrounding the CNS. More often, situations such as automobile accidents fracture or displace the bones protecting the CNS, and these fractures or displaced pieces compress, pierce, or shear sections of the CNS. Even if the bone itself is not displaced, it can still inflict damage on the CNS. For example, the skull is not simply a smooth, round case for the brain. It contains several bony projections that hold the brain in place. In the event of a sudden acceleration or deceleration (such as in an auto accident), the parts of the brain that are close to these protrusions often suffer injury from them because the brain has been displaced from its normal position and comes into forceful contact with these parts of the skull.

THE MENINGES. The CNS does not normally come into direct contact with bone. There are three protective layers, collectively called the **meninges,** which also protect the brain. The outmost layer (or **meanix,** which is singular for *meninges*) is called **dura mater.** Literally, this term means "hard mother," which is an appropriate description of this tough but somewhat flexible (sorry, Mom) membrane located closest to the bone. One layer closer to the brain is the **arachnoid mater,** which is a much thinner and weblike substance (hence the term *arachnoid,* meaning "spider"). Under this layer lies a fluid-filled space called the subarachnoid space (*sub* meaning "under"). The salty fluid in the subarachnoid space is called **cerebrospinal fluid (CSF),** which is found throughout the entire CNS. CSF fills a small canal running along the length of the spinal cord, and it fills four small pouches called ventricles within the brain. The innermost meanix is called the **pia mater,** a thin and very flexible layer that adheres to the surface of the brain and spinal cord.

CSF has a primarily protective function: it both supports and cushions the brain. The brain is extremely soft and fragile (the consistency is a little stiffer than toothpaste). If you have seen or touched a brain that was fixed in a solution such as formaldehyde, the consistency of the brain was probably much stiffer than normal, unfixed brain tissue. CSF protects the brain by suspending it in fluid. Essentially, your brain is floating inside your head. An average brain weighs about 1300–1400 grams, but it is not strong enough to support its own weight very well. In fact, it is extremely difficult to remove an unfixed brain from a skull without seriously damaging it. Fortunately, the brain does not normally need to support its own weight. Because it is floating, its net weight is reduced to only about 5% of its weight outside of the fluid bath. In addition to supporting the brain, CSF serves to help with excretion of waste products, maintaining the chemical environment for the CNS. CSF can also act as an additional channel for chemical communication within the CNS (Martin, 1996).

THE VENTRICULAR SYSTEM. In addition to the CSF in the subarachnoid space, the four internal ventricles also contain CSF for support (see Figure 2.20). The two largest ventricles are the **lateral ventricles** (ventricles 1 and 2), which are connected to each other and the **third ventricle** through the **interventricular foramen** (sometimes called the foramen of Monroe; *foramen* means "opening"). The third ventricle is located right at the brain's midline, and the massa intermedia passes through the middle of the ventricle. CSF from the third ventricle flows to the fourth ventricle through the **cerebral aqueduct** (sometimes called the aqueduct of Sylvius), and the **central canal** extends

Figure 2.20 **The Ventricles**

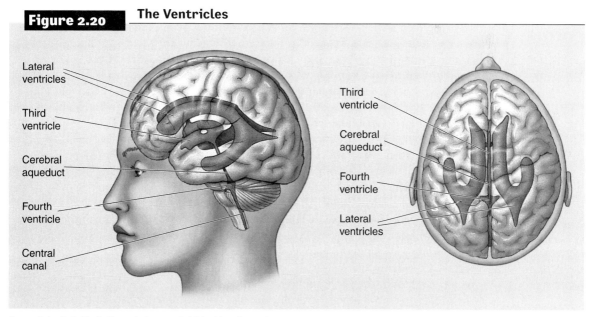

Source: John P. J. Pinel, *Biopsychology,* 5e. Published by Allyn and Bacon, Boston, MA. Copyright © 2003 by Pearson Education. Reprinted by permission of the publisher.

from the fourth ventricle into the spinal cord. The CSF itself is actually produced along the floor of the lateral ventricles and the roof of the third and fourth ventricles by cells and networks of blood vessels called **choroid plexuses.** CSF is absorbed by small protrusions into the superior sagittal sinus called **arachnoid granulations.** Reabsorption of CSF is critical because CSF is constantly being produced by the choroid plexuses, especially by the choroid plexus of the third ventricle. Collectively, the choroid plexuses can produce about 500 milliliters of CSF every day; that is enough to fill all the cavities in the nervous system four times over!

Given this rate of production, maintaining a balance between the rate of production and absorption of CSF is absolutely critical. When production exceeds absorption or some obstruction (such as the growth of a tumor or an undersized cerebral aqueduct) restricts the flow of CSF, a condition called hydrocephalus (which means "water-head") can result. If it is left untreated, tremendous pressure can build within the ventricular system, and the CSF, which normally protects the brain, can actually exert too much pressure on the brain and injure it. The resultant damage can be permanent, even fatal. This damage can be averted by using a surgical procedure to regulate the pressure. Essentially, it involves the installation of a shunt that drains CSF from the ventricular system into the abdominal cavity, where the fluid can be easily and safely absorbed.

THE BLOOD–BRAIN BARRIER. Bone, membranes, and fluid protect the brain from mechanical damage. However, it is necessary that the brain is also protected from damage from chemicals. Nobel Prize winner, Paul Ehrlich, who won the prize in 1908, dramatically demonstrated this in his dissertation work, which involved the staining of animal tissues. During his research, Ehrlich noticed that after he injected a certain blue dye (derived from aniline) into an animal's bloodstream, the dye colored all the animal's tissues except for the CNS. Wondering whether this could be due to some special property of the CNS, Ehrlich tried injecting the same dye directly into the CNS—into the CSF to be more precise. Injected this way, the blue dye was absorbed by the CNS, although no peripheral tissues were dyed. These results collectively suggested that the CNS is protected from the passage of some substances from the bloodstream, by a **blood–brain barrier** (Bradbury, 1979).

The blood–brain barrier is composed of two layers of cells that limit the flow of substances between the blood and neural tissue. Blood vessels in the CNS have a slightly different structure from that of blood vessels found elsewhere: They have a tightly packed layer of cells that can block the passage of many larger molecules (such as proteins) while allowing other large molecules (such as glucose) to pass. The blood–brain barrier is not equally effective everywhere in the brain. One of the more vulnerable areas, the **area postrema,** is a region of the medulla oblongata that can induce vomiting. This vulnerable area of the blood–brain barrier can actually serve to protect the CNS better, because an injected toxin can be detected and vomited, thereby protecting the rest of the CNS (and the person).

In addition to protecting the brain, the blood–brain barrier can be quite problematic for health researchers and practitioners. Many drugs that can be administered orally or intravenously do not cross the blood–brain barrier. In fact, most drugs do

Current Controversy

Are You Really Born with All the Neurons That You Will Ever Have?

The regeneration of damaged cells is something that we take for granted. A small cut on the hand typically heals quickly and without incident, leaving the hand fully functional. Even major injuries such as broken bones have a remarkable ability to heal. It seems as though damage to virtually any part of the human body can be repaired, provided that the damage is not too severe. However, people who are rendered paraplegic after spinal cord injuries do not typically regain full sensory and motor function. Similarly, a person who develops aphasia after a left hemisphere injury is not just temporarily aphasic. The person might exhibit some recovery of function over time, but this is often because the functions are assumed by new interconnections between the remaining intact structures. Why can the CNS not form new neurons to recover from injury? What property of the CNS makes regeneration impossible?

For years, the dogma in neuroscience has been that the human brain does not produce new, fully functional nerve cells throughout the lifespan. Instead, it has been claimed that humans are born with all the CNS cells that they will ever have, and if the cells are damaged, they are gone forever. This position no longer appears to be correct. In fact, there is one site in the adult human brain, the hippocampus, that appears to generate new neurons regularly (Eriksson et al., 1998). As you learned earlier in this chapter, the hippocampus appears to play an important role in memory, although it is not the storage site for memories. The hippocampus is also extremely vulnerable to damage from a stroke, so its capacity to repair itself is even more critical than is the case elsewhere in the CNS. Demonstrating that new neurons are formed in the brain is certainly exciting news, but the formation of the new cells (called neurogenesis) is good news only if the cells actually work. They must produce a functional benefit. Some of the investigations with rodents suggest that the new cells do in fact work. Just as in humans, the hippocampus of the rodent is capable of neurogenesis, and the formation of these new cells appears to produce measurable benefits in functions such as spatial memory (Nilsson, Perfilieva, Johansson, Orwar, & Eriksson, 1999).

These preliminary findings are extremely exciting. The knowledge that some areas of the CNS are capable of forming new cells suggests that new growth could occur if we knew how to trigger it and that future treatments of CNS damage could include the manipulation of these triggers. Treatments for neurodegenerative disorders such as Parkinson's disease and Alzheimer's disease could also be revolutionized as a result of this research.

---

not influence the CNS at all. As a general rule, if a substance is not soluble in fat (the cell membranes are composed of a lipid bilayer), it will not cross the blood–brain barrier. Some substances, such as nicotine, enter the brain by passing through the lipids in the walls of the capillaries. If one is developing drugs to treat a condition that also affects the CNS, the drugs have to be able to cross the blood–brain barrier. For example, most of the antiretroviral drugs that are used to treat HIV do not cross the blood–brain barrier and therefore do not protect the CNS from the disease.

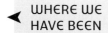 **WHERE WE HAVE BEEN**

In this chapter, we introduced the cells of the nervous system, described how they communicate with one another, and provided a taxonomy for the major divisions of the nervous system along with the structures associated with each division. Finally, we described how these structures are connected, how they are provided with nutrients, and how they are protected from damage.

Glossary

Absolute refractory period—The period after an action potential in which no additional action potentials can be produced.

Acetylcholine (ACh; cholinergic)—A neurotransmitter that is used by all motor neurons.

Action potential—The primary means of communication within the neuron. Action potentials are always the same size, they are propagated, and they are all or none. Action potentials result in the release of neurotransmitters.

Afferent—Moving information toward the nervous system or cell body.

Amygdala—Part of the limbic system that is involved with emotions.

Anterior—Toward the head (front of the brain, top of the spinal cord).

Anterior cerebral artery—Arteries that supply the medial frontal and parietal lobes.

Anterior commissure—Part of the commissural system that allows the two hemispheres to communicate. The anterior commissure connects olfactory areas of the brain with each other and the lateral temporal lobes with each other.

Anterior communicating artery—Joins the two carotid arteries together. Part of the circle of Willis.

Arachnoid granulation—Located in the superior sagittal sinus and involved in reabsorbing cerebrospinal fluid.

Arachnoid mater—The second layer of the meninges.

Area postrema—Part of the medulla that has a more permeable blood–brain barrier. The area postrema is involved with monitoring the blood for toxins and inducing vomiting if they are detected.

Astrocytes—Star-shaped glia that form the blood–brain barrier and have nutritive, metabolic, and storage functions

Autonomic nervous system (ANS)—Part of the peripheral nervous system (PNS) that is involved with regulating internal states, such as temperature.

Autoreceptors—Receptors that are located on the presynaptic neuron. Autoreceptors modulate and monitor the release of neurotransmitters.

Axodendritic—A synapse that is made up of an axon and a dendrite.

Axon—The component of the neuron that transmits the action potential and releases neurotransmitters.

Basal ganglia—The major division of the telencephalon that includes the caudate nucleus, putamen, and the globus pallidus. The basal ganglia are critically important for initiating movements and maintaining muscle tone.

Basilar artery—The two vertebral arteries join to form the basilar artery. The basilar artery supplies the pons, cerebellum, and midbrain.

Bell-Magendie Law—Description of the pairs of spinal nerves in which the dorsal projections entering the spinal cord (efferents) carry sensory information and the ventral projections from the spinal cord (afferents) carry motor information to muscles and glands.

Bipolar neuron—A neuron with two processes leaving the cell body.

Blood–brain barrier—Two layers of cells that limit the flow of substances between the blood and neural tissue.

Callosal agenesis—A genetic condition that describes a brain in which the corpus callosum is absent.

Carotid arteries—Arteries that supply each hemisphere with blood. The internal carotid artery divides into the anterior and middle cerebral artery.

Catecholamines—Neurotransmitters formed from tyrosine. There are three catecholamines: dopamine (DA), norepinephrine (NE), and epinephrine (E). All known catecholamine receptors are metabotropic and have numerous functions, including movement, reward, and emotion.

Caudal—Toward the tail.

Caudate nucleus—Part of the basal ganglia.

Central canal—The extension of the fourth ventricle that contains cerebrospinal fluid in the spinal cord.

Central fissure—The fissure in the brain that divides the frontal lobe from the parietal lobe.

Central nervous system (CNS)—The brain and spinal cord.

Cerebellum—The part of the hindbrain or metecephalon that is responsible for coordinating and initiating movement. It may be involved in learning and language processing.

Cerebral aqueduct—Connection between the third and fourth ventricles.

Cerebral cortex—The part of the telencephalon that included the frontal, parietal, occipital, and temporal lobes.

Cerebrospinal fluid (CSF)—A clear, nutrient-rich fluid that encases the brain and supports it. CSF is also found in the ventricles.

Cervical segments—The eight most anterior segments of the spinal cord.

Choroid plexus—Located on the floor of the lateral ventricles and the roof of the third and fourth ventricles and produces cerebrospinal fluid.

Cingulate cortex—Part of the limbic system, located at the anterior base of the fornix. May be involved in response selection, especially when there are two conflicting responses.

Circle of Willis—The basal and internal carotid arteries terminate in the circle of Willis, which is located above the pons. The circle of Willis may allow for compensatory flow among these arteries in case of damage.

Coccygeal segment—The thirty-first and lowest segment of the spinal cord.

Commissures—Tissues that connect structures in the two hemispheres.

Contralateral—On opposite sides.

Coronal section (frontal, transverse)—A brain slice taken parallel to the face.

Corpus callosum (includes the body, genu, rostrum, and splenium)—The largest of the commissures.

Cortex—The convoluted outer surface of the brain.

Dendrite—The component of the neuron that received information for other neurons.

Depolarization—Moving the electrical potential of the neuron to the positive. If there is sufficient depolarization, then an action potential will occur.

Diencephalon—The part of the forebrain that includes the thalamus and the hypothalamus.

Dorsal—Toward the back (top of the brain, back of the spinal cord).

Dorsal medial nucleus of the thalamus—The part of the thalamus that is responsible for relaying olfactory information.

Dura mater—The outermost layer of the meninges.

Efferent—Moving information away from the nervous system or cell body.

Endoplasmic reticulum—The organelle that is responsible for making, modifying, and sending proteins for packaging.

Endoskeletal—Having an internal skeleton.

EPSP—Excitatory postsynaptic potential; depolarization of the dendrite that, if sufficient, will result in an action potential.

Exocytosis—The process by which a vesicle of a neurotransmitter fuses with the axon terminal membrane and releases the neurotransmitter into the synapse.

Forebrain (prosencephalon)—The part of the brain that includes the diencephalon and the telencephalon.

Fornix—The part of the limbic system that connects the hippocampus to the mammilary bodies.

Frontal lobe—The frontmost part of the cerebral cortex; functions include motor, language, and inhibition.

GABA—Gamma-aminobutyric acid; the most common inhibitory amino acid neurotransmitter in the CNS.

Glia—Cells in the nervous system that are responsible for support and maintenance of neurons.

Globus pallidus—Part of the basal ganglia.

Glutamate—The most common excitatory amino acid neurontransmitter in the CNS.

G-protein-coupled receptors (metabotropic)—The most common type of neurotransmitter receptor in the CNS. These receptors are linked to G-proteins, which can control ion channels, but they can also influence gene expression. Activation of these receptors tends to have long-lasting responses.

Gray matter—Description of parts of the cortex that are made of cell bodies.

Gyrus (plural: gyri)—A ridge on the surface of the cortex.

Gemisphere—If the brain is divided along the longitudinal fissure, the two halves are the right and left hemisphere.

Heterotopic—Projecting from or connection two different areas.

Hindbrain (rhombencephalon)—Made up of the metencephalon and myelencephalon, including the medulla oblongata, pons, and the cerebellum.

Hippocampal commissure—The commissure that connects the right and left hippocampus.

Hippocampus—Part of the limbic system in the temporal lobe; involved in learning and memory but not the storage of memories.

Homotopic—Projecting from or connecting the same areas (right and left).

Horizontal section—A brain slice taken parallel to the ground.

Hyperpolarization—Moving the electrical potential of the neuron to the negative.

Hypothalamus—Part of the diencephalon and made of many nuclei, which are involved with feeding, hormone regulation, and sex.

Indoleamine (serotonin, 5-HT)—A neurotransmitter formed from tryptophan. The only indoleamine is serotonin (abbreviated as 5-HT), which is involved in eating, sleep, and mood.

Inferior—Below or bottommost.

Inferior colliculus—Part of the tectum involved in hearing.

Interventricular foramen—The small openings that connect the third ventricle with the lateral ventricles.

Ion channels—Channels in the membrane of the neuron that can open and close to allow movement of ions across the membrane.

Ipsilateral—On the same side.

IPSP—Inhibitory postsynaptic potential; hyperpolarization of the dendrite that will inhibit an action potential.

Lateral—Away from the middle (toward the outside).

Lateral fissure—A fissure on the side of the brain that separates the temporal lobe from the frontal and parietal lobes.

Lateral geniculate nucleus—The part of the thalamus that is involved in vision.

Lateral nuclei of the hypothalamus—Part of the hypothalamus involved in satiety, the feeling of having had enough to eat.

Lateral posterior nucleus of the thalamus—Part of the thalamus involved in relaying sensory information.

Lateral ventricles—The first and second ventricles located in the right and left hemispheres.

Lentiform nucleus—Part of the basal ganglia, it is the collective term for the globus pallidus and the putamen.

Limbic system—Part of the telencephalon, largely located in the temporal lobes. The limbic system is made up of the amygdala, hippocampus, fornix, cingulate, and mamillary bodies. Functions of the limbic system include learning, memory, and emotion.

Lobe—A subdivision of a part of the brain; the term is most often used to describe the four lobes of the cerebral cortex.

Longitudinal fissure—The fissure that runs from the pole of the occipital lobe to the pole of the frontal lobe that divides the brain into right and left hemispheres.

Lumbar segments—Segments 21–25 of the spinal cord.

Magnetic resonance imaging—A noninvasive imaging technique that uses the magnetic properties of blood or water to allow soft tissue such as the brain to be observed.

Mamillary bodies—Part of the limbic system that is thought to be involved in memory.

Massa intermedia—Located in the third ventricle, the massa intermedia performs a commissural role in connecting the right and left thalamus.

Medial—Toward the middle or neuraxis.

Medial geniculate nucleus—Part of the thalamus that is involved in relaying auditory information.

Medulla oblongata—Part of the hindbrain that is involved in vegetative functions such as breathing.

Meninges (singular: meanix)—Protective coverings of the brain. From the outermost to the innermost, they are the dura mater, the arachnoid mater, and the pia mater.

Metencephalon—The hindbrain portion of the brain that includes the pons and cerebellum.

Microglia (phagocytes)—Glia that have a housekeeping function, microglia are phagocytes as they remove dead tissue and have been implicated in some neurodegenerative disease states (e.g., Alzheimer's disease).

Midbrain (mesencephalon)—Contains the tectum and tegmentum.

Middle cerebral artery—The branch of the carotid artery that provides blood to the lateral frontal, temporal, and parietal lobes.

Mitochondria—The organelle that is responsible for providing the neuron with energy.

Monoamines—Neurotransmitters that are formed from a single amino acid.

Multipolar neuron—A neuron with more than two processes leaving the cell body.

Muscarinic receptors—A subtype of ACh receptor that is metabotropic and binds the ligand muscarine. It is found widely in the CNS and in smooth muscle.

Myelencephalon—The posterior portion of the brainstem.

Myelin—Insulation covering most axons in the CNS, made by oligodendrocytes.

Neuraxis—An imaginary line between the spinal cord and the front of the brain.

Neuron—Cells in the nervous system that are responsible for communication and therefore behavior.

Neurotransmitter—Chemicals that are released by the neuron (in the axon) that are used to communicate between neurons (over the synapse).

Nicotinic receptors—A subtype of ACh receptor that is ionotropic and binds the ligand nicotine. Although it is not common in the CNS, it is found widely in the PNS.

Nodes of Ranvier—Breaks in the myelin of an action potential that contain sodium–potassium pumps. Action potentials jump from node to node along the length of an axon.

Nuclei—Name for a group of neurons that have a similar structure and function.

Nucleus—The organelle that contains and processes the information contained in the DNA.

Occipital lobe—Lobe of the cerebral cortex at the back of the brain that is responsible for vision.

Oligodendrocytes—Glia that make myelin.

Parasympathetic nervous system—The part of the autonomic nervous system that is involved with nonemergency behaviors.

Parietal lobe—The cortical area that is between the occipital and frontal lobes. The parietal lobe has spatial cognition, vision, and somatosensory functions.

Parkinson's disease—A motor disease that results from destruction of the basal ganglia and loss of dopamine.

Periaqueductal gray—Part of the tegmentum that is important for pain perception.

Peripheral nervous system (PNS)—The parts of the nervous system other than the brain and spinal cord; the nerves that run through most of the body.

Pia mater—The innermost layer of the meninges.

Pituitary gland—The master endocrine gland, controlled by the hypothalamus and located just ventral to the hypothalamus.

Plasma membrane—Covering of the neuron, made of a lipid bilayer studded with proteins and channels.

Pons—Part of the metencephalon involved with transmitting information from the spinal cord to the rest of the brain.

Posterior—Toward the tail (back of the brain, bottom of the spinal cord).

Posterior commissure—Part of the commissural system.

Posterior communicating artery—The arterial link between the middle cerebral artery and the posterior cerebral artery; part of the circle of Willis.

Postsynaptic—In an axodendritic synapse, events occurring in the dendrite.

Presynaptic—In an axodendritic synapse (a synapse between an axon and dendrite), events occurring in the axon.

Primary visual cortex—Cortical area involved with processing visual information.

Pulvinar nucleus—Part of the thalamus involved in relaying somatosensory information.

Putamen—Part of the basal ganglia.

Red nucleus—A motor nucleus in the tegmentum.

Resting potential—The initial electrical charge that a neuron has across its membrane. In most neurons, the resting potential is ~ – 70 mV.

Ribosomes—The organelle that is responsible for manufacturing the proteins that are coded for in the DNA.

Rostral—Toward the nose.

Sacral segment—Segments 26–30 of the spinal cord.

Sagittal section (midsagittal)—A brain slice taken parallel to the side of the brain; *midsagittal* refers to sections taken through the center of the brain dividing it into the right and left hemispheres.

Saltatory conduction—The jumping of the action potential from one node of Ranvier to the next.

Satellite cells—Cells in the PNS that have functions similar to those of the glia.

Satiety—A feeling of being full after eating.

Schwann cells—Cells in the PNS that make myelin.

Sensory cortex—Cortex that is involved in sensory processing.

Serotonin—A neurotransmitter involved in the regulation of mood, sleep, and appetite.

Sodium–potassium pump—An active transport mechanism that is employed by the neuron to ensure that there are high concentrations of sodium in the extracellular fluid and high concentrations of potassium in the intracellular fluid. It moves three sodium ions out for every two potassium ions in.

Soma—The body of the neuron that contains the machinery for metabolic function.

Somatic nervous system—The part of the peripheral nervous system that is involved with interacting with the external environment.

Striatum—A collective term for the caudate nucleus and the putamen.

Sulcus (plural: sulci; fissure)—Similar to a fissure, though more shallow. Sulci are depressions in the cortex.

Superior—Above or topmost.

Superior colliculus—Part of the tectum involved in vision.

Sympathetic nervous system—The part of the peripheral nervous system involved in preparing the body for action.

Synapse—The gap between neurons.

Tectum—Part of the midbrain that contains the inferior and superior colliculus.

Tegmentum—Part of the midbrain that contains a number of motor nuclei, including the red nucleus and the substantia nigra.

Telencephalon—Part of the forebrain that includes the cerebral cortex, limbic system, and basal ganglia.

Temporal lobe—The lobe of the cerebral cortex that is bounded by the lateral fissure and the occipital lobe. The functions of the temporal lobe include language, memory, and emotion.

Terminal button—The end of the axon, where neurotransmitters are released.

Thalamus—Part of the diencephalon that is primarily responsible for relaying sensory information between the cortex and sensory organs.

Third ventricle—The midline ventricle.

Thoracic segments—Segments 9–20 of the spinal cord.

Transmitter-gated ion channels (ionotropic)—Receptors of neurotransmitters that control ion channels and result in fast responses.

Unipolar neuron—A neuron with only one process leaving the cell body.

Ventral—Toward the front (bottom of the brain, front of the spinal cord).

Ventral posterior nucleus—The somatosensory nucleus of the thalamus.

Ventricles—Four hollow areas in the brain that are filled with cerebrospinal fluid.

Ventrolateral nucleus of the thalamus—The motor nucleus of the thalamus.

Vertebral arteries—Arteries that provide blood to the ventral areas of the brain.

White matter—Tissue in the brain that appears white. Typically, white matter consists of myelinated axons.

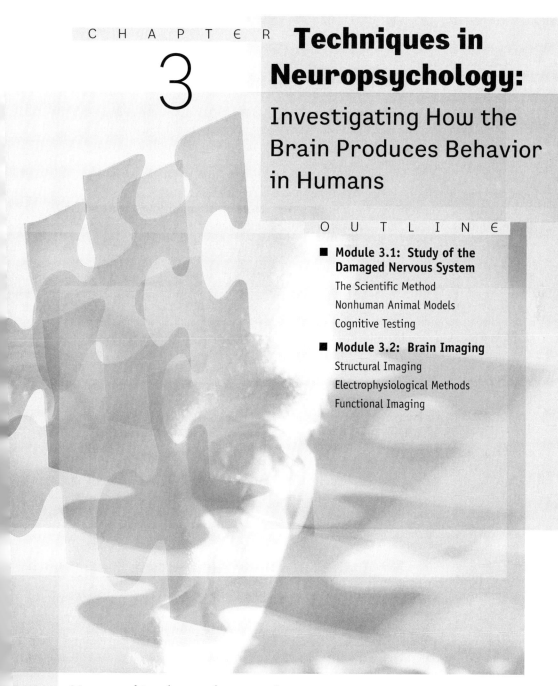

Techniques in Neuropsychology:

Investigating How the Brain Produces Behavior in Humans

Not everything that can be counted counts,
And not everything that counts can be counted.
—ALBERT EINSTEIN

MODULE **3.1**
Study of the Damaged Nervous System

Much of what we know about the human brain is the product of research performed with two populations of participants: humans who have sustained damage to the nervous system or who are remarkable in some way and nonhuman animals. Many of the studies of nonhuman animals have also investigated how behavior was affected by central nervous system damage. It may not be obvious, but depending on the damaged nervous system to tell us about the intact nervous system makes some critical generalizations (which may or may not be true). The process of imaging the nervous system and its activity and relating this to behavior in neurologically intact individuals is really the new kid on the block (which is the focus of Module 3.2). It remains to be seen whether these newer techniques, which allow us to investigate the intact nervous system, will supplant the older techniques that we will discuss in this module.

This module will focus on the study of the damaged brain and how it has contributed to our understanding of how the brain produces behavior. This chapter may also give you an appreciation of the multidisciplinary nature of neuropsychology.

The Scientific Method

As we will see in this chapter, the study of neuropsychology requires information from a number of different sources. Typically, the focus of the research that defines cognitive neuroscience/neuropsychology is on the relationship between brain and behavior. However, brain and behavior can be described at a number of levels and at a variety of complexities and time scales, which depend primarily on the question that is being investigated. For instance, depending on the interests of the researcher, something as simple as a memory can be described as "a change in individual dendritic spines, requiring the participation of various chemicals, a result of patterned action potentials, critically dependent on the integrity of specific areas of the brain, a function of a specific part of the brain," or as "that which is stored among the various parts of the brain that encoded it." Which level is right? The answer is a terrible one: It depends on the question. Some questions are better answered by an investigation of the minutiae of the properties of the phenomena; other questions are, by their nature, more globally focused.

However, despite the variety of methods that neuropsychologists use, there are some common principles (called the scientific method) that neuropsychologists follow. The scientific method has at its roots in the principles of objectivity and replication or confirmation of results. As researchers, we must strive to be as objective as possible, often using standardized tests or measurements. This level of objectivity is often referred to as the **empirical method** (*empirical* means "observation"). Associated with objectivity is **replication** of the results so that they can be confirmed (often by other researchers). When possible, neuropsychologists attempt to replicate their results so that they can be sure that their initial observations were not a fluke. Furthermore, because most research (including the materials in this book) is published, other researchers attempt to replicate (and extend) these results. Replication by other researchers is important as it ensures that the effects in the study are generalizable to people beyond those who participated in the first study. Although much of the research in neuropsychology relies on studying people who have had some type of neurological injury, one of the goals of neuropsychology is to understand how the neurologically intact brain produces behavior.

There is probably no single term that characterizes the scientific method better than **control.** First and foremost control refers to the ability to manipulate something of interest to determine the effects. In the studies that you will read in this book, control also includes the ability to exclude unwanted variables from the study. These **confounding variables** may affect the outcome of the study, leading a researcher to make false conclusions about the effects observed. Finally, control refers to having an appropriate comparison sample so that deviations from this sample can be observed.

Beyond the principles of control, replication, and the empirical method, there are some other common features of research studies. The first is that research is directed by a prediction, which determines the methods that we use. This prediction, or **hypothesis,** is often formed as a statement that can be rejected (e.g., "Performance on a word-learning task will be better when participants are tested in the morning than when they are tested at midnight"). This helps us to avoid asking questions that are so vague that they cannot be answered by any one study (e.g., "How does the brain produce consciousness?"). However, perhaps what is more important is that hypotheses help us to avoid questions that cannot be disproved. You should be able to see that the first hypothesis ("Performance of a word-learning task will be better when participants are tested in the morning than when they are tested at midnight") can be easily tested and either confirmed or rejected depending on the performance of the participants.

We also define how we will study our question, including definitions of what variables are of interest to us. The **independent variable** is the one that the researcher manipulates to determine how the behavior is affected. In the hypothesis above, the independent variable is time of day. The **dependent variable** is the response or behavior that the experimenter measures. These behaviors should be directly related to the manipulation of independent variable. In the hypothesis above, the dependent variable is how well the participant performed a word-learning task (perhaps the number of words that the participant was able to recall).

The following paragraph is a simple research study:

> I am interested in observing how listening to music affects memory for words. In a testing room in my lab, I have individual participants sit down and read a list of fourteen words. Each participant receives the same list of words. Half of the participants wear headphones and listen to white noise (which sounds like static on a television) while they are reading the words. The other half of the participants wears headphones and listen to music while they are reading the words. Both groups are given two minutes to read the words. Once my stopwatch shows that the two minutes are up, the list and the headphones are removed, and the participants tell me as many words on the list as they can remember. In case I miss some of the words, I record their answers with a tape recorder.

What is the hypothesis? (*"Listening to music affects memory for words." Notice that it does not say whether memory for words will be better or worse.*) What is the independent variable(s)? (*Listening to either music or white noise.*) What is the dependent variable(s)? (*The number of words that the participant is able to tell the researcher.*) What control measures has the researcher employed? (*Some of the control methods are having the same list of words, recording the responses of the participants with a tape recorder, using a stopwatch, having half of the group listen to nonmusical noises, and testing all of the participants in the same environment.*) What are some potential confounding variables? (*Maybe some participants do not like the choice of music and are distracted by it; maybe some participants are huge fans of the group playing the music and are distracted by it.*)

Finally, as we will see throughout the book, much of the research in neuropsychology is only quasi-experimental. That is, ethically and practically, we cannot manipulate the independent variable directly (e.g., we cannot give half of our participants frontal lesions while employing the appropriate control procedures with the other half). Or it may be that there are only a few people in the world that have the abilities in which you are interested. Additionally, unlike many studies with nonhuman animals, there may be inherent differences in our sample due to variables out of our control, such as environment, education, or nutrition. In quasi-experimental designs, our ability to reach a conclusion about a phenomenon under question sometimes does not result from observations in a single experiment. Instead, we must rely on the method of **converging operations.** That is, a common conclusion is reached by examining a number of studies that approach the question from a variety of different perspectives. If there is a consensus about the results of these studies, then researchers can be relatively confident that they have learned an important feature of how the nervous system produces behavior.

Nonhuman Animal Models

Many neuroscientists spend their entire careers studying nonhuman animals. In fact, from 1930 to 1965, much of psychology (not just neuropsychology) was dominated by the study of the white laboratory rat. During that period, researchers presumed that there were minimal basic differences (behavioral and neural) among most mammalian species. It was thought that the study of nonhuman animals would provide important information about important psychological constructs, such as learning, memory, and emotionality. Researchers such as Thorndike, Morgan, and Watson recognized early on that unlike research with human participants, research using nonhuman animals afforded greater objectivity and precision and allowed the researcher to control all of the aspects of the life cycle. We now know that there are important differences among mammalian species, especially with respect to brain and behavior, and these differences are also a source of important information regarding how the brain produces behavior.

Nonhuman animals that are raised in controlled conditions afford the researcher greater control. Furthermore, using nonhuman animals that have been raised in controlled conditions reduces the variability that is attributable to extraneous factors. This degree of homogeneity allows the experimenter to randomly assort the subjects into various treatment groups, a critical factor in performing experimental protocols. Moreover, because experiments can be performed by using nonhuman animals that have been raised in controlled conditions, researchers can actually isolate causal conclusions. In effect, the ability to study animals that have been raised in controlled

Neuropsychological Celebrity

Phineas Gage

On Wednesday, September 13, 1848, there was a terrible and remarkable accident in New England. Phineas Gage was a 25-year-old railway construction foreman who was very well liked by the men in his charge (or "gang," as it was called). He was an easygoing, responsible, and pious man. The railway was expanding across Vermont, and as the construction neared the town of Cavendish, the terrain became especially treacherous: It was filled with rock. Rather than circumventing the rock, the gang was blasting through it. This required drilling holes, putting in an explosive powder, inserting a fuse, and covering the powder with sand. The sand was then tamped in with a few careful strokes of an iron rod before the fuse was lit. On one such occasion, Phineas accidentally started tamping before the sand was in place, which prematurely ignited the charge. The explosion projected his four-foot-long, thirteen-pound tamping rod through his left cheek, penetrating the base of his skull and exiting through the top of his head, eventually landing more than forty feet away. Phineas fell to the ground, but he didn't even lose consciousness—he even spoke a few minutes later. His men carried him to a cart, on which he rode (sitting erect) for almost a mile before receiving treatment from Dr. John Harlow (Damasio, 1994).

The survival of Phineas Gage is probably the most remarkable part of this story, but that is not why it is told in more than 60% of all introductory psychology textbooks (Macmillan, 2000). He was "pronounced cured" in less than two months (on the basis of his physical recovery), but his personality had changed dramatically. In the words of his gang, "Gage was no longer Gage." In Dr. Harlow's words, Gage was now "fitful, irreverent, indulging at times in the grossest profanity (which was not previously his custom), manifesting but little deference for his fellows, impatient of restraint or advice when it conflicts with his desires, at times pertinaciously obstinate, yet capricious and vacillating, devising many plans of future operation, which are no sooner arranged than they are abandoned in turn for others appearing more feasible" (Harlow & Miller, 1993, p. 277). These changes rendered him virtually unemployable—not for lack of ability, but because of his new personality. The discovery that focal brain damage can alter one's personality while leaving other aspects of intellect intact was big news. Keep in mind that the year was 1848. Phrenology was dying away after becoming more of an entrepreneurial enterprise than a scientific one, and Broca had not yet presented his seminal work on the localization of language processing. The considerable interest in the case was probably also due to the spectacular nature of the accident.

Gage's case became more difficult to follow when he moved to Chile, subsequently returning to the United States, this time settling in California. Although his death is not well documented, it appears that he died of an epileptic fit on May 21, 1861 (over twelve years after the accident). Immediately after Phineas died, there were no postmortem studies of his brain. However, his body was later exhumed, and his skull (Figure 3.1) and the tamping iron were sent to Dr. Harlow, who then reported his findings. Gage's skull was later reexamined using modern neuroimaging techniques to model the probable lesion location, identified as involving both left and right prefrontal cortices (Damasio, Grabowski, Frank, Galaburda, & Damasio, 1994). The skull and tamping iron are currently on display at Harvard's Countway Library of Medicine.

Figure 3.1   **Phineas Gage's Skull**

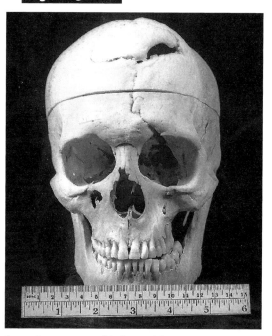

Source: Image courtesy of Anthony Walsh.

laboratory conditions affords a degree of precision that is not available to researchers who study human participants.

To some extent, these advantages are still very important considerations. Research has shown that wide-ranging variables, such as early environmental (prenatal and perinatal) conditions, genes, diurnal rhythms, and social influences, do affect both behavior and the nervous system. Examinations of the effects of discrete lesions on very precisely measured behaviors have provided tremendous insights into the relationship between brain and behavior. Species as diverse as geese and rats have contributed to our understanding of developmental neuropsychology in research including that performed by Tinbergen (who won the Nobel Prize for his research) on imprinting in avian species and that of Diamond on the effects of enriched environments on rats. Much of what is known about the teratogenic and behavioral effects of alcohol was first done in nonhuman animals. Furthermore, animal models of neurological diseases have provided a means by which these diseases can be investigated and perhaps eradicated.

However, there are a number of important limitations of this type of research. First and foremost, many research questions focus on only one facet of an organism and ignore other important factors. For instance, a common technique in learning theory is known as **delayed nonmatching to sample task.** Typically, this task involves a food reward and a food-deprived nonhuman animal. The animal observes the food reward paired with stimulus A; then the animal is required to pick the novel stimulus B to receive the reward. Certainly, researchers have discovered many important principles involved in learning and memory by using such tasks, and many species have been successfully tested with this technique. However, for a number of species, this technique has questionable ethological validity. In other words, it is unclear whether animals (human or otherwise) ever exhibit this type of behavior in naturalistic settings. As a further complicating factor, some species (e.g., rats) are neophobic (that is, they do not eat novel foods), further complicating interpretation of this task. Simply put, if the rat does not perform the task correctly, can we necessarily conclude that the deficit is related to learning, or should we conclude that this species does not interact with novel food items? Furthermore, some laboratory tasks are so artificial that they may not provide data that tell us about real-world function. Importantly, these considerations are also limitations of some research involving human participants.

Another limitation of research utilizing nonhuman animals is that this research might not be easily generalizable to other species. At one level, this argument has validity. For instance, no one would argue that the nervous system of nonhuman animals is identical to that of humans. However, the study of simpler systems can offer important insights. For instance, many neuroscientists study how the brain of nonhuman animals encodes, retains, and retrieves information. As we will see in other chapters, searching for these changes within the human brain is like looking for a needle in a haystack. Therefore, many researchers have chosen to either examine learning and memory in simpler systems (e.g., *Aplysia*, studied by the Nobel Laureate Eric Kandel). From a technical standpoint, it is doubtful that these experiments could have been performed initially on the human brain. From an ethical standpoint, many of these experiments could have never been performed on the human brain. Thus, non-human animal experimentation in laboratory settings has provided critical information regarding how, why, and where psychological phenomena such as learning occur within the nervous system.

At another level, the argument about generality is falsely simplified. Some critics suggest that nonhuman animals are not sufficiently behaviorally sophisticated to be useful in understanding the principles of human behavior. This viewpoint assumes that nonhuman animals are very simple creatures and ignores the rich, complex behaviors that nonhuman animals produce and their great behavioral flexibility in responding to novel situations. Furthermore, many mammalian systems are remarkably conserved. That is, there is a great degree of overlap among the basic properties of the nervous system, including chemical and electrical means of information transfer, metabolism, and even, in a very general sense, the layout of the nervous system. Even the code that makes us unique individuals is conserved across species. The same series of nucleotide bases in DNA code for the same amino acid proteins in everything from bacteria to us (with the exception of a few types of protozoa). Thus, at the most basic level of life—DNA—there is remarkable conservation of systems across species, and the understanding of how one species solves a problem posed by the environment may lead to understanding other solutions to the same problem. At a behavioral level, we also appear to be largely conserved. For instance, the principles of learning that we observe in dogs, cats, and pigeons are important primarily because they do generalize to other species, including humans. Some cognitive skills (e.g., language) may be so different in nonhuman animals (as compared to humans) that the usefulness of such research may relate only to understanding how the nonhuman animal perceives and symbolically represents the world (rather than providing a direct window onto human cognition).

Although we may be limited in our ability to study some forms of cognitive skills, it is possible to study some forms of higher cognitive function in some nonhuman animals. Importantly, their differences in these situations provide important insights into human cognition. Skills as uniquely human as semantic categorization and language can be studied in nonhuman animals and provide important and illuminating results. Pigeons, rats, chimpanzees, gorillas, and parrots can categorize objects into semantic classes that are typically linguistically related by humans. Moreover, members of these species appear to be able to generalize these categories to novel stimuli and in novel situations, observations suggesting that this is not a manifestation of some principle other than semantic categorization. These observations provide important evidence to suggest that language developed out of other cognitive capabilities that are present in nonhuman animals. Furthermore, these observations suggest that it is highly unlikely that language developed in complete ontogenetic and phylogenetic isolation from other cognitive abilities, such as memory or motor skill. However, this does not mean that gorillas (or other nonhuman animals) use language in the same way humans do.

However, there remain some important limitations to research with nonhuman animals. The first limitation is that although there are many similarities among mammalian species, there are also important differences. One obvious difference between

Table 3.1

A Summary of the Strengths and Limitations of Nonhuman Animal Research

Strengths	Limitations
Can control extraneous variables	Some topics may not be suitable
Can perform experiments	There are striking differences between human and nonhuman nervous systems
Can conclude causality	Might study one behavior/brain area in isolation
Can look for mechanisms in a simpler system	Might be very artificial
Can model disease processes	Human brain has functional diversity

humans and most other mammals is the complexity of the central nervous system. It is quite apparent that humans are capable of a number of behaviors that are unique to humans, including language and memory systems. For instance, although the hippocampus appears to be related to spatial learning in chickadees, humans, and rats, it is also clear that the hippocampus mediates broader behaviors in humans. In other instances, even this level of similarity is not conserved. For instance, when humans ingest the neurotoxin MPTP, they develop a permanent syndrome resembling Parkinson's disease, presumably the result of problems with the basal ganglia. However, when rats ingest MPTP, the results are quite strikingly different, as the rats eventually recover from the frozen state. These results suggest that there are important differences between rats and humans, especially in the basal ganglia. Such comparisons between human and nonhuman animals can be informative, although care needs to be taken to ensure that differences are not minimized. Finally, there are a number of questions that remain quite difficult to examine in humans, not to mention nonhumans (e.g., human consciousness, or is language represented phonemically in the brain?). As such, it may be that the study of nonhuman animals with topics such as these is impractical or impossible.

Table 3.1 summarizes both the strengths and the limitations of research using nonhuman animals.

Cognitive Testing

As we mentioned in the previous two sections, neuropsychologists examine the behavior of the people in whom they are interested. People with injury to the nervous system often have their first behavioral test in the emergency room in the form of a neurological exam, which examines the person's reflexes, cranial nerve functioning, and medical history. The physician also examines the person's muscle tone and abilities to make gross movements and to perceive stimuli. Often, a neurological exam includes an exam known as the Mini-Mental State Exam (Folstein, Folstein, & McHugh, 1975) or the Modified Mini-Mental State Exam (Teng & Chui, 1987). Both tests look at how well people can answer a series of questions, which are designed to briefly examine cognitive functions such as language (listening to the people speak as they tell the physician their medical history), orientation to location ("Do you know where you are?"), attention ("Can you count from 100 backwards by threes?"), and orientation to time ("Do you know what day it is?"). Although a neurological exam is not as detailed as a neuropsychological exam, it does provide important insights into the functioning of the person. Perhaps more important, physicians can perform these tests quickly to get a gross appreciation of the degree to which nervous system functions are involved in any injury. Although this is a generalization, a preliminary neurology exam is primarily interested in determining the degree to which any nervous system injury (or disease) affects basic neurological functions.

Neuropsychological testing is the detailed examination of higher cognitive functions. Because there is a whole chapter (Chapter 15) that describes this process in detail, we will describe a neuropsychological consultation very briefly here. Typically, a neuropsychological consult begins with a personal interview that is followed by a series of tests. In the personal interview, the client discusses his or her medical history and describes any problems or concerns. Neuropsychologists typically use a series of standardized cognitive tests. These tests are standardized in two ways: They are always given to participants in the same way, and they are always scored in the same manner. Theoretically, if a person were to be given the same test by two different neuropsychologists, that person should receive the same score on both tests and should not notice any deviation in how the test was delivered. (I say "theoretically," because there are always small differences in test procedures and in performance from day to day.) Typically, testing begins with some tests of general cognitive function, and then, depending on the results of these tests, tests of more specific cognitive function will be given. Together with the medical history and the neurologist's report, the results of the neuropsychological testing are used to help with diagnosis, intervention, and rehabilitation.

However, behavioral testing has flaws. For instance, if the person giving the test deviates from standard delivery or scoring procedures, the results obtained may be meaningless. Furthermore, although most neuropsychological tests have been widely validated, some tests may have problems with being generalized beyond the sample with which they were developed. For instance, a number of tests of general intelligence may be biased and may produce invalid test results in participants who do not belong to the dominant linguistic or cultural group. In addition, many people may have other coincident diseases or disorders (e.g., depression) that may affect their performance on neuropsychological tests. These coexisting conditions make it difficult to determine the degree to which any deficit results from the lesion in the nervous system or from the other condition. (For instance, depression can impair the person's desire to perform optimally on the tests.)

Table 3.2 summarizes both the strengths and the limitations of behavioral testing.

Self-Test

1. What is the largest weakness of case studies in general?

2. What are the advantages and disadvantages of studies of nonhuman animals? Could a cognitive psychologist spend his or her entire career studying nonhuman animals? Would this information be relevant to understanding how the human brain produces behavior? Why or why not?

3. What elements are surveyed in a typical neurological exam? How does that differ from a neuropsychological exam? Why do they differ?

Table 3.2

**A Summary of the Strengths and Limitations
of Behavioral Testing**

Strengths	Limitations
Standardized testing procedures	Small variations in test presentation and scoring
Standardized scoring procedures	Lack of cultural sensitivity
Identification of specific cognitive impairments	Degree to which other existing conditions may alter a cognitive profile
Validity of measurement of cognitive domain	

◄ **WHERE WE HAVE BEEN**   So far in this section, we have focused on how neuropsychologists, neuroscientists, and cognitive neuroscientists approach the study of damaged nervous systems to learn about brain and behavior. Included within this section was a discussion of how the study of nonhuman animals can inform our knowledge of brain and behavior systems.

WHERE WE ARE GOING ►   The chapter would not be complete without a discussion of one of the major groups of people studied in neuropsychology: the introductory psychology student. Included within the upcoming section are descriptions of the techniques that are used to visualize the intact human brain and relate brain and behavior in neurologically normal individuals.

MODULE **3.2**
Brain Imaging

Given that relating behavior to brain function is the central goal of neuropsychology, imagine the impact of being able to tell exactly what brain areas are being used (and how much) during any given task. Would that make neuropsychology's goal easy to obtain? Of course it would—wouldn't it? Functional neuroimaging provides the researcher with in vivo (live) pictures of the brain areas that are most active during a cognitive task. When this type of imaging was just starting to become popular, some people predicted that it would rapidly put an end to experimental neuropsychology. It most certainly has not. The task of human brain mapping has been revolutionized by neuroimaging, but the job of mapping the human brain is far from over, and current imaging methods have a number of technical and methodological limitations. Just as in any science, discoveries in neuropsychology lead to more questions. As Jules Sagaret described it, "The greater becomes the volume of our sphere of knowledge, the greater also becomes its surface of contact with the unknown." (This quote is often incorrectly attributed to Albert Einstein.)

This module explores the various means by which neuropsychologists measure (or at least infer) activity in the human brain. In learning about each new method, it is difficult not to compare them, describing one as better than another, or perhaps

Current Controversy

Can We Understand Normal Brains from Studying Abnormal Ones?

One of the most common critiques of case studies of people with brain damage is that we are merely inferring the function of the formerly intact brain. Specifically, we are inferring from the lack of brain tissue and the corresponding lack of function that the two went together in the intact brain. It is actually a large leap to suggest that a behavioral deficit can be related to the lack of a particular brain site.

A common analogy illustrates the point that I am trying to make. Think about an old radio that uses vacuum tubes rather than transistors. When all the tubes are in place, the radio works well and produces music. When you take out one of the tubes, the radio only makes a howling noise. Following the logic utilized in case studies of people, we would have to conclude that the function of the tube is to suppress howling. However, given what we know about how radios function, it is unlikely that there is a howling suppression tube. We know that the radio could be howling for a number of reasons, the primary one being that we have removed a tube that is critical for the normal functioning of the radio. (The howling is a symptom of the malfunction that does not normally occur when the radio is intact.)

What can we then conclude about the relationship between deficits in behavior and lesions? In the most restrictive sense, we can only observe how the rest of the brain performs any given task without that part of the brain. From these observations, we may be able to deduce what parts of the brain are critical for the performance of this function, although this conclusion is far from guaranteed. However, we cannot conclude with certainty that the lesioned area performs the task. Why? What if the part of the brain that is lesioned performs a connective function or contains within it axons (sometimes known as **fibers of passage**) that connect one part of the brain with another. As such, we can see that damage to these fibers of passage would result in the disconnection of the two areas (outside the damaged area) and that disconnecting these two parts could result in a deficit in that cognitive ability that did not directly relate to the function of the lesioned area.

Furthermore, as you will see in the following chapters, there is more than one way for someone to perform a task. For instance, next time you are in a classroom, look around at the variety of ways in which people in your class are taking notes. Some will hold their pen in their right hand, some will print, some may be using laptop computers, and yet others may be recording the lecture. If a task is sufficiently complex (and most are), there is surely more than one way to accomplish the goal. Thus, the failure to observe a deficit in a specific behavior following brain damage, does not guarantee that the lesioned section plays no part in the function. It may be that following the brain injury, the person modifies his or her strategy, allowing the person to compensate for deficits that resulted from the lesion. In this case, if we were to simply record how well a person could perform a task, we would underestimate the importance of the lesioned area in producing the behavior of interest.

So can we understand normal brains from abnormal ones? Yes, of course we can. However, we must ensure that we are observing the behavior carefully, that the task is carefully designed, and that we are careful not to generalize beyond what we were able to observe. Furthermore, as long as we rely on converging evidence for producing our conclusions, we will be able to learn important information from damaged brains.

---

even attempting to identify the "ultimate" investigative tool. There is no such tool. As you will discover in the following sections, different tools are better for different jobs. A $1000 table saw will not help you drive a nail. For that, you need only a $5 hammer. Similarly, in diagnosing epilepsy, functional magnetic resonance imaging (fMRI) is not the first choice because an electroencephalograph (EEG), which incidentally is much cheaper to perform, does an excellent job. The type of tool that is used must suit the problem to be solved.

One problem plagues all of the imaging tools, at least when they are used for research purposes. Everyone's brain is different. Because there is no average brain, this creates a serious challenge for researchers who wish to use neuroimaging. What then does one do with functional neuroimaging from a group of ten people? Most of the people (say, eight out of the ten) might demonstrate similar patterns of activation (such as posterior parietal cortex activation), but the boundaries of functional brain areas are not in exactly the same location for each of the ten people. So what should the researcher do? Researchers have not come to a consensus on how to report the data. For instance, some researchers choose to describe each person separately, whereas others advocate creating an average and composite image from the ten people. Still other researchers try to categorize the people into groups and then create average composite images of the two groups. The problem explodes from there. For instance, what if it looks as though there are more than two groups? There are no easy answers to these questions. If you spend some time reading current neuropsychology journals, you should have no trouble finding examples of each one of the strategies described above. The controversy over the use of single-case studies versus group studies in neuroimaging is far from resolved.

Structural Imaging

Structural neuroimaging provides an image of the structure of the brain. Before such methods were readily available, clinical neuropsychologists assessed individuals who had brain damage using long, complicated test batteries (described in Chapter 15) that helped to identify the person's behavioral deficits. On the basis of the pattern of these deficits, the neuropsychologist would attempt to localize the lesion. This is no longer necessary in most cases. Structural neuroimaging can usually inform clinicians about the precise location of abnormalities. This has not made the clinical neuropsychologist obsolete; behavioral assessments meant to identify deficits are still performed. However, these assessments are done with the goal of rehabilitation or at least management of the deficits. This paradigm shift in neuropsychology was initiated in the late 1960s when traditional X-ray imaging methods were combined with computers.

X-RAYS. Neuroradiology (studying the nervous system with imaging) was made possible because of a serendipitous discovery made by a physicist, Wilhelm Conrad Röntgen (1845–1923). While studying cathode rays, he noticed a glowing fluorescent screen on a nearby table. He quickly deduced that the fluorescence was coming from his partially evacuated glass Hittorf-Crookes tube and that the rays from the tube could penetrate the thick black paper that was wrapped around the tube. Röntgen was rewarded for his discovery with the first Nobel Prize in Physics in 1901.

As you most likely know, **X-rays** cannot pass through all materials with the same ease. The more dense the material, the less penetrable the substance is to X-rays, which makes X-rays useful for medical imaging. Less dense parts of the body (soft tissue, such as muscles) absorb relatively few X-rays, whereas higher-density areas (such as those containing bones) absorb more X-rays. Thus, the amount of radiation (X-rays) that passes through a region provides a measure of the density of the structures within the region. The principle is quite simple: Send a beam of X-rays into a structure, and see how many "stick" by detecting the ones that pass through on a photographic plate. Very dense structures (such as bone) appear bright on the resultant image, whereas lower-density structures (such as a crack in a bone) appear dark. This is how X-rays can provide a two-dimensional (2-D) representation of density.

The discovery of X-rays had a tremendous impact on medicine. It allowed physicians to look for pathology in a relatively noninvasive way. However, X-rays are radiation and therefore can be dangerous. High levels of X-rays can actually destroy tissue. Ironically, this feature of X-rays has also proved useful to medicine. X-rays can be used therapeutically to destroy unwanted tissues, such as cancerous growths. Much lower levels are used for diagnostic procedures, but repeated exposure can still be harmful. How many times have you gone for an X-ray and the attendant draped you in a lead gown and left the room before pressing the "on" button? Having one or two X-rays a year might not do much harm, but you would not want to get one every hour or two!

Conventional X-rays have not proved to be very useful for neuroimaging, largely because the brain is soft tissue encased in bone. Although X-rays are useful when looking for bone fractures, a 2-D X-ray of the skull does not provide much information about what damage has occurred inside the skull. When an individual has a penetrating (i.e., puncturing the skull) wound to the head, an X-ray primarily describes the nature of the entry wound, with little information about anything else. To make matters worse, X-rays cannot differentiate between cerebrospinal fluid and brain structures very well. Although X-ray machines are relatively inexpensive and are a fast way to get good structural information about the integrity of the skull, their ability to image the structures within the skull is limited.

COMPUTED TOMOGRAPHY (CT). **Computed Tomography** (CT) scans were the first good means available to noninvasively image live brain tissue. The method was developed out of research in the late 1960s and early 1970s that combined X-ray technology with the rapidly emerging field of computing (Raju, 1999). As was the case with the original discovery of X-rays, this research resulted in a Nobel Prize; physicist Allan Cormack and engineer Godfrey Hounsfield were awarded the Nobel Prize for Physiology or Medicine in 1979.

Technically, CT scanning is not much different from taking an X-ray. Both methods use the same types of radiation and measures, but CT scanning involves the projection of X-rays from multiple angles followed by the computerized reconstruction of the measures into three-dimensional (3-D) images. In principle, this is similar to examining an object from multiple angles (all of which are 2-D) and constructing an inferred three-dimensional (3-D) image from these multiple views. These views can be combined to provide a reasonably accurate 3-D representation despite the large differences among the appearance of the object from the various views. The brain images are typically constructed in a number of "slices," typically ranging between nine and twelve per scan. Just as conventional X-rays provide measurements of the densities of various tissues, so too does a CT scan. Highly dense areas (such as the skull) appear bright, whereas areas of lower density (such as CSF and brain matter) appear relatively dark. The spatial resolution provided by CT scanners is often adequate for clinical purposes (between 0.5 and 1.0 centimeters), but its differentiation between white and gray matter is rather poor (see Figure 3.2).

Figure 3.2   **A Sample CT Scan of the Brain**

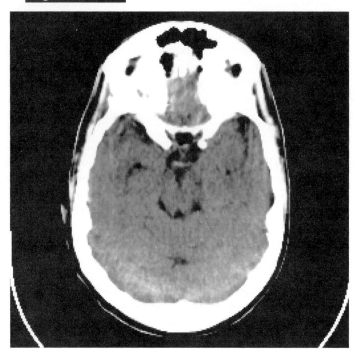

A CT scan is painless, takes relatively little time (less than half an hour), and can be performed on an unconscious individual. The person to be scanned typically lies flat on a bed that slides into the scanner's X-ray source and detector array. During the scan, this array rotates, delivering X-rays from all angles. A computer then combines and interprets these images, producing computed images in any of three planes. You have probably heard the term *CAT scan,* referring to computed axial tomography. The term *axial* refers to images being constructed in one plane, the **axial plane** (also referred to as the *horizontal plane* because they run in parallel with the horizon). Most early CT images were constructed in this plane, but now they are often constructed in two other planes as well (see Figure 3.3), which is why CT has become the more common term. Images in the **coronal plane** show slices perpendicular to the horizon, taken along the superior–inferior axis. Images in the **sagittal plane** are also perpendicular to the horizon, but they are taken along the dorsal–ventral axis.

CT scans are useful for both research and clinical applications. When used for clinical purposes, they help to identify anatomical abnormalities or acquired injuries,

Figure 3.3   **The Three Planes of Neuroimaging**

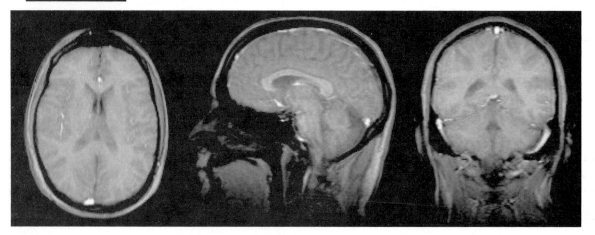

provided that these changes are reflected in changes in tissue density. This is not always the case; some brain tumors can have densities very similar to those of the surrounding tissues, making them difficult to detect on CT scans. However, the emergence of CT scanning technology suddenly enabled the diagnosis of a number of conditions that were previously identifiable only at autopsy. For example, multi-infarct dementia (described more thoroughly in Chapter 14) was rarely diagnosed before the advent of the CT scanner. This imaging method also had a profound impact on research. Correlating behavioral deficits with acquired brain injury no longer required postmortem examination, and more general brain atrophy could also be quantified in vivo.

Schematic of the Changing States of Hydrogen Atoms during Magnetic Resonance Imaging

Figure 3.4

Normal, random state

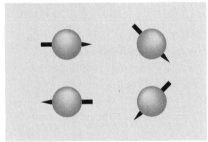

Polarized in a magnetic field

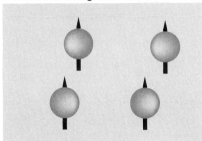

Radio frequency pulse is applied

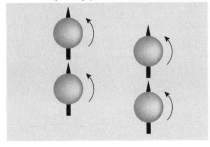

MAGNETIC RESONANCE IMAGING (MRI). Magnetic resonance imaging (MRI) is a technique based on the Nobel Prize–winning (Physics in 1952) research of Felix Bloch and Edward Purcell, who developed methods for nuclear magnetic precision measurement. Some twenty years later, their discoveries were applied to medical imaging. It was initially called "nuclear magnetic resonance imaging" (nMRI), but the term *nuclear* was dropped from the name because many people find references to radiation unsettling (Maier, 1995). Although people often confuse MRI scans with CT scans (presumably because they can produce a similar-looking product), the two methods image the brain in fundamentally different ways. MRI scanners are now widely regarded as a replacement for antiquated CT scanners because of their superior resolution, although CT scanners are still preferable in some situations.

As its name implies, MRI exploits the fact that many elements (such as hydrogen) can be influenced by magnetic fields. Hydrogen is an incredibly common element in the body, present in water, blood, tissue, bone—you name it. Think of these hydrogen atoms as little globes with north and south magnetic poles. Normally, these atoms are not polarized. In other words, the north pole on one hydrogen might point up, whereas the south pole on another hydrogen might point up (see Figure 3.4a). However, when placed in a strong magnetic field, the atoms become aligned—the north poles on all the atoms point in the same direction (see Figure 3.4b). Once they are aligned, the atoms can be perturbed in a uniform direction through the application of a radio frequency pulse (see Figure 3.4c). Different pulse frequencies are better at perturbing hydrogen atoms within different types of substances, depending on what you want to image (such as water or deoxygenated blood). What the MRI machine actually measures is the **relaxation time** that follows the pulse, which is the time taken by the atoms to return to their normal, random state. The MRI's **receiver coil** measures the information about the intensity of the signal, but the spatial information is provided from variations in the **gradient field** over the imaged area. The combination of these two types of information allows the construction of 3-D images of the brain (Perani & Cappa, 1999).

Unlike CT scans, these images are not measures of brain density (electron density, to be exact). Instead, they are usually representations of hydrogen density. However, there are two other properties of the tissues that can influence the MRI signal. The relaxation time can reflect the return to a random state along the longitudinal axis (called T1 relaxation time, or spin-lattice relaxation) or along the horizontal plane (called T2 relaxation time, or spin-spin relaxation). Different substances relax at different rates along these dimensions. Therefore, images of T1 relaxation look different from images of T2 relaxation and provide different information. On T1 images of the brain, bone, air, and water appear to be dark. On T2 images, air and bone still appear dark, but fluid appears to be quite bright (see Figure 3.5 for T1 and T2 MRI images of a tumor). The type of relaxation that one chooses to image depends on what one is looking for. Some conditions (such as Alzheimer's disease) are more easily detected on T1 images; other conditions (such as Parkinson's disease and arteriosclerosis) are more clearly visible on T2 images (Ketonen, 1998; Perani & Cappa, 1999; Vymazal et al., 1999).

MRIs contain extremely strong magnets, and their magnetic strength can be measured in units of **Tesla (T)**. The earth's magnetic field is roughly 0.00005 T, whereas an everyday refrigerator magnet is some 100 times stronger: 0.005 T. Most MRIs that are done for clinical purposes are another 300 times stronger, ranging from 0.5 T to

| **Figure 3.5** | **Contrast between T2 and T1 MRI Imaging** |

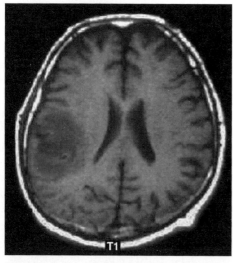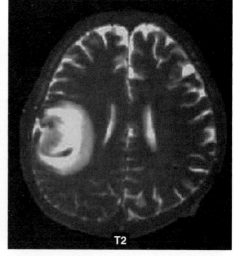

Note that fluid is bright and bone is dark for T2 images, but that the opposite is true for T1 images.

Source: Image courtesy of Leonard J. Tyminski.

1.5 T, whereas MRIs used for research purposes on humans can create strengths of 3.0 T to 8.0 T (Novak et al., 2001). (As an aside: In 2000, the engineers of Berkeley Lab's Superconducting Magnet Group set the world record for the strongest dipole electromagnet ever built. Their electromagnet attained a field strength of 14.7 Tesla— over 300,000 times the strength of the earth's magnetic field.)

Unlike CT scanning, which exposes an individual to X-ray radiation, MRI scans are generally considered to be almost completely noninvasive. However, this does not mean that they are 100% safe. Placing people in such strong magnetic fields can be very dangerous if they have pieces of metal in their body that can be attracted to a magnet. For example, if an individual with a metallic, magnetic aneurysm clip on a blood vessel in his or her head underwent an MRI, this could dislodge the clip. Heart pacemakers are also incompatible with MRI scanners. Surgical pins that are used to help set bones can also be problematic, but most metallic dental work (such as a filling) is magnetically inert. You might be surprised to learn that tattoos can also be problematic in an MRI. Some tattoo inks contain metal salts (which are attracted by the magnet). In an MRI, this can produce a burning sensation. Another potential hazard for individuals with tattoos who undergo MRIs is the fact that small metal shards can come off the needle during the tattooing process, becoming lodged in the skin of the recipient. These shards can then be attracted (and possible excised) by the magnetic force. Did your mother warn you against getting that tattoo? She might have been right.

The MRI's very strong magnetic fields can also be dangerous if magnetic objects are brought into the scanning area. For example, with a 3.0 Tesla MRI, a 10-pound hammer would get sucked into the magnet, striking the machine as hard as if it had the force of a half-ton object. The first photograph in Figure 3.6 illustrates what can

Examples of What Can Go Wrong When Metal Objects Are Used Too Close to the Strong Magnetic Fields Generated by MRI Scanners

Figure 3.6

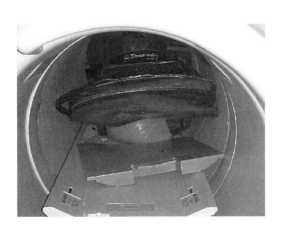
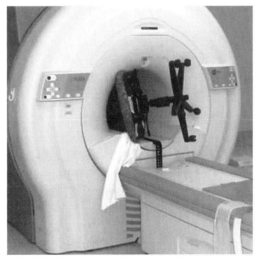

Source: Images courtesy of Moriel NessAiver, www.simplyphysics.com.

Self-Test

1. What is the howling radio analogy, and how is it relevant to interpretation of the effects of brain damage?

2. What property of X-rays makes them useful for both medical imaging and radiation therapy?

3. How can 3-D images be generated when only 2-D information is available?

4. What are the three planes of neuroimaging?

5. In what way is MRI imaging less invasive than CT scanning, and in what way is it actually more dangerous?

happen if one attempts to clean an MRI scanning room floor with a conventional metal floor polisher. The custodian who normally cleaned the MRI suite was away, and his replacement chose not to use a wooden mop. As you might suspect (but he did not), his metal floor cleaner was promptly pulled from his grasp. You can perhaps imagine a scenario that led to the situation in the second photograph.

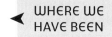

We have examined the ways in which neuropsychologists, neuroscientists, and cognitive neuroscientists image the structure of the living brain.

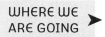

The following two sections describe methods of measuring the functioning brain. The first section details methods of measuring electrical potentials and magnetic fields that originate in the brain and are detectable on the scalp. The second section describes methods of measuring changes in blood flow in the brain.

Electrophysiological Methods

Electrophysiological methods of investigating brain–behavior relationships involve measuring the electrical and/or magnetic currents that are generated by brain activity. These methods are typically described separately from functional imaging methods (such as PET and fMRI, described in the next section), yet many argue (and rightfully so) that electrophysiology is also functional imaging. Traditional electrophysiological methods were focused less on localizing the source of the activity than on describing the nature of the activity (usually in terms of frequency, amplitude, and regularity). As you will see in the following sections, this focus is changing, blurring the line between electrophysiology and other functional imaging methods. However, the functional imaging methods that will be described are qualitatively different from the electrophysiological methods that are described in this section. Measuring changes caused by differences in blood flow is often considered a nuisance in electrophysiology, but it is the *goal* of a variety of other functional imaging methods (e.g., rCBF, SPECT). Furthermore, the weaknesses of most electrophysiological methods (such as poor spatial resolution) are the strengths of most other functional imaging methods, whereas their strengths (such as excellent temporal resolution) are weaknesses of the other methods.

ELECTROENCEPHALOGRAM (EEG). Electrophysiological measures of brain activity were recorded as early as 1875. Richard Caton, a British physician and physiology lecturer, recorded changes in electrical potentials from exposed brains of a number of animals.

His work had little impact at the time; it was repeated and republished by Adolph Beck of Poland some fifteen years later. Austrian psychiatrist Hans Berger became aware of Caton's work and attempted some similar experiments with nonhuman animals. After limited success, Berger decided to attempt to record the activity of human brains through the intact skull. In 1929, he published the results that he had obtained five years earlier using his son, Klaus, as his participant. Berger also tested a number of other people (including himself) and discovered regular waves (roughly ten cycles per second = 10 Hz), which he termed **alpha waves** because they were the first waves that he isolated. Berger was quite concerned that blood circulation might be creating harmonics in the recordings, but he also recorded blood pressure from the head to control for that possibility. Despite these careful measures, Berger's work was not well accepted at the time. This lack of acceptance might have been related to the scientific goal underlying Berger's recordings: He was searching for physiological evidence of telepathy (a person communicating with another through extrasensory means; Zillmer & Spiers, 2001). Berger did not receive a Nobel Prize (unlike the scientists who helped to develop X-ray, CT, and MRI technology), but he was considered for the award twice. After a series of personal and professional setbacks, he committed suicide in 1941.

Berger developed a technique that is now called *electroencephalography*. In practice, electroencephalography results in an **electroencephalogram** (EEG). To record an EEG, small metal disks are attached to the scalp (usually using a paste), and the small changes in electrical potentials are amplified and recorded (either on paper or in digital form). The locations of the electrodes are standardized and are generally organized in a symmetrical pattern, allowing the comparison of two analogous electrodes on opposite sides of the brain. One common standardized system for placing electrodes is called the 10-20 International Placement System. The "10" and "20" do not refer to the number of electrodes specified. Instead, they refer to the relative distances between the electrodes (10% or 20% of distances between landmarks on the skull), and these distances must be calculated on the basis of the head size of the person being tested. Even-numbered electrodes have right hemisphere placements (centrally placed electrodes are denoted with z's).

Berger's original system for describing the brain waves recorded during an EEG is still the best-known system. **Alpha waves** occur regularly at 8–13 Hz, and **beta waves** refer to activity faster than 13 Hz (some now describe $beta_1$ as 13–16 Hz, $beta_2$ as 16–20 Hz, and $beta_3$ as >20 Hz). **Theta waves** are relatively slow, at 4–8 Hz, and **delta waves** are the slowest at <4 Hz. In addition to describing these wave types, an EEG record might also include descriptions of synchronization or desynchronization between analogous sites (some degree of desynchronization is considered normal). Some EEG patterns are good indicators of convulsive disorders, such as epilepsy. One such pattern is spike and wave activity, wherein a short spike of high amplitude is immediately followed by a slow but high-amplitude wave (Rippon, 1999).

Older EEG output was not very flashy to look at. It usually consisted of a long printout of about twenty wiggly lines, one from each electrode (see Figure 3.7 for some examples). The output tended to be read in a qualitative manner, with the investigator looking for abnormal patterns of activity at one or more of the recording sites. Quantitative EEG methods are quite different: They rely on computers to analyze the

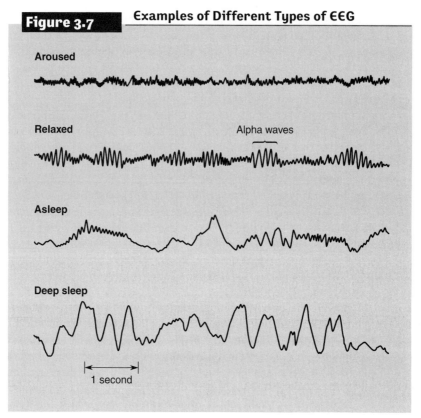

Figure 3.7   **Examples of Different Types of EEG**

Aroused

Relaxed   Alpha waves

Asleep

Deep sleep

|← 1 second →|

Source: John P. J. Pinel, *Biopsychology,* 5e. Published by Allyn and Bacon, Boston, MA. Copyright © 2003 by Pearson Education. Reprinted by permission of the publisher.

incoming data. Relatively recent developments in EEG have led to the spatial mapping of the source of electrical signals in EEG signal based on mathematical models. Advances in computer technology have largely driven this change. Improvements in the recording apparatus and refinements in the analyses of the data have led investigators to use increasing numbers of recording electrodes (up to 256). This has allowed much greater precision in localizing the source of neural activity in addition to describing its frequency and amplitude. However, even the latest and greatest EEGs can localize activity only within approximately 1 centimeter, and the accuracy of the localization decreases as the focus gets farther away from the scalp.

EVENT-RELATED POTENTIALS (ERPs). Recording event-related potentials (ERPs) (also called evoked potentials) is a procedure very similar to recording EEGs. The two methodologies use mostly the same equipment, and the measurement from the scalp is the same: small changes in electrical activity. The single biggest difference between recording EEGs and ERPs is that in an EEG, the person being recorded typically is not presented with any stimulation or cognitive task. The recordings are taken while the person is at rest, essentially measuring the "idling brain." If a person were to hear a loud noise during an EEG recording session, though, the perception of that noise would be reflected in the recording. However, because there is so much variability present in EEG recordings, these changes are often very difficult (or impossible) to observe—there is too much background noise in the recording.

ERP is an attempt to solve that problem. To study the brain's response to stimulation, a stimulus is presented repeatedly (sometimes hundreds of times) while an EEG is recorded. The resultant EEG does not look much different from one without a stimulus, but if one looks at the average difference that follows the stimulation, a characteristic, slow waveform usually emerges (see Figure 3.8). These waveforms are the "event-related" or "evoked" response, and they typically last for less than 1 second after the presentation of the stimulus. The various components of the waveform (changes that indicate increases or decreases in voltage) are then named according to their polarity (positive or negative) and time of onset. An N100 component refers to a negative change occurring 100 milliseconds after the stimulus presentation, whereas

Example of the Averaging of an Evoked Potential, Which Helps Increase the Signal-to-Noise Ratio, Producing Waveforms Characteristic of Particular Events

Figure 3.8

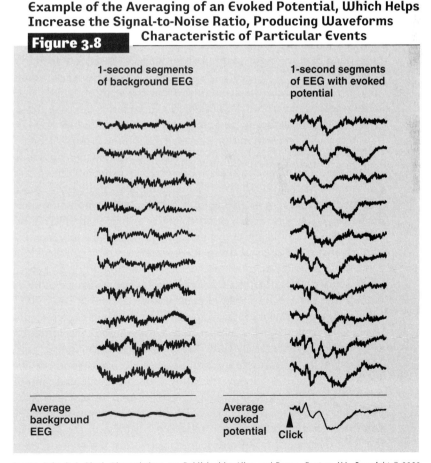

1-second segments of background EEG

1-second segments of EEG with evoked potential

Average background EEG

Average evoked potential

Click

Source: John P. J. Pinel, *Biopsychology,* 5e. Published by Allyn and Bacon, Boston, MA. Copyright © 2003 by Pearson Education. Reprinted by permission of the publisher.

a P300 component would be a positive change after 300 milliseconds (sometimes the two zeros are dropped, and the components are called N1 or P3).

These waveform components are often categorized into two types. **Exogenous components** are those associated with the physical characteristics of the stimulus. Therefore, altering the stimulus presented should alter the exogenous components of the waveform. **Endogenous components** are less dependent on the physical nature of the stimulus; instead, they appear to be determined largely by the cognitive task or context in which the stimuli are presented. As you might expect, these components are typically later in the waveform—after the initial sensation and perception of the stimulus. The distinction between endogenous and exogenous components of the waveforms is not always clear. Further, the source of the waveforms is often quite difficult to localize. The technique is good for studying relatively fast cognitive processes, such as attention and memory. It is also used to help diagnose conditions such as multiple sclerosis, Alzheimer's disease, and Korsakoff's disease.

MAGNETOENCEPHALOGRAPHY (MEG). Magnetoencephalography (MEG) is a very recent noninvasive technique for taking electrophysiological measures of the brain. However, unlike EEG and ERP, MEG does not measure the electric fields at the scalp. Instead, MEG measures the magnetic fields that are generated by the brain. According to the right-hand rule in physics, every current has an associated magnetic field that travels perpendicular to the current. These magnetic fields are very small, hard to measure, and normally difficult to distinguish from the small magnetic fields that are generated by nearby electronic devices (such as light bulbs or computers) or even the fields in the earth. For example, the magnetic field generated by the earth is more than a billion times stronger than those recorded from the brain's surface. To overcome this interference, MEGs are housed in rooms with thousands and thousands of pounds of shielding. The magnetic fields are detected by using a biomagnetometer, which contains many small coils. The brain's magnetic fields induce tiny currents in these coils, and these currents create magnetic fields in a **superconducting quantum interference device (SQUID)**. The SQUIDs work only at ridiculously low temperatures. They are kept at $-269°C$ by using liquid helium. As you might imagine, building and maintaining such a device are extremely expensive, even by medical imaging standards.

MEG's primary advantage over other functional imaging methods is its temporal resolution: It is able to detect changes over periods as short as 1 ms. The technique's speed is not due to the expensive computers that run it; it is the nature of the response being measured. As you will see in the next section, measures related to changes in cerebral blood flow have much less temporal resolution because the changes in blood flow are relatively slow. MEG measures the magnetic fields associated with the firing neurons in the brain, and because electricity (and the associated magnetic fields) can change so quickly, this allows for unprecedented temporal resolution.

The spatial resolution provided by MEG imaging can also be impressive, but unlike other methods (such as CT, MRI, PET), its resolution degrades significantly as you infer function from deeper and deeper centers in the brain. One the surface of the brain (between 1 and 3 centimeters), MEG can resolve to a few millimeters. However, deeper structures (e.g., subcortical structures) cannot be measured with nearly that accuracy; the resolution is roughly ten times worse. MEG's excellent temporal resolution and good spatial resolution for cortical structures toward the outer surface of the brain make it an excellent tool for studying primary sensory and motor cortical activity.

Functional Imaging

The functional imaging methods that are described in the next section infer brain activity without using measures of electrical currents or magnetic fields. For the most part, these methods are used to measure changes in local blood flow. The brain does not store any oxygen, and it stores very little glucose. Therefore, neural activity must be supported by local blood supply. As energy demands increase, so does blood flow. It would be ideal for researchers if there were a perfect relationship between energy metabolism and blood flow, but that is not the case. Supply tends to exceed demand. As energy requirements in a region of the brain rise, increases in local blood flow tend to exceed those requirements. Fortunately, this oversupply phenomenon makes measures of blood flow very sensitive to changes in metabolism, perhaps even more sensitive than more direct measures (Frith & Friston, 1996).

REGIONAL CEREBRAL BLOOD FLOW (rCBF). In the 1940s, researchers developed a technique to measure the overall **regional cerebral blood flow (rCBF)** (Kety & Schmidt, 1945). First, a participant must inhale a known quantity of nitrous oxide (N_2O), a metabolically inert substance that is freely diffusible. The substance would then circulate throughout the brain. After roughly 10 minutes, the scientists could then calculate the rCBF on the basis of the clearance of the substance. However, this technique had serious drawbacks. In addition to being invasive, it could provide only overall measures of the blood flow rather than a localized measure (Perani & Cappa, 1999; Zillmer & Spiers, 2001).

The technique was refined in 1961 when Lassen and Ingvar reasoned that the N_2O could be replaced with a isotopic tracer that could be measured externally, allowing inferences about changes in local concentration, not just overall blood flow (Lassen & Ingvar, 1961). By using a radioactive substance such as xenon 133 (^{133}Xe) instead of N_2O, the low levels of gamma radiation emitted by the substance over a period of 15 minutes could be measured with an array of detectors. Initially, researchers used relatively few detectors (eight), but adding more and more detectors to the array (up to 254) allowed for greater localization of the source of the radiation (Zillmer & Spiers, 2001). This technique could provide a crude measure of localized metabolism, but the invasive nature of the technique coupled with its poor spatial and temporal resolution limited its usefulness.

SINGLE PHOTON EMISSION TOMOGRAPHY (SPECT). Single photon emission tomography (SPECT) is similar to the ^{133}Xe method of measuring rCBF. However, it provides one major advantage. Similar to the difference between conventional X-rays and CT scans, SPECT involves the tomographic assessment of local changes in blood flow, allowing 3-D imaging. Inhaled ^{133}Xe can be used for SPECT imaging, but a variety of other commercially available gamma radiation–emitting tracers are usually used instead (Perani & Cappa, 1999). Most of these tracers are administered intravenously, and their half-life (time to reach a nonradioactive state) can be as long as 3 days. Just as in rCBF, an array of detectors is used to measure the local levels of gamma radiation. After the tracer is administered (inhaled or injected), local blood flow is inferred by measuring the single photons (or gamma rays) emitted from the brain.

SPECT has been used clinically to help identify regions with low metabolic activity following damage. For example, SPECT has been able to identify larger dysfunctional areas than were visible by using conventional CT scanning (Perani, Di Piero, Lucignani, et al., 1988). It has also been used to study the anatomical course of Alzheimer's disease (Perani, Di Piero, Vallar, et al., 1988). For example, Alzheimer's disease is characterized by a reduction in more posterior (temporal–parietal) metabolic activity (Perani & Cappa, 1995). SPECT has also proved to be useful for research, although the long half-life of the tracers that are used can be problematic. If one wishes to study a particular mental state (such as selective attention to written words such as the ones you are reading now), it is difficult to keep the participant in that state of mind for a very long time while the recordings are being made. After all, the changes in blood flow that are measured by these techniques are not just the changes that are induced by what the person is asked to think about—they are influenced by every thought the person has.

POSITRON EMISSION TOMOGRAPHY (PET). Positron emission tomography (PET) is a very flexible means for visualizing brain function. The other two functional neuroimaging methods that we have discussed in this section provide measures of local blood flow. PET scans are also capable of such measurements (with greater spatial and temporal resolution than the other two methods), but PET technology can also be used to study the brain's utilization of other substances, such as dopamine. PET imaging involves a series of steps. First, one must label a compound with a positron-emitting radionuclide. The substances that are most often labeled for psychology experiments are oxygen, water, and glucose. Second, the substance must be administered (injected or inhaled) to the person to be scanned. Third, the positrons emitted from the person's brain are scanned while the person is in the scanner, and tomography is used to construct a 3-D image of the activity. It sounds simple, doesn't it? Now, some more of the details.

The types of radioactive substances that are used in PET imaging are different from those used in SPECT in several ways. The tracers that are used in SPECT are commercially available and have relatively long half-lives (up to 3 days). The tracers that are used in PET have relatively short half-lives. The main radionuclides used in PET are carbon 11 (^{11}C), nitrogen 13 (^{13}N), and oxygen 15 (^{15}O); their half-lives are 20 minutes, 10 minutes, and 2 minutes respectively—orders of magnitude shorter than the half-lives of the substances used in rCBF or SPECT. This allows for greater temporal resolution in imaging changes in blood flow. However, this comes at a cost. Because the tracers do not last very long, they need to be manufactured on-site using a machine called a **cyclotron**. This is a particle accelerator that can generate the tracers. Cyclotrons are not cheap, which makes PET scanning much more expensive than SPECT. (The SPECT machine is sometimes called "the poor person's PET scanner.")

Example of an Annihilation Reaction That Gives Rise to the Photons Detected during Positron Emission Tomography

Figure 3.9

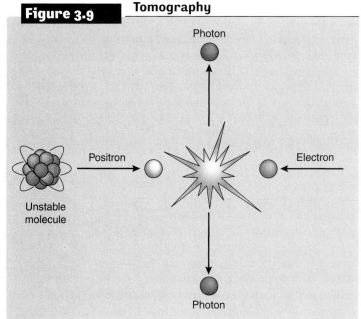

In addition to its greater temporal resolution, PET imaging is capable of better spatial resolution than SPECT. Part of its advantage is due to the physics (or chemistry, depending on your bias) of the reactions being measured. For an example, consider the most widely used tracer for PET imaging: $^{15}O_2$ (oxygen with one electron removed). $^{15}O_2$ is not a stable substance; sooner or later, it will release a positron to stabilize itself. Positrons are very rare, and they tend not to last very long; as soon as they come into contact with a free electron (which are common), they are annihilated. This process is fast; the average lifetime of a positron is a few hundred picoseconds (0.0000000003 second). There are two byproducts of the annihilation: two photons (also called *gamma rays*) that leave the scene of the collision in opposite directions at the speed of light 299,792,458 meters per second (see Figure 3.9). The photons are then detected by using a system of detectors, and, as is the case with SPECT imaging, computerized tomography is used to construct a 3-D representation of the functioning brain. However, unlike the single photons emitted and detected in SPECT imaging, each positron emission in PET results in the generation of two photons traveling in opposite directions, further enhancing the spatial resolution of the method.

PET imaging has a number of advantages over rCBF and SPECT. In addition to its better spatial and temporal resolution, it can be used to study a wider variety of substances. However, PET imaging has some major drawbacks. It is somewhat invasive, exposing participants to radiation. Because of this exposure, people should not get many (more than five) PET scans within a given year. Another drawback is that PET images of single participants tend not to be very reliable, perhaps in part owing to poor signal-to-noise ratios. Therefore, using PET for research purposes usually requires averaging responses across individuals. (This too can cause problems— remember the issue of single-case versus group studies.) This feature of PET scanning also makes it less useful for clinical purposes.

FUNCTIONAL MAGNETIC RESONANCE IMAGING (fMRI). The method for obtaining structural MRI images (imaging proton density) was described in the structural images section, but one important fact was omitted from the discussion: The structural images that are obtained in conventional MRI are not purely structural. Any modification in the brain's metabolic activity (such as performance of a visual task leading to increased blood flow to the occipital cortex) leads to changes in the distribution of hydrogen atoms (protons). The hydrogen atoms are virtually everywhere; they are located in membranes and cell bodies (both of which remain relatively still during normal brain activity) but also in water and blood (both of which move about quite a bit). The changes in proton density are small and short; in the early days of MRI imaging, they were not readily detectable. However, as MRIs became capable of faster image acquisition (using a technique called **echo-planar imaging, or EPI**), what was previously a relatively *structural* imaging method could now be used for *functional* imaging (Perani & Cappa, 1999; Stehling, Turner, & Mansfield, 1991). The EPI technique involves ultrafast alternating magnetic gradients, using only one spin excitation per image acquired. It requires special equipment that rarely used to be installed on MRIs used in clinical settings, but EPI-capable MRIs are becoming much more common now.

Functional magnetic resonance imaging (fMRI) uses much of the same equipment and methodology as does structural MRI. It also exploits the fact that many elements can be influenced by magnetic fields. After the participant's head is placed in a strong magnetic field, which polarizes the atoms, the atoms of interest are perturbed in a uniform direction through the application of a radio frequency pulse. The very first fMRI study measured changes in blood flow (the hemodynamic response) after participants were given intravenous injections of a paramagnetic contrast agent. The agent's concentration was detectable by using T2-sensitive EPI sequences. This allowed the investigators to track local changes in blood flow using MRI imaging. When the participants were exposed to visual stimulation, a localized increase in blood flow to the primary visual cortex was observed (Belliveau et al., 1991).

However, fMRI imaging is also possible without injecting any foreign agents. Hemoglobin is the substance that carries oxygen in blood. Oxygenated blood (containing oxyhemoglobin) and deoxygenated blood (containing deoxyhemoglobin) have different magnetic properties. By using fMRI, the relative ratios of oxyhemoglobin and deoxyhemoglobin can be compared. Recall that local increases in metabolic activity are accompanied by local increases in blood flow, and these increases generally exceed the demand of the tissues being supplied. Therefore, areas that exhibit increases in oxyhemoglobin are probably also exhibiting increases in metabolic activity (see Figure 3.10). This relationship may seem counterintuitive. One might expect that highly active areas would require a lot of oxygen and glucose, resulting in higher concentrations of deoxyhemoglobin. If this is what you would have predicted, you too are correct. There *is* a very brief period wherein active areas lead to local levels of oxygen depletion, but this period is so short and small in magnitude that the dominant hemodynamic response (and the one mostly measured in fMRI) is the local increase in oxygenation. The change in the relative concentration oxyhemoglobin to deoxyhemoglobin is often called the **blood oxygen level dependent (BOLD)** response.

fMRI has several advantages over SPECT or PET imaging. It can be performed on relatively common MRI equipment (available in the hospitals of most major urban centers in North America), it does not require exposure to radiation or the injection or inhalation of tracers, it typically costs less than PET imaging, and the

Diagram of the Oversupply of Oxygenated Blood That Gives Rise to the BOLD Signal Detected during Functional Magnetic Resonance Imaging

Figure 3.10

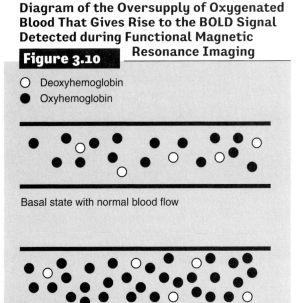

○ Deoxyhemoglobin
● Oxyhemoglobin

Basal state with normal blood flow

Activated state with increased blood flow

functional images can be superimposed over highly detailed anatomical images (allowing precise localization of the activity). Its temporal resolution is also far superior to those of SPECT or PET because the acquisitions can be as short as 100 milliseconds apart, allowing much more precise mapping of the time course of patterns of activation across a network of interconnected nuclei.

However, fMRI also inherits the disadvantages of MRI. Individuals are subjected to very strong magnetic fields, making it impossible to scan individuals who have pacemakers or other pieces of metal that are not magnetically inert. In fact, the magnetic field exposure in fMRI is even greater than that of MRI: In addition to agitation of the hydrogen atoms for the structural imaging, other molecules (such as deoxyhemoglobin) are also agitated. The procedure is presumed to be safe, but the long-term effects of exposure to such magnetic fields are unknown. The technology is simply too new for such effects to be detected.

◄ **WHERE WE HAVE BEEN**

We have examined the ways in which neuropsychologists, neuroscientists, and cognitive neuroscientists obtain structural and functional images of the brain for clinical and research purposes. The various methods differ in term of their spatial and temporal resolution, making some methods better suited for some situations. A summary of these methods is provided in Table 3.3 on the next page.

1. What advantage does CT scanning provide over conventional X-rays?

2. What is the difference between SPECT and PET?

3. What is the difference between EEG and ERP?

4. EEG and MEG are both electrophysiological measures, but they measure different phenomena. What do they measure?

5. What is the difference between MRI and fMRI? What do the two methods measure?

Self-Test

Table 3.3

Summary of Imaging Methods

Name	Type	Advantages	Disadvantages
X-ray	Structural	Cheap Fast	Little visualization of the brain No 3-D imaging
CT	Structural	In vivo measure of brain density Can scan metal objects Relatively noninvasive Relatively cheap	Poor spatial resolution Strictly structural image
MRI	Structural	Good spatial resolution Noninvasive	Cannot scan magnetic objects Expensive
EEG	Electrophysiological	Excellent temporal resolution	Poor spatial resolution
ERP	Electrophysiological	Excellent temporal resolution	Poor spatial resolution
MEG	Electrophysiological	Excellent temporal resolution Good spatial resolution for outermost structures	Expense Poor localization of noncortical structures
rCBF	Functional	Measures local changes in blood flow	Very poor spatial and temporal resolution
SPECT	Functional	Allows 3-D imaging of function	Very poor spatial and temporal resolution
PET	Functional	Many compounds can be imaged	Poor temporal resolution
fMRI	Functional	Good spatial resolution	Poor temporal resolution

Glossary

Alpha waves—Brain waves that occur regularly at 8–13 Hz.

Axial plane—Shows slices of the nervous system parallel to the horizon. Also referred to as the horizontal plane.

Beta waves—Brain waves that are faster than 13 Hz. $Beta_1$ as 13–16 Hz, $beta_2$ as 16–20 Hz, and $beta_3$ as >20 Hz.

Blood oxygen level dependent (BOLD) response—The change in the relative concentration of oxyhemoglobin to deoxyhemoglobin.

Computed tomography (CT)—A means of imaging live brain tissue that combines X-ray technology with computing. Involves the projection of X-rays from multiple angles followed by the computerized reconstruction of the measures into three-dimensional (3-D) images.

Confounding variables—These are unwanted variables that may affect the outcome of the study, leading a researcher to make false conclusions about the effects observed.

Control—This refers to the ability to manipulate something of interest to determine its effects. Control also includes the ability to exclude unwanted variables from the study. Control also refers to having an appropriate comparison sample, so that deviations from this sample can be observed.

Converging operations—The use of a number of studies that approach the question from a variety of perspectives, and the examination of the results to support a common conclusion.

Coronal plane—Shows slices of the nervous system perpendicular to the horizon, taken along the superior–inferior axis.

Cyclotron—A particle accelerator that can generate tracers.

Delayed nonmatching to sample task—After observing reward paired with stimulus A, then one is required to pick a novel stimulus to receive the reward.

Delta waves—Brain waves that are the slowest at <4 Hz.

Dependent variable—The response or behavior that the experimenter measures. These behaviors should be directly related to the manipulation of the independent variable.

Echo-planar imaging (EPI)—A technique that allows MRIs to became capable of faster image acquisition. EPI allowed what was previously a *structural* imaging method to be used for *functional* imaging. The EPI technique involves ultrafast alternating magnetic gradients, using only one spin excitation per image.

Empirical method—The word empirical literally means observation, and the method refers to the way scientists gather information, using standardized tests or measurements with a high level of objectivity.

Endogenous components—Those components of a brain wave that are less dependent on the physical nature of the stimulus. Instead, they appear to be determined largely by the cognitive task or context in which the stimuli are presented. These components are typically later in the waveform—after the initial sensation and perception of the stimulus.

Exogenous components—Those components of a brain wave associated with physical characteristics of the stimulus. Altering the stimulus presented should therefore alter the exogenous components of the waveform.

Functional magnetic resonance imaging (fMRI)—Allows for the relative ratios of oxyhemoglobin and deoxyhemoglobin to be compared.

Gradient field—Variations in this field provide spatial information in the construction of 3-D images of the brain area.

Hypothesis—The question that directs research. Formed as a statement that can be falsified.

Independent variable—The researcher manipulates this factor to determine how the behavior of interest is affected.

Magnetic resonance imaging (MRI)—A method for studying tissues using magnetic fields and radio receivers.

Magnetoencephalography (MEG)—A very recent non-invasive technique for taking electrophysiological measures of the brain. MEG measures the *magnetic fields* that are generated by the brain.

Neuroradiology—The study of the nervous system using imaging.

Positron emission tomography (PET)—A technique used to provide measures of local blood flow and study the brain's utilization of other substances, such as dopamine. This technique records the positrons emitted from the person's brain while they are in the scanner and uses tomography to construct a 3-D image of the activity.

Receiver coil—This unit measures the information about the intensity of the signal in the construction of 3-D images of the brain area.

Regional cerebral blood flow (rCBF)—Provides overall and localized measures of blood flow.

Relaxation time—The time interval that follows the pulse, which is the time taken by the atoms to return to their normal and random state.

Replication—A technique employed by researchers to ensure that initial observations did not occur by chance. Replication also ensures that effects in the study are generalizable to people beyond those who participated in the first study.

Sagittal plane—Show slices of the nervous system perpendicular to the horizon, taken along the dorsal–ventral axis.

Single photon emission tomography (SPECT)—A technique where local blood flow is inferred by measuring the "single-photons" (or *gamma rays*) emitted from the brain. This technique involves the *tomographic* assessment of local changes in blood flow, allowing 3-D imaging.

Superconducting quantum interference device (SQUID)—A device that allows for the creation of magnetic fields from currents. Work at ridiculously low temperatures—they are kept at –269°C using liquid helium.

Tesla (T)—A unit that measures magnetic strength.

Theta waves—Brain waves that are relatively slow at 4–8 Hz.

X-rays—Rays capable of penetrating solid materials, including wood, metal, and human tissue.

4

Laterality

Is the brain, which is notably double in structure, a double organ, 'seeming parted, but yet a union in partition'?
—H. MAUDSLEY

Most of us have two hands, two feet, two eyes. In fact, our bodies are fairly symmetrical—we have distinct right and left sides. This symmetry is mirrored in our brains. As you learned in Chapter 2, the brain has two hemispheres, and although they share many aspects, they are also distinct. Broca was the first to popularize the functional specialization of each hemisphere (although in Chapter 1, you learned that others observed this phenomenon first). In fact, if there is one take-home message from Chapter 1 it is that the observations of functional specialization of the brain led to the development of modern neuropsychology. To date, much of the research in neuropsychology has been done to deal with the topic of **laterality,** the functional specialization of the right and left hemispheres.

Early studies of the brain demonstrated that the left hemisphere (LH) is specialized for language and the control of the right hand and fingers. Although the functions of the right hemisphere (RH) were not readily understood, Hughlings-Jackson suggested that it played a role in visual identification of objects. As you will see, the RH is specialized for music, emotion, and spatial abilities as well as control of the left hand and fingers. Understanding the functions of the RH took longer, partly because the linguistic ability of the RH is rather poor, so the cognitive deficits resulting from RH damage tend to be subtle in comparison to the significant linguistic impairments that follow LH damage. In addition, the poor linguistic ability of the RH tends to make it difficult to obtain information regarding its function. For instance, try to think of a way to give a test that requires answers that cannot involve either spoken or written language. In developing your answer, remember that the RH controls the movements of the left hand and fingers and that most people are right handed. Therefore, tests that require drawing or sketching may also be rather difficult. If you have come up with a way to test the functions of the RH that requires little linguistic or right-hand motor skill, you have done well. Much of the first module in this chapter will examine tasks that were designed to test the functions of the two hemispheres separately.

It is important to remember that although much of this chapter will consider laterality of the two hemispheres separately, in reality, neurologically normal brain function relies on constant communication between the RH and the LH. Our experience is shaped by the complementary activity of the two hemispheres. Furthermore, as you will learn in this chapter, both hemispheres have some degree of competency for most functions. Language is a great example to illustrate these points. When you hear someone say the words "nice shoes," you instantly understand it as a compliment. However, when someone says the same words in a sarcastic tone, you no longer think that it was a compliment. What has just occurred? In most people, the LH interpreted the sound waves that made up the speech and interpreted it as the words "nice shoes." The RH interpreted the sound waves that composed the emotional tone of the speech (**prosody**) and allowed you to interpret the comment as either a compliment or an insult. The failure of the RH or the LH to communicate with one other becomes especially essential in ambiguous situations, when interpretation of stimuli is important to come to a correct conclusion.

WHERE WE ARE GOING ➤ The right (RH) and left (LH) hemispheres of the brain are specialized for distinctive functions. The first module of this chapter will examine the techniques that are used to explore the functions of each hemisphere. The second module will explain the neuroanatomical bases of laterality. The third module will discuss current theories as to why the brain is lateralized.

MODULE **4.1**
Methods

Split Brain

In the intact brain, the RH and LH communicate with each other using commissural systems. As you learned in Chapter 2, the commissures include the anterior and posterior commissures, the corpus callosum, the habenular commissure, and the hippocampal commissure. Much of what we know about the function of the commissures is based on work begun in the 1940s by Roger Sperry and Ronald Myers, who examined the effects of severing the corpus callosum in cats. Interestingly, the cats exhibited no obvious deficits following the surgery. However, they did not perform the same as cats with intact commissural systems when they were required to perform tasks of visual discrimination learning. In intact cats, a stimulus was presented a number of times to the left eye. When the cat saw the stimulus, it had to make a response to obtain a reward. When the eye that was stimulated was switched, no further learning was required. That is, the cat correctly reacted to the stimulus when the stimulus was presented to the right eye, despite having no experience with it. Commissurized cats by contrast, exhibited no transfer between the eyes. That is, when the left eye had been trained to a specific stimulus, the right eye no longer exhibited any recognition of the stimulus and had to be trained separately. Why was this so?

When the corpus callosum is severed, the information that is received from the right visual cortex can no longer be integrated with that of the right visual cortex. Recall from Chapter 2 that the corpus callosum is the largest in the commissural system and plays one of the largest roles in ensuring the transmission of information between the hemispheres. In essence, severing the corpus callosum results in a brain that is split into two separate halves that can no longer communicate with each other. Information received by one hemisphere can no longer influence the other hemisphere. In the example with the commissurized cats, the learning that had gone on in one hemisphere could no longer influence the activity of the other hemisphere.

However, sometimes the commissures transmit pathology. For instance, one form of epilepsy uses the commissural systems to involve both hemispheres in the production of severe seizure activity. The work of Sperry and Myers suggested that the severing of the commissures would improve the prognosis for individuals with this type of epilepsy. Although early studies did not find that commissurotomy resulted in fewer seizures, Phillip Vogel and Joseph Bogen, two neurosurgeons, suggested that not enough of the commissures had been cut and that the two hemispheres were still communicating. In the 1960s, they began to perform complete commissurotomies (cutting the corpus callosum and all of the other forebrain commissures) on individuals with intractable epilepsy. Vogel and Bogen observed that complete commissurotomy was a successful treatment and that the frequency and severity of seizures were reduced.

Individuals who have had a commissurotomy have two hemispheres that are intact but separate. That is, the motor, visual, auditory, and somatosensory abilities of

Figure 4.1   **An Example of a Chimeric Face**

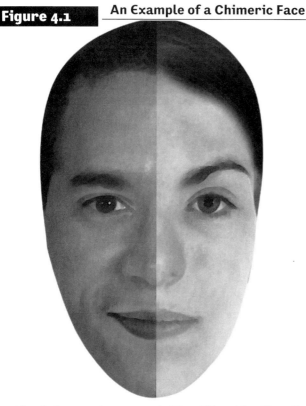

Often chimeric faces can be composed of two different hemifaces that are fused to make a novel face, although chimeric faces that are composed of one hemiface and its mirrored reflection are also used.

each hemisphere are intact. Sperry began to study Vogel and Bogen's patients as a means of understanding the cognitive abilities of the two hemispheres separately, without the confounding cross talk that occurs in neurologically intact brains. Sperry, along with Michael Gazzaniga, observed the surprising result that the RH was capable of comprehending spoken and written words. In fact, the result was so surprising that Vogel refused to put his name on the first sets of papers. Although the RH is largely unable to either speak or write, it is capable of arranging letters to spell three- or four-letter words (e.g., Gazzaniga, Bogen, & Sperry, 1965, 1967; Gazzaniga & Sperry, 1967).

Although the RH has some capability for language, it appears that the RH is specialized for other functions. For instance, Levy and colleagues (Levy, Trevarthen, & Sperry, 1972) observed that the RH played a special role in the recognition of faces. In this study, Levy used two different halves of faces that were combined to make one face (known as *chimeric* faces, as in Figure 4.1). After brief exposure to the chimeric faces, participants had to pick out which whole face they had observed. Because the visual input from the right eye is now separate from that from the left eye, the two hemispheres "saw" different faces. (Indeed, most of the participants did not appear to be aware that two faces were present!) Most of the time, the participants picked the face that had appeared in the left visual field (which sends information to the RH). Studies of individuals with split-brain commissurotomies continue to this day and provide important insights into the functions of the two hemispheres (e.g., Bogen, 2000; Gazzaniga, 2000; Walsh, 2000). In recognition of his ground-breaking work in understanding hemispheric functions, Roger Sperry received the Nobel Prize in Physiology or Medicine in 1981 (along with David Hubel and Torsten Wiesel, whom you will learn about in the next chapter).

Intracarotid Amobarbital Testing

Intracarotid amobarbital testing (IAT) is also known as the Wada test, reflecting the role of the neurosurgeon Juhn Wada, who pioneered its use in the late 1940s (Wada & Rasmussen, 1960). IAT is commonly used to assess the laterality of language in

Table 4.1				
Speech Lateralization and Its Relationship to Handedness				
		Cerebral Dominance for Language		
Handedness	**No. of Cases**	**Left (%)**	**Bilateral (%)**	**Right (%)**
Right	140	134 (96)	0 (0)	6 (4)
Left	122	86 (70)	18 (15)	18 (15)

Source: Adapted from Rasmussen and Milner (1977).

individuals who will be undergoing brain surgery. In this test, sodium amobarbital (a short-term anaesthetic) is injected into either the right or left internal carotid artery. The injection anaesthetizes the hemisphere ipsilateral to the injection; thus, an injection into the right carotid artery results in the right side of the brain "going to sleep." Typically, the individual receiving IAT has his or her contralateral arm in the air. When the injected hemisphere becomes anaesthetized, it no longer maintains motor control over the contralateral limb, and the arm drops. Once the hemisphere is anaesthetized, a neuropsychologist assesses the cognitive functions of the individual. Typically, the goal of IAT is to assess the language and memory capabilities of the two hemispheres independently of each other.

Anaesthesia tends to last for a period of minutes, during which the cognitive functions of the unanaesthetized hemisphere can be examined. Although there are many variations of the IAT, most attempt to measure expressive and receptive language ability, as well as long-term and short-term memory. Studies using IAT have revealed that most individuals exhibit LH dominance for speech, although some individuals exhibit either bilateral or RH dominance for language (see Table 4.1) (Rasmussen & Milner, 1977).

Interestingly, language functions of the brain may vary with hand dominance, RH language occurring more frequently in left-handers. Although about 4% of right-handers exhibited RH dominance for language, none exhibited bilateral representation of language (compared to approximately 15% of left-handers). Remember that bilateral representation of speech does not mean that language function is dispersed equally across the two hemispheres. Rather, these individuals exhibit some type of interference with different language functions (e.g., naming difficulties after IAT to the RH versus ordering difficulties after IAT to the LH). Most individuals, regardless of handedness, exhibit LH dominance for language. Finally, IAT is a very invasive procedure. Much of the research involving IAT as a means of understanding laterality relies on brains that have experienced significant pathology, which may exhibit significant differences from the neurologically intact brain.

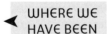

WHERE WE HAVE BEEN Techniques that are used either to assess or treat individuals with epilepsy have provided us with valuable insights into the independent capabilities of the two hemispheres of the brain. Split-brain surgery has provided us with an understanding of the linguistic abilities of the RH. In addition, IAT has been critical in demonstrating that there are individuals who exhibit RH dominance for language.

WHERE WE ARE GOING The two previous techniques for understanding laterality rely on individuals who have severe pathology, as no one would undergo split-brain surgery or IAT without having a good reason. The next two sections will investigate two common techniques that are used to understand laterality in neurologically intact individuals. Following that, the next two modules will explain the neuroanatomical bases of laterality and current theories as to why the brain is lateralized.

Before we can discuss techniques that are used to investigate laterality in neurologically intact individuals, we need first to review the sensory systems on which each task relies. Dichotic listening is a task that relies on the auditory system, whereas tachistoscopic presentations rely on the visual system. Inherent in both of these techniques is the assumption that the hemisphere that is specialized for a particular function will perform better than the other hemisphere.

VISUAL SYSTEM. The visual system (Figure 4.2) sends information from receptors located in the retina of both eyes to both hemispheres. However, this information is segregated with respect to where the item was viewed in space. For instance, visual information that is presented in the left side of space (or the left visual field, LVF) is transmitted to the primary visual cortex of the RH from the **nasal hemiretina** of the left eye (the half of the retina that is closest to the nose) and the **temporal hemiretina** of the right eye (the half of the retina that is closest to the temples). Conversely, visual information that is presented in the right side of space (or the right visual field, RVF) is transmitted to the primary visual cortex of the LH from the temporal hemiretina of the left eye and the nasal hemiretina of the right eye. Information that is perceived in the visual cortex of one hemisphere is communicated to the other hemisphere via the corpus callosum.

It is important to remember that the division of information between the hemiretinas occurs only in the periphery of the retina. For instance, the fovea (the center of the retina that is used for fine detail and color vision) automatically transmits information to both the right and left visual cortex. Thus, techniques that investigate the laterality of visual functions must take care to present stimuli peripherally and not to allow the fovea to observe the stimulus. Typically, this is achieved by having the participant stare at a point at the center of the screen

The Segregation of Information in the Visual System

Figure 4.2

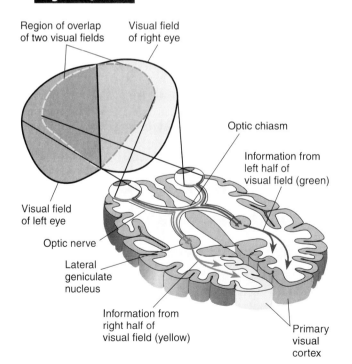

- Region of overlap of two visual fields
- Visual field of right eye
- Optic chiasm
- Information from left half of visual field (green)
- Visual field of left eye
- Optic nerve
- Lateral geniculate nucleus
- Information from right half of visual field (yellow)
- Primary visual cortex

Source: Neil R. Carlson, *Physiology of Behavior,* 8e. Published by Allyn and Bacon, Boston, MA. Copyright © 2004 by Pearson Education. Reprinted by permission of the publisher.

Segregation of Information in the Auditory System

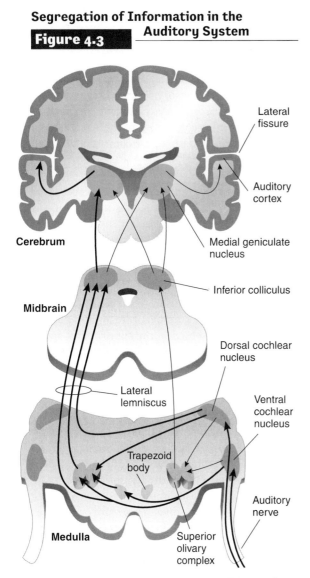

Figure 4.3

Lateral fissure

Auditory cortex

Cerebrum

Medial geniculate nucleus

Inferior colliculus

Midbrain

Dorsal cochlear nucleus

Lateral lemniscus

Ventral cochlear nucleus

Trapezoid body

Auditory nerve

Medulla

Superior olivary complex

Source: Neil R. Carlson, *Physiology of Behavior,* 8e. Published by Allyn and Bacon, Boston, MA. Copyright © 2004 by Pearson Education. Reprinted by permission of the publisher.

while keeping the stimulus away from the center of the visual fields (more than 1 degree from the center). Stimuli are also presented very briefly (less than 150 milliseconds). When stimuli are presented in such a fashion, your eyes have no chance to make movements from the center of the screen, thereby preventing the fovea from viewing the stimulus and sending the information to both hemispheres (McKeever, 1986).

AUDITORY SYSTEM. The auditory system (Figure 4.3) is not as segregated as the visual system, as all receptors in the cochlea send projections bilaterally. As such, auditory information that is received in one ear is sent to both hemispheres. However, projections to the ipsilateral hemisphere are weaker and less numerous and send information more slowly than projections to the contralateral hemisphere do (Kimura, 1967). Thus, although both hemispheres can attend to stimuli presented to either ear, situations in which information must compete result in the domination of contralateral projections. For instance, when competing stimuli are presented to the two ears simultaneously, the RH will preferentially attend to the input from the left ear, and the LH will preferentially attend to the input from the right ear (Kimura, 1967). As was the case with the visual system, information from either hemisphere is sent to the other via the commissural systems.

Dichotic Listening

Dichotic listening takes advantage of the suppression of the ipsilateral projections that takes place when stimuli compete with each other. Typically, dichotic listening tasks present different stimuli to each ear (Figure 4.4). These stimuli can be words, music, emotional tones, or even phonemes. Participants are then asked to either report what they heard or to listen for a target (e.g., the word *cat*) and to indicate whether the target was present or not. The number of correct responses is then tallied for each ear, and an asymmetry score is computed.

Dichotic listening tasks that use words or phonemes as stimuli tend to result in an asymmetry score that favors the right ear (e.g., Kimura, 1967). That is, participants tend to report more correct responses for stimuli that are presented to the right

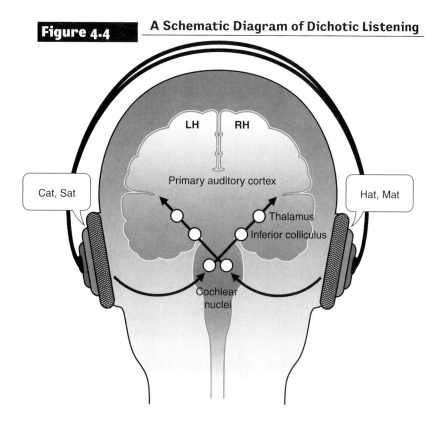

| Figure 4.4 | A Schematic Diagram of Dichotic Listening |

ear. This asymmetry presumably reflects the transmission of the stimulus from the right ear over the stronger, larger, and faster contralateral pathway to the LH. Most people exhibit LH language functions, and for them, the LH is better able to comprehend and report word or phoneme stimuli. However, some people with RH language functions exhibit asymmetries that favor the left ear.

It is interesting to note that dichotic listening studies tend to report that there are more people who have RH language functions than either IAT or split-brain studies do (approximately 20% of right-handers exhibit an asymmetry favoring the RH). Some critics suggest that the overrepresentation of RH language is an artifact of the testing conditions. That is, IAT is typically used to determine which hemisphere is responsible for the production of speech sounds, whereas dichotic listening typically requires the perception of speech sounds. In addition, we must remember that split-brain and IAT studies examine the laterality of individuals with pathology, and it may be that neurologically intact individuals exhibit greater variation in laterality. However, others suggest that most dichotic tasks are not pure measures of laterality and that overrepresentation of RH language reflects the impurities in the task. For instance, it has been demonstrated that when individuals are directed to attend to a specific ear, they can modify their asymmetry scores (e.g., Asbjornsen & Bryden, 1996).

Dichotic listening tasks that use music, environmental sounds (e.g., a dog barking), or emotional tones as stimuli tend to result in an asymmetry score that favors the left ear (for a review, see Springer, 1986). That is, participants tend to report more correct responses for stimuli presented to the left ear. This asymmetry presumably reflects the transmission of the stimulus from the left ear over the stronger, larger, and faster contralateral pathway to the RH. These results suggest that the RH is specialized for the processing of nonlinguistic sounds, such as music and prosody.

Tachistoscopic Presentations

Tachistoscopic presentations take advantage of the segregation in the visual system. Typically, tachistoscopic tasks involve the rapid presentation of stimuli to either the RVF or the LVF, using either a tachistoscope (a specialized piece of equipment that allows the rapid presentation of stimuli to either the RVF or LVF) or a computer screen. These stimuli can be words, letters, faces, or even spatial locations. Participants are then asked to report what they observed. The number of correct responses is then tallied for each visual field, and an asymmetry score is computed.

Tachistoscopic tasks that use words or letters as stimuli tend to result in an asymmetry score that favors the LH (for a review, see McKeever, 1986). That is, participants tend to report more correct responses for stimuli that are presented to the RVF. As was the case for dichotic listening, most people exhibit LH language functions, and for them, the LH is better able to comprehend and report visual stimuli that are words or linguistic in nature. However, as was the case for dichotic listening, some people exhibit asymmetries that favor the LVF, presumably reflecting RH language function.

Tachistoscopic tasks that require facial recognition, detection of emotional expression, or judgments about spatial location tend to result in an asymmetry score that favors the RH (for a review, see McKeever, 1986). That is, participants tend to report more correct responses for stimuli that are presented to the LVF. As was the case for dichotic listening, most people exhibit RH superiority for spatial information, including discrimination of spatial locations, identity of faces, and identity of emotional expressions. For them, the RH is better able to comprehend and report visual stimuli that are spatial in nature.

Self-Test

1. Circle the hemisphere that is most likely to demonstrate an advantage for the processing of the following stimuli in left-handed individuals:

   a. Tachistoscopic presentation of faces — RH   LH

   b. Dichotic words — RH   LH

   c. Dichotic melodies — RH   LH

   d. Tachistoscopically presented emotions — RH   LH

   e. Dichotic syllables — RH   LH

2. Circle the visual field that is most likely to demonstrate an advantage for the processing of the following stimuli in right-handed individuals:

   a. Faces — RVF   LVF

   b. Words — RVF   LVF

   c. Spatial location — RVF   LVF

   d. Emotional expression — RVF   LVF

3. Circle the ear that is most likely to demonstrate an advantage for the processing of the following stimuli in left-handed individuals:

   a. Melodies — Right   Left

   b. Words — Right   Left

   c. Environmental sounds — Right   Left

   d. Emotional expression — Right   Left

4. Why is there a discrepancy between the incidence of RH language reported for split-brain, IAT, and dichotic listening studies?

◄ **WHERE WE HAVE BEEN** As was the case for IAT and split-brain studies, the LH appears to be specialized for linguistic functions and the RH for prosody, facial recognition, spatial ability, and music. Although there is a tendency for left-handed individuals to exhibit atypical laterality, most left-handed individuals exhibit the same laterality as do right-handed individuals.

WHERE WE ARE GOING ► The next two modules will explain the neuroanatomical bases of laterality and current theories as to why the brain is lateralized.

MODULE 4.2
Neuroanatomical, Neurochemical, and Behavioral Findings

The human brain is physically and functionally asymmetric. At first glance, the two halves look roughly equivalent. However, given a closer look, even with the naked eye, some of the asymmetries between the two cerebral hemispheres are clearly noticeable. For example, the left frontal lobe extends farther forward than the right does, but the right occipital lobe extends farther back than the left does (Figure 4.5). As you will discover later in this module, some of the most influential research reports about neuroanatomical asymmetries were published in the 1960s and 1970s, but brain asymmetries were described as early as the second half of the nineteenth century. We have grouped the differences into two categories: general anatomical trends between the hemispheres and asymmetries in specific structures within the hemispheres.

Asymmetry of the Brain, Demonstrating the Rightward Torque

Figure 4.5

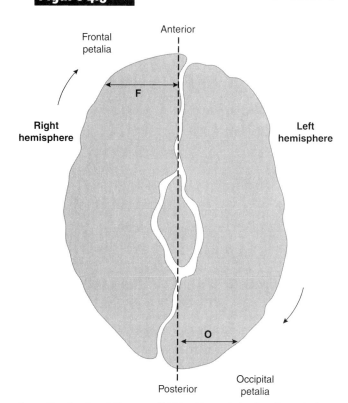

Source: Based on Toga & Thompson (2003), with permission from *Nature Reviews Neuroscience, 4,* 37–48, Macmillan Magazines Limited, and the author.

Neuroanatomical Asymmetries

GENERAL ANATOMICAL TRENDS

1. *Rate of maturation:* According to Hughlings-Jackson, French scientist Louis Pierre Gratiolet (1797–1851) was the first to observe that the gyri and sulci develop earlier in the LH (Kolb & Whishaw, 1996). Anatomical and functional asymmetries can be modified after birth (although there is little flexibility after puberty), but

Table 4.2

Postmortem Differences in Weight between the Hemispheres

Source	N	LH	RH	Right–Left Difference
Broca (1875)	19	530.84 g	531.31 g	0.47 g
Henderson (1986)	18	574.39 g	575.83 g	1.44 g
Crichton-Browne (1880)	18 males	616.1 g	618.2 g	2.1 g
	18 females	556.7 g	558.0 g	1.3 g
Brauen (1891)	100	549.7 g	551.2 g	1.5 g
Weighted averages		557.8 g	559.3 g	1.4 g

Source: Based on Miller (1996).

asymmetries are clearly visible before birth. As you will see in the following sections, many of the asymmetries within the hemispheres are also present at or before birth.

2. *Size of complete hemispheres:* Gratiolet was also the first to report that, overall, the RH is both larger and heavier than the left (Finger, 1994). This does not mean that every part within the RH is larger than its analogue on the left, but given the sum of all of the anatomical asymmetries between the hemispheres, the right has greater volume and mass (see Tables 4.2 and 4.3).

3. *Ratio of gray to white matter:* The relative distribution of gray matter (composed mostly of cell bodies) versus white matter (composed mostly of myelinated axons) is also different across the hemispheres. The gray matter/white matter ratio is usually higher in the LH (Gur et al., 1980). In other words, the LH contains more gray matter relative to white matter than does the right.

Table 4.3

Mean Hemispheric Volume ± Standard Deviation

Source	Sample	LH	RH	Z
Kelsoe et al. (1988)	14	392 ± 89.8 cm^3	402 ± 89.8 cm^3	0.045
Weis et al. (1989)	29	534.4 ± 50.6 cm^3	538.2 ± 49.2 cm^3	0.076
Gur et al. (1991)	23 male	575.46 ± 47.74 cm^3	580.69 ± 47.03 cm^3	0.055
	20 female	529.28 ± 57.89 cm^3	532.76 ± 59.42 cm^3	0.059
Kertesz et al. (1990)	50 male	88.59 ± 7.05	90.39 ± 6.46	0.266
	53 female	81.02 ± 7.16	82.90 ± 6.92	0.267
Heckers et al. (1991)	23	531.1 ± 79.8 cm^3	546.6 ± 75.0 cm^3	0.200
Salerno et al. (1992)	17	544 ± 61 cm^3	545 ± 58 cm^3	0.017
	18	548 ± 117 cm^3	551 ± 112 cm^3	0.026
Murphy et al. (1993)	19	36.9 ± 0.89	37.2 ± 0.89	0.337
Weighted average				0.167

Source: Based on Miller (1996).

4. *Density of neural tissue:* In part because of the differences in gray matter/white matter ratios, the LH also exhibits greater cell packing density than does the right (Miller, 1996).

Therefore, generally speaking, the LH matures earlier, it contains more gray matter relative to white matter, and it exhibits higher cell packing density than does the RH. However, the RH is generally larger and heavier.

ASYMMETRIES IN SPECIFIC STRUCTURES WITHIN THE HEMISPHERES. Perhaps the most easily identified asymmetry in neuroanatomical landmarks is the fact that the sylvian fissure usually extends farther (horizontally) toward the occipital lobe in the LH, whereas it ascends at a greater angle in the RH (Galaburda, 1995; Hochberg & Le-May, 1975). There is some evidence to suggest that this asymmetry emerged relatively early in hominid evolution: 60,000-year-old Neanderthal fossils appear to demonstrate the same asymmetry, as do some 3.5-million-year-old australopithecine fossils (Holloway, 1980, 1981; Holloway & De La Coste-Lareymondie, 1982; LeMay, 1976).

A related asymmetry has possibly received the most experimental attention over the past forty years. The region of the temporal lobe that lies under the posterior tip of the sylvian fissure is called the **planum temporale** (see Figure 4.6). In 1968, Norman Geschwind and Walter Levitsky published a paper in the journal *Science* in which they reported their investigation of 100 autopsied human brains (Geschwind & Levitsky, 1968). They found that 65% of the brains studied had a significantly longer planum temporale in the LH. In some cases, it was ten times larger. Only 11% of the sample exhibited a longer planum temporale in the RH, whereas 24% did not exhibit a significant asymmetry. This result was replicated by a number of investigators (Campain & Minckler, 1976; Wada, Clarke, & Hamm, 1975; Witelson & Pallie, 1973) and was extended by Tezner and colleagues, who also studied the brains of newborns, finding the same asymmetry (Tezner, Tzavaras, Gruner, & Hecaen, 1972). A similar (and

Figure 4.6   **The Planum Temporale and Heschl's Gyrus**

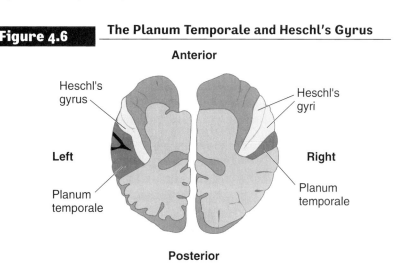

Source: John P. J. Pinel, *Biopsychology,* 5e. Published by Allyn and Bacon, Boston, MA. Copyright © 2003 by Pearson Education. Reprinted by permission of the publisher.

Table 4.4

Neuroanatomical Asymmetries That Typically Favor the LH

Asymmetries That Favor the LH	Reference
Longer Sylvian fissure	LeMay (1976)
Planum temporale	Geschwind & Levitsky (1968)
Wider occipital lobe	Galaburda, LeMay, Kemper, & Geschwind (1978)
Occipital lobe extends farther to the back	LeMay (1977)
Inferior parietal lobule	LeMay & Culebras (1972)
Globus pallidus	Kooistra & Heilman (1988)
Mesial temporal lobe	Good, Johnsrude, Ashburner, Henson, Friston, & Frackowiak (2001)
Anterior cingulate sulcus	Good et al. (2001)
Area 44 (of frontal operculum)	Galaburda (1980)
Pars opercularis	Stengel (1930)
Lateral posterior nucleus of the thalamus	Eidelberg & Galaburda (1982)
Medial cerebellum	Good et al. (2001)

related) asymmetry favors the RH. In the LH, there is usually a single Heschl's gyrus. However, in the RH, there are usually two. Some of the other neuroanatomical asymmetries are summarized in Tables 4.4 and 4.5.

Some of these neuroanatomical asymmetries are clearly visible with the naked eye. For example, the collective effect of having a left occipital lobe extending farther back and a right frontal lobe extending farther forward (see Figure 4.5) gives the brain the appearance of counterclockwise torque (Bradshaw & Nettleton, 1983). However, some of the asymmetries are less obvious, and discovering them has required more rigorous investigation. Many of the anatomical asymmetries described above exist for areas related to language processing (such as the planum temporale or area 44). Given the well-established functional asymmetries for language processing, these physical asymmetries are not particularly surprising. However, it is also possible that these asymmetries are so well documented because these are the areas on which investigators have focused.

Table 4.5

Neuroanatomical Asymmetries That Typically Favor the RH

Asymmetries That Favor the RH	Reference
Two Heschl's gyri instead of one	von Economo & Horn (1930)
Wider frontal lobe	LeMay (1977)
Frontal lobe extends farther forward	Galaburda et al. (1978)
Medial geniculate nucleus of the thalamus	Eidelberg & Galaburda (1982)
Calcarine sulcus	Good et al. (2001)
Anterior cingulate	Good et al. (2001)
Anterior insular cortex	Watkins et al. (2001)
Lateral cerebellum	Good et al. (2001)

CONNECTIONS BETWEEN THE TWO HALVES OF THE BRAIN. There are a number of structures that link the two halves of the brain. As we discussed in Chapter 2, the largest of the commissures is the corpus callosum. It is a large white matter structure consisting of approximately 200 million fibers connecting cortical centers in similar locations between the two hemispheres (e.g., connecting areas along the superior temporal gyrus of the LH to the same area in the RH). Recall from Chapter 2 that the corpus callosum has both **homotopic** and **heterotopic** connections between the hemispheres. Anatomically, there are four main regions of the corpus callosum. The most posterior area is called the **splenium.** Anterior to the splenium lies the **body of the corpus callosum,** and the bend at the anterior tip of the corpus callosum is called the **genu** (meaning "knee"). The portion of the corpus callosum inferior to the body at the end of the bend of the genu is called the **rostrum.** The two halves of the brain are also connected through the **massa intermedia,** which connects the two thalami. There is also a structure that links the two hippocampi, called the **hippocampal commissure.** There are also two structures that connect cortical areas between the two hemispheres: the **anterior commissure** and the **posterior commissure** (Figure 4.7).

Figure 4.7 — Commissural Systems

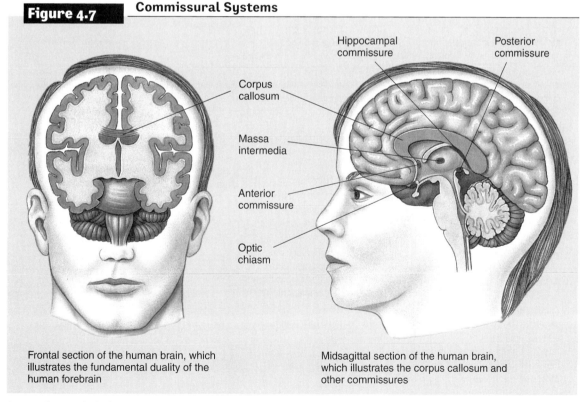

Frontal section of the human brain, which illustrates the fundamental duality of the human forebrain

Midsagittal section of the human brain, which illustrates the corpus callosum and other commissures

Source: John P. J. Pinel, *Biopsychology,* 5e. Published by Allyn and Bacon, Boston, MA. Copyright © 2003 by Pearson Education. Reprinted by permission of the publisher.

Neurochemical Asymmetries

In comparison to the investigation of neuroanatomical asymmetries, relatively little is known about asymmetries in neurochemistry. Interpreting the results of most of the research in this area is complicated by a number of factors. First of all, most of the work has been conducted on nonhuman animals, so how well these results generalize to humans is unknown. Furthermore, when neurochemical asymmetries exist, they often apply only to a particular region of the brain rather than to the entire hemisphere. Tables 4.6 and 4.7 summarize some of the major neurochemical asymmetries.

Table 4.6

Neurochemical Asymmetries That Favor the LH

Classification, Name, Location, and Function of Neurotransmitter	Asymmetry	Type of Participant or Subject	Reference
Small-molecule neurotransmitter/ acetylcholine	Temporal cortex contains higher levels of choline acetyltransferase (ChAT)	Humans	Sorbi, Amaducci, Albanese, & Gainotti (1980)
Located in all motor neurons in the brain and spinal cord.	Greater activity of ChAT	Humans	Amaducci, Sorbi, Albanese, & Gainotti (1981)
Acetylcholine interacts with dopamine pathways in the motor readiness system (McGuinness & Pribram, 1980).	Greater activity of ChAT in first temporal gyrus and cortical layers II and IV of Brodmann's area 22	Humans	Amaducci et al. (1981)
Small-molecule neurotransmitter/ monoamine, catecholamine, dopamine (DA)	More dopamine terminals in left basal ganglia (in humans, as shown through PET scanning)	Humans	Wagner et al. (1983)
Located in areas of the brain involved with movement and reward.	More DA in left globus pallidus	Humans	Glick, Ross, & Hough (1982)
	Schizophrenia is marked by abnormally high DA functioning (Meltzer, 1979). Schizophrenics demonstrate higher left hemisphere activation.	Humans	Mintz, Tomer, & Myslobodsky (1982)
	Pharmacologic stimulation of DA pathways produces asymmetric turning in circles. Group data reveal a general right turning preference, indicating left lateralization of DA.	Rats	Denenberg (1981)
Small-molecule monoamine, catecholamine, norepinephrine (NE)	More NE in left striatum	Rats	Rosen et al. (1984)
Involved in brain systems that regulate movement, mood, motivation, and attention. Many adrenergic neurons originate in the locus coeruleus.			

Table 4.7

Neurochemical Asymmetries That Favor the RH

Classification, Name, Location, and Function of Neurotransmitter	Asymmetry	Type of Participant or Subject	Reference
Small-molecule neurotransmitter/ monoamine, indoleamine, serotonin (5-HT)	More 5-HT in right accumbens	Rats	Rosen et al. (1984)
	Greater 5-HT in right amygdala relates to greater anxiety	Rats	Andersen & Teicher (1999)
Involved in brain systems that regulate eating, sleep, and emotional behavior	Higher 5-HIAA in mediofrontal region	Humans	Arato, Freckska, MacCrimmon, Guscott, Saxena, Tekes, & Tothfalusi (1991)
5-HT interacts with NE to control arousal (McGuiness & Pribram, 1980)	Administration of lithium, which is thought to stabilize serotonergic mechanisms (Treiser, Cascio, O'Donohue, Thoa, Jacobowitz, & Kellar, 1981) produces more profound EEG changes in RH	Humans	Flor-Henry & Koles (1981)
Small-molecule neurotransmitter, monoamine, catecholamine, norepinephrine (NE)	Pulvinar region of thalamus rich in NE	Humans	Oke, Keller, Mefford, & Adams (1978)
Involved in brain systems that regulate movement, mood, motivation, and attention.	Concentration of NE greater in areas of right thalamus that are responsible for somatosensory functions (namely, the ventrobasal complex)	Humans	Oke et al. (1978)
Many adrenergic neurons originate in the locus coeruleus.	LTP rats demonstrate greater uptake of NE in right hippocampus	Rats	Valdes et al. (1981)
	Higher NE levels in right thalamus, particularly in somatosensory nuclei	Humans	Oke et al. (1978)

Functional Asymmetries

Functional cerebral asymmetries have traditionally been reported for "higher" functions, such as the processing of language, space, or emotion. Some have claimed that functional asymmetries emerge only at higher levels of information processing (Moscovitch, 1979). Luria (1973) claimed that the more abstract a function is, the more asymmetric is its cerebral basis. However, as you will see in the following paragraphs, processing differences between the hemispheres have been identified for much "lower" perceptual tasks.

VERBAL/NONVERBAL. Perhaps the first functional (and still the most famous) dichotomy between the hemispheres was proposed by a country doctor in France named

Marc Dax, who published his father's claim that aphasia was associated with left hemispheric lesions after Broca's similar claims were made public. It is not doubted that LH is superior at linguistic processing. However, claiming that all tasks that are dominated by the LH are attributable to its verbal processing is a gross oversimplification. Similarly, claiming that the RH functions in a predominantly nonverbal manner is also not true. As you discovered in the previous module, the RH is very much involved in verbal communication. It is not primarily responsible for initiating speech or selecting meaningful words, but it does dominate the manner in which the words are spoken (prosody). As you will discover in the following sections, the manner in which the LH dominates the processing of stimuli is not strictly dependent on whether or not they are linguistic. Under the correct conditions (depending on the context, size, or speed of presentation), the LH will also dominate the processing of nonlinguistic stimuli.

LOCAL/GLOBAL PROCESSING. In 1977, David Navon of the University of Haifa developed a new task for studying how people process the hierarchical structure of stimuli. Navon created stimuli wherein the local elements of the stimulus do not always correspond with the global elements. Consider the example in Figure 4.8. The larger

Neuropsychological Celebrity

E.C.

E.C. was a 47-year-old man who started experiencing attacks of speechlessness and right-sided motor problems in November 1964. In March 1965, E.C. had a tumor close to his primary sensory and motor areas removed from his LH. This relieved some of his symptoms, but he still exhibited some language disturbances following the surgery. Unfortunately, his tumor came back. In December of that year, E.C.'s physicians decided that extreme measures were necessary. To ensure that the potentially fatal tumor would not come back yet again, they elected to remove the entire LH of E.C.'s brain. E.C. survived this radical procedure and exhibited some predictable symptoms following the surgery. For example, he was unable to move or feel tactile sensations from the right side of his body. He also had major language disturbances, including severe expressive (Broca's) aphasia. However, if the RH cannot normally initiate any speech, E.C. should not have exhibited apha-

sia at all—he should have been completely unable to speak. Although he had obvious difficulty speaking, he could produce words and short phrases such as "yes," "no," or "don't know." These words and phrases were almost always used appropriately, and they were voiced with the appropriate prosody. Sometimes, E.C. would utter longer (and usually emotionally expressive phrases) such as "Oh my God!" or "God damn it, yes" (Smith & Burtelund, 1966).

Therefore, E.C. provides clear evidence that the RH *can* produce meaningful speech—or does he? Despite these observations, it might be tempting to conclude that the RH cannot normally initiate speech. After all, E.C. was not neurologically normal before his surgery. The fact that his RH could initiate speech could be the result of his pathology and not indicative of normal cerebral lateralization. Although this is certainly a possibility, the fact that E.C.'s LH tumor produced aphasia before his first surgery suggests that he initially had left hemispherically dominated speech. Therefore, the speech functions that were later subserved by his (sole) RH are more convincing evidence that the RH can subserve at least some speech production.

**A Sample Stimulus Showing Both Global
and Local Features**

Figure 4.8

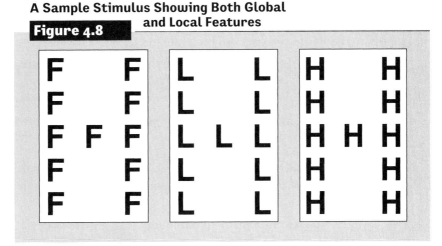

Source: Adapted from Navon (1977).

letter H can be composed of the smaller letters F, L, or H. In the two conditions using Fs or Ls, the local elements (the smaller letters) do not correspond with the global element (the large letter H). However, in the third condition, the two types of elements match. At first, Navon used these types of stimuli to discover that people tend to process the global elements of a visual scene before analyzing the local elements. When his research participants were instructed to identify the local elements, they exhibited much longer reaction times than when they made comparable judgments about the global elements. Further, when the two types of information conflicted, this slowed people's ability to correctly perceive the local elements (the global information provided interference). This effect was not present when participants were instructed to identify the global elements (the local information did not provide interference). Before completing the experiment, Navon had assumed that a single system was responsible for processing both the local and global elements. However, his results suggested that two different processing systems could be involved (Navon, 1977).

Subsequent studies of people who have suffered lateralized brain damage support the possibility that local processing and global processing are accomplished by anatomically and functionally distinct systems. Figure 4.9 summarizes the performance of two brain-damaged (out of twenty-five) individuals studied by Delis and colleagues (Delis, Robertson, & Efron, 1986). When a patient with LH damage was presented with incongruent global and local stimuli (not necessarily verbal stimuli), the LH damage impaired their ability to process the local elements, but their reproduction of the global elements was relatively intact. Conversely, RH damage impaired processing of the global elements, but the ability to reproduce local elements was spared. Navon's original paper on the hierarchical processing of stimuli using these types of figure was entitled "Forest before Trees. . . ." To use the same analogy in interpreting Delis and colleagues' results, the LH is specialized for processing the trees, whereas the right processes the forest.

Performance of Two Patients on a Figure-Copying Task with Both Global and Local Elements

Figure 4.9

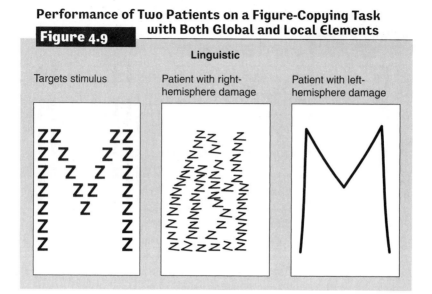

Linguistic

Targets stimulus | Patient with right-hemisphere damage | Patient with left-hemisphere damage

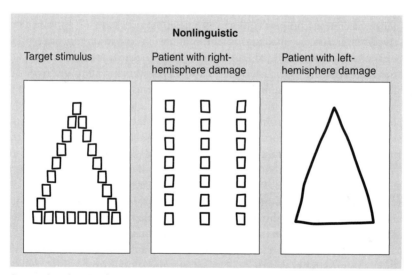

Nonlinguistic

Target stimulus | Patient with right-hemisphere damage | Patient with left-hemisphere damage

One patient has RH damage and the other has LH damage.

Source: Reprinted from *Neuropsychologia, 24,* D. C. Delis, L. C. Robertson, & R. Efron, "Hemispheric specialization of memory for visual hierarchical stimuli, pp. 205–214. Copyright 1996, with permission from Elsevier.

HIGH SPATIAL FREQUENCY/LOW SPATIAL FREQUENCY. The global/local processing advantages that are exhibited by the two hemispheres can also be explained by a different theory. The **spatial frequency hypothesis** of hemispheric specialization claims that the two hemispheres differ in their ability to process the basic sensory attributes of various stimuli. Before describing the theory, we must explain the concept of spatial frequency. Look at the alternating black and white stripes in Figure 4.10. There are two gratings, and the spatial frequency of each grating is a function of the number of light–dark changes that happen over a given amount of space. In this example, the gratings are the same size. Therefore, the grating with more light–dark changes (Figure 4.10a) exhibits higher spatial frequency, whereas the grating with fewer light–dark changes (Figure 4.10b) exhibits lower spatial frequency. Therefore, when you are examining an object such as a tree, the general contour of the tree (or its silhouette) is defined according to changes in luminance that are low in spatial frequency, whereas the more specific features of the tree (such as the individual leaves) are defined by changes that are relatively high in spatial frequency. For a crude demonstration of what the world looks like when your visual system has access only to visual information that is low in spatial frequency, try squinting as you look at this page. You should still be able to perceive the general outlines of the objects, but the fine details (defined by changes that are high in spatial frequency) are lost (Banich, 1997).

Justine Sergent (1983) argued that the LH is more sensitive to high spatial frequencies, whereas the RH is more sensitive to low spatial frequencies. However, this is not to claim that the two hemispheres differ in their ability to detect this information at a basic sensory level. Instead, Sergent argued that the hemispheric asymmetries emerge at a later stage of cognitive processing. This opinion was supported by subsequent experimental work (Kitterle, Christman, & Hellige, 1990). Sergent's theory can explain a number of experimental findings in addition to her own. Reconsider the global/local differences between the hemispheres that were discovered by using stimuli similar to Navon's. If a large letter H is composed of small letter Ls, are the local elements of the stimulus high or low in spatial frequency? How about the global aspect of the stimulus? Global elements are defined according to low spatial frequencies (preferentially processed by the RH), whereas local elements are defined according to high spatial frequencies. The spatial frequency hypothesis does not compete directly with the global/local hypothesis. Instead, it explains the effect at an even lower level of processing. Since Sergent first proposed it, the spatial frequency hypothesis has been tested extensively. Most experimental work has provided additional support for her hypothesis, but there certainly are exceptions. Although a detailed discussion of this issue is beyond the scope of this chapter, it should be noted that some of the findings are probably due to the possibility that hemispheric differences in the processing of spatial frequency are more related to the *relative* spatial frequency of

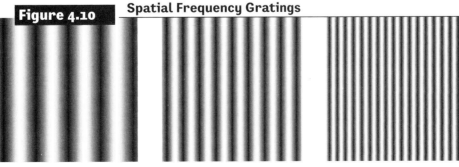

Figure 4.10   **Spatial Frequency Gratings**

Low spatial frequency   Medium spatial frequency   High spatial frequency

objects in a visual scene than their *absolute* spatial frequency (Ivry & Lebby, 1993; Kitterle, Hellige, & Christman, 1992).

HIGH TEMPORAL FREQUENCY/LOW TEMPORAL FREQUENCY. The preceding section characterized processing differences between the hemispheres in terms of their relative ability to process objects on the basis of their spatial frequency. Similarly, the two hemispheres can be characterized in terms of their ability to process stimuli presented rapidly. The experimental work is still relatively recent, but a consensus is building that the LH is better at processing rapid events, regardless of the modality of presentation. In the visual modality, there is a LH/RVF advantage for a wide variety of tasks requiring the processing of rapidly presented (but not necessarily linguistic) stimuli. For example, when a light flashes quickly enough, it no longer appears to be flashing (such as the screen in a movie theater). However, your ability to detect rapid flashes is not equal in the two visual fields. The critical rate at which the flicker of a light appears to fuse into the percept of a continuous light (i.e., when the light no longer appears to flicker) is higher for the LH (Goldman, Lodge, Hammer, Semmes, & Mishkin, 1968). Another task that illustrates the LH's superiority at detecting rapid visual events is the inspection time paradigm described in Figure 4.11 (Elias, Bulman-Fleming, & McManus, 1999; Nicholls & Atkinson, 1993; Nicholls & Cooper, 1991). The LH's superiority at detecting rapid changes in stimuli is also apparent in the auditory modality. There is a right ear advantage for the perception of temporal order (Mills & Rollman, 1980), perceiving differences in duration (Mills & Rollman, 1979), and detecting gaps of silence in short bursts of noise (Brown & Nicholls, 1997; Vroon, Timmers, & Tempelaars, 1977). There is even some evidence that the LH is more capable of processing rapidly presented tactile information (Bakker & Van der Kleij, 1978; Guylee, Elias, Bulman-Fleming, & Dixon, 2000; Hammond, 1981; Nicholls, 1996).

Although a consensus is building that such low-level asymmetries exist across modalities, relatively little is known about their implications. A common but largely untested interpretation is one in which the LH is generally superior at processing all temporally rapid stimuli, predisposing it to dominate tasks that require great temporal precision, such as linguistic tasks and skilled unimanual behavior (Calvin, 1983;

Figure 4.11   **Sample of an Inspection Time Paradigm**

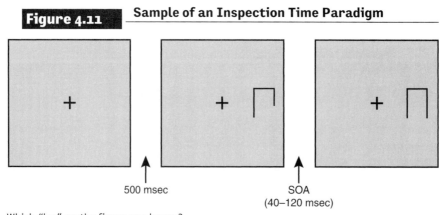

500 msec   SOA
(40–120 msec)

Which "leg" on the figure was longer?

Self-Test

1. List three anatomical asymmetries that favor the LH and three that favor the RH.

2. How is dopamine distributed asymmetrically in the normal human brain?

3. Which structures connect the two halves of the brain?

4. What is the spatial frequency hypothesis? How does it differ from the proposed global/local dichotomy?

5. Which hemisphere is better at processing rapid events? How could this advantage be related to functional asymmetries for higher functions?

Mills & Rollman, 1979; Tallal, Miller, & Fitch, 1993). If this position is correct, with use of a within-subjects experimental design, the hemisphere that is superior at perceiving rapid temporal events should be the same hemisphere superior at linguistic tasks and skilled unimanual behaviors. There is some evidence to support this position but also some evidence against it (Elias, Bulman-Fleming, & McManus, 2000; Elias, Bryden, & Bulman-Fleming, 1998; Guylee et al., 2000).

◀ **WHERE WE HAVE BEEN**

The previous section described some of the dichotomies that have been used to characterize the functional asymmetries between the hemispheres. The verbal/nonverbal dichotomy fails to describe many of the verbal functions that are subserved by the RH and nonverbal tasks that are dominated by the left. The global/local dichotomy helps to account for functional differences between the hemispheres in the visual modality, but it does not generalize well beyond this. The spatial frequency hypothesis is compatible with the global/local dichotomy, but it generalizes better to nonlinguistic visual tasks such as facial recognition. The position that the hemispheres differ in their ability to perform temporal processing has been supported by most of the experimental evidence, but the implications of this difference have yet to be fully explored.

WHERE WE ARE GOING ▶

Whereas the previous sections focused on describing the types of tasks that demonstrate functional asymmetries, the following sections detail some hypotheses about why these asymmetries developed in the first place. The explanations come from a number of perspectives, including positions that laterality is caused by the environment, genetics, asymmetries, or other events during prenatal development, as well as accounts of why hemispheric specialization might be adaptive. Although all these theories might appear to be competing with one another, many of them are not mutually exclusive. It is entirely possible that more than one of these accounts is an accurate description of why hemispheric specialization exists.

MODULE **4.3**
Why Is There Hemispheric Specialization?

What causes hemispheric asymmetry? Scientists have been studying hemispheric specialization for well over a hundred years. Although a great deal has been learned about anatomical and functional asymmetries across species, we know very little about the possible causes of such deviations from symmetry. There are many theories, most of which focus on the development of handedness. Some assume that laterality is learned and that an exclusively environmental explanation can account for the phenomenon; others take a more biological perspective. The following sections will critically review the theories that have been popular over the last century. If you are interested, Harris (1980) provides an excellent review of earlier theories.

Environmental/Psychosocial Theories

JACKSON'S PARENTAL PRESSURE THEORY. Some scientists have claimed that handedness is determined entirely by the environment of a child. For example, Jackson (1905) proposed that most humans are right-handed because their parents were right-handed and that any given child can be right-handed, left-handed, or even ambidextrous given the appropriate environment. Because of this flexibility, Jackson (1905) claimed, all children should be taught to use either hand interchangeably.

BLAU'S PSYCHODYNAMIC THEORY. Within a psychoanalytic framework, Abram Blau (1946) also argued that a child's handedness was the result of his or her environmental circumstances. Left-handedness was claimed to be the result of emotional negativism, having no biological basis whatsoever.

PROBLEMS WITH ENVIRONMENTAL/PSYCHOSOCIAL THEORIES. Following are some problems with Jackson and Blau's theories:

1. Handedness runs in biological families, regardless of the handedness of those who parent the child. Adoption studies have shown that a child's handedness is more closely related to that of the biological parents than to that of the adoptive parents (Carter-Saltzman, 1980; Hicks & Kinsbourne, 1976).
2. Left-handedness has persisted across the centuries (see Coren & Porac, 1977). If handedness is determined by environmental influences, why would it persist against sometimes violent opposition for so many years?
3. Siblings in a given family (even identical twins) do not always exhibit uniform handedness, despite very similar, if not identical, environmental circumstances (see McManus, 1980).
4. The newborn fetus exhibits structural asymmetries in the brain's hemispheres long before any parental or other environmental influence could have taken place (see Previc, 1991).

Genetic Theories

There is little doubt that handedness runs in families, but the extent to which this effect is due to environmental pressure (parents purposefully or accidentally teaching their children to be right- or left-handed) is unclear. According to a recent meta-analysis by McManus and Bryden (1992), two right-handed parents have a 9.5% chance of having a left-handed child. The chances rise to 19.5% if one parent if left-handed (and this effect appears to be driven primarily by left-handed mothers), and 26.1% of the children from two left-handed parents are also left-handed. Taken alone, these statistics do not necessitate a genetic conclusion, for the effect could be driven entirely by parental pressure. However, genetic arguments become much more convincing when one notes that even adoption studies suggest that handedness is under genetic control. The handedness of adopted children is more likely to follow that of their biological parents than of their adopted parents (Carter-Saltzman, 1980; Hicks & Kinsbourne, 1976).

Most early genetic theories proposed that handedness is a recessive trait, following the laws of Mendelian genetics (Chamberlain, 1928; Falek, 1959; Hudson, 1975; Jordan, 1911, 1922; Newman, 1931; Ramaley, 1913; Rife, 1940; Schott, 1931; Trankell, 1955; see Hardyck & Petrinovich, 1977, for a review). However, the pattern of inheritance followed by left-handedness appears to be far too complex for this type of genetic model. Specifically, the proportion of left-handed children born of one or two left-handed parents is too low to support such a simple model. As a result, more recent genetic theories such as that of Annett (1972), McManus (1985), and Klar (1996) have postulated an element of chance within the genetic model. Unfortunately, all of these models have some problems:

1. It is very difficult to evaluate (and therefore falsify) genetic theories of lateralization. With the exception of adoption studies, it is very difficult to separate environmental effects from genetic effects. Even in adoption studies, the environments of North America and Europe are very similar.
2. Different theorists define handedness according to different criteria. For example, Annett (1972) defines handedness in terms of relative hand skill (how well one can perform a task), whereas McManus (1985) defines it in terms of hand preference (which hand one prefers to use).
3. Genes code for the production of proteins, not behaviors. Although genes could be the mechanism of lateralization, genes do not provide information regarding why lateralization provides an adaptive advantage.

Anatomical Theories

The anatomical asymmetries that the brain exhibits pale in comparison to those that are found in other internal organs. The leftward displacement of the heart is arguably the most dramatic asymmetry, but even paired organs such as the lungs, kidneys, ovaries, and testes exhibit obvious and reliable lateralization (Bisazza, Rogers, & Vallortigara, 1998; Bogaert, 1997; Gerendai & Halasz, 1997; McCarthy & Brown, 1998). Some early investigators claimed that these asymmetries are causally related to cerebral asymmetries.

THOMAS CARLYLE'S SWORD AND SHIELD THEORY. The sword and shield theory was first put forward by Sir Thomas Carlyle. Carlyle claimed that handedness had its origins in early warfare, when combatants who held their sword in their right hand and shield in their left (and therefore better protected their heart) were more likely to survive in battle. The greater mortality of the left-handers in battle, then, was proposed as the mechanism driving the higher prevalence of right-handedness today.

Although the theory is appealing in its simplicity, the theory is also fraught with problems, including the following:

1. Right-handedness was the norm far before the Bronze Age, as suggested by the hunting style of Australopithecus (Dart, 1949), stone implements constructed by

Peking Man (Black, Young, Pei, & de Chardin, 1933), paintings of hands by Cro-Magnon (Magoun, 1966), examination of North American aboriginal art (Brinton, 1896), the hand used for skilled activities depicted in paintings in the tombs of Beni Hasan and Thebes between 2500 B.C. and 1500 B.C. (Dennis, 1958), and large-scale studies of ancient artworks (Coren & Porac, 1977). In all of these studies, the estimated distribution of hand preference is similar to the prevalence that we observe today.

2. The theory predicts that men would be more likely to be right-handed than women (because, after all, men were usually the ones fighting with swords). The data indicate the opposite: Males are more likely than females to be left-handed by a ratio of 5:4 (Gilbert & Wysocki, 1992).

3. Those very rare cases of **situs inversus,** in which asymmetries, including those of the heart and other organs, are reversed from left to right, do not exhibit left-handedness more frequently than expected (Cockayne, 1938; Torgerson, 1950; Wilson, 1872). For example, in a sample of 160 people with situs inversas, Torgerson (1950) found that only 6.9% were left-handed.

SALK'S PARENT HOLDING BABY THEORY.   Another cardiac theory claims that population-level right-handedness is a result of how we hold babies (Salk, 1966). More specifically, the theory claims that infants are more easily comforted when they are cradled in the parent's left arm, keeping the head of the baby closest to the parent's heart, because the sound of a heartbeat is known to soothe infants (Salk, 1973). Furthermore, holding the baby with the left arm leaves the parent's right hand free to perform more complex tasks. Because the adult's right hand would benefit from more practice in manipulating objects, right-handedness could have become the norm.

Although this theory correctly predicts the greater prevalence of right-handedness among females (who have traditionally performed more of the child-rearing duties) and the tendency for both left- and right-handed people to cradle babies using the left arm, it also has some serious flaws, including the following:

1. It is assumed that a left-sided carrying arrangement would have more influence on the handedness of the parent than it would on that of the child. Because carrying an infant with one's left hand leaves the infant's left hand free, this leftward carrying arrangement should have much greater influence on the handedness exhibited by the child than that exhibited by the parent.

2. The direction of this influence should favor left-handedness, not right-handedness.

Developmental Theories

Developmental theories of cerebral lateralization have an advantage over environmental, anatomical, and genetic theories in that they often incorporate influences from all of these factors. These theories also help to account for the fact that infants are lateralized (structurally at least, if not functionally) at birth.

GESCHWIND AND GALABURDA'S TRIADIC THEORY.   The Geschwind-Galaburda theory (G-G theory) has been extraordinarily popular, despite its flaws. In its most simplified form, the theory claims that elevated levels of testosterone are responsible for deviations from the "normal dominance pattern" (i.e., right-handed with left-hemispheric linguistic dominance) (Geschwind & Galaburda, 1987). The wide appeal of the theory is attributable both to the charismatic manner in which Geschwind popularized the theory and to its ability to account for a vast number of previously unrelated and inexplicable correlations.

These correlations include a number of reliable sex differences in the literature, such as a higher prevalence of left-handedness in males (Gilbert & Wysocki, 1992; Oldfield, 1971), higher prevalence of immune disorders in males, higher prevalence of language disorders in males (Taylor, 1974), the well-established cognitive sex differences such as male superiority in visuospatial and mathematical tasks and female superiority in linguistic tasks (Benbow & Stanley, 1980; Mann, Sasanuma, Sakuma, & Masaki, 1990), the different maturational rates of the sexes (females tend to mature faster than males) (Taylor, 1969), and the numerous neuroanatomical sex differences in the literature (Bishop & Wahlsten, 1997). The G-G theory also attempts to explain the relationship between behavioral laterality and developmental disorders, many of which are summarized in Table 4.8.

The G-G theory focuses on the role that the hormone testosterone has on tissue growth. Testosterone can affect the growth of many tissues, including an inhibitory effect on the growth of immune structures such as the thymus gland. Testosterone can affect the structure of specific nuclei in the hypothalamus and limbic system. Testosterone also has major effects on the development of other neural tissue, in part because sex hormone receptors are widely dispersed in the brain (Gorski, Harlan, Jacobson, Shryne, & Southam, 1980). According to the G-G theory, if effective testosterone levels are higher than normal during pregnancy owing to genetic factors, increased sensitivity to testosterone, the presence of a male co-twin, or an anomalous endocrine environment during pregnancy, this increase in testosterone levels is responsible for a myriad of consequences. These consequences include masculinization, early puberty, general growth retardation, a smaller left hemisphere, postpubertal thymus suppression, abnormal neural crest development, and atypical metabolism.

Table 4.8	
Associations between Indirect Measures of Stressors and Elevated Prevalence of Left-Handedness	

Condition or Group	References
Babies with low birth weight	O'Callaghan et al. (1993); Powls et al. (1996); Ross et al. (1992); Ross et al. (1987); Saigal et al. (1992); Segal (1989)
Babies with low APGAR scores	Schwartz (1988); but cf. Olsen (1995)
Offspring of smoking mothers	Bakan (1991); but cf. Olsen (1995)
Perinatal birth stress	Bakan et al. (1973); but cf. Ehrlichman et al. (1982); van Strien, Bouma, & Bakker (1987)
Premature birth	Ross et al. (1992); Ross et al. (1987)

More central to the theory is testosterone's ability to produce a condition termed *anomalous dominance* through its delay of LH growth. Anomalous dominance can be characterized by left-handedness, RH language dominance, and LH visuospatial dominance or reduced degree of handedness, language dominance, or visuospatial dominance. By slowing the growth of the LH, testosterone somehow results in a disruption of the normal cortical architecture of the LH. Furthermore, because of the LH growth delay, the G-G theory proposes that the RH compensates for this growth delay, with corresponding regions of the RH developing more quickly. This compensatory growth is the mechanism proposed by Geschwind and Galaburda (1987) to account for the overrepresentation of left-handed people in "right-hemispheric" vocations. This effect is also presumed to be responsible for left-handers' relative superiority at mathematics, visual arts, athletics, and music.

The G-G theory also accounts for the correlation between handedness and immune disorders. Because elevated testosterone levels are said to be responsible for both immune disorders and anomalous dominance, this relationship is responsible for the correlation between the two.

Some problems with the G-G theory include the following:

1. The theory does not explain why testosterone slows only the growth of the LH (and not the RH as well) in the neonate.
2. Some direct tests of the model have failed to support the G-G theory. For example, a study by Grimshaw, Bryden, and Finegan (1995) measured prenatal testosterone levels (in amniotic fluid) and compared these levels to the behavioral indicators of lateralization (e.g., handedness and language lateralization) in the same children ten to fifteen years later. The results were exactly the opposite of what would be predicted by the G-G theory: Children with high levels of prenatal testosterone were *more* likely to be right-handed and to have LH language lateralization.
3. Many of the correlational studies on which the theory has been based have not been successfully replicated, such as those that associate left-handedness with a number of diseases.

THE PATHOLOGICAL LEFT-HANDEDNESS THEORY. According to Peters (1995), there are three variants of the pathological left-handedness (PLH) theory. The first and most extreme variant is that proposed by Bakan and colleagues (Bakan, Dibb, & Reed, 1973), who claimed that right-handedness is the norm and that left-handedness is always the result of some sort of brain injury. A second and less extreme variant is that proposed by Satz and his colleagues (see also Dellatolas et al., 1993; Satz, 1972; Satz, Orsini, Saslow, & Henry, 1985), who maintain that sometimes left-handedness is normal and sometimes it is pathological. A third and even less extreme variant is the position that left-handedness itself might not be pathological but serves as a marker for other pathologies (Coren & Halpern, 1991; Geschwind & Behan, 1982; Geschwind & Galaburda, 1985c; Kinsbourne, 1988; Manoach, 1994).

Supporting the position that left-handedness might be caused by birth stress, there is a higher prevalence of left-handedness among groups of infants who appear (as assessed by indirect measures) to have been exposed to stressors (see Table 4.8).

Current

Controversy

Do Left-Handers Die Sooner Than Right-Handers?

One of the most popular and controversial issues in the handedness literature is the question of whether left-handers die sooner than right-handers. This might seem like an easy hypothesis to test experimentally, but the intricacies in interpreting the results of some recent studies might surprise you. The results of cross-sectional studies are very clear: If you sample a large group of people of a variety of ages, such as the more than 1 million people sampled by Gilbert and Wysocki (1992), you will find that the proportion of left-handers is much higher among younger people than it is among older people.

Does this mean that the prevalence of left-handedness has been suddenly increasing over the past fifty years after remaining relatively stable over the past fifty centuries? A more sensible conclusion might be that the left-handers simply are not living as long as the right-handers, which is referred to as the elimination hypothesis. However, the fact that there are fewer left-handers among older people does not necessarily imply that the left-handers are dying earlier. Instead, this trend could simply indicate the lessening of social pressure against left-handedness. It is quite possible that more people born in the 1930s and 1940s would have become left-handed if there had not been cultural pressure against it.

However, the story does not end there. Some longitudinal studies (in which the same individuals are tracked across a period of time) have also indicated decreased longevity among left-handers. Longitudinal research of this type is very difficult. It requires an accurate and complete record of both handedness and mortality statistics for large groups of people. These records are rare, but they do exist. In a very clever series of studies, Diane Halpern and Stanley Coren studied the longevity of left-handed and right-handed pitchers in major-league baseball (Coren & Halpern, 1991, 1993; Halpern & Coren, 1988). Just as was indicated in the cross-sectional studies, it appeared that the left-handed baseball pitchers were not living as long as their right-handed cohorts. A similar result has been observed in cricket players (Aggleton, Kentridge, & Neave, 1993). However, a number of other studies have failed to find similar effect (Hicks, Johnson, Cuevas, Deharo, & Bautista, 1994; Persson & Allebeck, 1994; Wolf & Cobb, 1991), and still others have criticized the methodology used in these studies (Harris, 1993; Hugdahl, Satz, Mitrushina, & Miller, 1993).

In addition to claiming that left-handers die sooner, Coren (1989) has proposed a mechanism for the decreased longevity. He claims that left-handers are more prone to accident-related injuries. These claims of increased accident rates among left-handers (referred to as the *clumsy hypothesis*) have also garnered mixed support. Some studies find relatively elevated accident rates among left-handers (Aggleton, Bland, Kentridge, & Neave, 1994; Coren, 1989; Graham & Cleveland, 1995; Graham, Dick, Rickert, & Glenn, 1993; MacNiven, 1994; Taras, Behrman, & Degnan, 1995; Wright, Williams, Currie, & Beattie, 1996), whereas others do not (Merckelbach, Muris, & Kop, 1994; Peters & Perry, 1991). Others have even suggested that it is not left-handers who exhibit elevated accident rates, but those with mixed handedness (Hicks, Pass, Freeman, Bautista, & Johnson, 1993). In any event, the jury is still out on Coren's elimination hypothesis and its corollary, the clumsy hypothesis. Coren has successfully replicated his own findings, but some other investigators have not.

Supporting the second and third variants of the theory (that left-handedness might be pathological or serve as a marker for other pathologies), there is a higher prevalence of left-handedness among people with a number of pathological conditions (see Table 4.9 on pages 128–129).

There are some serious problems with all three variants of the PLH model, including the following:

1. The birthing process (and the amount of money and technology available to support it) varies tremendously among cultures, but the prevalence of left-handedness

Table 4.9

Associations between Elevated Prevalence of Left-Handedness and Pathological Conditions or Circumstances That Could Lead to Pathology

Condition or Group	References
Albinism	Murdoch & Reef (1986)
Alcoholics	Bakan et al. (1973); Biro & Novotny (1991); London (1987); London (1989); London, Kibbee, & Holt (1985); McNamara, Blum, O'Quin, & Schachter (1994); Nasrallah, Keelor, & McCalley Whitters (1983)
Allergies	Coren (1994); Geschwind & Behan (1982); Geschwind & Behan (1984); but cf. Gilger, Pennington, Green, Smith, & Smith (1992); Pennington, Smith, Kimberling, Green, & Haith (1987); Smith (1987); Steenhuis, Bryden, & Schroeder (1993); but cf. van Strien et al. (1987); Bulman-Fleming, Bryden, & Wyse (1996)
Autism	Boucher (1977); Colby & Parkison (1977); Geschwind (1983); Gillberg (1983); Laxer, Rey, & Ritvo (1988); Leboyer, Osherson, Nosten, & Roubertoux (1988); Lewin, Kohen, & Mathew (1993); Pipe (1988); Soper et al. (1986); Tsai (1982); but cf. Barry & James (1978); Boucher, Lewis, & Collis (1990)
Autoimmune thyroid disease	Wood & Cooper (1992)
Breast cancer	Kramer, Albrecht, & Miller (1985); London (1989); London & Albrecht (1991)
Children with hydrocephalus	Lonton (1976)
Cerebral palsy	Galliford, James, & Woods (1964); Keats (1965)
Coronary artery disease	Lane et al. (1994)
Criminality	Ellis & Ames (1989); but cf. Hare & Forth (1985)
Criminals	Lombroso (1903)
Crohn's disease	Geschwind & Behan (1982); Persson & Ahlbom (1988); Searleman & Fugagli (1987); but cf. Meyers & Janowitz (1985)
Deafness	Arnold & Askew (1993); Bonvillian, Orlansky, & Garland (1982)
Delinquency	Ellis & Ames (1989); Gabrielli & Mednick (1980); but cf. Feehan, Stanton, McGee, Silva, & Moffitt (1990)
Depression	Bruder, Quitkin, Stewart, Martin, Volgmaier, & Harrison (1989); but cf. Clementz, Iacono, & Beiser (1994); Moscovitch, Strauss, & Olds (1981)
Down syndrome	Lewin et al. (1993); Pipe (1988)
Dyslexia	Annett & Kilshaw (1984); Bemporad & Kinsbourne (1983); Eglinton & Annett (1994); Geschwind (1983); Strehlow, Haffner, Parzer, Pfuller, Resch, & Zerahn-Hartung (1996); Tonnessen, Lokken, Hoien, & Lundberg (1993)
Early-onset Alzheimer's disease	Seltzer, Burres, & Sherwin (1984)
Eczema	see Bishop (1986); Smith (1987); Stanton, Feehan, Silva, & Sears (1991)
Epilepsy	Lewin et al. (1993)
Epileptic schizophrenia	Oyebode & Davison (1990)
Immune disorders	Geschwind (1983); Geschwind & Behan (1982); Tonnessen et al. (1993)

Table 4.9

(Continued)

Condition or Group	References
Learning-disabled children	Geschwind & Behan (1982); but cf. Gilger et al. (1992)
Mental retardation	Geschwind & Behan (1982); Lucas, Rosenstein, & Bigler (1989); Morris & Romski (1993); Soper, Satz, Orsini, Van Gorp, & Green (1987)
Migraine headaches	Bishop (1986); Geschwind (1983); Geschwind (1984); Geschwind & Behan (1982); Guidetti, Moschetta, Ottaviano, Seri, & Fornara (1987); but cf. Hering (1995); van Strien et al. (1987)
Myasthenia gravis	Geschwind & Behan (1982); but cf. Bryden, McManus, & Bulman-Fleming (1994); Cosi, Citterio, & Pasquino (1988); McManus, Naylor, & Booker (1990)
Posttraumatic stress disorder	Spivak, Segal, Mester, & Weizman (1998)
Prisoners	Andrew (1978)
Psychoticism	Clementz et al. (1994); Taylor & Amir (1995)
Rett syndrome	Olsson & Rett (1986)
Schizophrenia	Manoach, Maher, & Manschreck (1988); Piran, Bigler, & Cohen (1982); Taylor & Amir, 1995, but cf. David, Malmberg, Lewis, Brandt, & Allebeck (1995); Shimizu, Endo, Yamaguchi, Torii, & Isaki (1985)
Severe sleep apnea	Hoffstein, Chan, & Slutsky (1993)
Skeletal malformations	Geschwind & Behan (1982)
Sleep difficulties	Coren & Searleman (1987); but cf. Hoffstein et al. (1993)
Smoking	Harburg (1981); Harburg, Feldstein, & Papsdorf (1978); London (1989)
Strabismus	Holman & Merritt (1986); Lessell (1986); Niederlandova (1967)
Students who worry too much	Dillon (1989); but cf. Mueller, Grove, & Thompson (1993)
Stuttering	Christensen & Sacco (1989); Dellatolas, Annesi, Jallon, Chavance, & Lellouch (1990); Geschwind (1983); Hatta & Kawakami (1994); Records, Heimbuch, & Kidd (1977); but cf. Webster & Poulos (1987)
Thyroid disorders	Geschwind & Behan (1982)
Ulcerative colitis	Bryden et al. (1994); Geschwind & Behan (1982)

in different cultures is remarkably similar. One would expect greater prevalence of left-handedness among cultures that experience relatively more "stressful" births.

2. The prevalence of left-handedness has not decreased across time, despite marked improvements in medical science. Now that obstetricians have much better training and technology, according to the PLH theory, one would expect the prevalence of left-handedness to decrease. In fact, the prevalence of left-handedness appears to be increasing, if it has changed at all (Brackenridge, 1981).

3. The presence of direct birth stressors (such as anoxia) have not been linked to left-handedness (Ehrlichman, Zoccolotti, & Owen, 1982; see Previc, 1996, for a review).

4. Left-handedness has often been linked with various professional groups and groups of the intellectually gifted (see Table 4.10).

PREVIC'S VESTIBULAR-MONOAMINERGIC THEORY. Whereas the G-G theory focused on a possible chemical mechanism for creating functional lateralization, Previc (1991, 1996) proposed a more mechanical model involving fetal position. Although fetal position is relatively flexible throughout the first two trimesters of pregnancy, during the final trimester, two thirds of fetuses are confined to the leftward fetal position (see Figure 4.12), with their right side facing outward (Taylor, 1976). Just as two thirds of all fetuses remain in the leftward position during the third trimester, two thirds of all humans display a slight enlargement of the left portion of their face (Kirveskari & Alanen, 1989). Because the fetus usually has the right ear facing outward, this causes asymmetries in auditory experience. There is some experimental evidence suggesting that fetuses can hear language sounds in utero and recognize those sounds. Therefore, lateralization of language perception may be a function of both asymmetrical auditory experience and the physical constraints on the left side of the face.

Previc (1991, 1996) postulates separate mechanisms to account for motoric lateralization and perceptual lateralization. The vestibular experience of the fetus during the final trimester is also asymmetrical. During normal walking, people usually spend more time in the acceleratory phase (although the rate of acceleration is less) than in the deceleratory phase (Smidt, Arora, & Johnston, 1971). When the fetus is confined to the leftward position, the acceleratory component of the maternal walk is registered as rightward movement, producing asymmetric shear forces in utero. There is considerable evidence that the left otolith (part of the inner ear) dominates

---

Table 4.10

Professional and Intellectually Gifted Groups Associated with a Higher Prevalence of Left-Handedness

Group	References
Architects	Gotestam (1990); Peterson (1979); Peterson & Lansky (1977)
Children of professional parents	Annett (1978)
Children with superior mathematical ability	Annett & Manning (1990); Benbow (1988)
Creative thinkers	Coren (1995); Newland (1981)
Divergent thinkers	Coren (1995)
Gifted children	Hicks & Dusek (1980)
Lawyers	Schachter & Ransil (1996)
Musicians	Gotestam (1990); but cf. Hering, Catarci, & Steiner (1995); Oldfield (1969)
Professional baseball players	McLean & Cuirczak (1982)
Students of the visual arts	Mebert & Michel (1980); Peterson (1979)
The intellectually precocious	Benbow (1986)

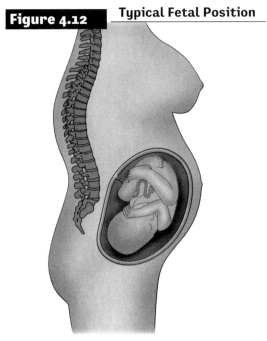

Figure 4.12 | **Typical Fetal Position**

In the third trimester, most fetuses are confined to the leftward fetal position with the right ear facing outward.

over the right in two thirds of the population. There is a rightward deviation of the body axis in most people, while 25% demonstrate a leftward tilt, and 12% do not appear to show any significant deviation (Kohen-Raz, 1986). Furthermore, there is a preference for turning to the right in the normal population, and after unilateral damage to the vestibular system, people prefer to turn toward the involved side (Peiterson, 1974).

In a more recent formulation of his theory, Previc (1996) also postulates a role for monoamines in the incidence of non-right-handedness. Specifically, he claims that non-right-handedness is associated with impaired noradrenergic function and, to a lesser extent, impaired serotonergic function. Given these associations, Previc (1996) proposes that vestibular projections to the locus coeruleus (which produces norepinephrine) and raphe nucleus (which produces serotonin) are critical for the lateralization of motor dominance and monoaminergic activity.

Problems with the Previc theory include the following:

1. Perhaps the most daunting failure of the Previc theory is some of the statistical data used to support it. Two thirds of all fetuses are confined to the leftward fetal position, so the theory would predict that one third of all babies would be left-handed. In fact, the prevalence of left-handedness is much lower than that, namely 10–13%, a far cry from the 33% predicted by Previc.
2. Another problem with Previc's theory is his attempted explanation of the dissociation between motoric and sensory lateralization of function. An example of the dissociation is the lack of a perfect relationship between handedness and linguistic hemispheric dominance. Although Previc proposes different mechanical rationales for these two types of lateralization, both the asymmetrical auditory experience and asymmetrical shear forces on the vestibular system are presumably caused by fetal position. Unless a fetus can be positioned in such a manner that allows asymmetrical stimulation of the vestibular system in one direction while allowing the opposite pattern of asymmetrical auditory stimulation, dissociations between motoric and perceptual laterality should not occur.
3. Previc's claim that fetal position at birth is related to functional laterality has not always been borne out by experimental evidence. For example, Searleman found that left-handedness was related not to birth position, but to birth stress (Searleman, Porac, & Coren, 1989). Goodwin found that fetal position was not related to head-turning or reaching behaviors (Goodwin & Michel, 1981). Vles also found that fetal position was not related to handedness (Vles, Grubben, & Hoogland, 1989).

THE DEVELOPMENTAL INSTABILITY THEORY. The developmental instability (DI) theory (Gangestad & Yeo, 1994; Markow, 1992) differs from most genetic theories of lateralization in that it proposes that variations in functional/anatomical asymmetries are outcomes of DI. DI is characterized by reduced canalization or even incorrect expression of a genetic sequence as a result of pathogens, toxins, or mutations. According to the theory, people with disturbances in laterality should also show both minor physical anomalies (MPAs), such as widely spaced eyes, multiple hair whorls, or low-set ears, and fluctuating asymmetry (FA), characterized by individual differences in the bilateral symmetry of physical features.

Support for the theory comes from the relationship between measures of DI and functional lateralization. Individuals with greater DI composite scores exhibit atypical lateralization scores, not just in the opposite direction from the normal asymmetries but also with more severe deviations than normal in the predicted direction (Yeo, Gangestad, Thoma, Shaw, & Repa, 1997). The theory is also attractive in that it provides a relatively simple account for the association between atypical laterality and developmental disorders such as skeletal malformations (Geschwind & Behan, 1982).

Some problems with the DI theory include the following:

1. The principal problem with the DI theory is that none of its variance can ever be accounted for by genetics (McManus, 1985). There is clearly a genetic influence on cerebral lateralization, and the DI theory cannot account for this influence.
2. Even if the DI theory proves useful for describing individual differences in cerebral lateralization, the theory is not informative about population-level asymmetries. If symmetry is the norm, why are 90% of all people right-handed and left-hemispheric dominant for language?

THE VANISHING TWINS THEORY. Despite its popular appeal (in part attributable to a program on the Learning Channel and an article in the *New Yorker*), references to the vanishing twin theory are rare in the academic literature. The theory ties two previously unrelated phenomena together into a model of laterality. The first phenomenon is the mirror-imaging that is occasionally seen in twins. Second, the majority of pregnancies that are initially diagnosed with multiple gestations produce only one viable child (see Landy, Keith, & Keith, 1982). Taken together, some people have argued that all left-handers (approximately 13% of the population) once had a twin, but only one embryo survived to full term. By the same logic, it is also claimed that the other half of the surviving twins (another 13%) should be right-handed.

Tracking the source of this theory has proven to be very difficult. Some attribute it to Charles Boklage for his comment that "the numbers are such that it is entirely possible that every non-right-hander in the world is a product of twin embryogenesis" (Boklage, 1997, personal communication). However, he has never published this theory in any scientific journal, and he appears to have mixed feelings about the position: "I don't think of vanishing twins as a 'cause' of left-handedness" but "I have no reason even to dilute that idea, let alone to retract it" (Boklage, 1997, personal communication). Others, such as Wright (1995), have claimed that the theory was suggested by Luigi Gedda of Rome's Gregor Mendel Institute.

The vanishing twin theory certainly has some empirical support. Approximately 1/80 (1.25%) of all births are twins (Jeanty, Rodesch, Verhoogen, & Struyven, 1981), and of those, approximately one third are monozygotic (from a single egg and sperm). However, many more than 1.25% of all pregnancies have multiple gestations before six weeks. Because ultrasound is getting better (achieving higher resolution) and becoming more common, we now know that multiple gestations are more common than was once thought. In a classic study by Levi (1976), 1.7% of pregnancies in a sample of 6990 showed evidence of multiple gestations. A few years later, Varma estimated the prevalence to be slightly higher: 2.0% in a sample of 1500 (Varma, 1979). More recent estimates range between 3.3% and 5.4% (Landy, Weiner, Corson, Batzer, & Bolognese, 1986).

Of these multiple gestations, how many fetuses survive? Levi (1976) reported that a shocking 71% of the multiple gestations "disappeared," meaning that most pregnancies ended in births of singletons. In a review of the literature, Landy et al. (1982) reported a 43–78% disappearance rate before six weeks. More recently, in a sample of eighty-eight multiple gestations, Blumenfeld and colleagues (Blumenfeld, Dirnfeld, Abramovici, Amit, Bronshtein, & Brandes, 1992) reported a 49% disappearance rate. Therefore, the viability of multiple gestations does not appear to be very high. Approximately 3% of all pregnancies have multiple gestations before six weeks, and fewer than half of these pregnancies result in multiple births (which approximates the 1.25% prevalence of twinning among viable births).

The second phenomenon that is invoked in the vanishing twin theory of handedness is the mirror-imaging phenomenon exhibited by 15–22% of monozygotic twins (Gedda et al., 1984; Golbin, Golbin, Keith, & Keith, 1993). In extremely rare cases, complete situs inversus is reported in one twin (Gedda et al., 1984). Most commonly, dental abnormalities are reported as evidence of mirror-imaging, but other physical

Figure 4.13   **Hair Whorl Asymmetry**

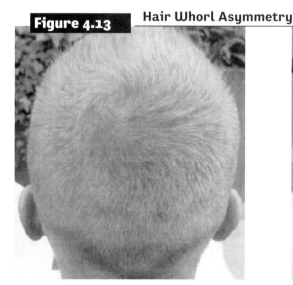 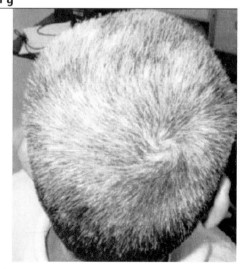

These two individuals have hair whorls that radiate in opposite directions.
Source: Images courtesy of A. Klar.

markers such as hair whorls (see Figure 4.13), fingerprints, and facial dysmorphologies have also been noted.

It is very unlikely that the vanishing twin theory can account for all cases of left-handedness. Assuming that left-handed fetuses are just as viable as right-handed fetuses, for every left-hander who is the survivor of a "right-handed, vanished twin," there should also be a right-hander that survived a "left-handed, vanished twin." Approximately 13% of the North American population is left-handed. Even if all monozygotic twins exhibited mirror-imaging, 26% (13% + 13%) of all pregnancies would need to have multiple gestations at one point to account for the current prevalence of left-handedness. This value is far greater than the current estimates of 3%. Furthermore, only 15% of twins who survive to term exhibit mirror-imaging. Taking this value into account, the prevalence of multiple gestations would have to be far greater than 26%.

Despite its apparent inability to account for the prevalence of left-handedness, the theory is consistent with a number of other findings. Left-handedness is more common among twins (Coren, 1994; Davis & Annett, 1994), and both twinning and handedness appear to run in families. Furthermore, the theory also predicts an association between left-handedness and relatively harsher uterine environments, possibly resulting in only one twin surviving to term. Also, left-handedness is associated with low APGAR scores (Schwartz, 1988; but cf. Olsen, 1995), premature birth (Ross, Lipper, & Auld, 1992, 1987), skeletal malformations (Geschwind & Behan, 1982), and low birth weight (O'Callaghan, Burn, Mohay, Rogers, & Tudehope, 1993; Powls, Botting, Cooke, & Marlow, 1996; Saigal, Rosenbaum, Szatmari, & Hoult, 1992; Segal, 1989), all of which appear to be more common in twins as well.

Evolutionary Theories

Although some evolutionary theories focus on potential benefits of lateralization in general (and sometimes right-handedness in particular), others have put forth the "suggestion that the left-handed represent an evolutionary retrogression (Levy, 1969; Miller, 1971; Nebes, 1971)—a phylogenetic step backward" (Hardyck & Petrinovich, 1977, p. 386). Some theories attempt to account for the interspecies laterality effects (MacNeilage, 1991), whereas others simply focus on the advantage that cerebral lateralization might provide for tool- and language-using humans.

CORBALLIS'S FINE-MOTOR CONTROL THEORY. Corballis (1991) proposed that handedness and language are lateralized to the same hemisphere because both require similar fine-motor control. Motor innervation of both hands and feet is primarily under the control of the contralateral hemisphere, and the hemisphere that is usually preferred for skilled motoric activities has been assumed to be responsible for language (which also requires fine motoric activation). The theory states that as early hominids learned to make and use more and more sophisticated tools, they developed more skilled motor control, lateralized to the LH. This practice with fine-motor sequences predisposed the LH to take on subsequent language functions, which also require very fine-motor control. A similar view was put forward by Kimura and Archibald (1974), who claimed that left speech lateralization developed from manual asymmetry, perhaps through the left hemisphere's superiority for controlling sequences of rapid movements.

There are some problems with this evolutionary scenario, including the following:

1. Why is the LH usually (90% of the time) primarily responsible for both skilled unimanual activities and linguistic processing? The theory gives a cogent account of why both language and handedness should be dominated by one hemisphere (within the individual)—but why the LH?
2. Left-handers do not usually demonstrate the opposite (i.e., RH) pattern of language dominance, as the theory predicts.
3. Linguistic lateralization appears to be more related to lateral preference for ballistic tasks (such as kicking and throwing) than for fine-motor tasks such as writing and manipulating tools (Day & MacNeilage, 1996; Elias & Bryden, 1998).

THE INTERHEMISPHERIC CONDUCTION DELAY HYPOTHESIS. Ringo and colleagues (Ringo, Doty, Demeter, & Simard, 1994) suggest that laterality provides a general advantage to organisms with relatively large brains. They propose that "specialization comes about because the temporal delay in conducting nerve impulses back and forth between the two hemispheres is simply too long in many instances to permit interhemispherically integrated neuronal computations" (Ringo et al., 1994, p. 331). They support this argument by comparing the time required for interhemispheric communication to the temporal specificity required for tasks that normally exhibit functional lateralization. The average interhemispheric transmission takes almost 30 milliseconds. For tasks that do not require great temporal precision, an **interhemispheric conduction delay (ICD)** of 30 milliseconds might be tolerable. However, tasks such as linguistic perception appear to require temporal precision greater than 30 milliseconds. "Elementary speech sounds (vowels and consonants) are temporal patterns whose components may last 50–200 milliseconds" (Miller, 1996, p. 5). The just-noticeable-difference for a single phonetic segment is on the order of 10–25 milliseconds (Miller, 1996). The temporal precision required for language production appears to be even greater. The intervals between movements that are required to produce different phonemes vary between 12 and 23 milliseconds (Gracco & Abbs, 1986; Miller, 1996). Skilled unimanual behaviors appear to require even greater temporal precision.

Consider the temporal precision required in making a relatively simple throw. Calvin (1983) calculates that the launch window (the time during which a thrown object can be released and still successfully hit the target) is substantially below Ringo and colleagues' (1994) estimated ICD of 30 milliseconds. Assuming a target of a rabbit at a distance of 4 meters (Figure 4.14), the launch window is 6–7 milliseconds. Calvin (1983) argues that the selection pressure favoring encephalization and lateralization of function was primarily due to the adaptive advantage of accurate throwing during hunting and warfare.

The Ringo and colleagues (1994) theory has some of the same weaknesses as the other theories, including the following:

1. Although the theory offers a plausible explanation about why lateralization provides an adaptive advantage, it does not explain population-level asymmetries. Why does the LH dominate linguistic processing for 90% of the population? The Ringo et al. (1994) theory simply predicts that one hemisphere or the other should dominate.

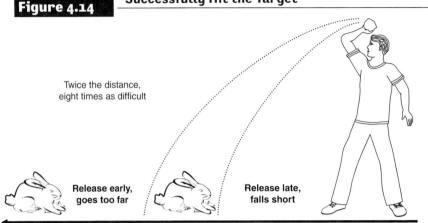

| Figure 4.14 | Time during Which a Thrown Object Can Be Released and Still Successfully Hit the Target |

Source: Image courtesy of W. H. Calvin. Copyright © 2004.

2. The theory does not address the relationship between linguistic lateralization and handedness. As it is currently formulated, the theory would predict independence between lateralization for various functions.

3. The theory does not address the sex difference in the handedness literature, nor is it informative about the correlations between atypical lateralization and various conditions discussed previously.

Summary

The theories that we reviewed in this module come from a variety of different perspectives, some of which are incompatible with one another. For example, the position that handedness develops entirely as a consequence of one's environment is not compatible with the position that laterality is under some sort of genetic control. However, the genetic theories of lateralization do not necessarily compete with the developmental and evolutionary theories discussed here, because they address a different level of explanation. Genes code for the production of proteins, not behavioral traits. Therefore, even if lateralization is entirely controlled by genetic processes and we successfully identified all genes that are relevant to its expression, we still would not necessarily know what developmental mechanisms are critical or why lateralization is advantageous to the individual. Similarly, isolating the genes that are responsible for the growth of feathers in birds would not be informative about why feathers are adaptive. Even if the developmental theories of Previc (1991, 1996) or Geschwind and Galaburda (1985a, 1985b, 1985c, 1987) prove to be completely correct, it is quite possible that the mechanisms they propose are controlled through the expression of genes.

1. What are two environmental explanations for the cause of hemispheric specialization?

2. Why must handedness be influenced by genetics? Why cannot strictly environmental explanations account for it?

3. Previc argues that laterality is caused by asymmetries in fetal position. How could fetal position in the third trimester influence the development of motoric or linguistic laterality?

4. The vanishing twin theory of left-handedness depends on the fact that some monozygotic twins demonstrate mirror-imaging. What is this, and how often does it happen?

5. The interhemispheric conduction delay hypothesis claims that laterality evolved because as brains grew larger, the delay associated with sending signals between the hemispheres grew too long. Why should the delay matter? For which tasks would the delay matter?

◀ **WHERE WE HAVE BEEN**   The previous module detailed some hypotheses about the cause of cerebral asymmetries. The explanations came from a number of perspectives, including positions that laterality is caused exclusively by the environment, by genes, or by factors that are present during prenatal development as well as accounts of why hemispheric specialization might have been adaptive. Although all these theories may appear to be competing with one another, keep in mind that many of them are not mutually exclusive. It is entirely possible that more than one of these accounts is an accurate description of why hemispheric specialization exists.

Glossary

Anomalous dominance—Refers to those people in whom the pattern of cerebral dominance differs from the "standard" form.

Anterior commissure—Connects cortical areas between the two hemispheres.

Body of the corpus callosum—Area anterior to the splenium.

Developmental instability theory—Proposes that variations in functional/anatomical asymmetries are outcomes of developmental instability (DI). DI is characterized by reduced canalization or even incorrect expression of a genetic sequence as a result of pathogens, toxins, or mutations.

Genu—The bend at the anterior tip of the corpus callosum.

Heterotopic—Connections between dissimilar cortical areas.

Hippocampal commissure—Links the two hippocampi.

Homotopic—Connecting cortical centers in similar locations between the two hemispheres.

Interhemispheric conduction delay (ICD)—Measurement that results from comparing the time required for interhemispheric communication to the temporal specificity required for tasks that normally exhibit functional lateralization.

Laterality—The functional specialization of the left and right hemispheres of the brain.

Massa intermedia—Connects the two thalami.

Nasal hemiretina—The half of the retina closest to the nasal passage.

Planum temporale—The region of the temporal lobe that lies under the posterior tip of the Sylvian fissure.

Posterior commissure—Connects cortical areas between the two hemispheres.

Prosody—The manner in which the words are spoken.

Rostrum—The portion of the corpus callosum inferior to the body, at the end of the bend of the genu.

Situs inversus—Asymmetries in which the heart and other organs are reversed from left to right compared to normal.

Spatial frequency hypothesis—This hypothesis of hemispheric specialization claims that the two hemispheres differ in their ability to process the basic sensory attributes of various stimuli.

Splenium—The most posterior area of corpus callosum.

Tachistoscope—A machine designed to present images at varying rates and locations on a screen.

Temporal hemiretina—The half of the retina closest to the temple.

5

The Sensorimotor System

Never confuse movement with action.

—ERNEST HEMINGWAY

MODULE **5.1**
Sensorimotor System

I vividly remember sitting in a lecture one day listening to a professor state that the brain was primarily for movement and, in my not-so-clever way, writing a note to my friend that said, "If the brain is for moving, why are we stuck here listening?" I say "not-so-clever" because at the time, my brain was performing quite a number of movements, including the obvious acts of tearing off a piece of paper, writing on it, and passing the note, but also the more subtle movements associated with sitting and remaining upright and the automatic movements that my eyes make whenever I am viewing the world. As it turns out, much of our brain is for moving us through the world. However, accurate movements depend on our ability to monitor the position and placement of our body and its parts, which relies on **somatosensory feedback** from our joints, tendons, muscles, and skin.

As you read this chapter, keep in mind that movement utilizes a parallel and hierarchical system that relies heavily on functional segregation. As we will see, if our brains did not organize movements in this fashion, almost all of our time would be spent programming out the sequences of movements rather than actually moving. Think for a moment about writing your name. For you to write your name, you must coordinate the activity of your arm, wrist, hand, and fingers, which requires the coordinated flexing and relaxing of over thirty-eight muscles. The sheer number of calculations that you would have to make to program the activity of each muscle is staggering, even without taking into account the calculations that must be made to modulate the force and location of the activity.

> WHERE WE ARE GOING ➤ The first module of this chapter will explore how the brain produces movements and the role of sensation in producing accurate movements. The second module will discuss disorders of movement that result from brain damage.

Why Sensorimotor?

In Chapter 2, you learned that the anaesthetic you get at the dentist works due to its ability to block sodium channels in the trigeminal nerve (cranial nerve V), thus preventing them from opening. Of relevance to this chapter is what happens to your ability to move your tongue when you can no longer feel it. Those of you who have had this experience know that it is very easy to bite your tongue while you are speaking (or eating) and more difficult to speak clearly. This is because the accurate and automatic motor programs that you use for eating or speaking require detailed sensory feedback from your mouth. Although anaesthetic is good for stopping pain sensations, it also stops all somatic sensation from your mouth and nearby face. The somatosensory information that your skin, joints, and muscles provide ensures that your brain makes accurate movements; and without it, you risk making inaccurate movements that increase your risk of biting your tongue.

The role of somatosensory feedback in the production of movements is illustrated by a former darts champion known as G.O., who experienced almost complete destruction of the somatosensory nerves in both arms due to an infection (Rothwell, Traub, Day, Obesso, Thomas, & Marsden, 1982). G.O. could still display a wide array of fine-motor skills with his fingers, and he was able to make shapes in the air with his fingers (with or without visual feedback). On the surface, then, very little was wrong with G.O.; he could perform complex motor movements, and he could easily demonstrate that he could still move his fingers. However, he stated that his hands were virtually useless to him (Rothwell et al., 1982).

In everyday life, he was unable to perform intricate motor skills, such as picking up spilled cereal or fastening buttons. He was also unable to hold a pen or write or even to hold a coffee cup for very long. These difficulties were exacerbated when G.O. was unable to use visual feedback to monitor his movements. The problem that G.O. faced was that he was no longer able to use somatosensory feedback to monitor the position of his hands. That is, without seeing it, he could no longer tell how strongly he was grasping an item (or whether he was grasping it at all), nor could he monitor the position of his hands to correct his movements. Furthermore, without sensory feedback from his hands, he was unable to know whether he was maintaining a constant level of muscle contraction, which resulted in his dropping objects (Rothwell et al., 1982).

Many of the adjustments that we make to our movements are guided by somatosensory feedback. For instance, when we reach out to grasp a cup of coffee, we immediately stop our movement forward when our hand touches the cup. We also use information from the muscles and joints of our arm to judge the position and force with which we are moving our arm. G.O. would be unable to use either tactile feedback to stop his movements or position/force information from his muscles and joints to judge the speed and direction of his grasp and therefore would be more prone to spilling the coffee. G.O.'s inability to correct this deficit, despite knowing about his inability to feel his arms, illustrates that many of the automatic adjustments that we make to movements occur unconsciously. That is, these adjustments are made without the involvement of higher cortical areas and are relatively resistant to interference from higher cortical areas.

Somatosensory Receptors

Much of the somatosensory information that we receive about the world comes from sensory receptors in the skin. We can feel a number of different sensations, including vibration, pressure, pain, and touch, suggesting that there are a variety of different sensory receptors present in the skin. The types of receptors are usually functionally grouped into three types of somatic information: **nociception,** which are the sensations of pain and temperature; **hapsis,** which are the sensations of fine touch and pressure; and **proprioception,** which is awareness of the body and its position in space. Regardless of function, most of the sensory receptors in the skin are **mechanoreceptors,** which react to distortion such as bending or stretching. There are also mechanoreceptors that wrap around the hairs that cover our body, which is why we can "feel" our hair. When hair is moved, it stretches or deforms the follicle from which it grows,

the **Real** world

Chicken Pox, Shingles, and Dermatomes

Unless you had a vaccination, there is a good chance that you had chicken pox when you were a child. Although the sores produced by the virus *Herpes varicella zoster* eventually went away, the virus did not. Instead, it is living in your cranial and spinal nerves (Kleinschmidt-DeMasters & Gilden, 2001). In most people, the virus is dormant, although in adulthood, stress, fatigue, or other events that compromise the immune system (e.g., HIV) may trigger the virus to become active again, resulting in a condition known as shingles. Typically, the virus becomes active in only one dorsal root ganglion, leading to hyperexcitability of that dorsal root ganglion. The increased sensitivity of the affected dorsal root ganglion leads to excessive firing, which is often perceived as a burning sensation or sharp stabbing pain. Shingles is an interesting condition to study because the virus maps the dermatome of the affected dorsal root by producing blisters on the skin along the nerve endings. Although shingles usually affects only the dorsal root of a spinal nerve, typically in the torso or face, there are cases in which the virus becomes active in other nerve tissue and can result in stroke or blindness. Regardless of the site of infection, immediate medical attention is required for shingles, as treatment may help to prevent chronic **neuralgia** (pain that does not result from any obvious lesion). Treatments for shingles might include drugs that stop the virus from reproducing (e.g., Acyclovir) and steroids to reduce inflammation.

which then activates the mechanoreceptors. There are many different types of mechanoreceptors throughout the body, although most are axons that have mechanosensitive ion channels on them. Although not much is known about how these mechanosensitive ion channels work, the axons that contain these ion channels are primary afferent axons that enter the spinal cord through the dorsal roots. The cell bodies of the primary afferent axons reside in the dorsal root ganglia of the spinal cord.

The spinal cord is organized into dorsal and ventral root ganglia; the **dorsal root ganglia** are somatosensory, and the **ventral root ganglia** are motor. There are thirty pairs of spinal nerves, each of which is made up of dorsal and ventral roots that exit the spinal cord through a notch in the vertebrae of the spine. These spinal segments can be divided into four groups on the basis of where the nerves originate (Figure 5.1): cervical (C) 1–8, thoracic (T) 1–12, lumbar (L) 1–5, and sacral (S) 1–5. Each of the thirty dorsal roots of the spinal cord innervates different areas of the skin referred to as **dermatomes.** Maps of dermatomes (see Figure 5.1) really reflect the areas of skin that are served by the dorsal roots of a specific spinal nerve. When a dorsal root is cut, the spinal cord can no longer obtain information from that nerve. However, not all sensation from that dermatome is lost, as there is extensive overlap between dermatomes. In fact, to lose complete sensation in one dermatome, you must cut three dorsal roots: the one serving the dermatome and the dorsal roots above and below it.

Somatosensory Pathways in the Brain

There are a number of sensory pathways in the brain, and they are often divided into two main pathways, which are named for their position in the spinal cord and the

The Four Sections of the Spinal Cord (Cervical, Thoracic, Lumbar, and Sacral), Which Innervate Dermatomes

Figure 5.1

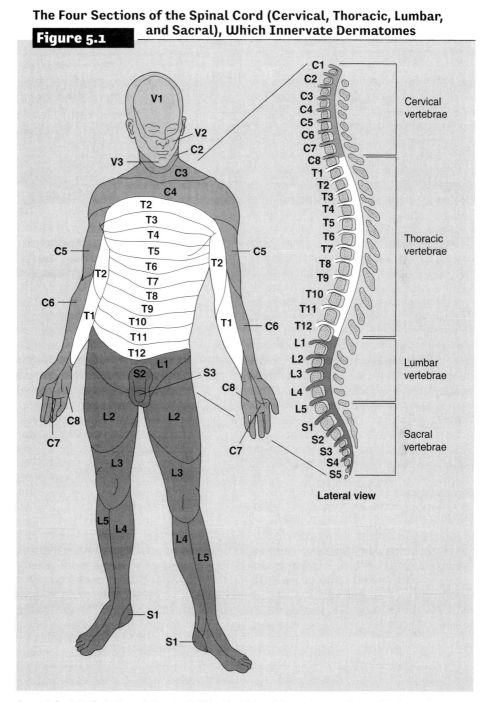

Lateral view

Somatosensory Pathways (Dorsal Spinothalamic Tract and Ventral Spinothalamic Tract) from the Spinal Cord to the Somatosensory Cortex

Figure 5.2

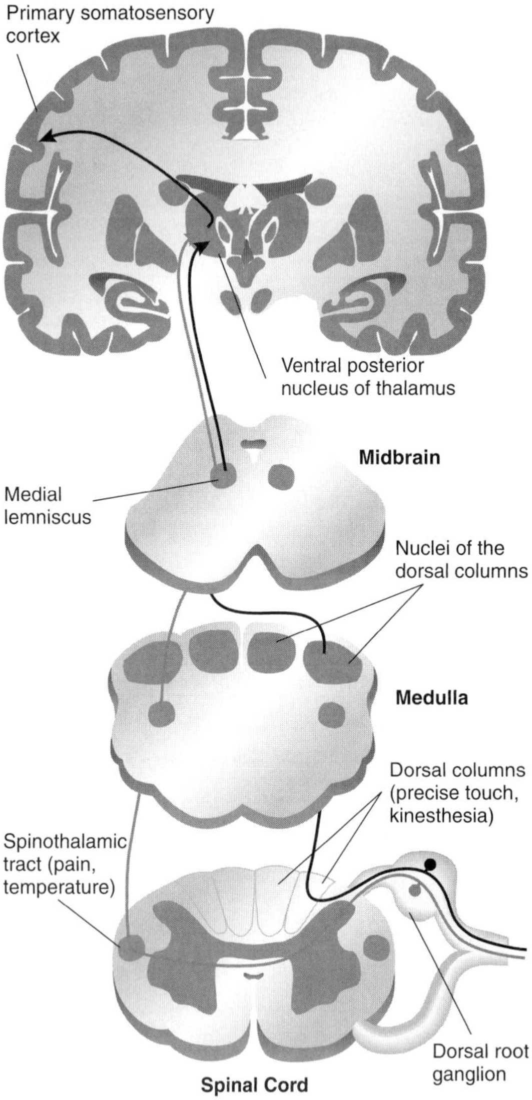

Source: Neil R. Carlson, *Physiology of Behavior,* 8e. Published by Allyn and Bacon, Boston, MA. Copyright © 2004 by Pearson Education. Reprinted by permission of the publisher.

connections made: the dorsal spinothalamic tract and the ventral spinothalamic tract. The **dorsal spinothalamic tract** (Figure 5.2), which is responsible for transmitting information about proprioception and hapsis, enters the spinal cord through the dorsal root ganglion and synapses ipsilaterally in the dorsal column nuclei of the spinal cord. The axons of the dorsal column nuclei ascend through the spinal cord until the brainstem, where they decussate or cross, and continue to ascend through the brainstem in a pathway called the medial lemniscus. The axons of the medial lemniscus synapse in the ventrolateral thalamus, which sends projections to both the motor and somatosensory cortex. Nociceptive information travels separately in the **ventral spinothalamic tract** (see Figure 5.2), which enters the spinal cord through the dorsal root ganglion and ascends the spinal cord contralaterally. In the brainstem, these axons join the medial lemniscus and ascend to the ventrolateral thalamus. As was the case for the dorsal spinothalamic tract, some of these neurons send projections to the somatosensory cortex.

Although somatosensory information for hapsis and nociception is transmitted separately, because they send information through the same pathways to the same destinations, damage to the brainstem or thalamus results in equal loss of both hapsis and nociception. However, damage to the spinal cord can result in different patterns of deficits. As you most likely know, damage to the spinal cord results in a loss of sensorimotor function below the site of injury. However, if the spinal cord is not completely **transected** (cut through), nociception is lost for the side of the body contralateral to the injury, and hapsis is lost for the side of the body ipsilateral to the injury.

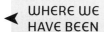

WHERE WE HAVE BEEN Somatosensory information plays an essential role in the production of movements, primarily by providing critical feedback to the brain about the position of the body. Somatosensory information can be divided into three separate functions: proprioception, nociception, and hapsis. Hapsis and proprioception are mediated by the dorsal spinothalamic tract, and nociception is mediated by the ventral spinothalamic tract.

WHERE WE ARE GOING The next section of this module will explore how the brain produces movements and how sensation is integrated in the production of accurate movements. The second section will discuss disorders of movement that result from brain damage.

Association Cortex

Control of voluntary behavior is organized like a business. There is a boss at the top, who gives out commands (often without doing much of the work directly), and there are various levels of workers with different functions, who are goal directed and fairly autonomous. In the case of the sensorimotor control, the two different areas of association cortex are at the top of the hierarchy (Figure 5.3). As we will see, the secondary and primary motor areas actually carry out the commands fairly independently, sending their commands to the muscles through the descending motor pathways. Rather than playing a direct role in voluntary movements, the basal ganglia and cerebellum modulate motor responses, the independent contractors in the organization. Critical feedback, both somatosensory and motor, is achieved through the ascending sensorimotor pathways.

Hierarchical Organization of the Sensorimotor System

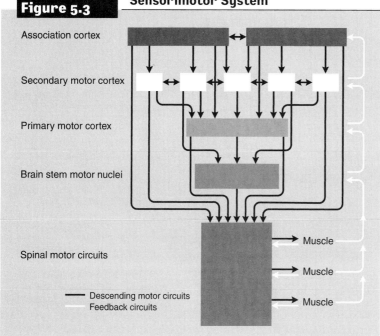

Figure 5.3

Source: John P. J. Pinel, *Biopsychology*, 5e. Published by Allyn and Bacon, Boston, MA. Copyright © 2003 by Pearson Education. Reprinted by permission of the publisher.

POSTERIOR PARIETAL ASSOCIATION CORTEX. The parietal lobes tend to be active whenever the brain is interacting with space or with spatial information (how the brain perceives and interacts with space is the focus of Chapter 10). As such, the posterior parietal association cortex plays (Figure 5.4) an important role in determining both the original position of the body and objects around the body in space. If you think about it, any movement through space requires extensive knowledge about the spatial relations of the objects in the space, including your own body. If you want to do anything that actually contacts other objects, such as picking up a cup of coffee, you need to correctly estimate the distance between your hand and the cup. In addition you need to compute the angle and size of the handle in order to pick the cup up efficiently. Thus, knowledge of the spatial arrangement and position of the body is required to effectively move through the world. (In the example at the beginning of the chapter, the failure of the anaesthetized tongue to provide information about its

Figure 5.4 | Input and Output Pathways of the Posterior Parietal Association Areas

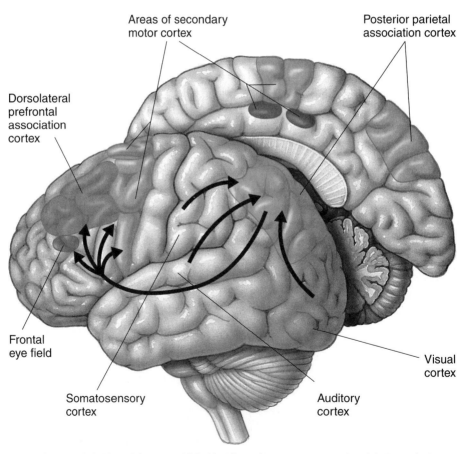

Source: John P. J. Pinel, *Biopsychology,* 5e. Published by Allyn and Bacon, Boston, MA. Copyright © 2003 by Pearson Education. Reprinted by permission of the publisher.

position can result in unintentional injury to the tongue.) However, knowledge of the body is not enough for accurate purposeful movements, such as catching a ball. To accomplish these types of movements requires precise knowledge of the spatial relationships between external objects and the body.

The posterior parietal association cortex is an association cortex because it receives input from a variety of sensory systems, including proprioception, hapsis, and vision. Using this information, the posterior parietal association cortex is responsible for creating a mental picture of the body in space. Within the posterior parietal cortex, Brodmann's area 5 (BA5) receives inputs from primary somatosensory cortical areas, whereas BA3, BA1, BA2, and BA7 receive higher-order visual information. As you will see in Chapter 10, individuals with damage to these areas of the parietal lobes tend to have difficulties with spatial relations, but they also tend to have disturbances of body image. It is as if individuals with parietal damage fail to recognize parts of their body as belonging to themselves. The posterior parietal lobes are involved in the processing of spatial relations of both the body and objects surrounding the body, which plays a critical role in the production of accurate movements. However, it is the extensive interconnections between the posterior parietal association cortex and the dorsolateral prefrontal association cortex that allow this information to guide movements. In addition, the posterior parietal association cortex has extensive reciprocal connections with areas that are lower in the motor hierarchy, such as secondary and primary motor cortex.

DORSOLATERAL PREFRONTAL CORTEX. The dorsolateral prefrontal association cortex (Figure 5.5) is thought to be involved with the decision to execute voluntary movements. In a series of experiments performed by using monkeys, Patricia Goldman-Rakic and colleagues demonstrated that the dorsolateral prefrontal association cortex actively directs lower areas in the motor hierarchy, such as the secondary and primary motor cortex (Goldman-Rakic, 1987). Furthermore, activation in the dorsolateral prefrontal association cortex occurred before the monkey began to pick up an object, suggesting that the decision to make the movement to pick up the object is initiated by the dorsolateral prefrontal association cortex (Goldman-Rakic, Bates, & Chafee, 1992). Neuroimaging studies in humans have observed that when neurologically intact participants were asked to make a series of movements with their fingers or toes, activation was observed in the dorsolateral prefrontal cortex (BA8) and the secondary (BA6) and primary motor cortex (BA4) (Rolani & Zilles, 1996). Interestingly, when participants were asked to only imagine moving their fingers similar levels of activity were observed in these areas, except for the primary motor cortex.

Given the large interconnections between the dorsolateral prefrontal association cortex and the posterior parietal association cortex, it seems likely that the sensory information that is provided to the dorsolateral prefrontal association cortex by the posterior parietal association cortex plays a large role in the decision to make the movement. However, given the large role that the frontal lobes play in memory (Chapter 8) and attention (Chapter 11), it is likely that the dorsolateral prefrontal lobe also is assessing the likely outcome of planned movements. The dorsolateral prefrontal association cortex sends extensive projections to the secondary and primary motor cortex. As we will see in the next sections, the dorsolateral prefrontal association cortex is specifying

Output and Inputs of the Dorsolateral Prefrontal Association Cortex

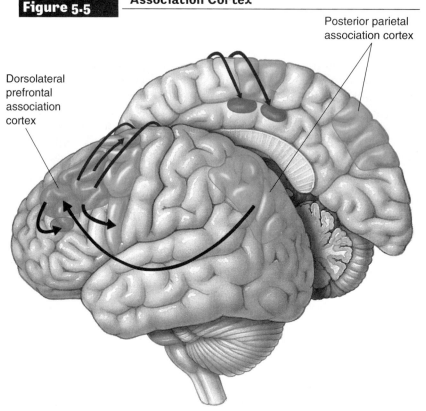

Figure 5.5

Dorsolateral prefrontal association cortex

Posterior parietal association cortex

Source: John P. J. Pinel, *Biopsychology,* 5e. Published by Allyn and Bacon, Boston, MA. Copyright © 2003 by Pearson Education. Reprinted by permission of the publisher.

what movement to make, and the lower levels are specifying *how* the movements will be made.

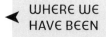

WHERE WE HAVE BEEN

The sensorimotor system can be divided into independent and parallel components, which are hierarchically organized. At the top of this hierarchy are the posterior parietal association cortex and the dorsolateral prefrontal association cortex, both of which play important roles in the generation of voluntary movements. The posterior parietal association cortex is involved with generating a mental image of the body and judging the relative position of the body with respect to external objects. The dorsolateral prefrontal association cortex is involved with the decision to initiate movements. Both areas of association cortex have extensive interconnections with each other and with lower levels of the motor hierarchy.

WHERE WE ARE GOING

Although the dorsolateral prefrontal association cortex gives the signal to engage in a movement, it is the lower levels of the hierarchy that are involved in producing these movements. The subsequent sections of this module will examine each level of the hierarchy and its role in the production of movement. The second module will discuss disorders of movement.

Secondary Motor Cortex

Areas of the secondary motor cortex include the supplementary motor area, the premotor cortex, and the cingulate motor areas (Figure 5.6). Regardless of the specific site, all areas of the secondary motor area are reciprocally connected to each other. In addition, the secondary motor cortex sends direct projections to brainstem nuclei. Electrical stimulation of any of these areas results in complex motor movements, suggesting that they all play a role in voluntary motor production. Interestingly, all areas of the secondary motor cortex appear to be bilaterally active before and during voluntary movements (Seitz,

Figure 5.6 **Secondary Motor Cortex**

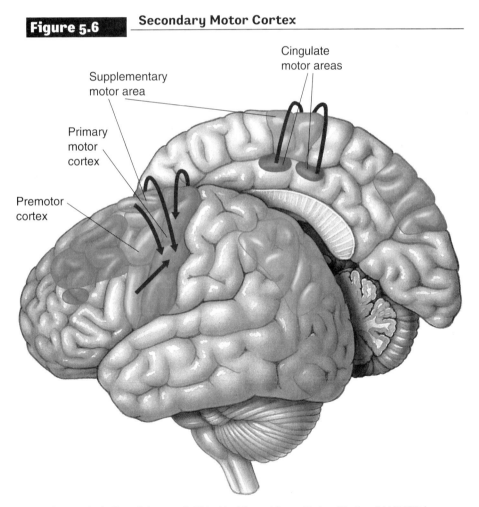

Source: John P. J. Pinel, *Biopsychology,* 5e. Published by Allyn and Bacon, Boston, MA. Copyright © 2003 by Pearson Education. Reprinted by permission of the publisher.

Stephan, & Binkofski, 2000), suggesting that these areas are involved in the planning and execution of motor movements. However, there are a number of reports of increased activation in the cingulate, premotor cortex, and supplementary motor area in response to imagined movements (Decety & Jeannerod, 1995; Jeannerod & Decety, 1995), so there is no evidence that these motor programs must actually occur (Roth et al., 1996).

Although large similarities are observed between areas of the secondary motor cortex, it is still assumed that each has a unique role in the programming and execution of motor programs (Rizzolatti, Luppino, & Matelli, 1998). For instance, it appears that activation of the supplementary motor area is associated with self-generated movements, whereas activation of the premotor cortex is associated with externally generated movements (Deiber, Passingham, Colebatch, Friston, Nixon, & Frackowiak, 1991). Self-generated movements are typically controlled by internal feedback (e.g., rhythmic tapping of the finger), which is consistent with the large connections of the supplementary motor area with somatosensory areas in the parietal lobe. Externally generated movements are typically externally controlled or triggered (e.g., tapping the finger at the same speed as a metronome), which is consistent with the large connections of the premotor cortex with visual and auditory cortical areas. Less is known about the role of the cingulate, although cingulate activation is often observed when there is conflict about whether or not action should be taken.

Primary Motor Cortex

Primary motor cortex controls the movements of the muscles, and it plans out the coordinated activity of the muscles. As you can see in Figure 5.7 (pages 152–153), the primary motor cortex is the area of the brain that is directly in front of the central fissure (precentral gyrus), which is right next to the primary somatosensory cortex (postcentral gyrus). There are heavy interconnections with the somatosensory cortex, suggesting that there is the ability to modify motor programs on the basis of sensory feedback. In fact, **stereognosis,** the ability to identify objects by touch, is most likely mediated by the connections between the primary motor cortex and somatosensory areas. Interestingly, damage to the primary motor cortex does not lead to limb paralysis; rather, it reduces the speed, accuracy, and force with which an individual makes a movement, along with causing astereognosia (described later in this chapter) (Schieber, 1990; Valenza, Ptak, Zimine, Badan, Lazeyras, & Schnider, 2001).

As you learned in Chapter 1, Penfield and Jasper mapped the primary somatosensory and primary motor cortex. Their observations led them to conclude that both the primary somatosensory cortex and primary motor cortex are organized somatotopically, or with respect to the layout of the body. When the somatotopic map of the sensorimotor or primary motor cortex is mapped graphically, the result is the homunculus in Figure 5.7. These drawings illustrate the parts of the body in different sizes, depending on how much cortical area is devoted to sensation from that area. As you can see, some relatively large body parts (e.g., trunk, leg) have little cortical representation, whereas other, smaller body parts (e.g., hand, mouth) have extensive cortical representation. The somatosensory and motor representations for the same body part are side by side; that is, representation of the sensory properties of the left hand is next to the motor representation of the left hand.

Although Penfield and Jasper's original findings are largely considered to be correct today, there have been some modifications. For instance, representation of the hand is not as simple as was first thought. Rather than there being a specific area for each component of the hand (e.g., index finger) there appears to be a network of neurons distributed throughout the premotor cortex that become active when the index finger is moved (Schieber & Hibbard, 1993). That is not to say that there is no somatotopic representation of the hand; recent research has suggested that there is representation of individual fingers that overlaps representation of adjacent fingers (e.g., the representation of the middle finger overlaps the representation for the ring and index fingers) (Beisteiner et al., 2001). This overlapping representation of fingers is not confined to the primary motor cortex; it has been observed in the primary somatosensory cortex as well (e.g., Krause et al., 2001). In addition to problems with the hand, there is some suggestion that the homunculus as presented in Figure 5.7 may have the face presented upside down (Servos, Engel, Gati, & Menon, 1999).

◄ **WHERE WE HAVE BEEN**   The secondary motor cortex takes the goal that was directed by the cortical association areas and plans out the actions that must be taken. Using these plans, the primary motor cortex determines the sequence of muscle movements to be made. Each area of the secondary motor cortex has its own unique function. Given the functional and organizational similarities and the degree of interconnection between the primary motor cortex (precentral gyrus) and the primary somatosensory cortex (postcentral gyrus), it is clear that voluntary movement is sensorimotor in nature.

WHERE WE ARE GOING ►   The basal ganglia and cerebellum play critical roles in movement. Furthermore, damage to these areas results in a number of movement disorders. The next section of this module will examine the role of the basal ganglia and cerebellum in the production of voluntary movement in neurologically intact individuals. In addition, the spinal motor circuits will be examined. The next module will examine disorders of movement and the brain damage that is associated with each disorder.

Basal Ganglia and Cerebellum

The **basal ganglia** are a subdivision of the telencephalon, and they are composed of three structures: the **caudate nucleus,** the **putamen** (collectively referred to as the **striatum,** meaning "striped structure"), and the **globus pallidus.** The globus pallidus and putamen can be collectively called the **lentiform nucleus.** The globus pallidus looks similar in shape and size to the thalamus; just lateral to the egg-shaped thalami (plural of *thalamus*) are the two globus pallidi. These egg-shaped structures are encased in the putamen, and the caudate extends from the putamen in a C-shaped curling, taillike structure. All three structures are named after their appearance: globus pallidus means "globe," putamen means "shell," and caudate means "nucleus with a tail." See Figure 5.8 (page 154) for a summary of the structures of the basal ganglia.

The basal ganglia are critically important for initiating movements and maintaining muscle tone. The caudate and putamen (striatum) receive the vast majority of the

Figure 5.7 — Primary Somatosensory and Motor Cortices

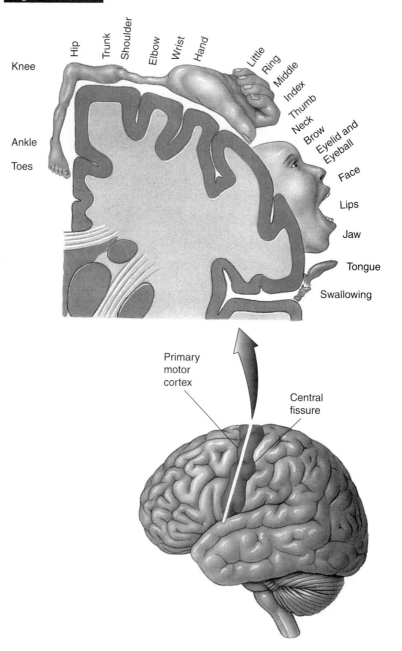

Figure 5·7 (continued)

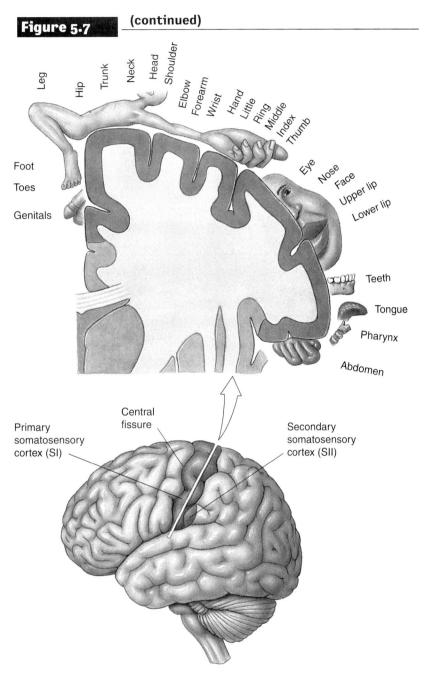

Leg

Hip

Trunk

Neck

Head

Shoulder

Elbow

Forearm

Wrist

Hand

Little

Ring

Middle

Index

Thumb

Foot

Toes

Genitals

Eye

Nose

Face

Upper lip

Lower lip

Teeth

Tongue

Pharynx

Abdomen

Primary
somatosensory
cortex (SI)

Central
fissure

Secondary
somatosensory
cortex (SII)

Source: John P. J. Pinel, *Biopsychology,* 5e. Published by Allyn and Bacon, Boston, MA.
Copyright © 2003 by Pearson Education. Reprinted by permission of the publisher.

Figure 5.8	**Structures of the Basal Ganglia**

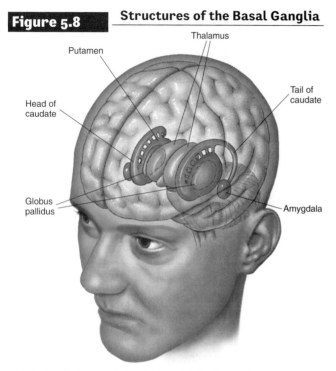

Source: John P. J. Pinel, *Biopsychology,* 5e. Published by Allyn and Bacon, Boston, MA. Copyright © 2003 by Pearson Education. Reprinted by permission of the publisher.

Figure 5.9	**Zones of the Cerebellum**

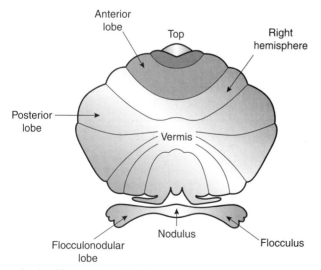

Source: Reprinted by permission of Paul Janzen.

cortical inputs to the basal ganglia as well as the projections from the substantia nigra. As you will discover later in this chapter, the substantia nigra is perhaps best known because it degenerates selectively in Parkinson's disease. However, another common motor disorder also involves the basal ganglia. Huntington's chorea results from damage to the striatum—both the caudate nucleus and the putamen. The striatum receives most of the motor input for the basal ganglia, and the globus pallidus serves as the primary output. Most of these connections are with the thalamus, which in turn connects to motor and nonmotor structures, such as the cingulate cortex and prefrontal cortex, both of which are presumed to be involved in response selection.

The cerebellum plays a very important role in the modulation of motor movements and the acquisition of motor skill. It is a very dense and complicated structure (it is widely claimed that the cerebellum contains 50% of the brain's neurons while representing only 10% of its weight), but for the purpose of our discussion here, we will discuss it in terms of three zones (see Figure 5.9). The cerebellum can be described in terms of three zones: the **lateral zone,** the **intermediate zone,** and the **vermis.** Both the lateral zone and the intermediate zone are represented in each cerebellar hemisphere, but the vermis lies between the hemispheres. Within these zones are three nuclei of the cerebellum, collectively referred to as the **deep cerebellar nuclei.** The **fastigial nuclei** receive projections from the vermis, the **interpositus nuclei** receive projections from the intermediate zone, and the **dentate nuclei** receive projections from the lateral zone. As one might expect, the different regions of the cerebellum are functionally as well as anatomically distinct. The vermis is involved with maintaining posture and coordinating whole-body movements. The intermediate zone is specialized for guiding skilled limb movement (particularly targeting movements, such as reaching and grasping). The lateral zone of the cerebellum is involved in coordinating multijoint movements, including ballistic movements such as swinging a bat. It also appears to play an important role in the acquisition of motor skills (not just multijoint ballistic ones), and its role in "higher" cognitive functions such as language are currently being explored.

Spinal Motor Pathways

There are two main systems of motor projections that descend from the brain to the spinal cord to initiate and control movement. Both systems have projections that originate in the cortex, along with projections originating in brainstem structures. The first system of projections is the **ventromedial system.** The brainstem projections of this system form three tracts: the **vestibulospinal tract** (important for maintaining balance), the **reticulospinal tract** (important for maintaining posture), and the **tectospinal tract** (important for controlling the head and eye movements). The cortical projection of this system forms the **ventral corticospinal tract** (important for controlling the muscles of the trunk and upper legs, collectively used in tasks such as walking). The points of origin and pathways of these tracts are illustrated in Figure 5.10. The other system of motor projections is called the **lateral system** (illustrated in Figure 5.11). It has one tract projecting from the brainstem and one tract projecting from the cortex. The brainstem projections form the **rubrospinal tract** (important for making movements of the limbs and hands), and the cortical projections form the **lateral corticospinal tract,** which is also important for controlling limb movement and the extremities such as fingers and toes.

MODULE **5.2**
Sensorimotor Disorders

Now that we have reviewed the components of the sensorimotor system and the connections that allow these components to interact, we are going to review what happens when part of the system is not working properly. Some conditions arise from primarily cortical damage. These conditions include apraxia, astereognosis, phantom sensation, and alien limb. Other disorders arise from relatively selective damage to subcortical structures. These disorders include Parkinson's disease, Huntington's Chorea, Gille de la Tourette syndrome, and tardive dyskinesia.

Cortical Sensorimotor Disorders

APRAXIA. **Apraxia** is a difficult term to define. Taken literally, the word refers to a lack of action. However, apraxic individuals are still capable of action, but their actions are often unorganized and inappropriate. Like a number of other neuropsychological disorders, apraxia is defined by exclusion. In addition to detailing what functional difficulties an individual might have, one must also describe some functions that are left intact for the definition to be useful and accurate. For example, consider

Figure 5.10   The Ventromedial Motor System

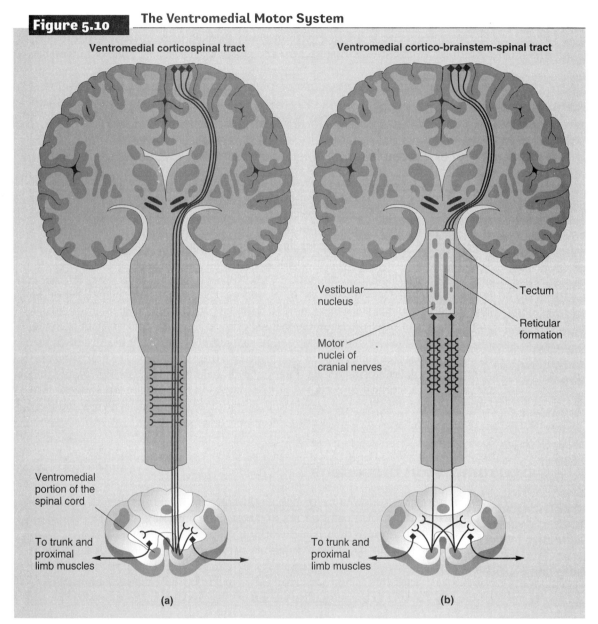

Ventromedial corticospinal tract

Ventromedial cortico-brainstem-spinal tract

Vestibular nucleus

Tectum

Reticular formation

Motor nuclei of cranial nerves

Ventromedial portion of the spinal cord

To trunk and proximal limb muscles

To trunk and proximal limb muscles

(a)

(b)

Source: John P. J. Pinel, *Biopsychology,* 5e. Published by Allyn and Bacon, Boston, MA. Copyright © 2003 by Pearson Education. Reprinted by permission of the publisher.

the term **alexia,** used to describe a deficit in reading. If the term were defined simply as "an inability to read text," someone who is illiterate could be considered alexic. Even if it were defined as "an acquired inability to read," someone who was rendered blind from an accident could be considered alexic. Instead, the disorder must be defined with a description of the functional problem (inability to read) and a descrip-

| Figure 5.11 | The Dorsolateral Motor System |

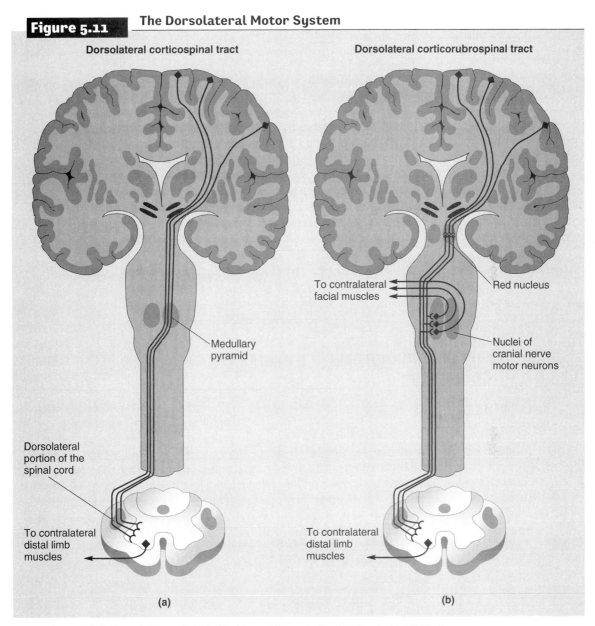

Source: John P. J. Pinel, *Biopsychology*, 5e. Published by Allyn and Bacon, Boston, MA. Copyright © 2003 by Pearson Education. Reprinted by permission of the publisher.

tion of the functions remaining intact, such as intact primary visual functions and object recognition.

Apraxia is a deficit in performing skilled voluntary movements. However, the motor deficits that are apparent in apraxia cannot be attributable to primary sensory problems, paralysis or muscle weakness, or some other motor disturbance (such as tremor). The term *apraxia* was used as early as 1871 by Steinthal to describe the inability to perform purposeful movements in response to a command (Rogers, 1996). Liepmann is often credited with being the first to describe apraxia, but this is not the case. Early opinion about the mechanism of apraxia differs significantly from what is generally believed about the disorder today. Most early investigators who noted apraxia in their patients attributed the inability to produce purposeful movements to the person's inability to fully recognize the objects or tools to be incorporated in the movement. It was assumed that the problem was not the sequencing and production of the movement itself, but rather a problem associating objects with movements. Similar to the visual agnosias described in the previous chapter, this type of agnosia could be considered "motor agnosia."

Today, apraxia is generally regarded as a disorder of motor planning. This position was clearly articulated by Liepmann in 1900 (Brown, 1988). Contradicting the thirty years of discussion of apraxia as a recognition disorder, Liepmann presented a case of apraxia in which the observed deficits were clearly not due to problems with object recognition.

Apraxia can be expressed in a wide variety of forms. In fact, the term has been used to describe a wide variety of disorders, some of which barely resemble the dis-

Neuropsychological Celebrity

Mr. T.

Those of you who spent much of the 1980s glued to the television probably associate the name "Mr. T." with the image of a large African American man with a Mohawk haircut and countless gold chains around his neck. Mr. T.'s contributions to the A-Team were mostly physical. Other members of the team supplied the brains while Mr. T. supplied the brawn. Liepmann (1900, 1905) describes the case of a different Mr. T.: a 48-year-old civil servant whose impact on the development of neuropsychology was related to his inability to perform physical tasks correctly. Liepmann described Mr. T.'s movements as "bizarre and distorted," and when commanded to perform actions, he "failed in almost everything." For example, Liepmann asked Mr. T. to pour water from a jug held in his left hand to a glass held in his right hand. In response, Mr. T. attempted to pour with his left hand, but simultaneously lifted the empty glass in his right hand to his mouth. According to Liepmann's earlier

physical examination, Mr. T. did not exhibit paralysis on either side of his body, so his incorrect movements could not be attributed to an inability to move. Even the example above illustrates that he could manipulate objects with either hand.

The prevailing opinion among neuroscientists at the time was that apraxia was the result of a failure in recognition. Liepmann tested this position with Mr. T. by reasoning that the apraxia should be present on all commands relating to a potentially unrecognized object. On further testing, Liepmann made the remarkable discovery that Mr. T.'s apraxia was present only when he attempted to complete purposeful movements with the right side of his body (arms or legs), but when Mr. T. responded with his left, he could comply with commands both quickly and accurately. This lateralized deficit (now called *unilateral apraxia*) could not be explained in terms of a recognition failure. Further, Liepmann discovered that Mr. T.'s deficits were not restricted to a single modality. He exhibited apraxic right limb movements in response to verbal commands, written commands, gestures, or tactile information, such as a tickle in his right ear.

order first described by Steinthal. In any event, it is generally accepted that there are four major classes of apraxia: ideomotor, ideational, constructional, and oral (described in detail in the following subsections). Across these types, some cases of apraxia, such as the one of Mr. T. just described, involve movements of one side of the body. It is normally the right side that is affected, and the deficit is called **unilateral apraxia.** However, apraxia can also impair movements on both sides of the body. This is described as **bilateral apraxia.** Three other types of apraxia are also discussed later in this chapter: limb apraxia, dressing apraxia, and callosal apraxia. We have included these disorders in this section on cortical motor disorders, but as you will see, there is debate about whether these three varieties of apraxia should really be described with the term *apraxia* at all (Rogers, 1996).

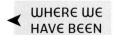

WHERE WE HAVE BEEN After reviewing both the subcortical and cortical components of the sensorimotor system, we have introduced a class of cortical motor disorders that fall under the name *apraxia*. These movement disorders are characterized by deficits in performing skilled voluntary movements, but these deficits are not attributable to sensory problems, paralysis, or muscle weakness.

WHERE WE ARE GOING In the following sections we detail the symptoms of ideomotor, ideational, constructional, and oral apraxia in light of a more general definition of apraxia. Then we describe some less common and more controversial variants of apraxia, including limb apraxia, oral apraxia, dressing apraxia, and callosal apraxia.

IDEOMOTOR APRAXIA. In **ideomotor apraxia,** an individual cannot execute or imitate simple gestures in response to a command. One can test for ideomotor apraxia by asking an individual to wave goodbye, salute, beckon "come here," or pretend to hitchhike. In all of these gestures, the individual is being asked to make gestures that are intransitive. In intransitive gestures, one does not manipulate (or pretend to manipulate) an object. Ideomotor apraxia can also impair one's ability to perform transitive gestures—gestures that involve manipulating (or pretending to manipulate) an object. For example, one can also test for ideomotor apraxia by asking an individual to show how he or she would flip a coin, use a hammer, use a screwdriver, open a screw-topped bottle, or unlock a door. One can also test an individual's ability to complete relatively complicated serial acts, such as putting a letter in an envelope and preparing it for mailing (folding the piece of paper, placing it in the envelope, sealing the envelope, and stamping it). When administering these tests in a clinical setting, neuropsychologists typically assess the individual's ability to imitate these gestures as well. Remember that apraxia typically occurs following left hemisphere damage, and this type of damage can also compromise language functions. Therefore, if an individual is asked to demonstrate how he or she would unlock a door, the inability to do so could be due to a motor sequencing problem or to difficulty understanding the terms used in the request.

IDEATIONAL APRAXIA. Liepmann first distinguished between ideomotor and **ideational apraxia,** and this distinction has been maintained over the past 100 years. However, the distinguishing characteristics between ideomotor and ideational apraxia are still fodder for debate today, making the distinction less useful. Some have proposed that ideomotor apraxia is an inability to correctly form single movements, whereas ideational apraxia is the inability to correctly sequence a series of movements (Rothwell, 1994). An alternative distinction contrasts the two types rather differently. Ideomotor apraxia can be characterized as "an impairment in knowing *how*, rather than *what*, to do" (Bradshaw & Mattingley, 1995). Therefore, the individuals do not exhibit impairments with the concepts that are required to form the movements, but the implementation of the concepts is impaired. In contrast, ideational apraxia is characterized by confusion or loss of knowledge about an object's use. The person remains capable of completing the individual elements of the required movement, but the logical ordering of the movements is impaired. Because ideational apraxia can involve the loss of knowledge about how an object should be manipulated, the deficit also impairs one's ability to identify whether another person is using the object appropriately (e.g., hammering a nail with a screwdriver).

Some claim that ideational apraxia is present only for transitive gestures, such as manipulating tools. Others argue that ideational apraxia cannot be reliably distinguished from ideomotor apraxia and that it is simply a more extreme form of the latter. In practice, the distinction is a very difficult one to make. Reconsider the example of using a screwdriver as a hammer. If you were assessing someone with left hemisphere damage and the person made this error, how would you interpret it? Is the person misidentifying the screwdriver as a hammer? Is he or she correctly identifying the screwdriver but forgetting the correct movement pattern associated with the tool? Dissociating ideational and motor programming problems is extremely difficult, but most neuropsychologists agree that the disorders result from different functional deficits (Heilman & Rothi, 1993).

CONSTRUCTIONAL APRAXIA. Constructional apraxia was described as early as the beginning of the twentieth century by Rieger (1909), although the term itself was coined later by Kleist (1934) (Rogers, 1996). **Constructional apraxia** is an inability to construct a complex object, wherein one cannot arrange the elements of the object correctly. It is a deficit in processing the spatial aspects of the task, but the movements that are required can be performed correctly. The deficit is not caused by a problem in perceiving the objects, nor is it a problem in performing voluntary actions. Instead, the deficit seems to stem from the inability to use visuoperceptual information to guide voluntary action.

ORAL APRAXIA. **Oral apraxia** is an inability to perform skilled movements of the face, lips, cheeks, tongue, pharynx, or larynx following a command (Rogers, 1996). This disorder (also called *buccofacial apraxia*) was first described by Hughlings-Jackson (1870). His patient was unable to stick out her tongue or cough when asked to do so by the examiner, but she could perform all of these movements when eating normally (Martin, 1998). Other tests that are used to detect oral apraxia include asking the person to pretend to suck on a straw, blow a kiss, yawn, or clear one's throat. Many of these oral gestures have meanings, but if individuals with oral apraxia are asked to mimic meaningless oral gestures, they are just as impaired. However, when objects are introduced (such as a straw) as props for the commanded movement, their performance improves (Heilman & Rothi, 1993).

LIMB APRAXIA. **Limb apraxia** is an impairment in fine or precise movements of the limbs. Tasks such as coin flipping, alternately tapping a stylus on two sides of a line, or repeatedly tapping a finger are all extremely difficult for someone with this disorder (Martin, 1998). In more practical terms, individuals with limb apraxia are impaired when using common objects such as scissors or screwdrivers. The types of actions that are affected can be relatively complex or simple. For example, one task that is problematic for limb apraxics is maintaining a fist with one hand and an open palm with the other, then alternating which hand holds which position (Luria, 1966). The ability to make more complicated movements, such as imitating meaningless hand gestures or novel hand positions, is also impaired (Lehmkuhl, Poeck, & Willmes, 1983; Pieczuro & Vignolo, 1967). The types of errors that are committed by a person with limb apraxia vary considerably, but one common type of error involves the substitution of a body part for the object whose use is being mimicked. For example, when asked to pantomime stirring a cup of tea with a spoon, the individual might extend the index finger (representing the absent spoon) followed by a stirring motion rather than mimicking grasping a spoon and stirring the liquid with it (Banich, 1997).

Because limb apraxia shares some symptoms with paresis (in which movement is impaired for a specific region of the body), some question whether limb apraxia is a genuine apraxia (Rogers, 1996). Remember that our definition of apraxia specified that the disorder cannot be attributable to primary sensory problems, paralysis or muscle weakness, or some other motor disturbance (such as tremor).

DRESSING APRAXIA. As you might guess from its name, **dressing apraxia** is a deficit in dressing oneself. The difficulties appear to stem both from problems in orienting limbs correctly while dressing and from problems in manipulating the clothes themselves. Remarkably, an individual who exhibits dressing apraxia does not normally exhibit other apraxic symptoms typical of ideomotor or ideational apraxia (Krasyuk & Rivchina, 1968; Mendez, 2001; Morera, Gonzalez-Feria, Valenciano, & Sabat, 1989). Assessing dressing apraxia can be difficult. Different people wear different kinds of clothes, and some clothes are much easier to manipulate than others. In addition to socioeconomic variables that influence what people wear, there are also (decreasingly obvious) sex differences. Women's clothing tends to be more complicated than that of men. Another complication is that the neuropsychological examination typically does not involve undressing and dressing, unlike the typical physical examination performed by a physician. To address these problems, Morera and colleagues (1989) developed a standardized test of dressing apraxia that requires individuals to put on a cardigan-style garment. There is little doubt that Mr. Rogers would have performed well on this test!

I am somewhat hesitant to include a discussion of dressing apraxia in this module on sensorimotor disorders because there is currently a debate about whether the disorder is primarily motor or spatial. It typically emerges following *right* parietal lobe lesions (in contrast to the forms of apraxia just described, which typically emerge following *left* hemisphere damage), but it is usually expressed bilaterally (Morera-Fumero

& Rodriguez, 1990; Takayama, Sugishita, Hirose, & Akiguchi, 1994). Because dressing apraxia can be accompanied by disorders of attention (such as hemispatial neglect) and visual attentive or constructive disorders (Mendez, 2001), some have argued that it is primarily a disorder of spatial attention rather than controlling movement.

Another aspect of dressing apraxia that makes it relatively unique is the fact that the movements we make while dressing tend to be relatively automatic. Of course, the act of dressing oneself was not automatic at first. Seeing the frustration on the face of a child who is trying to tie his or her shoes or remove a heavy coat is evidence of how effortful dressing can be. However, as we acquire practice, these behaviors become so well learned that we lose our conscious memory of all the little steps that are required. Can you describe, in words, exactly how to tie your shoes? Can you describe it without acting it out first? If not, you probably rely heavily on implicit memory to do it (we will discuss implicit memory in Chapter 8). In contrast, most of the apraxic behaviors described previously concern consciously controlled, explicit memory-driven movements.

CALLOSAL APRAXIA. More than thirty people have exhibited left-hand apraxia following damage to the corpus callosum (DeRenzi & Faglioni, 1999; Faglioni & Basso, 1985). Unlike most apraxias, which produce bilateral symptoms, **callosal apraxia** is the selective impairment in performing skilled left-hand movements or manipulating objects with the left hand in response to a command. (Recall that Liepmann's patient Mr. T. was apraxic for *right* limb movements.) Callosal apraxia is characterized by both ideational and ideomotor symptoms, although the deficit is most severe when left-hand movements must be evoked rather than imitated (Graff-Radford, Welsh, & Godersky, 1987). Some have suggested that this disorder is the result of a disconnection between the left hemisphere, which is specialized for fine-motor sequencing (particularly in response to linguistic commands), and the right hemisphere, which controls the left hand (Banich, 1997; Rubens, Geschwind, Mahowald, & Mastri, 1977).

These two regions are normally connected through the corpus callosum. However, in a group of people suffering very similar corpus callosum lesions, only some developed callosal apraxia. Epileptic patients who have had their corpus callosum severed to treat their seizures sometimes develop some degree of callosal apraxia, but the deficit emerges only when the instruction or relevant information is presented to the left hemisphere. When the right hemisphere receives the information directly, the left-hand movements are appropriate and accurate (Gazzaniga et al., 1967; Risse, Gates, Lund, Maxwell, & Rubens, 1989; Volpe, Sidtis, Holtzman, Wilson, & Gazziniga, 1982; Zaidel & Sperry, 1977). Studies of people born without a corpus callosum (a condition called **callosal agenesis,** described in detail in Chapter 4) are difficult to reconcile with the results described above. When the corpus callosum is damaged, left-hand apraxia often (but not always) results. However, in individuals who have never had a corpus callosum, there might be some evidence of impairments in transferring learned motor skills from one hand to the other, but these individuals do not appear to exhibit callosal apraxia (Ettlinger, Blakemore, Milner, & Wilson, 1972; Lassonde, Sauerwein, & Lepore, 1995; Rogers, 1996).

GAZE APRAXIA. Gaze apraxia (also called *ocular apraxia*) is apraxia specific to eye movements. It is just one of the symptoms of a syndrome called the **Bálint–Holmes syndrome** (discussed in detail in Chapter 11). Although people with gaze apraxia can move their eyes in any direction, they cannot shift their gaze *intentionally* to fixate on an object or point in space. When given instructions to look at a specific location, they might make random eye movements or even look in the wrong direction. If they eventually manage to fixate on the object, the fixation is very difficult to maintain and can be lost quickly. Bálint–Holmes syndrome is typically caused by bilateral lesions to the parieto-occipital junction (posterior parietal lobe and lateral occipital lobe). These lesions are often caused by **ischemia,** but individuals in the early stages of Alzheimer's dementia can also exhibit Bálint–Holmes syndrome. When people in the early stages of dementia exhibit the syndrome, functional imaging shows a selective bilateral reduction in metabolism by parietal and occipital cortical regions (Pietrini et al., 1996).

ALIEN LIMB SYNDROME. The **alien limb syndrome** (often referred to as *alien hand syndrome* because it usually affects one of the hands) is one of the strangest disorders in neuroscience. Here, the individual believes that one of the limbs is acting out of his or her control. The affected limb makes complex but involuntary movements, many of which are quite disturbing to the affected individual. The movements can even be dangerous and hurtful. In one case of an 81-year-old woman, the alien limb made choking and striking movements toward the neck and head region (Ay, Buonanno, Price, Le, & Koroschetz, 1998). In an effort to control these involuntary movements, people with alien limb syndrome adopt all sorts of behavioral strategies. One such strategy is to instruct the limb verbally (in the second person), or even berate it for its irreverent actions. Another strategy is to restrain the alien limb with the other, "good" limb, resulting in bilateral competition, also called *intermanual conflict.* Damage to the right parietal lobe has been associated with alien limb syndrome (Dolado, Castrillo, Urra, & De-Seijas, 1995). However, a number of cases have also been presented in which the damage is clearly to regions of the corpus callosum (Chan & Liu, 1999; Geschwind et al., 1995) or mesial frontal regions (Chan & Liu, 1999).

◀ **WHERE WE HAVE BEEN** We reviewed the features of several cortical motor disorders. Apraxia is a deficit in performing skilled movements that is not attributable to primary sensory problems, paralysis or muscle weakness, or other primary motor problems. The four major classes of apraxia are ideomotor, ideational, constructional, and oral.

WHERE WE ARE GOING ▶ In the following sections, we detail some cortical disorders that are primarily somatosensory in nature, including astereognosia (a deficit in perceiving objects by touch) and phantom sensation (in which an individual perceives a form of tactile hallucination.

ASTEREOGNOSIA. **Astereognosia** is characterized by a deficit in perceiving (recognizing, naming) objects through tactile stimulation, but basic tactile sensation remains intact (Gordon, 1926; Guillain & Bize, 1932; Stolboun, 1934). Object recognition is something we rarely do on the basis of touch alone, but the recognition of some common objects (such as a pen or spoon) using touch alone is relatively easy for neurologically normal individuals. This is not so for individuals with astereognosia. The disorder should remind you of the visual agnosias that we discussed in Chapter 4, and it should not surprise you that astereognosia is also called *somatosensory agnosia*. To make matters even more confusing, the disorder also goes by the names *tactile asymbolia* and *tactile agnosia* (Reed & Caselli, 1994). In terms of its clinical features, object recognition using other sensory modalities remains relatively intact, and people with astereognosia can rely on these other sensory modalities to perform some object recognition tasks. For example, an individual who is allowed to explore an object using touch alone might be able to identify the object by drawing a picture of what he or she can feel and then identify the item on the basis of the picture. Recognition of the basic features of an object by touch, such as size, weight, and texture, remain intact, but recognition of the object is impaired. The disorder is thought to be caused by parietal lobe (somatosensory cortex) lesions (Binkofski, Kunesch, Classen, Seitz, & Freund, 2001). However, these lesions tend to be located in the association cortex (such as Brodmann areas 39 and 40 in the inferior parietal lobe) rather than the primary sensory cortex. This is consistent with the behavioral observations that people with astereognosia exhibit a high-level recognition disorder but no primary sensory problems.

PHANTOM SENSATION. The brain is an extraordinarily flexible organ, capable of substantial physical and functional changes following injury to the brain or the rest of the body. Many of these transformations are beneficial, compensatory changes that help to lessen the impact of injury. However, not all of the changes that the brain is capable of making are good. One such example is that of **phantom sensation.** Phantom sensation is not "real" in that it exists without primary sensory input. However, it is quite real in that the perceiver cannot distinguish between phantom sensations and normal sensations. This description might remind you of hallucinations; phantom sensations resemble hallucinations in a variety of ways. Someone who is experiencing a visual hallucination "sees" stimuli that are not present. The most common type of phantom sensation is **phantom limb pain,** which follows the amputation of part (or all) of a limb. The perceived pain is not concentrated at the point of amputation, but rather inside the body part that is no longer present. For example, after amputation of one's hand at the wrist, one might experience strong pain in the thumb of the missing hand. The pain exists without sensory input, just as a visual hallucination is perceived without visual stimulation. Unfortunately, phantom limb pain is not an extremely rare disorder. In fact, over two thirds of all amputees experience it after the surgery (Gallagher, Allen, & MacLachlan, 2001).

One important clue about the cause of phantom sensations came from a study by Professor Vilayanur Ramachandran and colleagues at the University of California at San Diego (Ramachandran, Stewart, & Rogers-Ramachandran, 1992). In this study, the sensory abilities of several people were tested by stroking parts of their bodies with cotton swabs and then asking them to identify which body part was being

the **Real** world

Grow Your Own Phantom Hand!

It takes only a few minutes to "grow" your own phantom hand. Try the following demonstration, described by Haseltine (2002). You will need the following items:

- A partner
- This textbook
- A desk or table
- A wire coat hanger that you don't mind wrecking

Step 1. Bend the hanger in the middle into a two-pronged fork.

Step 2. While seated at your desk or table, open this book to the page with the picture of the full-size hand (p. 523). (Figure 5.12 serves as a model.)

Step 3. Place your left hand next to the hand in the picture, in the same orientation. Cover your real hand with the cover of the book, such that you can see only the model hand (p. 523).

Step 4. Have your partner tap both your hand and the picture of the hand simultaneously. The tapping should be repeated, covering much of the area of the hand, but the pattern should not be too regular. Instead, try to tap using a random pattern. Continue this for a few minutes. During this period, you will probably start to sense your own hand shifting toward the hand in the book. Don't worry; this is normal. Your partner should continue the random tapping for another few minutes.

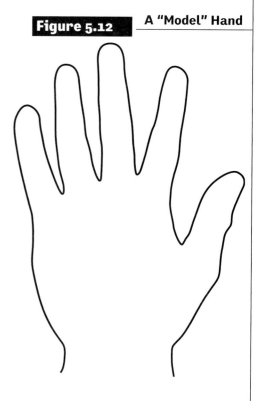

Figure 5.12   A "Model" Hand

Step 5. After you start to feel the sensation of the tapping of the drawing, your partner should try to tap *only* the drawing some of the time, without warning you. Even though the hanger is no longer touching your real hand on the taps, you should continue to sense the contacts.

Step 6. Reverse roles with your partner. Repeat steps 1–5. If you are feeling devious and you want to take out some of your academic frustrations on your textbook for this course, keep a sharp pencil nearby. Once your partner reports sensing contacts with the drawing, without warning take the pencil and stab the picture of the hand (not the real hand!). Your partner may not actually feel the pain of the contact, but the act should really get his or her heart racing! Repair the damage to your book, or buy another copy.

How does this work? According to Matthew Botvinick, who developed a procedure similar to this (Botvinick & Cohen, 1988), our awareness of our body parts is acquired knowledge rather than hard-wired knowledge that we are born with. The learning is accomplished through repeated sensory experiences, combining our tactile sensations with visual and auditory input. The more often the information from these different senses agrees, the stronger the association becomes. In the preceding demonstration, the tactile sensation of being touched with the hanger was linked with the visual sensation of the picture of the hand in this book being touched. Therefore, your brain learned to make an association between tactile feedback and the visual sensation of seeing the picture of the hand being touched.

touched. When examining one young man, Ramachandran touched him with the cotton swab, and the man replied, "Left finger." When touched in another spot, the man replied, "Left thumb." These answers might not seem remarkable to you, but they were truly amazing because the man no longer had a left arm. Ramachandran was stroking the left side of the man's face with the cotton swab.

This section on phantom sensation began with the statement that the brain is an extraordinarily flexible organ and that this flexibility is not always beneficial. Ramachandran's experiment details just how flexible the brain can be. Why would sensation on the face be interpreted as sensation from a missing limb? Take another look at Figure 5.7. Note the part of the cortex devoted to sensory input from the face, and then note the part normally devoted to sensation from the hand. They are adjacent to one another. The phantom sensations appear to be the result of cortical reorganization wherein areas that no longer receiving sensory input (e.g., areas devoted to a recently amputated arm) start to accept sensory input from adjacent projections. This finding has implications for the treatment of phantom limb pain. If the precise location of the remapping is known (e.g., the face–hand mapping described previously), one could reasonably speculate that pain-treating methods (such as acupuncture) could be applied to the remapped area in hopes of dampening the phantom pain.

Self-Test

1. What does it mean when a disorder is "defined by exclusion"?

2. What is the difference between ideomotor and ideational apraxia?

3. Was Mr. T. apraxic for movements of his left side, right side, or both?

4. What is alien limb syndrome?

5. What causes phantom sensations? Are they normal?

Subcortical Sensorimotor Disorders

PARKINSON'S DISEASE. In 1817, James Parkinson described a new movement disorder as follows:

> Involuntary tremulous motion, with lessened muscular power, in parts not in action . . . with a propensity to bend the trunk forward and to pass from a walking to a running pace, the senses and intellects being uninjured. . . . The first symptoms perceived are a slight sense of weakness, with a proneness to trembling . . . most commonly in one of the hands and arms. These symptoms gradually increase in the part first affected, and at an uncertain period, but seldom less than 12 months or more, the morbid influence is felt in some other part . . . or limb. (Parkinson, 1817, pp. 1–3, as quoted by Bradshaw & Mattingley, 1995, p. 290)

As it is described today, **Parkinson's disease** is characterized by four major symptoms. Perhaps the best-known symptom is **tremor at rest.** This type of tremor is caused by alternating contractions in musculature when the person is not initiating any movement. Typically, it first involves the shaking of the hands. As the disease progresses, tremor can also be evident in the lower limbs and the face. The tremors are most noticeable in a limb when it is supported. The tremors appear to get worse when an individual is under stress, and they cease during sleep. Because it is a rest tremor, the tremor subsides when an individual initiates movement (e.g., picking up a kettle to pour some tea). This is quite unlike the features of **action tremor,** in which the shaking is worse when movement is initiated. The second major symptom is **akinesia,** which refers to a general loss in movement (**bradykinesia** is a lesser form of akinesia, referring to a slowness of movement). People with Parkinson's disease have difficulty initiating movements, particularly whole-body movements such as getting up out of a chair. Akinesia can also be observed *during* a movement. For example, one typical symptom is the reduction or absence of normal actions such as the swinging of ones arms while walking. Akinesia also appears for relatively reflexive movements, such as eye blinking. The third hallmark feature of the disorder is **rigidity,** in which passive movement is resisted because of chronically contracted muscles. The affected individual tends not to notice this symptom as much as its result, which is a slowness of movement. The fourth feature of Parkinson's disease is a **disturbance of posture.** This feature is most noticeable in an individual's style of walking (called **gait**). People who have Parkinson's disease have difficulty maintaining their balance and tend to walk in very small steps, leaning forward slightly. The unsteadiness is particularly evident in turning.

In terms of its neuropathology, Parkinson's disease primarily affects subcortical structures. The first major breakthrough in understanding the neural basis of the disease came in 1919, when Treatikoff was working on his thesis for a doctorate in medicine (Treatikoff, 1974). He performed autopsies on nine people who died during the later stages of Parkinson's disease. He found that a part of the midbrain that is normally quite dark (an area called the *substantia nigra,* which means "dark substance") was not very dark in comparison to normal brains, suggesting that this region had degenerated. His suspicion of this target region grew even stronger when he examined the brain of a person whose Parkinson's disease was present only on one side of the body. In this case, only half of the substantia nigra showed signs of degeneration—the half on the side opposite to the symptoms. We now know that most of the neural degeneration in Parkinson's disease happens along the striatal dopamine pathway, which extends from the substantia nigra to the components of the basal ganglia (caudate, putamen, and globus pallidus). Although most of the degeneration is localized here, there also appears to be damage to the locus coeruleus.

Localizing the site of neurodegeneration in Parkinson's disease was certainly informative, but it was not very helpful for treating Parkinson's disease (at least not yet—more on that later in this section). The first major discovery that helped to inform the treatment of Parkinson's disease came in the 1960s. Also performing autopsies on people who died during the later stages of the disease, Ehringer and Hornykiewicz (1960) found that dopamine levels in the basal ganglia were far lower than normal. Therefore, the obvious therapeutic strategy would be to try to supplement the endogenous levels of dopamine. This strategy was also employed in the 1960s. Unfortunately, dopamine itself cannot be used as treatment because it does not cross the blood–brain barrier when administered orally. However, treating Parkinson's disease patients with L-dopa (a precursor of dopamine that is decarboxylated in the substantia nigra) reduces the symptoms dramatically (Cotzias, Papacasiliou, & Gellene, 1969; Tolosa, Marti, Valldeoriola, & Molinuevo, 1998). This type of treatment is initially effective in reducing the symptoms in 85% of people with Parkinson's disease, but the drugs become less and less effective with time, even when the dosage is increased.

In addition to drug therapies, two types of surgical treatments have also been developed. The more commonly used surgical treatment is to intentionally lesion another part of the motor system. It might sound crazy, but surgeons can facilitate movement and reduce unwanted movement by lesioning various parts of the brain. One such procedure is called a **thalamotomy** (also called a *stereotaxic coagulation*). It involves lesioning one side of the thalamus in hopes of reducing unilateral tremor, and it has proven to be effective in over 80% of operated cases (Dawson, 2000). Thalamotomies are not very effective at treating akinesia/bradykinesia or rigidity. For these symptoms, another surgical procedure, called a **pallidotomy,** is used. In this procedure, a lesion (typically a heat lesion) is created in the globus pallidus. As is the case with thalamotomy, over 80% of patients who receive a pallidotomy improve significantly. This procedure can be performed bilaterally or even in conjunction with a thalamotomy (Dawson, 2000; Obeso, Guridi, & DeLong, 1997).

Pallidotomy and thalamotomy were developed starting in the late 1950s, but another, much more controversial surgical strategy has been pioneered more recently. It involves the attempted replacement of the damaged or dead cells. Parkinson's disease is a relatively uncommon neurodegenerative disorder in that the cell death is very specific. Other conditions, such as Alzheimer's disease, are characterized by widespread cell loss, though some areas are more affected than others. In Parkinson's disease, the vast majority of the cell loss is in the 500,000 or so neurons located in the substantia nigra (compared to the 50 billion neurons elsewhere in the brain). This feature makes the disease amenable to cell transplants. A few different types of transplant have been investigated. One strategy has been to graft cells from the adrenal medulla to the substantia nigra in hopes that these cells will continue to produce dopamine. The people who have received this surgery so far have demonstrated very modest improvements (Ostrosky-Solis, Quintanar, Madrazo, Drucker-Colin, Franco-Bourland, & Leon-Meza, 1991). Another, more controversial strategy has been to transplant fetal tissue (obtained from voluntarily or spontaneously aborted fetuses) into the substantia nigra. The controversy that surrounds this procedure is largely an ethical debate about the abortion of human fetuses. That issue is certainly an important one, but it is beyond the scope of our discussion here.

The reported efficacy of fetal tissue transplantation has varied considerably but has mostly been positive. Some patients appear to be much better after the surgery; others do not. When benefits are detected, their longevity has also come into question (Hauser et al., 1999). Perhaps the new cells differentiate and become functional, only to succumb to the processes that killed the cells that were there in the first place. Some investigators have even questioned whether the perceived benefits of the surgery are due to a placebo effect (Hauser et al., 1999). In any event, if any neurodegenerative disorder can be treated by transplanting neural tissue, Parkinson's disease is the perfect test case for this procedure because of the extent to which its neurodegeneration is localized.

What causes Parkinson's disease? The short answer is that we do not know. There certainly appears to be a genetic component, at least in some cases of Parkinsonism. Gene mutations (missense mutations in the gene encoding the alpha-synuclein protein) have been found in families with a seemingly inherited form of Parkinson's disease, and various mutations of the *parkin* gene have been discovered in families with a rare juvenile form of Parkinson's disease (Haass & Kahle, 2001; Polymeropoulos,

Current Controversy

Designer Heroin and Parkinson's Disease

During the mid-1980s, seven young adults (20–30 years of age) were hospitalized in California because they were exhibiting the classic symptoms of the latter stages of Parkinson's disease. This was extremely puzzling to their attending physicians. How could they have Parkinson's disease? They were much too young. Furthermore, Parkinson's disease develops slowly; it does not appear suddenly. What was the matter with these patients? After very careful investigating, it was discovered that all seven people had injected some synthetic heroin that had been made in the same batch and sold on the streets during the summer of 1982. However, this was no ordinary batch of street heroin. This particular batch had

not been made correctly (the process was rushed), and it accidentally contained a compound called 1-methyl-4-phenyl-1,2,3,6-tetrahydropyridine, abbreviated as MPTP (Langston, 1985). When MPTP is metabolized by a primate (but not mice), it gets converted into methylphenylpyridinium (MPP+) which is toxic to dopamine-producing cells (Langston, 1985; Ricaurte, Langston, Delanney, Irwin, Peroutka, & Forno, 1986). Most of these cells are concentrated in the substantia nigra, so this chemical selectively destroys these cells. This discovery had a major impact on Parkinson's disease research. First, it provided researchers with an experimental model for the disease such that it could be simulated in nonhuman animals, further allowing the exploration of alternative treatments. Second, it highlighted the possibility that normally occurring Parkinson's disease was the result of an environmental toxin.

2000). It is possible that this gene leads to the formation of a substance that is particularly toxic for the substantia nigra. However, it is also possible that Parkinson's disease is caused by exposure to an environmental toxin. One of the strengths of these arguments is that Parkinson's disease appears to be a relatively new phenomenon. If one looks closely through historical medical records and detailed descriptions of behavior, one can find descriptions of most central nervous disorders (Huntington's disease, Tourettes syndrome, schizophrenia), even if they are not named as such. This is not the case for Parkinson's disease. Given its easily identifiable characteristics (such as rest tremor), one might reasonably expect to find a description that resembles Parkinson's disease from 300 or more years ago. The position that the disorder is caused by a new and prevalent environmental toxin (pesticides are one class of chemicals that have been implicated) is bolstered by the relatively recent emergence of the disorder (Koller, 1991). Other candidate causes for Parkinson's disease include syphilis, carbon monoxide poisoning, and the formation of tumors. It is widely suspected that Parkinson's disease usually results from the combination of a genetic predisposition and an as yet unidentified environmental trigger (Hubble et al., 1998).

HUNTINGTON'S CHOREA. George Huntington studied a degenerative motor disorder that appeared in families in Long Island, New York. Huntington first saw the disease long before he published his paper "On Chorea" in 1872. When he was 8 years old, he was driving with his father when he saw two thin, tall women twisting and grimacing from "that disorder." His memory of that day had such an impact on him that when he became a physician (like his father and grandfather), Huntington went on to study the disorder. He was only 22 years of age when he published his first complete description of the disorder in 1872 (Huntington, 1872; Kolb & Whishaw, 1996).

The disorder now called **Huntington's chorea** is characterized by dancelike, writhing movements and intellectual deterioration resulting from a genetic abnormality. The term *chorea* is from the Greek word meaning "to dance," and it helps to characterize the jerky and apparently coordinated yet involuntary movements that unceasingly plague individuals with the disorder (Banich, 1997). These abnormal movements are not present early in life. The gene that causes the disease always expresses itself (it is dominant), but it typically does not do so until the affected individual is 30 or 40 years of age. Once symptoms appear, the disease tends to progress for ten to fifteen years before eventually resulting in death. Initially, the involuntary movements are very slight and often consist of incessant fidgeting. The movements themselves do not involve single muscles. Instead, they typically involve entire limbs. As the disease progresses, sustaining muscular contractions (such as sticking out one's tongue) becomes impossible. Eventually, purposeful movement (including speech) becomes severely impaired. In addition to the motor symptoms, the disease produces changes in personality, memory, and processing speed.

The cerebral changes associated with Huntington's chorea are extensive. We placed our discussion of the disorder in this section on subcortical motor disorders because the most obvious deterioration is in the GABAergic neurons of the striatum (midbrain) and the basal ganglia. Functional imaging has also confirmed that basal ganglia activity is abnormal in Huntington's chorea (Harris et al., 1996). However, the disease also results in widespread cortical damage, particularly during its latter stages. The extent of these structural changes appears to correlate positively with the extent of functional abnormalities, including basic movements, complex fine-motor tasks (such as writing), and other cognitive impairments (Starkstein et al., 1988; Webb & Trzepacz, 1987).

The HD gene (whose mutation results in Huntington's chorea) was mapped to chromosome 4 in 1983 (Gusella et al., 1983). The mutation itself is called a *nucleotide triplet repeat,* and the DNA affected codes for the protein huntingtin. Too many copies of a sequence of nucleotides result in Huntington's chorea. An absence of the gene entirely results in a condition called *Wolf-Hirschhorn syndrome.* In the case of Huntington's chorea, as the number of repeated triplets of nucleotides (e.g., cytosine, adenine, guanine = CAG) increases, the earlier the age of onset for the disease. To make matters worse, the relatively unstable trinucleotide repeat can actually get longer when it is passed from parent to child, progressively decreasing the age of onset as the disease is handed down from generation to generation. The discovery of the HD gene paved the way for the development of a new test that allows those with Huntington's chorea in their family to determine whether they carry the gene. As is the case with so much modern genetic research, this development led to a complicated debate on how (if at all) this test should be used. The late age of onset for the disorder (30–40 years of age) complicates matters even further because most people who become parents have children before they develop any symptoms of the disease. If the parent develops the disease, his or her children have a 50% chance of also developing the disease. This pattern of inheritance has made Huntington's chorea relatively easy to trace back through the centuries. It was not recognized as a distinct medical condition before Huntington identified it, but there certainly are behavioral descriptions that match Huntington's chorea that predate Huntington. Vessie has traced the disease to the village of Bures, England, in 1630 (Vessie, 1932). Some people have even suggested that the infamous witches of Salem may have suffered from Huntington's chorea, and that the disease led to their persecution.

GILLES DE LA TOURETTE SYNDROME. The syndrome first described by George Gilles de la Tourette in 1885 and now known as **Gilles de la Tourette syndrome** (also called *Tourette's syndrome*) is characterized by **motor tics** and **vocal tics.** The motor tics are involuntary and often repetitive movements such as head jerking, blinking, shrugging, grimacing, or spastic movements of the hands and arms. Typical vocal tics include the repetition of words (called *palilalia*), compulsive repetition of words spoken by others (*echolalia*), uttering obscenities (called *coprolalia*), and various nonlinguistic vocalizations such as sniffing, snorting, or crying. Before Tourette's description of the disorder (Gilles de la Tourette, 1885), symptoms such as these were often viewed as symptoms of hysteria. Unlike the two subcortical motor disorders that we have already discussed in this module, the symptoms of Tourette's syndrome emerge relatively early in life. The disorder often emerges before 11 years of age, and it is three times more common in males than in females. As people with Tourette's syndrome age, it is quite common for the tics to increase in complexity. What may start out as a repetitive and spastic gesture may evolve into a gesture that appears to be more purposeful. For example, a spastic hand movement toward the face might change into a grooming movement by which an individual adjusts his or her hair repeatedly. Most of these changes are probably purposeful strategies by the person with Tourette's syndrome to mask the disorder. Making the movements appear to be intentional and useful makes them less noticeable to others.

Although the genetic basis of Tourette's syndrome has not been as clearly identified as that of Huntington's chorea, Tourette's syndrome also appears to run in families. Over one third of people with the syndrome also have an afflicted family member. However, the pattern of inheritance is not clear, and like many other disorders, it might arise from a gene–environment interaction (State, Pauls, & Leckman, 2001). In terms of localizing the genetic abnormality, it appears to be sex-linked (remember that it is three times more prevalent in males), and some investigators have linked the disorder with a gene on chromosome 18. The neurological abnormalities that are associated with the disorder are largely (but not exclusively) subcortical. People with Tourette's syndrome tend to have reduced basal ganglia volume (Hyde, Stacey, Coppola, Handel, Rickle, & Weinberger, 1995; Singer et al., 1993), but recent work suggests that this difference is not present in females with Tourette's (Zimmerman, Abrams, Giuliano, Denckla, & Singer, 2000). Suspicion of basal ganglia involvement in the disorder has also been supported by studies of the effects of basal ganglia lesions. When these structures are damaged through other means (such as tumors or strokes), tics often result. In terms of treatment, Tourette's syndrome tends to be treated with drugs (such as haloperidol) that reduce dopamine and, to a lesser extent, norepinephrine transmission. However, drugs that act on other neurotransmitter systems, such as GABA agonists like Baclofen, have also been used to treat the disorder (Singer, Wendlandt, Krieger, & Giuliano, 2001).

Up to this point, we have been discussing Tourette's syndrome as if it appears in isolation. However, this is often not the case. Tourette's syndrome tends to be **comorbid** (i.e., to occur along with other disorders) with obsessive-compulsive disorder and attention-deficit hyperactivity disorder. Obsessive-compulsive disorder is characterized by unwanted obsessions and recurrent behaviors accompanied by an urge to do something to relieve the discomfort caused by the obsession. Although people with the disorder realize that their obsessions are excessive and/or unreasonable, the symptoms can be overwhelming, resulting in severe impairment and dysfunction. Half of all children with Tourette's syndrome exhibit some obsessive-compulsive behaviors; one quarter exhibit full-blown obsessive-compulsive disorder (Golden, 1990). Tourette's syndrome is also often comorbid with attention-deficit hyperactivity disorder (Jankovic, 2001). This condition is characterized by abnormal behavior in three categories: inattention, hyperactivity, and impulsivity. All three disorders (Tourette's syndrome, obsessive-compulsive disorder, and attention-deficit hyperactivity disorder) are associated with undesirable and nonintentional movements (such as tics). Further, all three disorder have been associated with basal ganglia dysfunction. However, all three disorders are also characterized by undesirable and nonintentional *thoughts*, suggesting that the basal ganglia are normally involved in behaviors that do not require movement.

TARDIVE DYSKINESIA. Unlike the disorders described previously, **tardive dyskinesia** is more of a side effect than a disorder. The drugs of choice for treating schizophrenia (such as haloperidol) block dopamine transmission. Although this is often an effective treatment for the condition, these drugs also have profound effects on the human motor system if they are taken over long periods of time. Tardive dyskinesia is a movement disorder that occurs in approximately 30% of long-term users of antipsychotic medications depending on their age and ethnic background (Chong, Mahendran, Machin, Chua, Parker, & Kane, 2002; Fenton, 2000; Glazer, 2000).

Given what you learned in the section on Parkinson's disease, you should reasonably expect that someone who is taking antidopaminergic medications should exhibit slow and laborious movements coupled with tremors. This is not the case. The symptoms of tardive dyskinesia do not look much like Parkinson's disease. Instead, the condition is characterized by an increase in spontaneous movement. Also unlike the case in Parkinson's disease, these movements tend to be most pronounced in the facial region (especially the mouth and lips), but more severe cases also exhibit symptoms in the limbs. The movements themselves resemble those produced by people with Huntington's chorea and the tics produced by people with Tourette's syndrome. At this point, you should be wondering why tardive dyskinesia is characterized by *increases* in movement rather than *decreases* in movement. Because the dopaminergic neurons in the substantia nigra are chronically understimulated when a person takes antidopaminergic medication for long periods, these neurons become supersensitive to stimulation. Therefore, when the receptors are stimulated, the result is unwanted movement.

The motor side effects of antipsychotic medications can be treated in a variety of ways. However, the most effective strategy in combating tardive dyskinesia is to avoid it in the first place. Once its symptoms develop, lowering the dose of the offending medication does not relieve the symptoms. Sometimes that even makes them worse. Therefore, first and foremost, the dosage of antipsychotic medications should be kept as low as possible such that the antipsychotic benefits of the drug can still be realized but the development of tardive dyskinesia is kept to a minimum. Once symptoms develop, they can sometimes be treated effectively with anticholinergic drugs.

Tardive dyskinesia is worrisome for a number of reasons. The fact that people develop permanent motor disorders as a side effect of their medication is clearly cause for concern. In response to these concerns, several new antipsychotic medications (such as risperidone) have been developed. Unfortunately, these newer-generation drugs are not without their risks. Even risperidone appears to contribute to the formation of tardive dyskinesia. The company that produces the drug was recently sued by a woman who developed the condition after a fourteen-month period on risperidone. The woman won a settlement of 6.7 million dollars. Another worrisome aspect of tardive dyskinesia is the fact that many schizophrenics refuse to take their antipsychotic medication out of fear that they will develop this disorder. Some of the newer drugs have certainly reduced the risk, but they have not eliminated it.

Curiously, tardive dyskinesia has also been observed in schizophrenics who have never been treated with any antipsychotic medications. McCreadie and colleagues (McCreadie, Thara, Padmarati, Srinivasan, & Jaipurkar, 2002) used MRI to study the neuroanatomical features of never-treated schizophrenic patients with dyskinesia compared with those who do not make abnormal movements. The group with dyskinesia exhibited more changes in the striatum compared with normal controls, whereas the schizophrenics without dyskinesia exhibited more global cortical atrophy.

Self-Test

1. What are the four major symptoms of Parkinson's disease?

2. What are some of the treatments for Parkinson's disease?

3. When do the symptoms of Huntington's chorea emerge? Why?

4. What are the features of Tourette's syndrome?

5. What causes tardive dyskinesia?

◀ **WHERE WE HAVE BEEN**

After reviewing the components and connectivity of the sensorimotor system, we reviewed some sensorimotor disorders caused by cortical disturbances. These conditions included apraxia, astereognosis, phantom sensation, and alien limb disorder. We also reviewed several motor disorders caused by subcortical disturbances including Parkinson's disease, Huntington's chorea, Gille de la Tourette syndrome, and tardive dyskinesia.

Glossary

Action tremor—Tremor that is worsened by the initiation of movements.

Akinesia—A general loss in movement; one of the four major symptoms of Parkinson's disease.

Alexia—A deficit in reading; an inability to read text.

Alien limb syndrome—A disorder that is characterized by an individual believing that one of his or her limbs is acting out of his or her control, because one of his or her limbs makes complex but involuntary movements; also known as *alien hand syndrome*.

Apraxia—A deficit in performing skilled voluntary movements that cannot be attributable to primary sensory problems, paralysis or muscle weakness, or some other motor disturbance; four major classes of apraxia are ideomotor, ideational, constructional, and oral.

Astereognosia—A disorder in which there is a deficit in perceiving (recognizing or naming) objects through tactile stimulation but basic tactile sensation remains intact; also known as *somatosensory agnosia, tactile asymbolia,* and *tactile agnosia.*

Bálint–Holmes syndrome—A syndrome that is typically caused by bilateral lesions to the parieto-occipital junction.

Basal ganglia—A subdivision of the telencephalon, which is divided into three components (caudate nucleus, putamen, and globus pallidus); an important component of the motor system that initiates movements and maintains muscle tone.

Bilateral apraxia—A deficit in performing skilled voluntary movements that affects both sides of the body and cannot be attributable to primary sensory problems, paralysis or muscle weakness, or some other motor disturbance.

Bradykinesia—A lesser form of akinesia that involves a slowness of movements.

Callosal agenesis—Being born without a corpus callosum.

Callosal apraxia—The selective impairment in performing skilled left-hand movements or manipulating objects with the left hand in response to a command.

Caudate nucleus—A component of the basal ganglia; along with the putamen, it is collectively known as the striatum and receives the vast majority of cortical inputs to the basal ganglia as well as projections from the substantia nigra.

Comorbid—When two or more diseases or disorders are diagnosed in one individual.

Constructional apraxia—A deficit that is characterized by an inability to construct complex objects, wherein an individual cannot arrange the elements of the object correctly.

Deep cerebellar nuclei—The collective term for the three nuclei of the cerebellum.

Dentate nuclei—Nuclei in the cerebellum that receive projections from the lateral zone.

Dermatomes—Different areas of the skin that are affected differently by each of the thirty dorsal roots of the spinal cord

Disturbance of posture—One of the four major symptoms of Parkinson's disease, in which the individual has difficulty maintaining his or her balance and tends to walk in very small steps, slightly bent over.

Dorsal root ganglia—Somatosensory nodules on dorsal roots that contain afferent spinal nerve neuron cell bodies; there is one dorsal root ganglion for each of the thirty pairs of spinal nerves.

Dorsal spinothalamic tract—Sensory pathway in the brain that is responsible for transmitting information about hapsis and proprioception; enters the spinal cord through the dorsal root ganglion and synapses ipsilaterally in the dorsal column nuclei of the spinal cord.

Dressing apraxia—A deficit that is characterized by an individual's difficulty with dressing himself or herself, which seems to stem from problems in orienting limbs correctly while dressing and problems in manipulating the clothes themselves while dressing.

Fastigial nuclei—Nuclei in the cerebellum that receive projections from the vermis.

Gait—An individual's style of walking.

Gaze apraxia—An apraxia that is specific to eye movements; it is a symptom of Bálint–Holmes syndrome and is also known as *ocular apraxia;* people who are diagnosed with gaze apraxia have the ability to move their eyes in any direction but cannot shift their gaze intentionally to fixate on an object or point in space.

Gilles de la Tourette syndrome (Tourette's syndrome)—A subcortical sensorimotor disorder first described by George Gilles de la Tourette in 1885, which is characterized by motor and vocal tics.

Globus pallidus—A component of the basal ganglia; acts as the primary output nucleus of the basal ganglia.

Hapsis—The sensations of fine touch and pressure; one of three types of somatic information, along with proprioception and nocioception.

Huntington's chorea—A subcortical sensorimotor disorder characterized by dancelike, writhing movements and intellectual deterioration that results from a genetic abnormality.

Ideational apraxia—A deficit that is characterized by an individual's confusion or loss of knowledge about an object's use, although the individual retains the ability to complete the individual elements required to perform the movement (e.g., hammering a nail with a screwdriver).

Ideomotor apraxia—A deficit that prevents an individual from executing simple gestures in response to a command or attempt to imitate (e.g., an inability to wave goodbye when asked).

Intermediate zone—One of the three zones of the cerebellum; similar to the lateral zone, it is found in both hemispheres of the cerebellum; it is specialized for guiding skilled limb movements (especially targeting actions, such as grasping or reaching).

Interpositus nuclei—Nuclei in the cerebellum that receive projections from the intermediate zone.

Ischemia—A condition caused by reduced or blocked blood flow to a tissue, which will lead to damage to that tissue.

Lateral corticospinal tract—One of two tracts in the lateral system; runs from the brainstem to the spinal cord to initiate and control movements; important for controlling limb movement and the extremities (e.g., fingers and toes).

Lateral system—One of two main systems of motor projections that descend from the brain to the spinal cord to initiate and control movement; consists of two tracts: one that runs from the brainstem (rubrospinal tract) and one that runs from the cortex (lateral corticospinal tract).

Lateral zone—One of the three zones of the cerebellum; similar to the intermediate zone, it is found in both hemispheres of the cerebellum; involved in coordinating multijoint movements, including ballistic movements (e.g., swinging a bat); also plays a role in the acquisition of motor skills and possibly involved in higher cognitive functions (e.g., language).

Lentiform nucleus—Collective term for the globus pallidus and the putamen.

Limb apraxia—An impairment in fine or precise movements of the limbs (e.g., flipping a coin).

Mechanoreceptors—Sensory receptors in the skin with many functions, including reacting to distortion and wrapping around the hairs that cover our bodies.

Motor tics—Involuntary and often repetitive movements (e.g., head jerking, blinking).

Neuralgia—Pain that does not result from any obvious lesion.

Nocioception—The sensation of pain and temperature; one of three types of somatic information, along with hapsis and proprioception.

Oral apraxia—A deficit that is characterized by an inability to perform skilled movements of the face, lips, tongue, cheeks, larynx, or pharynx following a command; also referred to as buccofacial apraxia.

Pallidotomy—A procedure that is used to treat the symptoms of akinesia or bradykinesia and rigidity,

in which a lesion is typically made in the globus pallidus.

Parkinson's disease—A subcortical sensorimotor disorder that is characterized by four symptoms (tremor at rest, akinesia, rigidity, and disturbance of posture).

Phantom limb pain—The most common type of phantom sensation; follows the amputation of part or all of a limb, and the perceived pain is not concentrated at the point of amputation but rather inside the body part that has been amputated.

Phantom sensation—Sensation that exists without primary sensory input; the perceiver has difficulty detecting which sensation is real and which is not.

Proprioception—Awareness of the body and its position; one of three types of somatic information, along with proprioception and hapsis.

Putamen—A component of the basal ganglia; along with the caudate nucleus, it is collectively known as the striatum and receives the vast majority of cortical inputs to the basal ganglia, as well as projections from the substantia nigra.

Reticulospinal tract—One of three tracts formed by the brainstem projections of the ventromedial system; important for maintaining posture.

Rigidity—Occurs when passive movement is resisted because of chronically contracted muscles; one of the four major symptoms of Parkinson's disease.

Rubrospinal tract—One of two tracts in the lateral system; runs from the brainstem to the spinal cord to initiate and control movements; important for making movements of the limbs and hands.

Somatosensory feedback—Information that is obtained from the sensory network that monitors the body's surface and its movements; the system includes joints, muscles, tendons, and skin.

Stereognosis—The ability to identify objects by touch; likely mediated by the connections between the primary motor cortex and somatosensory areas.

Striatum—Collective term for the caudate nucleus and the putamen; receives most of the motor input for the basal ganglia.

Tardive dyskinesia—A movement disorder in which an individual suffers from involuntary movements of the face and neck; more of a side effect than a disorder, it can occur after prolonged treatment of psychoses (e.g., schizophrenia) with antipsychotic medication.

Tectospinal tract—One of three tracts formed by the brainstem projections of the ventromedial system; important for controlling head and eye movements.

Thalamotomy—Also known as *stereotaxic coagulation*; a procedure used by surgeons to facilitate movement and reduce unwanted movements that involves lesioning one side of the thalamus in an attempt to reduce a unilateral tremor in Parkinson's disease patients.

Transected—Cut through.

Tremor at rest—Tremor caused by alternating contractions in musculature when an individual is not initiating any movement; it subsides once an individual initiates a movement; one of the four major symptoms of Parkinson's disease.

Unilateral apraxia—A deficit in performing skilled voluntary movements with only one side of the body that cannot be attributable to primary sensory problems, paralysis or muscle weakness, or some other motor disturbance; it normally affects the right side of the body.

Ventral corticospinal tract—The tract formed by the cortical projections of the ventromedial system; important for controlling the muscles of the trunk and upper legs, collectively used in tasks such as walking.

Ventral root ganglia—Motor nodules on ventral roots that contain efferent spinal nerve neuron cell bodies; there is one ventral root ganglion for each of the thirty pairs of spinal nerves.

Ventral spinothalamic tract—Sensory pathway in the brain that is responsible for transmitting nociceptive information; enters the spinal cord through the dorsal root ganglion, ascends the spinal cord contralaterally to the brainstem, where its axons join the medial lemniscus and ascend to the ventrolateral thalamus.

Ventromedial system—One of two main systems of motor projections that descend from the brain to the spinal cord to initiate and control movement; its brainstem projections form three tracts (vestibulospinal tract, reticulospinal tract, and tectospinal tract); its cortical projections form the ventrocortical spinal tract.

Vermis—One of the three zones of the cerebellum; it lies between the cerebellar hemispheres; involved with maintaining posture and coordinating whole-body movements.

Vestibulospinal tract—One of three tracts formed by the brainstem projections of the ventromedial system; important for maintaining balance.

Vocal tics—Repetition of words (palilalia), compulsive repetition of words spoken by others (echolalia), uttering obscenities (corprolalia), and various nonlinguistic vocalizations (e.g., sniffing, snorting).

Sensation and Perception:

Vision

Reality is merely an illusion, albeit a very persistent one.
—ALBERT EINSTEIN

Most of us take for granted our ability to see the world around us. Up appears to be up, water looks wet, and dogs do not look like cats. What if we were to tell you that much of what we "see" is in fact an illusion perpetrated by your brain? The complexity behind how our brain "sees" the world is overwhelming. Somehow, our brains take discrete wavelengths of light (sensation) and translate them into the phenomena that appears to us as the three-dimensional real world (perception). As we will see in this chapter, much of what we perceive as the real world is the result of an amazing series of transformations that begin at the eye and end in a variety of locations in the brain. The visual system does not produce an accurate internal copy of the external world. In fact, the visual system produces distorted, upside-down, backward, two-dimensional images that are interpreted by other parts of the visual system as the real world.

There are two basic aspects to the study of any sensory system: sensation and perception. **Sensation** refers to the detection of some aspect of a stimulus in the environment, whereas **perception** refers to the way in which we (or our brains) interpret the information that is gathered by the senses. In short, you sense the stimulus, although you perceive what it is. By necessity, perception relies on the information gathered by the senses, which include vision, audition, smell, taste, and proprioception. Sometimes perception can be fooled (such as with optical illusions), and the information that is provided by the senses affects perception. Sometimes, even when the sensation is correct, the perception will still be inaccurate. However, perception is not the simple translation of sensation into meaning, as context can affect these processes. For instance, have you ever watched a horror film and just about jumped out of your skin when an innocuous noise occurred (e.g., a telephone ringing)? Ordinarily, on hearing the ring of the telephone, you would have correctly interpreted the sound as a benign one. However, in the context of the horror film, the unexpected nature of the sound caused you to perceive the sound as a potential threat.

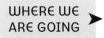
WHERE WE ARE GOING We are going to begin this chapter with a general examination of the organizing principles of sensory systems, followed by a specific discussion of how the visual system is organized. We will also discuss how disturbances in the visual system produce behavioral outcomes and what these behaviors tell us about the organization of the visual system.

MODULE **6.1**
Organization of Sensory Systems

Most sensory systems are organized in a similar fashion, and although this discussion will focus primarily on the visual system, for the most part these generalities also apply to the other senses. To understand organizational principles in sensory systems, the three main types of sensory cortex (primary, secondary, and association cortex) must be described first. The **primary sensory cortex** is the first part of the cortex that receives information relayed from the senses through the thalamus. Of the visual cortical areas, the primary cortex has the most direct access to the information provided by the sensory systems (e.g., eyes). The primary sensory cortex sends this information to secondary sensory cortical areas. As such, the **secondary sensory cortex** receives much of its information from the primary sensory cortex. Within each sensory modality, the secondary sensory cortex is highly interconnected, and thus the secondary sensory cortex also receives information from other areas of the secondary sensory cortex. The secondary sensory cortex sends its information to the association cortex. As you might guess by the name, the **association cortex** is any area of the cortex that receives information from more than one sense. As we will see, the regular manner with which information is received and disbursed through these three cortical areas suggests that sensory systems can be categorized into three organizing principles:

1. Sensory systems are characterized by hierarchical organization.
2. Each level of the organization contains functionally distinct cortical areas.
3. The processing of sensory information occurs in parallel throughout the cortex.

Hierarchical Organization

The first principle of sensory systems is that they are characterized by hierarchical organization. One way to understand this hierarchy is to use the example of the organization of a large business. In a large business, there may be one president. Often there are a number of vice presidents, each with a different responsibility (e.g., personnel, accounting). Below the vice presidents there may be a number of department heads, and below the department heads, the average working stiff. As we go down the hierarchy, the number of people increases, and the jobs become more and more specific. As we go up in the hierarchy, the jobs become more complex and involve the integration of more and varied information. However, regardless of where you look in the system, all jobs are important, and the loss of function at any level may result in chaos (which is why strikes by people who perform basic functions are so devastating).

This is also the way in which sensory systems are organized. At the level of the eye, there are a large number of very specialized receptors that have one function: to transform light into signals that are meaningful in the nervous system. At the level of the association cortex, the job is more complex: to integrate information from a number of sensory systems into a perception of the outside world. As we move from the lowest to the highest level of sensory systems, we also see that the neurons change from having simple on/off sensory functions to those that respond optimally to stimuli of greater complexity and specificity. The deficits that arise when the various levels are damaged are informative as to the function of each of the levels. If the eyes (basic sensory function) are removed (making the person unable to receive any visual sensory information), then the person is blind. However, as we climb the sensory hierarchy, we may see increasingly bizarre phenomena. For instance, damage to some areas of the visual association cortex in the temporal lobes may result in a person who can quite clearly see (the person can easily navigate through the environment) but who cannot provide verbal labels of the environment based on what he or she sees (Goodale, Milner, Jakobsen, & Carey, 1991).

Segregation by Function

Early reports of visual cortical function assumed that all areas at the same level of organization were performing the same functions (e.g., any area of the secondary visual cortex was equally involved in processing information from the primary visual cortex) (Figure 6.1). However, it now appears that all areas are *not* processing the same kind of information. In fact, within each of the three levels of the sensory cortex, there are specific areas that are involved in processing specific aspects of the same sensory stimulus. For instance, within the primary visual cortex there are cells that respond preferentially to color information and those that respond preferentially to specific orientations (e.g., Hubel, Wiesel, & Stryker, 1977). Although this feature of sensory system organization now seems obvious to us, this discovery about the visual cortex was sufficiently important to win a Nobel Prize (in 1981, in Physiology or Medicine) for researchers David Hubel and Torsten Wiesel. This type of functional segregation occurs at all three levels of the cortex in sensory systems (Figure 6.2).

Processing of Information in Parallel

Have you ever had a string of outdoor lights that would not light up if one bulb burned out? That string of lights was a serial circuit. If there was one break in the circuit (the burned-out bulb), none of the lights would turn on. Initially, sensory systems were viewed as serial circuits. That is, if one part of the circuit was missing, then the flow of information was stopped at the point at which the break occurred. However, as we will see in the next module, this is not how sensory systems transmit information.

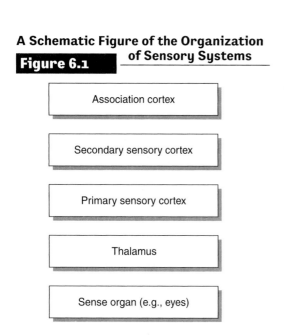

A Schematic Figure of the Organization of Sensory Systems

Figure 6.1

| Association cortex |
| Secondary sensory cortex |
| Primary sensory cortex |
| Thalamus |
| Sense organ (e.g., eyes) |

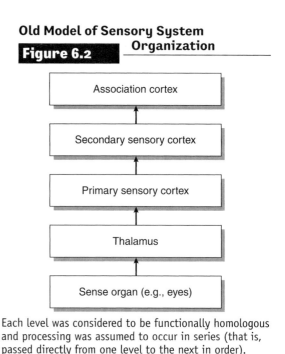

Old Model of Sensory System Organization

Figure 6.2

| Association cortex |
| Secondary sensory cortex |
| Primary sensory cortex |
| Thalamus |
| Sense organ (e.g., eyes) |

Each level was considered to be functionally homologous and processing was assumed to occur in series (that is, passed directly from one level to the next in order).

1. How are sensation and perception different? In what ways are they the same?

2. Does the brain produce a virtual representation of the outside world?

3. Are all areas within one level of sensory cortex processing the same information? Why or why not?

4. What do optical illusions tell us about sensation and perception?

Information is transmitted throughout the sensory system in parallel, each level receiving some information from the level immediately below it and some information from levels below that (Figure 6.3). When information is processed in parallel through multiple pathways, information flows through the levels of the sensory system rapidly and decreases the reliance of the system on any one level of processing. It is important to remember that the areas of sensory systems are very interconnected with each other (both within and between levels) and that although Figure 6.3 does not depict them, there are also descending connections between the levels.

◀ **WHERE WE HAVE BEEN**

We have distinguished between sensation and perception and have suggested that the brain does not simply reproduce the outside world inside your brain. We have also outlined the basic principles of all sensory systems, which are that sensory systems are organized hierarchically, that there is functional segregation within these levels, and that information is processed in parallel.

WHERE WE ARE GOING ▶

In the next module, we are going to examine the retino-geniculate-striate visual system and examine how this system is largely responsible for producing visual perception. We will also examine how the

A More Accurate View of the Organization of Sensory Systems

Figure 6.3

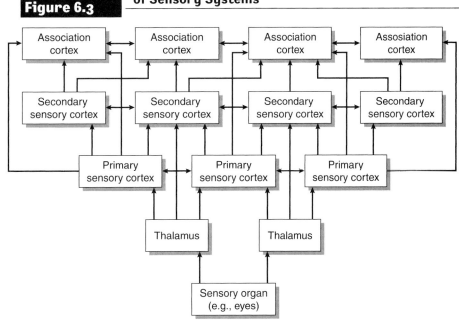

information is segregated beyond the primary visual cortex and examine the features of this segregation. In Module 6.3, we will examine disturbances in the visual system and how they produce their effects, as well as what these behaviors tell us about the organization of the visual system.

MODULE **6.2**
The Visual System

Light: Stimulus for the Visual System

Electromagnetic (EM) energy exists in a very wide range of frequencies. At very short wavelengths, EM energy forms high-energy gamma rays and X-rays; at very long wavelengths, it forms low energy radio waves. Somewhere in the middle (with wavelengths of about 400–700 nanometers), EM energy is visible to the human eye. Technically, all EM energy is "light," although the term *light* is usually used to refer to the relatively narrow band of EM energy that humans can sense with their eyes. The light that we see has two potential sources. We see either light coming directly from something that is producing it (such as the sun or a light bulb) or light that has traveled from a source to an object and is then reflected off the object or multiple objects. Perceptually, different wavelengths of light are perceived as different colors. Relatively short wavelengths appear violet, blue, or even green; longer wavelengths appear orange or red. Some other species can detect EM energy at higher or lower wavelengths than humans can. For example, a bee can detect lower frequencies of light (in the ultraviolet range) than humans can.

The Eye and Retina

Light enters the eye through the pupil and is focused on the **retina** by the curvature of the cornea and fine-tuned by the lens. The retina is a layered structure at the back of the eye that contains five different types of cells (receptors, horizontal cells, bipolar cells, amacrine cells, and retinal ganglion cells), each of which has a different function. **Receptors** are responsible for converting light energy into neural responses, which are then transmitted to the brain via the retinal ganglion cells. The receptors in the retina (rods and cones) are specialized and are active during different types of lighting conditions. Amacrine and horizontal cells are responsible for lateral communication between the various cells (e.g., communication between cones and other cones or retinal ganglion cells and other retinal ganglion cells). Bipolar cells synapse on the receptors, and they in turn synapse on the retinal ganglion cells, whose axons leave the retina via the optic nerve (Figure 6.4).

Rods are typically active in low light levels and are very sensitive to movement. Cones are typically active in medium to bright light and are responsible for high-acuity vision, or vision that provides rich details and color. Cones tend to synapse 1:1 on bipolar cells, which then synapse individually on retinal ganglion cells. As such, each retinal ganglion cell that synapses on a cone is quite sensitive to the activity of that cone. In contrast, although rods are exquisitely sensitive to small changes in the environment, they pay for this sensitivity by having low acuity. This presumably re-

Figure 6.4	A Schematic of the Five Kinds of Cells That Make Up the Retina

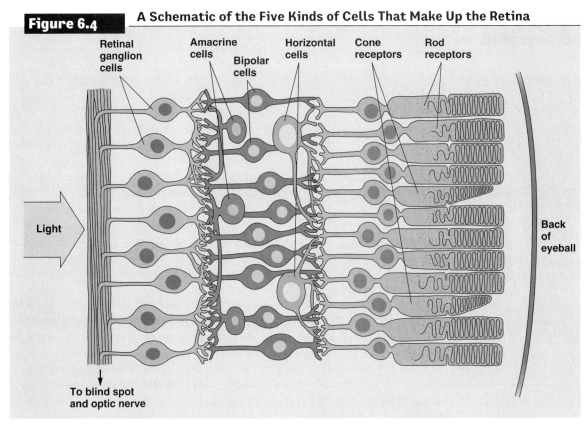

Source: John P. J. Pinel, *Biopsychology,* 5e. Published by Allyn and Bacon, Boston, MA. Copyright © 2003 by Pearson Education. Reprinted by permission of the publisher.

sults from having multiple rods synapse on one bipolar cell, which in turn converges on the same retinal ganglion cell with other bipolar cells. Table 6.1 offers a comparison of the features of rods and cones.

Table 6.1	A Comparison of Rods and Cones

Rods	Cones
Scotopic	Photopic
Active in dim light	Inactive in dim light
Inactive in bright light	Active in bright light
Very sensitive to small fluctuations in light	Insensitive to small fluctuations in light
Low acuity	High acuity
Insensitive to color and detail	Sensitive to color and detail
High convergence of information to retinal ganglion cells	Low convergence of information to retinal ganglion cells

Schematic Diagram of the Retino-Geniculate-Striate Visual Pathway

Figure 6.5

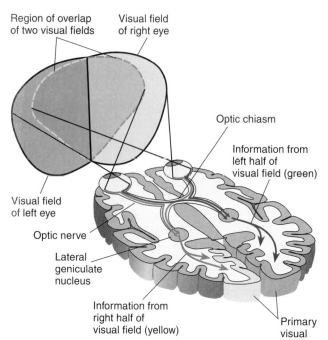

Information in the right visual field is transported via the LGN to the left primary visual cortex (V1). Notice that the nasal hemiretinas send projections contralaterally, whereas the temporal hemiretinas send projections ipsilaterally. This pattern of projections ensures that information about the right visual field is kept together.

Source: Neil R. Carlson, *Physiology of Behavior,* 8e. Published by Allyn and Bacon, Boston, MA. Copyright © 2004 by Pearson Education. Reprinted by permission of the publisher.

Light behaves in the eye as it does in air; that is, it tends to travel in straight lines. If we divide the space that we see into two halves, called the right and left visual fields, we can see that light reflecting off something on the right visual field winds up on the left side of the retina and vice versa (Figure 6.5). However, the right and left sides of the retina project (via the retinal ganglion cells that make up the optic nerve) to different hemispheres of the brain! This is a little different from what we saw in Chapter 4, in which the whole of the right hand (or right ear) projected to the left hemisphere.

Typically, we refer to the sides of the retina as either *nasal* (closest to the nose) or *temporal* (closest to your temples). The retinal ganglion cells in the nasal hemiretina project contralaterally to the **lateral geniculate nucleus** of the thalamus (LGN) and the retinal ganglion cells in the temporal hemiretina project ipsilaterally to the LGN (Figure 6.5). These projections to the LGN ensure that information about the right side of space from either eye stays together in the left LGN and that information about the left side of space from either eye stays together in the right LGN. Thus, the left and right visual fields are segregated into different hemispheres in the brain.

Retino-Geniculate-Striate System

The largest and most thoroughly studied visual pathway is the retino-geniculate-striate system. This system begins in the eye and ends in the primary visual cortex. Although the visual system conforms to the three principles of sensory organization outlined in the previous module, we perceive visual information as an integrated whole. Normally, we do not perceive the color of an object separately from its identity. This module will demonstrate how the brain integrates visual information to produce the perception of the object as an integrated whole. It is important to recognize that until recently, it was not possible to perform detailed examinations of the visual system in humans. Therefore, most of the research presented in this module has resulted from studying either cats or macaques (a type of monkey).

the **Real** world

Can You See Your Blindspot?

As a first insight into how the visual system is quite different from what you might think it should be, you should note that the receptors (which convert the light into action potentials) are on the innermost layer of the retina and the retinal ganglion cells (which exit the eye via the optic nerve) are on the outermost layer of the retina.

Light must pass through four layers of the retina before producing a response from the receptors. These receptors must then send their message to the retinal ganglion cells, which are on the outermost layer of the retina. The retinal ganglion cells then congregate and form the optic nerve, which then exits the eye. The point at which the optic nerve leaves the eye has no receptors and therefore, is blind. This point is called your blind spot. Why is it that when we look around the world, we do not notice this area of blindness?

To prove to yourself that you do have a blind spot, try the following exercise

1. Look at the cross below. Do not look at anything other than the cross. Now move the book back and forth until the black dot on the right disappears. It will disappear when it is on your blind spot.

2. Try the same activity but with these stimuli. Can you see the letters in the space, or does the bar appear to be whole? The phenomenon that you are experiencing is known as *completion*.

THE LATERAL GENICULATE NUCLEUS OF THE THALAMUS. The LGN is a six-layered nucleus of the thalamus that receives information from the retina. These layers receive different sensory information. The top four layers of the LGN are composed of neurons that have small cell bodies and are referred to as the **parvocellular** or **P layers** (*parvo* means "small"). The bottom two layers of the LGN are composed of neurons with large cell bodies and are referred to as the magnocellular or M layers (*magno* means "large").

The P pathway is composed of the parvocellular neurons in the LGN and the axons of the retinal ganglion cells that synapse on them. The P pathway is responsive to color, detail, and stationary or slowly moving objects. The M pathway is composed of magnocellular neurons in the LGN and the axons of the retinal ganglion cells that synapse on them. The M pathway responds to movement and orientation but does not respond to color or detail. Moving backward to the retina, you should be able to predict that the retinal ganglion axons of the P pathway belong to neurons that synapse on cones, whereas the retinal ganglion axons of the M pathway belong to neurons that synapse on rods. This is how the M and P pathways are segregated. Thus, information about the details and color of a moving object in the right visual field will be sent through the P pathway to the top four layers of the left LGN. The details about the movement of the same object will be sent through the M pathway to the bottom two layers of the left LGN.

STRIATE CORTEX. The visual cortex is also known as the **striate cortex,** because when it is viewed under a microscope it has a striped appearance. As you can see in Figure 6.5, information is transmitted ipsilaterally from the LGN to the **primary visual cortex (V1).** That is, the left LGN sends axons (via the optic radiations) to left V1, whereas the right LGN sends axons to right V1 (Figure 6.5). Although the striate cortex is not part of the retino-geniculate-striate pathway, notice that some of the retinal projections go directly to the superior colliculus, part of the tectum. This projection will become important in Module 6.3, where we will discuss a phenomenon known as *blindsight.*

The axons of the LGN project and synapse on layer 4 of the cortex (there are six layers to the striate cortex). From there, layer 4 cells send projections to the other five layers of V1, mostly with the layers either immediately above or below them. Many of the cells in V1 are functionally segregated and respond only to specific features of the stimulus (such as orientation or color). From V1, there are projections forward to the descriptively named areas of V2, then V3, then on to the V4 complex and then the **middle temporal region** (known as area MT). MT sends its projections dorsally to the parietal lobe, and the V4 complex sends its projections ventrally to the temporal lobe (e.g., DeYoe & Van Essen, 1988).

Rather than focusing on the wiring diagrams of these connections, let's focus on the functions of these higher cortical areas. V1 receives projections from both the M and P pathways and is, in a sense, the gateway to the higher cortical areas. However, please remember that not all visual information gets projected to V1. Much of V1 is concerned with responding to color, movement, orientation, and the other information that is passed on through the M and P pathways. Cells within V1 may respond to stimuli presented to either retina, and they appear to compare the position of the stimulus in the two eyes, which is called **binocular disparity.** You can demonstrate binocular disparity by focusing on an object 4–5 feet in front of you. Repeatedly close one eye, then the other. The object should appear to jump back and forth, reflecting the different position it occupies on either retina. Binocular disparity is one way in which our brains produce dimensionality.

V2 can be categorized into three layers: thick, thin, and pale. These names also reflect how the layers look under the microscope. The thick stripes on V2 receive information from the M pathway and are primarily concerned with movement. The thin stripes in V2 receive information about color, and the pale areas between the thick and thin stripes receive information about color and orientation. The cells in V2 that respond to movement do so in a special way. They appear to respond selectively when the stimulus is moving (but not when you are moving, which would also produce subjective movement on the retina; Galletti, Battaglini, & Fattori, 1990). V2 might also be sensitive to the depth of motion, or whether or not the object is moving away from or toward you (Cynader & Regan, 1978). Thus, V2 adds further information about the nature of the stimulus, possibly including addition of dimensionality that is not observed in the previous levels.

V3 is third in line. It receives information from the thick stripes in V2, and it receives some input directly from V1 (primarily from the M pathway). As such, it appears that V3 is responsive to movement and orientation and is functionally part of the M pathway. The preference for motion is even more complex in V3, in that it appears to prefer specific velocities of motion. It is hypothesized that V3 may be functionally involved in the tracking of moving objects through space (Galletti et al., 1990).

It appears that almost all visual input converges on the V4 complex (e.g., Zeki, 1983). The V4 complex receives information from V3 as well as V2 and the LGN (Lysakowski, Standage, & Benevento, 1988). It is thus responsive to color and orientation and sends its projections ventrally to the temporal lobes for further processing. Originally, it was thought that the V4 complex was one area and that its primary function was color processing, owing to the large number of color responsive cells that are found there. However, this conclusion ignored the large number of orientation selective neurons that are also found in V4. Thus, within the V4 complex, at least two functional systems are present: a color-selective system that probably plays a role in the perception of color and a spatially sensitive and orientation-sensitive system that plays a role in pattern recognition. Importantly, a pattern recognition function for V4 has been confirmed, as damage in V4 disrupts the ability of monkeys to discriminate among similar shapes (Merigan & Pham, 1998).

MT (which is sometimes known as V5) is responsive to movement and orientation and sends its projections dorsally to the posterior parietal cortex for further processing. Because of the high numbers of cells that are responsive to movement, it seems reasonable to suggest that MT is functionally relevant for analysis of movement. In fact, lesions to area MT appear to impair the ability of monkeys to visually track moving targets (Dursteller & Wurtz, 1988).

This section has exposed you to how light is converted to produce the world that we see around us through the visual processing that occurs in the retino-geniculate-striate pathway. This section has also illustrated the principles of sensory system organization. That is, the visual system is hierarchical (illustrated by the increasing complexity of responses as we go up in the system), there is functional segregation (as exemplified by the M and P pathways), and there is parallel processing (as demonstrated by the direct connections between the LGN and the various levels of cortex). It should be remembered that most cells are responsive to more than one dimension (e.g., color *and* orientation). In this sense, *responsive* means that AP potentials (sometimes in specific patterns) are produced by the neuron in response to a particular stimulus (which was encoded initially by the receptor cells).

Ventral and Dorsal Streams of Processing Visual Information

THE VENTRAL STREAM. Area V4 is the origin of the **ventral visual stream**. As you recall, area V4 is responsive to both color and patterns. The main output for neurons in V4 is the inferior temporal cortex, which, like V4, has more than one functional unit. Within the inferior temporal cortex, there are cells that are very complex and tend to be selective for shape, color, or texture (e.g., Desimone, Schein, Moran, & Ungerleider, 1985; DeYoe, Felleman, Van Essen, & McClendon, 1994; Elston & Rosa, 1998). Some researchers have suggested that neurons within the inferior temporal cortex are so specific for patterns that there may even be cells that are selective for specific faces (e.g., Perret, Rolls, & Caans, 1982; Tovee, Rolls, & Azzopardi, 1994). This has led to the ventral stream being labeled the "what" pathway.

To recognize objects, the brain must be able to distinguish complex objects from each other and to recognize them in different conditions, including changing lighting conditions or when viewed from alternative perspectives. It appears that the neurons in the inferior temporal cortex do just that: they respond selectively to the object and appear to be unaffected by changes in position or orientation (e.g., Desimone, Albright, Gross, & Bruce, 1984). Furthermore, as we move from the retina to the inferior temporal cortex, the size of the receptive fields increases. That is, the neurons are more receptive to the global features of objects (e.g., color and shape) rather than just to one feature (e.g., color or orientation). Thus, neurons in the inferior temporal cortex respond to the integrated features of entire objects, which aids in identification. Furthermore, neurons in the inferior temporal cortex can "see" color. The ability to distinguish among objects on the basis of color is an important adaptation, which among other things helps us to determine where one object ends and another begins (figure–ground separation). Figure–ground separation also provides us with important cues about object identity and helps the brain to construct a three-dimensional percept of the world.

THE DORSAL STREAM. Area MT is the origin of the **dorsal visual stream,** with exquisite sensitivity to movement, in both two-dimensional space and three-dimensional space. Again, you might recall that area MT is dominated by the M pathway; therefore, the features of the M pathway also dominate the dorsal stream. The main output for neurons in area MT is the posterior parietal cortex, an area that has been implicated in directing visual attention to specific points in space (e.g., Colby, Duhamel, & Goldberg, 1995). As such, the dorsal stream is often labeled the "where" pathway.

The cells in the posterior parietal lobes are specialized for processing spatial relations in a number of ways. That is, many neurons within the posterior parietal area are responsive to both visual fields, which allows for the computation of an object's exact position in space. These neurons also appear to be able to track moving objects and respond differentially to the direction and speed of the movement. Many researchers have suggested that the posterior parietal cortex is responsible for creating stable maps of the world and placing items within that map. Collectively, this results in knowledge of where an object is in space.

However, knowing where an object is in space is not enough for motor tasks that rely on the utilization of the object. For instance, reach out and pick up an object that is in front of you. If you completed this task, you not only needed to know the location of the object in space, you also needed to know how to position your fingers, where to grip the object, and the distance between your hand and the object. Goodale and Milner (1992) suggest that the dorsal stream is more likely a "how" pathway; that is, the role of the dorsal stream is to know *how* motor acts are to be performed so that accurate manipulation of objects is possible. In fact, it does appear that some neurons within the parietal lobes are specialized for integrating motor commands with spatial information (e.g., Mountcastle, Lynch, Georgopoulos, Sakata, & Acuna, 1975). Although the distinction between *where* and *how* is subtle, it does appear that *how*

Neuropsychological Celebrity

D.F.

While taking a shower one day, D.F. was overcome by carbon monoxide from a faulty chimney for a nearby water heater. As a result of carbon monoxide poisoning, D.F. suffered a large lesion to her lateral occipital region, including extensive damage to the ventral visual stream. As a result of this damage, she suffers from a condition known as visual agnosia, which is the inability to recognize objects based on visual information (Goodale et al., 1991). This damage is so severe that D.F. can no longer tell the size of objects using her sight. For instance, if she is shown a 2-centimeter cube and a 10-centimeter cube, not only is she not be able to tell you that they are cubes, but she is also unable to tell you which one is bigger. When D.F. is asked to name the subjects of line drawings of simple objects such as an apple, she cannot make a copy of them. When she is asked to draw a picture of an apple from memory, the drawing is good, although it is as if she were drawing with her eyes closed. That is, if in the middle of making the drawing she has to lift her hand from the page and then restart the drawing, she often ends up on a different part of the page.

However, D.F. is not blind. She can walk around just the same as anyone. What seems really amazing about D.F. is that she can accurately pick up the cubes described above. When we pick up large objects, we increase the distance between our thumb and index finger. When we pick up small objects, we decrease the distance between our thumb and index finger. This ability is referred to as *scaling*, and DF shows normal scaling.

In an interesting twist, Jakobson and colleagues (1991) report the case of V.K., who has lesions in the dorsal stream. V.K. is quite able to name line drawings, estimate size, and use visual information to identify objects in the environment. However, V.K. exhibits difficulties in scaling her grasp when reaching for objects and with aiming her hand at the object that she picks up.

---

encompasses both where an object is and how to use it and is thus a more complete description of the pathway.

INTEGRATION OF THE SYSTEMS. The dorsal and ventral streams may have different functions, but how do they interact to produce our normal visual experiences? After all, we do not usually say to ourselves, "Oh, there is my cat. Oh, and she is jumping off the chair." Our brains produce integrated knowledge of object identity and its location, whether the object is moving, and how to utilize it. Some of this unified percept comes from the rich interconnections between the two streams. Furthermore, both of these streams send projections to the prefrontal cortex, where much of this information is integrated. However, not all of the information that is encoded in these two streams may be available to conscious experience.

An interesting experiment by Pelisson and colleagues (Pelisson, Prablanc, Goodale, & Jeannerod, 1986) suggests that some aspects of vision are unavailable to conscious visual experience. In this experiment, neurologically normal participants were asked to point at a light. They began their task with their finger placed on a light directly in front of them. A short time later, a light would appear off to the side, and their task was to point at it. During half of the trials, the light would move position immediately after the first time the participant looked at it. Regardless of whether the light moved or not, participants were accurate at pointing to the light. So what?

Well, the interesting part of this experiment is that although they were accurate at pointing to the new location of the light that moved, none of the participants could reliably tell the experimenters whether the light had moved or not. Thus, much of what is encoded in the dorsal stream may not be available to consciousness, at least to the verbal centers in the brain, despite accurate guidance of motor movements.

As you can see, the visual system is incredibly complex, and every lobe in the cortex processes visual information. The amount of resources that the brain spends on processing visual information should give you some appreciation of how important vision is to us as a species. Although this is a simplistic formulation, there are two streams of visual information: one involved in the coding of what an object is and one involved in coding how to use the object. Deficits in these two streams provide an important insight into how the visual system (and other sensory systems) is organized.

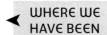 We have distinguished between sensation and perception and have suggested that the brain does not simply reproduce the outside world inside your brain. We have also outlined the basic principles of all sensory systems and the functional neuroanatomy of the visual system. Simply put, as we ascend in the visual cortex, the processing of information becomes more complex and attuned to the global features of objects and the environment.

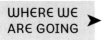 In the next module, we are going to examine disturbances in the visual system and how they produce their effects, as well as what these behaviors tell us about the organization of the visual system.

MODULE **6.3**
Deficits in the Visual System

This module explores the variety of difficulties people exhibit in perceiving and recognizing objects after suffering brain damage. These disorders vary tremendously, and the specificity of the impairments can be amazing. For example, a sheep farmer might suffer a stroke, lose his ability to recognize human faces (including that of his wife), but retain his ability to recognize the faces of sheep from his flock. As another example, a 43-year-old woman suffered brain damage because of a vascular abnormality. She can still recognize common objects and faces, but she cannot perceive movement. Previously simple tasks such as pouring tea have become very difficult because the fluid now appears to be frozen.

None of the disorders that we discuss below can be attributed solely to primary sensory problems such as blindness. Acquired blindness can arise from a wide variety of injuries: damage to the eye, optic nerve, optic chiasm, thalamus, or even the primary visual cortex. Damage to any of these structures causes impairments in the conscious sensation of visual information. Although disorders of visual perception are often accompanied by these more primary sensory problems, these problems are not the sole cause of the perceptual deficits.

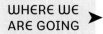 The following sections describe a variety of visual disorders. Some of these disorders appear to be failures in perception; others are deficits in associating intact perceptions with meaning. The last section in this module describes blindsight, a phenomenon that can be characterized as a deficit in conscious visual perception.

Agnosia

Most of this module focuses on forms of **agnosia,** a term that was first introduced by Sigmund Freud to describe a lack of "knowing" (recognition) that can occur in any sensory modality. However, *agnosia* is a term that must be defined in both positive and negative terms (DeRenzi, 1999). A person who demonstrates agnosia must demonstrate a deficit in recognition (the negative part of the definition) that is not due to impairments in sensation, attention, language, or general intelligence (the positive part of the definition). Therefore, to demonstrate an agnosia in visual object naming, an individual must demonstrate that he or she can in fact see the object, attend to it, display knowledge about the object's name (and perhaps function), and display adequate intelligence to perform the naming task. This definition does not mean that agnosic individuals do not also demonstrate sensory, attentional, and language deficits—they often do. However, these deficits alone are not sufficient to account for their perceptual deficit.

Certain visual agnosias have traditionally been divided into two forms: apperceptive visual agnosia and associative visual agnosia. Lissauer (1890) proposed this split at roughly the same time that Freud introduced the term *agnosia*. However, rather than using the term *agnosia*, Lissauer used the term *mindblindness*. This term has been abandoned because agnosias occur outside of the visual modality; as you will learn in later chapters, there are also auditory agnosias and tactile agnosias.

APPERCEPTIVE VISUAL AGNOSIA. The inability to recognize an object due to a problem perceiving it is termed **apperceptive visual agnosia.** Unlike the condition of associative visual agnosia (described in the next section), this deficit is not a problem associating perceptions with meaning. Instead, it is characterized by a problem grouping visual sensations into a unified percept (Vecera & Gilds, 1998). As you learned earlier in the chapter, perceptual grouping is not a simple task. Close your eyes and imagine looking at a bicycle from the side, then from the back, then from the front, then from the top. (If you are having trouble imagining one from these views, look at Figure 6.6, then consult your physician.) The visual form of the bicycle changes radically between these views, but its percept remains the same: It always looks like a bicycle. Even if you change the lighting, decorate the bicycle with ribbons, or put a man dressed in a bear costume on the bicycle, it still looks like a bicycle.

This is not so for an individual with apperceptive visual agnosia. If a usual object is displayed in an unusual orientation, this person will have trouble identifying it. Adding superfluous elements to an object also makes it much more difficult to identify (Warrington & Taylor, 1973) (see Figure 6.7). Similarly, shadows can sometimes provide enough distracting information to make an object unidentifiable (Warrington, 1982). The disorder is not caused by a primary sensory deficit; apperceptive agnosics

Figure 6.6	Different Views of an Object

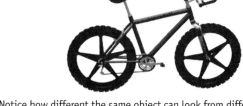

Notice how different the same object can look from different views. Although the visual form changes radically, the percept remains the same.

Source: Images provided courtesy of Michael J. Tarr, Brown University.

Figure 6.7	Apperceptive Visual Agnosia

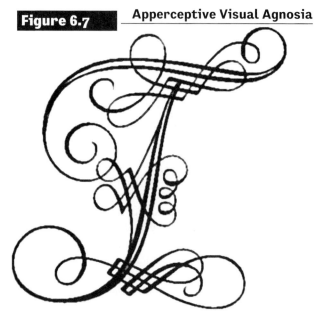

Adding superfluous elements to letters makes them more difficult to recognize, especially for apperceptive visual agnosics.

can usually discriminate among simple colors, and make brightness or form comparisons. However, sometimes even the simplest of form comparisons can be impaired. After suffering carbon monoxide poisoning, one individual was unable to reliably differentiate between centrally presented X's and O's (Benson & Greenberg, 1969).

There are a variety of measures that are capable of detecting apperceptive visual agnosia. One simple bedside test is to have an individual copy simple line drawings. Other standard measures include the presentation of objects in unusual views or figures containing superfluous information. Carbon monoxide poisoning, which damages posterior temporal and occipital cortices (usually bilaterally), often causes the lesions that give rise to apperceptive visual agnosia. Unlike the lesions that often give rise to associative visual agnosia, these lesions need not be localized within the left hemisphere (Jankowiak & Albert, 1994; McMullen, Fisk, Phillips, & Maloney, 2000). Circumscribed right hemisphere lesions can give rise to the condition (Heilman & Bowers, 1995; Shelton, Bowers, Duara, & Heilman, 1994; Warrington & Rudge, 1995).

ASSOCIATIVE VISUAL AGNOSIA. The inability to associate visual forms with meaning is termed **associative visual agnosia**. This disorder also must be defined in terms of positive and negative symptoms; the ability to perceive the objects as a whole is intact (unlike in apperceptive visual agnosia). Therefore, when given a line drawing to copy, associative visual agnosics are often able to produce faithful replicas. However, associating these percepts with meaning is impaired. When asked to name the object that they just copied or to identify its function, they display profound deficits. The disorder can also be detected when individuals are asked to draw pictures from memory or to describe the visual characteristics of objects.

Consider the drawing in Figure 6.8. A middle-aged male physician suffered brain damage and lost his ability to recognize common objects, faces, and text. He could still write but lost his ability to read (a condition called **alexia without agraphia,** described in detail in Chapter 8). When presented with line drawings of common objects and asked to name them, he performed very poorly. However, when asked to copy the picture of the object, he performed quite well (despite an inability to see in part of his visual field). His copy of a locomotive (Figure 6.8) was quite accurate in general form and in detail, but even after completing the drawing, he was not sure

Figure 6.8	**Associative Visual Agnosia**

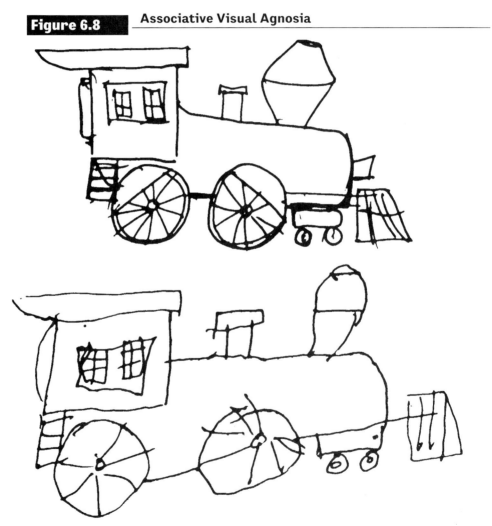

Despite being able to generate an excellent copy (bottom) of the original drawing of the locomotive (top), a man with associative visual agnosia could not identify the drawing he had made.

Source: Reprinted from *Cognitive Neuropsychology,* McCarthy & Warrington, p. 35, Copyright 1990, with permission from Elsevier.

what the object was. He described it as "a wagon or car of some kind. The larger vehicle is being pulled by the smaller one" (Rubens & Benson, 1971). In addition to problems identifying pictures of objects, he had trouble identifying real objects, even if they were very familiar to him. When asked to identify his own stethoscope, he described it as a "long cord with a disc at one end." Despite his inability to recognize objects on the basis of visual information, he remained capable of using tactile information to identify objects, demonstrating the modality specificity of his disorder.

Associative visual agnosia is not simply a memory deficit specific to objects. Shown a picture of an anchor, one such individual was unable to recognize the object but could copy the drawing well. After copying the drawing, the person still could not name the object. However, when he was questioned what an anchor is, his definition was "a brake for ships." Knowledge about the use of objects can also be displayed in other ways, such as asking the individual to mime the use of the object. When the judgment must be made on the basis of visual information alone, the mimed use will usually be incorrect. Conversely, when the information is provided in another modality (e.g., auditory, tactile), the mimed use should be correct. Therefore, when shown a visual representation of a spoon, an associative visual agnosic might not be able to identify it or mime its use. However, when the individual is told that the object is a spoon or is allowed to investigate it with his or her hands, the person can correctly mime its use.

Associative visual agnosia is not simply a naming disorder. If it was, individuals would be able to mime the use of objects after being provided with a visual representation of the object. There are case reports of such individuals, but they are not typical of the condition. For example, Sirigu and colleagues (Sirigu, Duhamel, & Poncet, 1991) described a 19-year-old male who suffered bilateral temporal lobe lesions and demonstrated profound impairments in naming visually presented objects. However, he could often demonstrate how to use the object or describe how it is normally manipulated despite an ability to describe its function. He frequently remarked, "I can tell you how to use it, but I have no idea what it is used for."

One clever test for the detection of associative visual agnosia is the "real or not" test (Kroll & Potter, 1984; Riddoch & Humphreys, 1987). A person is presented with line drawings of objects or animals and is asked to identify whether the drawing represents a "real" (plausible) object or not. The objects that are not "real" range from nonsensical shapes to hybrid objects composed of parts of real objects. For example, a hybrid "nonreal" animal drawing might have the head of an elk, the front legs of a polar bear, the back legs of a horse, and the tail of a kangaroo (see Figure 6.9). A nonliving hybrid object might be the handle of a kettle attached to a ruler. People with associative visual agnosia perform very poorly on this test.

Ironically, there is also a test for associative visual agnosia on which neurologically normal individuals perform worse than agnosic individuals. When presented with drawings of impossible figures (see Figure 6.10), associative visual agnosics have no more difficulty copying these figures than they do figures of "real" objects. In contrast, neurologically normal people have considerably more difficulty with the impossible objects, presumably because they are "being misled by the internal contradictions, associative agnosics have no such trouble, slavishly copying both types of material, line by line" (Bradshaw & Mattingley, 1995, p. 95).

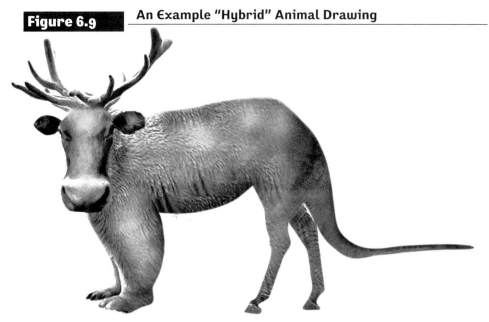

Figure 6.9   An Example "Hybrid" Animal Drawing

Associate visual agnosics have trouble determining whether such animals are real or not.

Lesions that produce associative visual agnosia are usually located along the posterior left hemisphere (DeRenzi, 1999), although lesions in a number of other loci have also resulted in the disorder (including some right hemisphere locations). One possible reason for this variability could be that the label *associative visual agnosia* refers to a class of related disorders. One can lose the ability to associate faces, words, or various categories of objects with meaning (Farah, 1990, 2000).

CATEGORY-SPECIFIC VISUAL AGNOSIA. Some associative visual agnosics display remarkably specific symptoms. Nielson (1946) described an agnosic individual who was profoundly impaired in identifying living things but relatively unimpaired with nonliving stimuli. McCrae and Trolle (1956) also observed a similar pattern, as they described an individual who was quite impaired in identifying animals (e.g., confusing a squirrel and a cat because they both have whiskers) but had no trouble identifying common

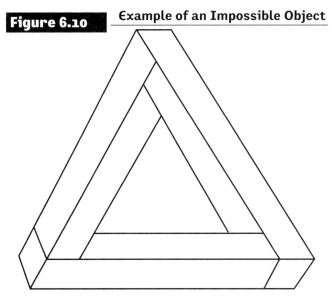

Figure 6.10   Example of an Impossible Object

Unlike normal controls, associative visual agnosics often have no more difficulty copying these impossible figures than they do figures of real objects.

objects or other classes of living things, such as trees or flowers. The opposite pattern of deficit, an impairment in recognizing nonliving things but relatively intact recognition of living things, has also been observed, but it is much less common (Funnell & Sheridan, 1992; Sacchett & Humphreys, 1992; Satori & Job, 1988; Warrington & McCarthy, 1994).

One of the most famous examples of a person with **category-specific visual agnosia** is J.B.R., first described by Warrington and Shallice (Warrington & Shallice, 1984). J.B.R. suffered damage to both temporal lobes as a result of herpes simplex encephalitis in 1980. This left him with a wide variety of impairments, including language problems (such as a word-finding deficit) and memory problems (amnesia). When given the standard tests of apperceptive visual agnosia, J.B.R. performed quite well. He seemed to have no trouble forming percepts of the objects that were presented to him. However, his associative visual agnosia symptoms were severe and highly specific. When identifying common nonliving objects, such as a calculator, chair, or pair of binoculars, J.B.R. had little trouble identifying the objects. He could answer about 90% of the questions correctly. However, when he was presented with line drawings of living things, such as a rabbit, sheep, or bear, his performance was terrible, dropping to about 5% correct (Warrington & Shallice, 1984). Another individual studied by Warrington and Shallice (1984) exhibited a similar pattern of deficit.

Clinical evidence of this type of agnosia has also been supported with functional imaging evidence. When neurologically normal individuals are asked to name people while undergoing a PET scan, activation of left anterior inferior temporal areas has been observed. When they name tools, the activation is more posterior along the left inferior temporal lobe. If they are asked to name animals, the activation is typically in between these two areas (Damasio, Grabowski, Tranel, Hichwa, & Damasio, 1996). These patterns of activation mirror the common lesion locations related to agnosias in these categories (Damasio et al., 1996). Functional neurosurgical evidence has also supported the position that one's ability to name living things can be selectively impaired, depending on the location of the lesion. Strauss et al. (2000) examined the naming ability of seventy-nine patients who had anterior temporal lobectomy surgery. Just as one would predict on the basis of PET imaging, this resulted in a selective impairment in the ability to name living things.

On the basis of this evidence, it is tempting to conclude that the brain organizes information into modules that are defined by these categories. However, the interpretation of these results can be considerably more complicated. Some suggest that category-specific visual agnosia is simply an artifact of uncontrolled differences between the categories of items used in assessing the condition (Takarae & Levin, 2001). Consider the following questions: Is it normally more difficult to name animals than nonliving things? Could people with brain injuries simply be worse at naming, regardless of the type of object being named? Are pictures of living things normally more complex than those of nonliving things, making them more difficult to recognize and name? Are different types of animals simply less familiar than the nonliving objects used in these tests? (After all, how many times have you seen a pair of scissors and how many times have you seen an elephant?) Is one class of objects more similar in appearance than another? Take a look at Figure 6.11, and notice some of the common features between the living things. They tend to have appendages (e.g., legs,

| **Figure 6.11** | **Examples of Common Living and Nonliving Things** |

Living things

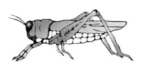 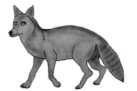 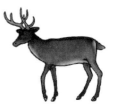

Nonliving things

 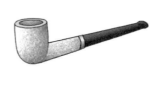 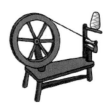

Some individuals are profoundly impaired at identifying living things, but relatively unimpaired with nonliving stimuli. The reverse pattern of deficit has also been observed.

Source: Images provided courtesy of Michael J. Tarr, Brown University.

wings), eyes, and rounded bodies. The nonliving things do not tend to look similar at all. These types of questions have been used to cast doubt on the conclusion that neural representations of living and nonliving things are functionally and anatomically distinct. However, these factors alone do not appear to be capable of accounting for the differences in naming performance across the two categories. When the tests are equated for name frequency, familiarity, and visual complexity, the living versus nonliving difference is still present (Strauss et al., 2000).

There is an interesting exception to the living/nonliving dichotomy that is often observed in category-specific visual agnosia. Individuals who demonstrate selective difficulties in naming living things also tend to exhibit deficits in naming musical instruments, a special class of nonliving objects (Dixon, Piskopos, & Schweizer, 2000). Musical instruments differ considerably in terms of their visual similarity, but their functions (in a broad sense) are all very similar: They all make music. The same can be said for many drawings of animals: In functional terms, they are quite similar (pet, food, pet food, etc.). This curious exception helped to develop a different interpretation of the category-specific deficits in visual agnosia.

Some researchers proposed that knowledge of visual object form and object function are represented differently in both functional and anatomical ways (Farah & McClelland, 1991). This requires the assumption that our knowledge of living things is highly dependent on our knowledge of their visual characteristics, whereas our knowledge of nonliving objects is less dependent on this information. Because the representations of living things tend to be visually similar but not very different functionally, becoming less able to access memory about visual object form should selectively impair ones ability to recognize living things. Conversely, if one is impaired in the ability to access functional information about objects, this should selectively impair the ability to identify nonliving things.

Computer simulations have provided support for this type of model (Dixon, Koehler, Schweizer, & Guylee, 2000; Farah & McClelland, 1991), but some confirmatory evidence is also provided from examinations of agnosics (Dixon, 1999; Dixon, Koehler, et al., 2000). Dixon and colleagues (Dixon, Bub, Chertkow, & Arguin, 1999) used novel computer-generated shapes (blobs) instead of line drawings (see Figure 6.12). This way, the visual stimuli could be controlled for visual similarity, complexity, and familiarity. These shapes were then paired with labels of tools or birds. When presented to a 71-year-old agnosic who was asked to remember the shape–name associations, the agnosic demonstrated difficulty associating the labels of birds with the shapes (i.e., labels that were high in functional similarity) but relatively little difficulty pairing names of tools (i.e., labels that were low in functional similarity). Similarly, in other experiments in which arbitrarily constructed blobs were paired with semantically close or semantically disparate labels, both neurologically normal and

Figure 6.12   Examples of Blob Stimuli Employed by Dixon and Colleagues

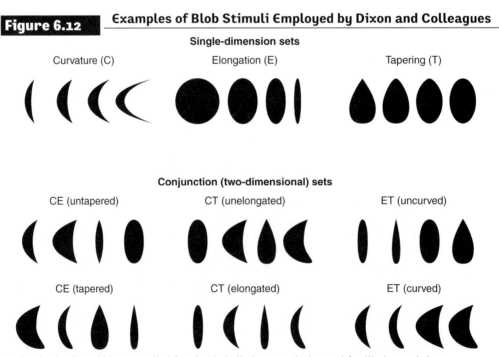

These visual stimuli could be controlled for visual similarity, complexity, and familiarity, and they were paired with labels of tools or birds.

Source: Dixon et al. (1997). Reprinted with permission.

agnosic individuals had trouble discerning between semantically similar items (Dixon, Bub, & Arguin, 1997). Therefore, category-specific visual agnosics might demonstrate deficits in memory for the semantic or visual properties of objects rather than a selective impairment in the identification of living or nonliving things.

PROSOPAGNOSIA. Imagine waking up in the morning, looking in the bathroom mirror, and not recognizing the face looking back at you. It sounds incredible, doesn't it? This scenario is a daily reality for many people. **Prosopagnosia** is the inability to recognize familiar faces that, like other agnosias, is not attributable to sensory problems (i.e., blindness) or more general intellectual deficits. The term is a combination of the term *prosop,* which is Greek for "face," and Freud's term *agnosia* (a lack of knowledge). A few such cases were described in the scientific literature before Bodamer coined the term *prosopagnosia* in 1947 (Ellis & Florence, 1990). As you will discover in the following paragraphs, there are a variety of reasons why face processing can be impaired, and it is quite possible that the term *prosopagnosia* describes a class of visual disorders. To further complicate matters, prosopagnosia can also be considered a variant of apperceptive visual agnosia, associative visual agnosia, or even category-specific visual agnosia.

Let's revert to the example of not recognizing your own face in the mirror. Even if you did not recognize the *face* in the mirror, it is unlikely that you would question the identity of the *person*. After all, the person is wearing your pajamas, moving when you move, and is *in the mirror*. Therefore, many other cues are available to help you identify the person. This is also the case for prosopagnosics identifying others. A prosopagnosic man might recognize his wife because of her clothes, shape, walk, or tone of voice or because she is the person sleeping next to him when he wakes in the morning. One prosopagnosia researcher, Dr. Mike Dixon, is a very tall man. Despite marked prosopagnosia, J.T., a man studied by Dr. Dixon, had relatively little trouble recognizing him when he walked into the room. If J.T. was in a university laboratory and a thin male over 6'4" with short hair walked in the room, J.T. would remark, "Hello, Dr. Mike."

Prosopagnosia is not a general loss of memory about people. One common test of prosopagnosia is the "famous faces test." The task of testing facial recognition is a little more challenging than testing other intellectual capacities, such as vocabulary. Most native English speakers can reasonably be expected to know many of the same words. The same is not true for knowledge of faces. An examining clinician cannot be expected to have pictures of your mother, neighbor, eighth-grade teacher, or best friend. Therefore, to test facial recognition, investigators generally use collections of famous people's faces, such as actors, singers, and politicians. When presented with a picture of Elvis Presley, a prosopagnosic person might not be able to identify him. However, if asked to describe Elvis, they might identify him as "the king of rock and roll" or perhaps even sing a measure of "Blue Suede Shoes."

Prosopagnosia can appear to result from *apperceptive* types of symptoms. For example, when asked to describe what faces looked like, a prosopagnosic patient described by Hecean and Angelergues (1962) remarked, "Faces don't look normal anymore, they are quite distorted and contorted like some sketches [by] Picasso." Most prosopagnosics who appear to have apperceptive symptoms also have difficulty with other perceptually challenging tasks, such as identifying pictures of objects taken from unusual angles or discriminating between overlapping figures (DeRenzi, 1999).

Prosopagnosia can also appear to result from *associative* types of symptoms. In these cases, performance on other perceptually challenging tasks is not typically impaired. Even face-matching tests can be completely accurately, but naming familiar faces is severely impaired. Despite the inability to name the familiar face, associative prosopagnosics retain their semantic knowledge of the person and can provide other identifying information (as in the Elvis example mentioned earlier). These two types

Controversy

Current

Are Faces Special?

You need not look any further than the table of contents of many neuropsychology books to notice the debate on the specificity of facial recognition. According to some, faces are recognized in a very different manner than are other objects. This position can be made evident by having different chapters on "Face Recognition" and "Object Recognition"—see McCarthy and Warrington's *Cognitive Neuropsychology* (1990) or Farah's *The Cognitive Neuroscience of Vision* (2000) for examples. Others view facial recognition as simply another example of object recognition, albeit a task that is quite difficult and possibly very sensitive to damage. This position can be reflected by including discussions of prosopagnosia within chapters on disorders of object recognition, such as in Bradshaw and Mattingley's (1995) *Clinical Neuropsychology: Behavioral and Brain Science*. They "argue for the conclusion that prosopagnosia may be one aspect of a more *general* alteration of perception" (p. 112). Our discussion of it is in the chapter on visual perception, placing us firmly on the fence between the two positions.

Arguing for the presence of a facial perception module seems quite counterintuitive at first. Neural real estate is precious. If an area was specialized for the recognition of objects, why would it not also assume the role of recognizing faces? Postulating an additional functionally and anatomically distinct system is not parsimonious. Some might even call it a waste of resources. However, the few reports of a highly selective disruption in the ability to recognize faces suggests that there may in fact be a facial perception module. Furthermore, developmental psychology has shown that babies are predisposed to treat faces differently from other

objects. As we suggested in the first module of this chapter, there might be neurons within the inferior temporal cortex that respond selectively to faces. Furthermore, although most objects are more difficult to recognize upside-down, inversion makes faces dramatically more difficult to recognize. Taken together, these findings suggest that facial recognition and object recognition are dissociable.

The position that disruptions in facial processing is a manifestation of a more general disruption is bolstered by the evidence that prosopagnosics often have difficulty discriminating among objects in other categories, such as car makes, mammals of similar form, or furniture of similar shape (DeRenzi, 1999). Some argue that prosopagnosia is a visual recognition disorder that is not specific to human faces. Instead, the deficit emerges whenever a discrimination of identity must be made on the basis of the unique features of an item within a given category. For example, Damasio, Damasio, and Van Hoesen (1982) detail deficits in a prosopagnosic birdwatcher who lost the ability to identify species of birds. They also describe a prosopagnosic farmer who was no longer able to determine which cow was which. Note that these individuals could identify line drawings as either cows or birds, but they could not identify specific cows or birds. This inability is very similar to problems in identifying faces in prosopagnosia. The fact that the visual stimulus is a face is evident, but the unique features of individual faces that indicate identity are no longer useful. Researchers such as Damasio therefore suggest that faces are *not* a unique class of visual stimuli and that the nature of the deficit in prosopagnosia is related to the ability to use unique visual features to identify individuals. Are faces special? Maybe.

of prosopagnosia might be occurring as a result of damage to two different stages of processing. If the face itself cannot be properly perceived (grouping the features into a unified percept), its recognition will be impaired. This is presumably what is causing apperceptive prosopagnosia. However, perceiving the face is not sufficient for recognition; the percept must be combined with the semantic, biographical memory, including the person's name, the relationship one has to the person, and so on. The biographical memories themselves are usually intact in prosopagnosia, so associative prosopagnosia might result from a disconnection between one's perception of the face and the semantic information about the person.

The biographical, semantic memories about people are not themselves impervious to damage. K.S., a 40-year-old woman, could not name famous or familiar faces after a right anterior temporal lobectomy. This was not due to a general intellectual impairment (her I.Q. after the surgery was 119) or visual problems (she performed well on object recognition tests). Instead, the deficit appeared to stem from a loss of her knowledge of information about people. Other cues, such as the voice of the person, were not helpful. K.S. also demonstrated impairments regarding famous animals (such as Moby Dick or Lassie), famous buildings (such as Big Ben), and even the names of common products (Ellis, Young, & Critchley, 1989). Despite her inability to recognize famous faces, K.S. should not be considered prosopagnosic: her impairments are not specific to the processing of faces, and her semantic knowledge regarding the previously familiar people is no longer intact (DeRenzi, 1999).

Given the variation in the symptoms that appear to underlie prosopagnosia, it should come as no surprise that lesions in a variety of locations can give rise to the disorder. Farah (1990) summarized the evidence from seventy-one prosopagnosics. Despite the wide variety in locations observed, two themes can be extracted from the information: First, when the lesion is unilateral, prosopagnosia is more likely to result from right (rather than left) hemisphere lesions. Second, prosopagnosics usually have occipital lesions, but temporal lesions are also quite common.

COLOR AGNOSIA. Color agnosia is a loss of knowledge about color that cannot be accounted for by an impairment of color discrimination, aphasia, or some general intellectual deterioration (Beauvois & Saillant, 1985). This definition may leave one wondering how such a deficit could ever be detected: If the person has lost his or her knowledge of colors, how can one assess the person's sensation of color? There are a variety of perceptual tests that force individuals to use color information, but they do not require the naming of the color (McCarthy & Warrington, 1990). Most current theory on color agnosia appears to have been based on Lewandowsky's original 1908 report on color agnosia (as cited in Davidoff, 1996).

One such method is the color-sorting test. In the first written account of color agnosia, Sittig (1921) described this test, in which he gave individuals color patches and asked them to sort the patches into groups that were alike, referring to grouping all shades of blue and so on. Because the patches differed in the brightness of color, individuals sorting by brightness would place all light colors in one pile and darker shades of the colors into other piles. As you might imagine, this abstract task can be performed in a number of ways (such as sorting by brightness), making the results difficult to interpret.

A second method is to ask individuals to color black-and-white line drawings (De-Renzi & Spinnler, 1967). Although some items have no "correct" color (such as a man's coat), other items (e.g., grass, sky) have fewer possible alternatives. To overcome any motor difficulties individuals might have in this task, it can be simplified such that they need to select only the appropriately colored crayon. However, this task also has its shortcomings. If the individual also has some deficits in recognizing line drawings of objects, this can seriously impair the person's ability to select the correct color. For instance, if a picture of a rabbit is perceived as a picture of a plum, the color purple is a perfectly sensible choice.

A third method is essentially a variant on the coloring method. Instead of being asked to color their own drawings, individuals are presented with precolored line drawings. Some of the items are colored appropriately (e.g., the sky is blue, the leaves are green), whereas other items are not (e.g., a blue lion, a red banana). The task is to indicate whether items are colored appropriately or not (Beauvois & Saillant, 1985).

Optic Aphasia

Similar to associative visual agnosia, **optic aphasia** is a disorder in which the naming of visual objects is impaired. However, unlike associative visual agnosia, the recognition of the objects (including information about the functions of the objects or descriptions of the circumstances in which one might find the objects) is intact. The condition is also similar to **anomia,** the inability to correctly name objects, except that optic aphasia is specific to visually presented stimuli. If information about the object is provided through another modality (e.g., showing a picture of a lion and telling the person that it is "king of the jungle"), the correct name can be retrieved.

In 1889, Freund described a 57-year-old man with this condition (Freund, 1991), but there is still no consensus as to whether optic aphasia is dissociable from associative visual agnosia. Some view the two diagnostic labels as indicative of two severities of the same condition; others believe that the disorders are qualitatively different (see Martin, 1998). The most compelling evidence that the two conditions are separable comes from asking affected individuals to pantomime the use of visually presented objects. Those who exhibit associative visual agnosia usually cannot correctly mimic the use of the object (indicating a problem associating the visual object with meaning), whereas those who exhibit optic aphasia usually *can* pantomime the object's use, despite their inability to name it.

For example, P.T. suffered a stroke that left his primary sensation, language, coordination, and general intellect intact. However, he lost his ability to name visually presented objects. When presented with a clarinet, he identified it as a flute. Despite getting the name of the instrument wrong, when he pantomimed playing the instrument, he positioned his hands as if it were a clarinet, not a flute. When instructed that "flute" was the incorrect answer, he changed his response to "clarinet," presumably guided by his own gestures. His response to a picture of a combination lock was similar. He named the object a "telephone" (presumably because of the numbers and dial, resembling an old rotary phone), but he correctly mimed the actions necessary to open a combination lock (Gazzaniga, Ivry, & Mangun, 1998).

Blindsight

Damage to the primary visual cortex normally results in a "blind" part of the visual field opposite to that of the damage. This blind spot is called a **scotoma.** When objects such as Xs and Os are presented within a person's scotoma, the person does not consciously perceive them. However, some people appear to retain their ability to make simple discriminations between stimuli, identifying form (such as X versus O), direction of movement, location, color, or even a combination of these features, despite subjective reports that they do not "see" the stimuli! For example, a figure of an X might be presented in someone's scotoma, and the person is asked whether he or she sees anything there. The person replies that he or she sees nothing, and the person is reluctant to make a response. When pressed, using a forced-choice paradigm (i.e., yes/no questions), the person often offers correct responses—sometimes as often as 90% of the time. When asked, people often report that their responses were "guided by a feeling," but not by conscious vision. For instance, if the task was discriminating between an X and an O, the participant might respond that the Xs felt "jagged," or the Os felt "smooth"; these feelings are nevertheless *not* subjectively visual. This is known as **blindsight.**

Imagine being the researcher or participant in a study of blindsight. If you are the researcher, you ask the participant to describe the visual properties of a stimulus that is deliberately placed where the participant cannot see it. (Doesn't this sound like an ESP experiment?) To participants who have insisted that they cannot see objects placed in their scotoma, the experiment might seem like a cruel joke. Indeed, some participants simply refuse to respond, skeptical of the usefulness of guessing. Those who actually choose to respond are "rewarded" by further questions about the visual properties of what they didn't see. Indeed, G.Y., a famous blindsighted individual, suggests that describing his deficit is the same as "trying to tell a blind man what it is like to see" (Weiskrantz, 1995).

Early explanations of blindsight suggested that there may be islands of residual visual cortex subserving the preserved percepts. However, functional neuroimaging studies of G.Y. found no activity within V1 during blindsight, although activity was detected in visual association areas and other brain regions. Thus, at least in G.Y.'s case, islands of activity in V1 cannot account for his correct responses. Other investigations have also failed to confirm the islands hypothesis (Barbur, Weiskrantz, & Harlow, 1999).

If blindsight is not mediated by the primary visual cortex, then what neural systems are involved? Others have suggested that intact projections from the retina to the superior colliculus (which projects to the pulvinar nucleus and visual association areas) may subserve visual function in blindsight (Cowey & Stoerig, 1991; Rafal, Smith, Krantz, Cohen, & Brennan, 1990). Cowey and colleagues also suggest that cortical mechanisms could account for blindsight. Recall that not all projections from the LGN go directly to V1. In fact, Cowey suggests that the projections from the LGN to the visual association cortex may be spared in individuals with blindsight, providing residual (but not necessarily conscious) visual function (Stoerig & Cowey, 1997). Indeed, it may be that the ability to make explicit judgments of the visual properties of stimuli depends on an intact visual association cortex (Stoerig & Cowey, 1997).

Even more surprisingly, these preserved visual abilities might not be limited to simple form and position information. For instance, Marcel (1998) studied two individuals with blindsight and demonstrated that words that were presented in the scotoma could influence subsequent behavior. If the word *river* was presented in the scotoma and participants were asked to define the word *bank*, they would define the word as the border of a river, even though the more common definition of the term is "a financial institution." Marcel (1998) suggests that blindsight may encompass more complicated visual perception than was previously recognized. Interestingly, there are also rare but analogous conditions in other modalities: "deaf hearing" in audition and numbsense/blindtouch in somesthesis (Garde & Cowey, 2000; Halligan, Hunt, Marshall, & Wade, 1995). These perceptual phenomena may also rely on similar intact subcortical and secondary cortical mechanisms. This would be consistent with a common organizational structure evident in all sensory systems.

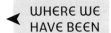 **◄ WHERE WE HAVE BEEN** We have investigated some common organizational features of sensory systems. We have detailed the functional neuroanatomy of the visual system, and described what happens when this system is damaged. Syndromes such as visual agnosia have taught us much about the organization of the visual system, as well as providing fascinating examples of disconnection syndromes.

Glossary

Agnosia—A deficit in recognition that is not due to impairments in sensation, attention, language, or general intelligence; can occur in any sensory modality.

Alexia without agraphia—A condition in which individuals lose the ability to read but retain the ability to write.

Anomia—The inability to correctly name objects.

Apperceptive visual agnosia—The inability to recognize an object owing to a problem in perceiving it; often results from damage to the posterior temporal and occipital cortices (usually bilaterally) and circumscribed right hemisphere lesions.

Association cortex—Cortex that receives information from more than one sensory modality.

Associative visual agnosia—Refers to a class of related disorders in which individuals lose the ability to associate visual forms with meaning; often results from damage to the posterior left hemisphere.

Binocular disparity—The difference in view caused by looking at an object first with one eye, then with the other eye.

Blindsight—A condition in which people are not consciously aware that they are perceiving visual stimuli but, when forced, often show evidence that the stimuli are being perceived.

Category-specific visual agnosia—A form of associative visual agnosia in which individuals display symptoms within a class of visual stimuli (such as an inability to name nonliving objects, such as a calculator).

Color agnosia—A loss of knowledge about color that cannot be accounted for by an impairment of color discrimination, aphasia, or some general intellectual deterioration.

Dorsal visual stream—The visual pathway that primarily processes information about object location.

Lateral geniculate nucleus (LGN)—A nucleus of the thalamus that receives information from the retina. It contains six distinct cell layers that receive different sensory information.

Middle temporal region (MT, V5)—An area of the visual cortex that projects dorsally to the posterior parietal lobes; is responsive to movement and orientation and may be functionally relevant for analysis of movement.

Optic aphasia—A condition in which individuals' ability to name visual objects is impaired but their ability to recognize objects is intact.

Parvocellular layers (P layers)—The name for the top four layers of the LGN, which are composed of neurons that have small cell bodies.

Perception—The way in which our brains interpret the information that is gathered by the senses (vision, audition, smell, taste, and proprioception).

Primary sensory cortex—Cortex that receives information relayed from the senses through the thalamus.

Prosopagnosia—The selective inability to recognize faces that cannot be attributable to sensory problems (i.e., blindness) or more general intellectual deficits.

Retina—Layered structure at the back of the eye that contains five different types of cells (receptors, horizontal cells, bipolar cells, amacrine cells, and retinal ganglion cells).

Scotoma—The "blind" spot that appears when the primary visual cortex is damaged; appears in the visual field opposite to where the damage has occurred.

Secondary sensory cortex—Cortex that receives much of its information from the primary sensory cortex.

Sensation—The detection of some aspect of a stimulus in the environment.

Ventral visual stream—A visual stream that primarily processes object identity.

CHAPTER

7

Memory

It isn't so astonishing the number of things that I can remember, as the number of things that I can remember that aren't so.

—MARK TWAIN

How would you define memory? When asked to provide a definition of memory, many people would simply provide a synonym for the ability to consciously recall specific events or facts. Does this definition adequately describe what you do when you look up a phone number? Most likely, when you look up a phone number, you forget the number immediately after you call it (unless you call the number a lot). How does your first definition fit the types of memories that we have for specific skills, such as riding a bicycle? What words would you use to tell someone else how to ride a bicycle? Do these words capture the essence of riding a bicycle? On top of it all, you are probably able to use skills that you cannot remember learning. For example, although you learned to speak a specific language as a child (e.g., English), you probably cannot remember ever learning how to speak this language despite the fact that you use it constantly. These examples illustrate that there are a number of different memory systems that underlie different types of memories. As we will see, one type of memory is easy to describe using language, whereas another type of memory is quite difficult to describe using language.

MODULE **7.1**
Types of Memories

If we were to describe memory as a unitary phenomenon, we would have to describe it as both permanent and erasable, as having both limited and unlimited capacity, as being both conscious and unconscious, and as having a duration limited to only a few seconds or lasting a lifetime. These contradictory features of memory form the basis of what we will investigate in this module. In fact, most memory researchers believe that memory is not a unitary phenomenon. As we will see, there are a variety of memory systems that are subserved by a number of different neural systems within the brain. The existence of multiple memory systems might account for these apparent discrepancies in how we describe memory.

WHERE WE ARE GOING ➤ This module will present material that will explain the position that there are multiple memory systems, using behavioral results that illustrate how the brain learns and remembers different types of information. Module 7.2 will present material examining what we know about memory by studying people with neurological deficits or impaired memory.

What Is Memory?

To examine what memory is, we need to briefly discuss learning. After all, try remembering something that you have not first learned or try demonstrating that you have learned something that you cannot remember. Very simply defined, **learning** is a relatively permanent change in behavior as a function of experience. Learning is typically demonstrated by having an organism demonstrate a change in behavior as a result of experience or showing that the organism recalls or remembers these experiences and changes its behavior accordingly. Learning and memory are the two sides of the same coin, which could be called *experience-dependent behavior*. It is important to note that studies of both learning and memory as phenomena are basically inferential; that is, we watch behavior and infer that someone is learning or remembering on the basis of what the person does. Thus, the distinction between learning and memory is somewhat artificial, as these two phenomena depend critically on each other.

Some memory researchers make a division of between learning and memory in the following way: Learning is concerned with attending to the information (**encoding**) and storing it for later use (**consolidation**); **memory** is concerned with retrieving the information from where it was stored (**retrieval**) in the brain (Figure 7.1). Problems with either the encoding, consolidation, or retrieval of information will result in an impairment in function, although unless you know where in the chain the problem occurred, you will not be able to tell whether the problem resulted from failure to learn or failure to remember. As we will learn in this chapter, good storage leads to good retrieval. Although encoding, consolidation, and retrieval are useful concepts, it is important to stress again that memory is not a unitary phenomenon. It is tempting to view memory as a filing cabinet or computer hard drive for experiences. However, as we will see, memory shares many similarities with these storage devices (including the ability to misplace important items). Unlike filing cabinets and computers, forgetting might actually serve an important function in your brain.

Figure 7.1   **Events Required to Produce a Memory**

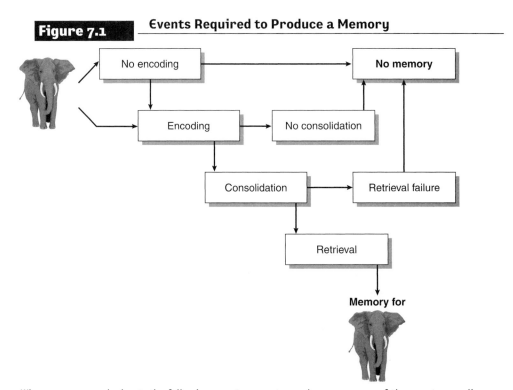

When you see an elephant, the following events occur to produce a memory of the event: encoding, consolidation, and retrieval. Interference at any one of these steps results in no memory for the event.

Sensory Memory and Short-Term Memory

Try this experiment: Turn a bright light on in a dark room. Look at the light, and then turn it off. How long can you "see" an image of the light? Does the image go away as soon as the light is turned off? Memory requires information that is gathered by the senses to be perceived and encoded. Neiser (1967) identified the phenomenon that you just experienced in the experiment as a type of sensory memory. He named these short-term **sensory memories** either **iconic memory** if they were visually based or **echoic memory** if they were sound-based.

Much of what we know about iconic memory relies on the use of a tachistoscope, which permits stimuli to be presented for extremely short periods of time. A researcher named Sperling (1960) performed a series of extremely interesting experiments investigating iconic memory (Figure 7.2). Sperling presented participants with three rows of four letters for 50 milliseconds. Participants were then asked to name all the letters that they could remember. In this first experiment, participants typically remembered about three or four of the twelve letters. However, in a second experiment, Sperling asked the participants to report the letters that were in either the top, middle, or bottom row, *after* the participants had viewed the array of letters. Interestingly, the participants tended to remember the same number of letters, three or four, only now they were specific to a particular row.

How do we interpret this evidence? If we were to take into account only the results from the first experiment, we might be tempted to say that participants remembered three or four letters and forgot the rest. The results of the second experiment suggest that participants can direct their remembering to a particular line of information. How is this possible? Because the participants did not know ahead of time which line they would be asked to remember, these results suggest that most of the twelve letters were in iconic memory and that participants can remember specific features of visual information for a short period of time. Sperling interpreted his results as evidence that his participants were "reading" their responses from a rapidly decaying visual trace.

Sperling introduced a delay between the viewing of the letter array and the reporting of the letters. He found that delays of approximately 500 milliseconds resulted in the largest decrease in iconic memory. This result is consistent with Sperling's hypothesis that the participants were reading from a decaying visual trace. Intriguingly, when a bright light follows the letter array immediately, it appears as if the bright light "erases" the letter trace, as participants cannot remember the usual three or four letters from the array. This suggests that iconic memory is very fragile and heavily reliant on peripheral stimuli. Furthermore, it appears that these letters are being rapidly

An Example of the Experiment Performed by Sperling

Figure 7.2

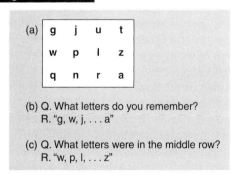

(a)
g	j	u	t
w	p	l	z
q	n	r	a

(b) Q. What letters do you remember?
   R. "g, w, j, . . . a"

(c) Q. What letters were in the middle row?
   R. "w, p, l, . . . z"

In (a) the three rows of four letters are presented briefly (50 milliseconds). When participants are asked to remember as many letters as they can—part (b)—they typically can remember three or four letters. When participants are asked to remember as many letters as they can from the middle row in (c), they typically can remember three or four of the middle row.

transferred to a more durable format (Sperling, 1963, 1967) in order for them to be able to be recalled a short time later. A number of subsequent experiments have demonstrated that color, motion, and shape can be stored in iconic memory. Interestingly, it appears that the two sides of the brain perform this task equally well (Marquez, Zubiaur, Serrano, & Delgado, 1989). Presumably, the advantage that the left hemisphere has for identifying letters and numbers is not due to differences in iconic memory.

Echoic memory has many of the same properties as iconic memory. For one thing, it is a very fragile and temporary memory store. To investigate echoic memory, participants are typically presented with a series of brief tones and asked to indicate when they hear a second tone. The loudness of the second tone is manipulated. When the second tone immediately followed the first tone, researchers found that the noise had to be very loud to be detected. When the second tone followed the first tone after a long delay, the detected noise could be much quieter. These results suggest that, like iconic memory, the echoic memory trace is much stronger immediately after the perception of a sound. There are a number of experiments that suggest that echoic memory appears to share many features with iconic memory, the major difference being the modality of the stimulus.

What happens to sensory memories? As we saw above, it appears that sensory memory is rapidly converted to a more durable form of memory, which is referred to as short-term memory. **Short-term memory** is responsible for holding information for periods beyond what can be stored by sensory memory, although like sensory traces, short-term memory is not permanent. Short-term memory can be in any sensory modality (visual, auditory, tactile, gustatory, or olfactory).

The differences between short-term visual memory and iconic memory were nicely illustrated by an experiment performed by Posner, Boies, Eichelman, and Taylor (1969). In this task, participants were asked to look at two letters and say "yes" if they had the same name and "no" if they did not (e.g., the stimulus *Aa* should result in a response of "yes," and the stimulus *Ab* should result in a response of "no"). They found that participants were faster when they were presented with letters that were of the same name and case (e.g., *aa* or *BB*). Curiously, the researchers also found that delays up to two seconds between the presentation of the first stimulus and the second stimulus (much longer than iconic representations) resulted in better performance for the congruent pairs. Posner and colleagues suggested that the comparisons made in this task with the short delay relied on the visual similarities between the pairs, whereas the comparisons made in this task with the longer delay (more than two seconds) relied on the verbal response made to the stimuli. However, visual short-term memory does not just process verbal material. Using the same paradigm, Phillips and Baddeley (1971) used complex visual stimuli that resembled checkerboards instead of letters. As before, participants had to state whether or not the two patterns were the same or different. Phillips and Baddeley obtained very similar results with one exception: They found evidence that this memory store lasted much longer than two seconds! Furthermore, following the initial stimulus with a distractor (another visual stimulus) did not affect performance of this task, which is unlike what is observed with iconic memory (for which distracting stimuli do interfere with performance). These results are evidence for a separate form of visual memory that differs from iconic memory and is responsible for holding relevant visual information for slightly longer periods. This type of memory is referred to as **short-term visual memory.**

The differences between **short-term auditory memory** and echoic memory can be illustrated by the double-take effect. Sometimes when you are speaking to someone, you do not always understand what the person is saying and you find yourself "replaying" a comment. Often, it seems as if you come to understand the comment during the replay. In a very elegant experiment, Glucksberg and Cowen (1970), studied participants who were wearing headphones and listening to a speech using only one ear (e.g., the right ear). To ensure that the participants were paying attention to the speech, the experimenter had them repeat it aloud. At the same time, a different speech was being presented to the other ear (in this example, the left ear), which the participants were supposed to ignore. Participants were really quite good at this task and repeated the correct speech back quite well. However, sometimes the ignored speech would contain a number. Randomly, the participants would have to report this number to the experimenter; interestingly, the participants were also good at this. Similar to the case with short-term visual memory, their performance was best when the interval between the number and the request from the experimenter was short (less than five seconds) and poorest when the interval was quite long (more than five seconds). Thus, it appears that, as with the visual system, there is evidence that there is a difference between sensory memory and short-term representations of auditory material.

Another important difference between short-term memory and sensory memory is that unlike sensory memory, there appears to be a limit to how much information short-term memory can store. Miller (1956) observed that short-term memory could hold about seven units of information. If you try to remember the list of numbers 1 3 0 6 8 6 7 5 3 0 9, you should be able to recall about seven of them. However, when the numbers are grouped as: 1 (306) 867-5309, you should be able to recall all ten. Thus, it appears that short-term memory does not care about the content of the information—people readily use short-term memory to hold seven letters, seven numbers, or seven words. When we reduce the number of pieces into chunks, such as the components of a long-distance phone number, we are reducing the load on short-term memory. Thus, **chunking** information improves your ability to hold larger sets of information in short-term memory.

Information in short-term memory is not a permanent store. There is evidence that much of what is held in short-term memory is rapidly forgotten, especially if there is a distraction (Brown, 1958; Peterson & Peterson, 1959). In a series of experiments, it was demonstrated that when participants were given two sets of information to remember (e.g., a consonant trigram such as BFN and a three-digit numeral such as 235) followed by a distractor task (e.g., counting backward from 100 by threes), the participants recalled very few of the letters in the consonant trigram (Figure 7.3). This experimental design came to be known as the **Brown-Peterson design,** and many experiments were conducted to determine why there was such rapid forgetting under these circumstances.

These results were interpreted in two distinct ways: interference effects and trace discrimination. Some researchers suggested that the disruption of the memory in the Brown-Peterson design was due to retroactive interference. **Retroactive interference** is inferred when the learning of new material interferes with the recall of previously

Figure 7.3 — The Brown-Peterson Design

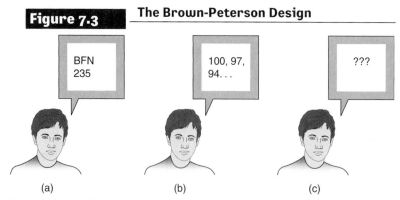

In part (a), participants are given a consonant trigram and a three-digit number to remember. In part (b), participants are asked to count backward by threes from 100. In part (c), participants are asked to remember the letters. Typically, performance on this task is very poor.

learned material (as compared to **proactive interference,** which occurs when new learning is disrupted by previously learned material). That is, keeping track of where you are in the counting task and performing the subtraction retroactively interferes with the ability to remember the consonant trigram. Others suggested that trace discrimination was at the root of the forgetting. **Trace discrimination theory** suggests that short-term memories begin to degrade spontaneously over time and that retrieval of short-term memory requires that the information be distinct from other pieces of stored information. That is, memory for the consonant trigram and the three-digit numeral

Current Controversy

Better Living through Modern Chemistry

Most of us experience forgetfulness in our everyday lives (Where did I put the remote? Where are the car keys?). Wouldn't it be nice to take a pill and ensure that we wouldn't forget? Nutriceuticals, the field in which nutritional supplements *(nutri-)* are used to treat disease *(-ceuticals),* is a burgeoning field, with estimated sales in the billions of dollars. Plants such as gingko biloba, kava kava, and red ginseng have all been suggested as supplements that can, among other things, improve memory. Components of food such as antioxidants (e.g., vitamin E) or coenzyme Q-10 are routinely ascribed properties related to relieving symptoms of dementia.

But what is the evidence that they actually work? In a meta-analysis, Beaubrun and Gray (2000) suggested that many of the forty studies that had been conducted on the effectiveness of ginkgo extracts in the treatment of dementia were flawed. For instance, a majority of the studies reviewed used nonrandom samples of individuals and/or did not control for placebo effects. However, Beaubrun and Gray (2000) acknowledged that, although they were few in number, in the studies that were well designed, it did appear that there was a reduction in cognitive decline among individuals with dementia who received gingko. Keep in mind, though, that gingko biloba is quite chemically complex, and no one is sure why it works or how (nor for that matter what the active component is). Furthermore, it is unclear whether or not more traditional treatments would have produced similar results.

You also need to take into consideration that the field of nutriceuticals is not regulated as the pharmaceutical industry is. Thus, unlike taking an aspirin, when you take a gingko biloba capsule, you might not be taking a uniform dose. The preparation of nutriceuticals is not standardized, nor is there any guarantee that you will be receiving the same amount of the preparation from capsule to capsule or between different manufacturers. Different manufacturers prepare their products differently, and this preparation is currently unregulated. Importantly, these preparations could have physiological effects that may make certain conditions worse, and they may interact with prescription medications. Finally, many of these supplements are part of a healthy diet, and you may already be getting them as an added benefit of what you eat.

begins to decay immediately. The numbers that the participant calculates in the subtraction task are also stored in short-term memory. Over the course of the subtraction task, the information from the subtraction task and the consonant trigram cannot be reliably distinguished. Unfortunately, neither hypothesis can completely explain the behaviors produced by the Brown-Peterson design. Although both hypotheses have their strengths, they both also have weaknesses. Currently, there is no better hypothesis regarding this phenomenon.

◄ **WHERE WE HAVE BEEN**   We have examined the properties of sensory memory and short-term memory. Although these memory systems share many facets, the evidence suggests that they are separable memory systems. These memory systems are concerned primarily with perceiving information and with maintaining the information over the short term.

WHERE WE ARE GOING ►   In the next section, we will investigate both working memory and long-term memory. We will investigate where in the brain these systems appear to be located in neurologically normal participants. Module 7.2 will present material examining what we know about memory by studying people with neurological deficits or impaired memory.

Working Memory

One way to characterize memory is by how long the information can be retained. As we have seen, sensory memory has a duration ranging from milliseconds to seconds, and short-term memory has a duration of only a few seconds. But what about other "short-term" memories that we can hold for minutes or even hours? For example, when you drive to a sporting event, you may have a choice of a number of locations in which to park your car. Most people can watch the event and then successfully return to their car. Once the car is located, they soon forget the information about where the car was parked. (Try remembering a parking spot that you used three games before last!) This example shares an important similarity with short-term memory: Once the old information (your parking spot three games ago) is replaced by new information (your current parking spot), retrieval of the old information is seriously impaired (as in the rapid forgetting that occurred in the Brown-Peterson design). Does this example suggest that some short-term memories might last for hours?

To deal with this observation and others similar to it, the concept of **working memory** was developed. Working memory contains information that is going to be acted on or used in some fashion. Unlike material in sensory memory and short-term memory, material in working memory does not have to come directly from the environment. That is, working memory can manipulate information that is retrieved from long-term memory stores and does not require that the event be physically present. For instance, think about calling a good friend on the telephone. If you were able to do this without looking up the phone number, your working memory retrieved the information from long-term memory stores so that you would be able to dial the number. Although the phone number requires the information to be held for only a relatively short period of time, the parking spot example (above) suggests that information

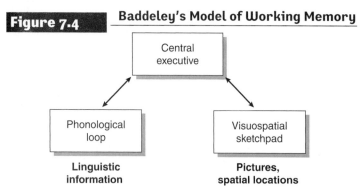

Figure 7.4 — **Baddeley's Model of Working Memory**

In this model, the central executive is responsible for allocating resources for processing the material. The phonological loop is responsible for handling information that is language-based, whereas the visuospatial sketchpad is responsible for handling information that is nonlinguistically based, such as pictures or locations in space.

can be held in working memory for relatively long periods of time. However, remembering a phone number and a parking spot might require different types of memory—one that is primarily visuospatial ("Where in space did I park?") and one that is primarily linguistic ("What is Molly's phone number?").

Baddeley and his colleagues have performed a number of experiments that have done much to illustrate the properties of working memory. Baddeley presents a three-component model of working memory with the primary component (or **central executive**) responsible for controlling attention and supervising the two "slave" subsystems (Figure 7.4). The two slave systems are known as the **phonological loop** and the **visuospatial sketchpad;** they are separate and are responsible for manipulating different types of information (Baddeley & Hitch, 1974). The phonological loop is responsible for the manipulation of linguistic information, whereas the visuospatial sketchpad is responsible for the manipulation of visuospatial information, such as mental imagery and spatial locations. Within the three-component model of working memory, the properties of the phonological loop are the best understood, followed by the visuospatial sketchpad, and then the central executive. Baddeley (1998) suggests that the wealth of information about the properties of the phonological loop might reflect the relative simplicity of the phonological loop compared to either the visuospatial sketchpad or the central executive. It is important to keep in mind that when this model was first developed, a large amount of research had already been performed on language and language processing. Before continuing on with the discussion of the properties of these components of working memory, try the experiment outlined in *The Real World.*

THE PHONOLOGICAL LOOP. The phonological loop consists of at least two components (Figure 7.5): a phonological store and a controller for inner speech, often referred to as an articulatory control process. The phonological store can hold linguistic information for no more than 2 seconds, unless it is refreshed by inner speech. The articulatory control process is used when nonverbal information (e.g., written words) is converted into the phonological sounds of language, thereby producing inner speech. These two components of the phonological loop work in tandem and are active whenever linguistic material is being manipulated by the phonological loop.

Many of the investigations of working memory have relied on a technique known as the **dual-task paradigm.** To interfere with the phonological loop, a participant is asked to perform two tasks at the same time, one of which is the primary task (e.g., list learning) and one of which is irrelevant (e.g., repeating the days of the week). This

the **Real** world

Can You Do Two Things at the Same Time?

Try this experiment and find out.

Read the following list of words and time how long it takes you to read it:

§

tomato	kiwi	lettuce	beans
carrot	pepper	okra	melon
lemon	cucumber	grapes	apple
pineapple	peach	figs	potato

§

Now flip over the book, and list as many of the words as you can (no peeking!).

Now trace the pattern on either side of the list with your index finger while you are reading this list. Time how long it takes you to read the list.

§

hammer	eraser	tack	putty
drill	nail	drywall	bolt
scissors	glue	paint	saw
pen	awl	calculator	screwdriver

§

Now flip over the book, and list as many of the words as you can.

Now, out loud, say the days of the week while you are reading this list. Time how long it takes you to read the list.

§

cow	goat	chinchilla	giraffe
sparrow	snake	kitten	agouti
orangutan	eagle	pig	chicken
sheltie	frog	monkey	salmon

§

Now flip over the book, and list as many of the words as you can.

What did you notice? Was one list harder than another? Did reading one list take you longer? Most people report that their recall of the list is poorer and that it takes longer to read the list when they are saying the days of the week. (On top of it all, most people can say the days of the week faster when they are not also reading another list.) This type of dual-task paradigm is frequently used in the investigation of the properties of working memory.

form of the dual-task paradigm is often called **articulatory suppression.** Articulatory suppression results in a disruption in the performance of a primary task, perhaps because the phonological loop has a limited store and the irrelevant task is using some of the resources available to the phonological loop. An interesting real-life example of articulatory suppression occurs when you are trying to conduct two conversations

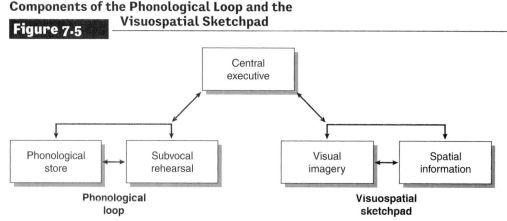

Components of the Phonological Loop and the Visuospatial Sketchpad

Figure 7.5

The phonological loop appears to consist of two components, one that acts as a phonological store and one for subvocal rehearsal. The visuospatial sketchpad appears to consist of at least two distinct components: one for creating visual imagery and one for manipulating spatial information. It is important to remember that in everyday life these components work together to provide a unified percept.

at the same time (e.g., you are using the telephone, and someone in the room is trying to carry on a conversation with you). If this has happened to you, you know that you often switch between the two conversations and that you often fail to attend to important features in one or the other conversation. These effects are likely due to the resources that are diverted from the phonological store. In articulatory suppression, the irrelevant word is repeatedly fed back into the phonological store through the articulatory control process. Furthermore, because the articulatory control process is repeatedly involved in producing the irrelevant word, there are fewer resources to encode the material from the primary task into phonology so that it can access the phonological store. Although many researchers have their participants say the irrelevant items aloud, disruption of the phonological loop can occur without overt speech.

Importantly, it does not appear that the effects that are observed with articulatory suppression result from divided attention. It seems reasonable to suggest that when you are doing any two activities at the same time, your performance on the primary task would be impaired. However, if participants perform a nonlinguistic secondary task (such as tracing a shape with their fingers), there does not appear to be a disruption of the primary linguistic task (e.g., Baddeley, Lewis, & Vallar, 1984). Thus, it appears that performing two tasks at once affects the phonological loop only when the secondary task requires the resources of the phonological store or the articulatory control process.

How big is the storage capacity of the phonological loop? If the phonological store can hold information for about two seconds, then it seems likely that the capacity of the phonological loop might be equivalent to the number of items that can be spoken in two seconds. In a series of very clever experiments performed by Zhang and Simon, this hypothesis was investigated. This series of experiments relied on features of the Chinese language that could be manipulated to test the capacity of the phonological loop. For instance, written Chinese is made up of about 200 components that are called *radicals* (similar to letters in English). These components make up the characters in typeset Chinese and are very familiar to people who read Chinese. However, unlike English letters, these radicals do not typically have oral sounds that go with them. When participants were asked to remember lists of Chinese radicals, a very interesting result was obtained (Zhang & Simon, 1985). Participants were not able to remember the lists of radicals very well. However, if the radicals were presented in pairs that, when combined, made a single speech sound (phoneme), participants were able to remember almost three times the number of radicals (even though there was, technically, more information to remember). When the radicals were combined to make multisyllabic words (but had the same number of radicals), performance was poorer than when the radicals were combined to make a single speech sound but better than when the radicals did not indicate a phoneme.

Zhang and Simon interpret this result as evidence that the storage capacity of the phonological loop is limited by the number of sounds that a participant can make in a brief period of time. The greatest number of radicals was remembered when the radicals were combined to form a single phoneme, then followed by combinations of radicals that indicated multisyllabic phonemes. Articulation of multisyllabic phonemes takes more time than uttering single phonemes, which, according to Zhang and Simon, is why performance on the multisyllabic task is relatively impaired. However, the poorest performance occurred when the articulatory control process could not be engaged (i.e., the radical did not indicate a sound), which would have prevented the radical from entering the phonological store.

In another experiment, Zhang and Simon investigated how homophones affected performance. Homophones are words that make the same sound when spoken but are spelled differently and have different meanings (e.g., *would* and *wood*). Oral Chinese has quite a large number of homophones, and in this experiment, participants were asked to remember lists of homophones (Zhang & Simon, 1985). Zhang and Simon found that participants did not perform very well when they had to write out as many of the words from the list as they could. Zhang and Simon interpret their results as indicating that, again, the articulatory control process did not provide discriminatory information to the phonological store. That is, because all the words were indicated by the same sound, performance on this task did not rely on remembering the sound of the word (which presumably is what is encoded by the phonological loop). Rather, performance on this task required a memory of the visual or semantic properties of the word (which apparently was not encoded very well).

THE VISUOSPATIAL SKETCHPAD. The visuospatial sketchpad (VSSP) is assumed to be responsible for the manipulation of visuospatial images. Research suggests that the VSSP is also composed of two subunits: one that is responsible for mental imagery and one that is responsible for spatial information (Figure 7.5). Information that is held in the VSSP can come either from the environment (primarily through visual perception) or from mental imagery. This is quite similar to the phonological loop, as the phonological loop can hold either overt speech (obtained through auditory perception) or covert speech (inner speech).

The VSSP shares a number of features with the phonological loop. For one thing, there is a limited store, and information in the store can be affected by the performance of a secondary, irrelevant task. In the studies that follow, you can see that mental imagery plays a large part in the VSSP. For instance, in one experiment (Brooks, 1967), participants were asked to remember a series of sentences. These sentences differed in the degree to which they provoked a mental image (e.g., "the 3 is to the right of the 7" versus "the 3 is to the slow of the 7"). Brooks observed that participants were better able to remember the sentences that were easily imageable. Furthermore, it appeared that participants were able to remember approximately eight of the imageable sentences. Concurrent performance of irrelevant spatial tasks (such as requiring the participants to press buttons in a pattern during the task) during a memory task for imageable sentences impairs the recall of the imageable sentences (e.g., Baddeley, Grant, Wight, & Thomson, 1975). Interestingly, it also appears that mental imagery does not require the participation of the visual system, as people who are blind can perform these types of tasks.

However, mental imagery is not all that the VSSP can manipulate. Although much less is known about it, it also appears that the VSSP is involved with the storage and manipulation of spatial information, such as the location of objects in space (such as when you try to recall the location of your keys). Shepard and Metzler (1971) asked participants to look for objects that were the same among groups of similarly (but not always identical) shaped objects that were presented in different orientations (Figure 7.6). They found that the time that it took participants to make their decisions depended on the degree to which the stimulus object (the one in the group of objects) was rotated from the target object (the one that they were asked to look for). That is, it took participants longer to determine whether the objects were the same if they were rotated 90 degrees from each other than if the angle was only 30 degrees. Shepard and Metzler interpreted this result as suggesting that the participants were mentally rotating the objects until both were in the same orientation and then making their decision as to their similarity. It appears that having to perform an irrelevant spatial task but not a verbal one also interferes with performance on tasks requiring spatial processing (e.g., Logie, Zucco, & Baddeley, 1990).

Figure 7.6 ——— **An Example of the Mental Rotations Test**

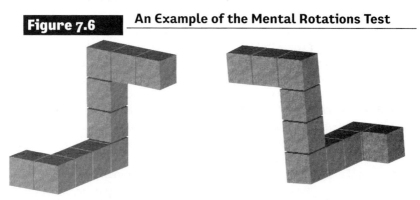

Are these two figures images of the same object in two different orientations, or two completely different objects? (Answer: Two different objects.)

Through the study of people with specific cognitive deficits, we can observe that working memory for spatial locations is separable from that of imagery. Martha Farah and her colleagues (Farah, Hammond, Levine, & Calvanio, 1988) describe an individual who was quite impaired at describing mental images. He was unable to describe what type of tail a monkey might have and how it would be different from that of a pig, how the color of a ripe versus unripe fruit might change, and so on. However, he did not have a problem with performing tasks that required the manipulation of spatial information, such as the mental rotations task or placing cities on a map. The opposite effect also has been observed. For example, Levine and colleagues (Levine, Warach, & Farah, 1985) studied a man who was quite able to give detailed descriptions of his mental images but was quite unable to point to locations within his room (or to point to the direction of familiar landmarks) when his eyes were closed. These deficits appear to be related specifically to the VSSP, as neither of these people had problems with language.

THE CENTRAL EXECUTIVE. When the tripartite model of working memory was first introduced in this chapter, the central executive was said to be responsible for controlling attention and supervising the two slave systems. However, there has been far less research on the central executive than on either of the two slave systems. One reason for this is that it is very difficult to study the central executive without involving either of the slave systems. The other reason is that the concept of the central executive is rather vague, and various definitions of the central executive include such functions as allocation of attention, integration of the information coming from two slave systems, and strategy selection.

One example of strategies that people use for solving problems is illustrated in the following example. Most keys look alike, and most people who work at any large institution have large numbers of keys. Although there are some differences (e.g., the keys for my university are golden and most house keys are silver), how do you remember which key goes in which door? Many keys at my university have numbers stamped on them. Several people I know remember which key is which by learning the number that corresponds to each door, whereas I remember the shape of the key that goes with each door and others put plastic tags on the keys and remember which color goes with which door. Regardless of how you remember keys, it is unlikely that you typically stand at a locked door and try all of your keys. When you encounter a problem, you must decide how to solve it (do you use a verbal or a spatial strategy?), you must allocate resources to it, and you must assess the information that is coming in to decide whether the problem has been solved. Perhaps one of the most important functions of the central executive is the ability to switch among strategies to find the best solution to the problem.

Another everyday example illustrates some other properties of the central executive: Have you ever been walking to class, thinking about a problem, and when you get there, you realize that you cannot remember the route that you took? Presumably, you took the correct spatial route through the campus, because you arrived at the correct classroom. Furthermore, you most likely performed a series of complicated motor movements, along with thinking about your problem. This task has become relatively automatic and caused little interference with other ongoing tasks. However, other tasks are more difficult to do at the same time, such as driving in rush hour traffic and speaking with a passenger. In this situation, it is quite common for the driver (and the passenger) to stop talking when passing other cars or when weaving in and out of traffic. Thus, it appears that the central executive is able to allocate attention so that, in some situations, more than one task can be done at one time and to shut down competing activity when situations require more attention.

Norman and Shallice (1986) proposed a model of how the brain controls both voluntary and habitual activity. They suggest that a supervisory attentional system is responsible for monitoring ongoing behavior and ensuring the correct outcome. The supervisory attentional system is particularly required in situations in which the routine selection of actions might result in a bad outcome, such as those involved in coping with novelty. Shallice and Burgess (1996) suggest that the supervisory attentional system is involved in the planning of actions and in producing multiple actions that are performed relatively independent of each other. Baddeley (1998) suggests that these features of the supervisory attentional system mirror the proposed functions of the central executive.

Burgess and Shallice (1996a, 1996b) suggest that there are a number of tests that rely primarily on the functions of the supervisory attentional system/central executive. The first test, known as the **Hayling test,** is a test in which participants are given a sentence with the last word missing. In the first part of the test, participants are asked to provide a word that would finish the sentence in a meaningful way. The sentences are constructed so that they produce highly cued or automatic responses (e.g., "The doctor stitched up the cut with a _____ " would lead to "The doctor stitched up the cut with a *needle*"). The second half of the test uses the same sentences, but now participants have to finish the sentence with a word that makes no sense (e.g., "The doctor stitched up the cut with a *pigeon*"). Thus, the second half of the test requires the participant to inhibit the automatic response and produce a novel one. Although the Hayling test undoubtedly relies on the phonological loop, the interesting comparison is between the automatic and the inhibition conditions, which relies primarily on the central executive. Another test that is used to test the properties of the central executive is the **Brixton test** (Figure 7.7), which consists of a series of plates on which ten dots are presented. One of the dots is colored and moves from plate to plate over successive trials. The dot moves from plate to plate according to very simple rules. Participants are asked to predict where the dot will be next. Again, although the test might involve the VSSP, correct prediction of the future location of the dot requires deducing rules and strategies, which are functions posited for the central executive. However, unlike the case with the other two components of working memory, despite these tests of central executive func-

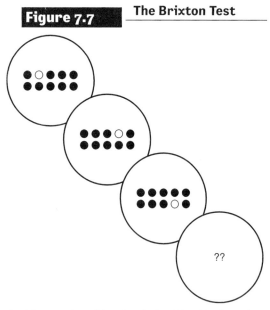

Figure 7.7   **The Brixton Test**

In this test, the subject is asked to identify where the white dot will be on the last trial.

tion, it is difficult to conceptualize what performance on these tasks means with respect to the capacity of the central executive. By its very nature, the central executive must be able to multitask, apportion resources for competing activities, and rapidly switch strategies. Good performance on these tasks therefore requires a number of skills all occurring at the same time, which tends to make the interpretation of the results difficult. Instead of looking at "normal" central executive function, much of the work using these tasks has focused on where in the brain central executive functions are located, using both imaging techniques and case studies.

WHERE IN THE BRAIN IS WORKING MEMORY LOCATED? On the basis of the functions of working memory components and the knowledge you have gained from previous chapters, you might be tempted to localize the phonological loop to Broca's area and the temporal lobes, the VSSP to the parietal lobes, and the central executive to the frontal lobes. For the most part, these assumptions have been shown to be correct, although as we will see, important contributions are made by other areas of the brain.

When participants perform tasks requiring the phonological loop, researchers tend to observe left hemisphere activation (Figure 7.8a), primarily localized within the left posterior parietal cortex (BA40), Broca's area (BA44), the left premotor area (BA6), and the left supplementary motor area (BA6). Broca's area, the left premotor area, and the left supplementary motor area are all known to be involved in the planning and production of speech and have been shown to be active in tasks that require covert speech (Smith & Jonides, 1998). When tasks are designed to reduce the utility of covert speech, only the frontal and parietal areas showed activation, suggesting that these areas are important for working memory tasks requiring the phonological loop.

If the phonological store can be anatomically distinguished from the controller for inner speech, we might predict that lesions of these areas might differentially affect phonological working memory. Indeed, lesions of Broca's area result in Broca's aphasia, a speech disturbance marked by serious difficulties with the production of speech. Broca's aphasics also have serious problems with phonological working memory tasks, especially when the delays are long and would typically elicit subvocal rehearsal. This problem with working memory appears to be selective for verbal materials, as Broca's aphasics are unimpaired in tasks of visuospatial working memory. Conversely, lesions of the left posterior parietal area produce deficits that are consistent with problems with the phonological store. That is, individuals with left posterior parietal damage often have a condition known as *conduction aphasia,* which is marked by an inability to repeat back verbal material, even when the delay is short. (Conduction aphasia is described in more detail in Chapter 8.) Conduction aphasics also show other language problems, such as the transposition of phonemes in a word, that are consistent with phonological store functions for the left posterior parietal area (Smith & Jonides, 1998). Again, the deficit that is observed with conduction aphasics is specific to verbal material, as working memory for spatial patterns is unimpaired.

When participants perform tasks requiring the VSSP in imaging experiments, researchers tend to observe increased right hemisphere activity (Figure 7.8b). Within the right hemisphere, the visuospatial working memory tasks have been reported to result in activations in the right dorsolateral prefrontal areas (BA48, 9), right premo-

Figure 7.8   Anatomical Correlates of Baddeley's Model of Working Memory

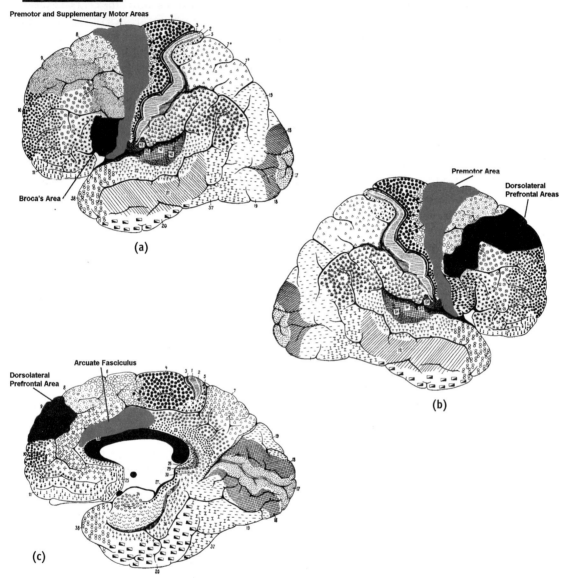

(a)

(b)

(c)

Part (a) shows localization of the phonological loop using results from imaging studies. Part (b) is localization of the VSSP using results from imaging studies. Part (c) is localization of the central executive using results from imaging studies.

Source: Figure 85 from *Brodmann's Localisation in the Cerebral Cortex,* translated and edited by Laurence J. Garey, p. 110. Copyright © 1999, World Scientific Publishing. Reprinted by permission.

tor areas (BA6), and right presupplementary motor areas (Smith & Jonides, 1999). However, as was the case with the behavioral results, the anatomy of the subsystems of the VSSP is not as well worked out as that of the phonological loop. It appears that tasks that rely heavily on the production of imagery are associated with increased activity within the right dorsolateral prefrontal cortex (BA46, 9) (e.g., Fletcher, Dennis, Shallice, Frith, Frackowiak, & Dolan, 1996), whereas tasks that rely heavily on judgments of spatial location are more consistently associated with increased activity within the right premotor cortex (BA6). However, some tasks, such as mental rotations, involve widespread activation throughout the brain, including increased activity within anterior parietal areas (BA7a, BA7b), middle frontal gyrus (BA 8), extrastriate areas (BAs 39 and 19), and somatosensory cortex devoted to the hand (Cohen, Kosslyn, Breiter, DiGirolamo, Thompson, Anderson et al., 1996). As you can tell, there is still much to be done with respect to localizing the components of the VSSP.

When participants perform tasks requiring the central executive in imaging experiments, researchers tend to observe that there are similar patterns of activation in frontal areas, regardless of whether or not the task also involves the phonological loop or the VSSP (Figure 7.8c). It appears that tasks that require attention and inhibition (e.g., the Hayling or Brixton test) consistently activate the anterior cingulate cortex (Figure 7.8c), whereas tasks that require the management of resources, such as dual-task performance, appear to consistently activate such frontal areas as the dorsolateral prefrontal cortex and the anterior cingulate (Smith & Jonides, 1999). Interestingly, as you will learn in Chapter 11, lesions of the frontal cortex are associated with problems with planning and other components of the central executive, such as allocating resources in dual-task paradigms (e.g., Allain, Etcharry-Bouyx, & Le Gall, 2001), inhibition of previous responses, and choosing strategies (e.g., Burgess & Shallice, 1996a, 1996b). However, the results from the imaging studies are still quite new, and some researchers question their validity (e.g., Andres & Van der Linden, 2001).

Thus, although our initial instincts to localize the phonological loop to Broca's area and the temporal lobes, the VSSP to the parietal lobes, and the central executive to the frontal lobes have some support, there are some large deviations from the expected pattern. It appears that areas of the brain that are involved in the planning of motor movements (e.g., supplementary motor area) and executing movements (e.g., cerebellum) also play a large part in working memory. It also appears that the demands of the task play a large role in the observed effects.

◄ **WHERE WE HAVE BEEN**   We have examined the separable memory systems that underlie sensory memory, short-term memory, and working memory. Working memory underlies many cognitive processes that require the manipulation and short-term retention of a variety of materials. The tripartite model of working memory has a central executive (responsible for attention and allocation of resources to the slave systems), the phonological loop (with a separate verbal store and subvocal rehearsal system), and the VSSP (with separate systems for the manipulation of imagery and spatial information). Although far from complete, imaging studies have done much to localize these hypothesized systems within the brain.

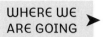

WHERE WE ARE GOING In the next section, we will investigate long-term memory, including where in the brain these systems appear to be located in both neurologically normal participants and those with brain damage. Module 7.2 will present material regarding a variety of disorders and their specific impacts on memory and memory functions.

Long-Term Memory

What is your grandmother's first name? What is the capital of Arkansas? What is 5 times 6? How do the answers to these questions differ from the other types of memories that we have discussed in the previous sections? One of the main differences is that you learned the answers to these questions many years ago. **Long-term memories** are those that you can recall days, months, and even years after they were stored. In contrast to the other forms of memory that we studied in the previous sections, it does not appear that there are limitations to the capacity of long-term memories (or if there are limitations, the capacity is extremely large). It is also quite interesting to realize that although some events were stored in long-term memory, they are no longer retrievable. For instance, I learned the state capitals in grade 6, and although I am fairly certain that I managed to pass the test, I most certainly cannot remember them anymore. Furthermore, some events, such as what you had for breakfast last Tuesday, appear never to make it into long-term memory.

A useful distinction can be made between types of long-term memories. Memories for events, such as "For my last birthday, my friends took me out for dinner," and memories for facts, such as "The capital of Arkansas is Little Rock," are typically called **explicit memories.** Memories for skills and habits, such as how to tie a bow in shoelaces are typically called **implicit memories.** However, just to be confusing, both explicit and implicit memories go by other names (perhaps because one way to become famous in psychology is to discover phenomena and name them), which might reflect the belief systems of the researcher and/or their training (see Table 7.1). This

Table 7.1

A Limited Sample of Terms Describing the Dichotomy between Implicit and Explicit Memories

Terms for Unconscious Memory	Terms for Conscious Memory
Implicit	Explicit
Semantic	Episodic
Procedural	Declarative
Skill	Fact
Habit	Memory
Reference	Working
Knowing how	Knowing that
Perceptual	Autobiographical
Taxon	Locale

Neuropsychological Celebrity

H.M.

In 1953, a man known by his initials—H.M.—underwent surgery to relieve epileptic seizures. He had been having seizures since he was about 10 years old. The severity of the seizures progressed as he aged, and drug treatments became ineffective. Therefore, at the age of 27, he underwent a bilateral medial temporal lobe resection, including the removal of the amygdala, the anterior hippocampus, and the cortex surrounding these structures. In many regards, the surgery was a success: The frequency of his seizures was reduced, his personality was unchanged, and his I.Q. actually increased to 118 (probably because during previous I.Q. tests, the seizures impaired his performance). However, H.M. is severely impaired, and his impairments are so striking that he may be the most studied person in all of neuroscience (Scoville & Milner, 1957).

Since 1953, H.M. has been largely amnesic for the events that occur around him—a deficit that is limited to explicit memory; that is, since his surgery, H.M. has learned no new facts, he cannot recall any personal experiences, nor can he recall the names of people that he has met since his surgery. The memory deficit that H.M. has is very specific: If you ask him about the events of his life before his surgery, he is able to provide details of songs, classmates, and "current events." This result suggests that his deficit is limited to encoding and/or storing new information, as he can retrieve items from his long-term store.

---

text will use the terms *implicit* and *explicit* to label these types of memories (which probably says something about my training and belief systems).

Generally, explicit memories are available for conscious recollection and can be verbally described, whereas implicit memories are not available for conscious manipulation and are very difficult to describe verbally (e.g., Moscovitch, 1994). For instance, I remember learning to drive a car with standard transmission (including hearing my dad scream, "Clutch!!! Clutch!!!"), and I certainly know that I know how to drive a standard (the explicit part of the memory). However, try telling someone who doesn't know how to drive a standard shift car exactly how to do it. (I seem to recall my dad telling me that "the clutch just 'feels' right when it is going to engage," which was far from helpful and quite hard on the transmission.) The actual motor activities that are involved in driving a standard shift car and using a clutch (the implicit part of the example) are very hard to describe verbally—it just seems that once you know how, you know how. As we will see, these differences are quite pronounced and appear to be functions of different parts of the brain. Furthermore, it is possible to have impaired explicit memory and still have normal implicit memory.

It has been said that H.M. is the most studied man in psychology; indeed, his contributions to our understanding and views about memory have been significant. Following surgery to treat intractable epilepsy, requiring the bilateral removal of the medial temporal lobes, H.M. shows a marked distinction between his abilities for implicit and explicit memory. Since his surgery in 1953, H.M. has been unable to keep track of daily events or to learn the names of new people (some of whom he has known for about fifty years). When H.M. is asked about personal events (such as the death of his father, his current age, or where he lives), he is quite unable to provide information. Remarkably, he has identified current pictures of himself as being of his father.

In addition, it appears that words that have appeared in the English language since his surgery, such as *fax* or *Jacuzzi,* are quite foreign to him, and he cannot retain them. The defining event of his generation—the assassination of President John F. Kennedy—is something that he does not recall. (Ask your parents and grandparents where they were when they learned about the Kennedy assassination.) Put simply, H.M. suffers from profound deficits in explicit memory, or **amnesia.**

H.M. has not suffered a loss of all explicit memories. He is still quite capable of recalling events that occurred before his surgery. He appears incapable of forming new explicit memories, regardless of the modality—words, text, names, tunes, anything that anyone has tried to test him with (e.g., Freed & Corkin, 1988). However, H.M. is quite capable of problem solving and spends his days watching television and solving crosswords (although he can work the same crossword again and again without appearing to notice, and commercials in the program cause him to forget the plot of the story). H.M. also shows normal working memory, sensory memory, and short-term memory.

Perhaps one of the most interesting observations about H.M. is that he shows normal implicit memory. One such task is called mirror tracing. In this task, participants are asked to trace shapes using visual feedback from a mirror. Most people find this task quite difficult initially, although they improve with practice. (Try it by using a mirror in your home.) H.M.'s performance on this task also showed improvement with practice. However, if H.M. is asked whether he has ever performed this task before, he will say that he has not, despite his almost perfect performance. Thus, H.M.'s deficit seems largely restricted to explicit memory.

Knowing what we know about H.M., it is hard to imagine why a surgeon would perform such a radical surgery. To appreciate some of the reasons why the surgery was performed in the first place, we need to look at the state of memory research in 1953. Two of the leading figures in the study of learning and memory were Karl Lashley at Harvard University and his former student D.O. Hebb at McGill University in Montreal. Although both were involved in the study of memory, they focused their search on different scales: Lashley in the search for the cortical location of memory and Hebb in the search for how the neuron encoded memories.

Lashley pioneered the search for the **engram** (physiological representation of a memory), beginning with his studies of rats in 1915. Much of Lashley's work revolved around lesioning various parts of the rat brain and studying how this affected memory. Of course, this methodology was complicated by the fact that one cannot ask rats to perform most tests of explicit memory, such as writing or vocalizing the correct answer. On the basis of hundreds of experiments, Lashley concluded that no one location in the brain was responsible for memory, although he did observe that the amount of cortex that was removed was related to deficits (i.e., the larger the amount of cortex that is removed, the greater the memory deficit). Lashley interpreted this result as suggesting that memories are stored diffusely throughout the cortex and that no one part of the brain is special for memory. In fact, Lashley said, "I have never been able by any operation on the brain to destroy a specific memory—even when the memory is elicited by electrical stimulation of the part of the cerebral cortex that is subsequently removed" (Lashley, 1952, as cited in Orbach, 1998). Thus, on the basis of Lashley's work, it did not appear feasible that bilateral removal of part of the temporal lobes would result in any memory impairments. (As an aside: It may be that Lashley did not observe these deficits because his tasks required implicit, not explicit, memory.) Furthermore, bilateral temporal lobectomies had been performed before the one done on H.M., with no obvious impairments. The majority of these people had undergone this treatment to try to treat schizophrenia. Their memory for events was not tested, and their behavior following the surgery was attributed to their psychosis. Only after the deficit was observed in H.M. were these other people tested, and it became evident that they experienced similar pathology.

On the basis of what we know about H.M., what can we say about the nature of memory? We know that the varieties of memory systems that we have discussed (e.g., implicit, explicit, working memory, and short-term memory) are not just distinct behaviorally. It appears that they might result from the functioning of distinct areas of the brain (as damage to the temporal lobes results in deficits in explicit memory and not short-term memory, implicit memory, or working memory). We know that the storage of explicit memories is not in the temporal lobes (e.g., H.M. can recall events that occurred before his surgery). Furthermore, it appears that H.M.'s deficit can be restricted to the encoding and/or storage of new explicit memories, as he is able to retrieve memories from his childhood. As you will see in Module 7.2, it appears that implicit memory function and explicit memory function rely on activity in very different parts of the brain.

Why are implicit and explicit memories so different? First, it appears that explicit and implicit memories are mediated by different parts of the brain. However, iconic and echoic memories share a remarkable number of features, despite the fact that they are encoded in the visual and auditory cortex, respectively. However, on close inspection, it appears that these parts of the brain are encoding quite different information.

Explicit memories are concerned with encoding what is different or novel in the environment. That is, explicit memories are concerned with recalling specific events, facts, or other information that is somehow unique. When you recognize a person from a photograph, you are discerning what is unique about the face and providing it with a name. This must be the case, because most faces are more the same than they are different—most faces (human or dog) have a nose, eyes, ears, and a mouth—yet if the face is known to us, we can quickly move past the similarities to provide the name of the person (which is probably not unique, either—how many Jennifers and Jasons do you know?). Furthermore, explicit memories might be processed by a variety of categories, and the data are searched until the correct item has been located. For instance, if you were trying to remember the name of the leading actor in a movie, you would not search through a phone book, which has many names in it; although the concept of name is engaged, this strategy is not one that will easily limit your search). Instead, you limit your search to names of actors that you know (the related concept). You might also try to name other shows or movies that the actor was in or name other actors that remind you of him or her.

This example illustrates another feature of explicit memory: typically, the encoding of the information is active, and the internal cues that were used to encode can be used to help with the retrieval of the memory (Loftus, 1997). Studies of eyewitness testimony have demonstrated that these cues can directly influence the subsequent recall of the information. When accidents are described as resulting from high speeds (e.g., "The car raced through the intersection and hit the bicycle"), people tend to estimate the speed as having been higher than when an accident is described as resulting from other factors (e.g., "The car nudged the bicycle"). This occurs despite the fact that participants viewed exactly the same tape of the accident (Loftus, 1998). Loftus suggests that these effects are due to the influence of the cues that are used to encode and retrieve the memory of the accident. She suggests that explicit memories are not "videotapes" of events; they are more like rough sketches of the events that can be colored by other, extraneous factors. Furthermore, encoding of explicit memories must occur rather rapidly, as many events that we recall only happened once.

Implicit memories are less driven by concepts, and more driven by the experience itself. The encoding of implicit memories is more passive and is more related to the sensory phenomena that occur during the event. In contrast with explicit memory, implicit memories are concerned with what is the same in the environment. That is, implicit memories are concerned with recalling procedures that must be performed in the same way each time. For instance, when you are learning to shoot a free throw in basketball, you are encouraged to take the same stance each time, to bounce the ball the same number of times, and to hold your shooting arm the same way each time. Some players take this to the extreme and have to wear the same socks or shoes every time. (Michael Jordan always had his University of North Carolina shorts under his Bulls uniform for good luck.) The value of exact repetition seems to be especially true with implicit memories, for which "if it ain't broke, don't fix it." If you think about it, it probably would not be a good strategy to switch the manner in which you do a number of implicit tasks—that is, of course, as long as your current method works. Again, in contrast with explicit memory, it appears that the encoding of implicit memories takes a number of trials. (Think about how difficult it is to learn a new implicit task, such as riding a bicycle or skating.) Although the encoding in implicit memory is more passive and requires more trials than explicit memory, implicit memory is also prone to error. For instance, not even Michael Jordan is perfect at the free throw line, despite thousands and thousands of practice trials and undoubtedly superior ability.

Self-Test

1. Why is it so difficult to define memory without referring to learning?

2. In what ways are working memory and short-term memory alike? In what ways are they different?

3. What are the limits of iconic memory? Are the same processes active in iconic memory as in echoic memory?

4. What are the components of the working memory model proposed by Baddeley? What evidence is there that the brain is organized in this fashion?

5. Implicit and explicit memory are good at recording specific types of information. What are these types of information?

6. What facets of implicit memory make it distinct from explicit memory?

WHERE WE HAVE BEEN We have examined the separate memory systems known as sensory memory, short-term memory, working memory, and implicit and explicit memory. We have shown that there are a number of factors that differentiate implicit and explicit memories. Implicit memories are formed slowly and are concerned with similarity of events. Explicit memories are formed quickly and are concerned with novelty. It appears that the two systems rely on different parts of the brain.

WHERE WE ARE GOING In Module 7.2, we will investigate the neurological bases of long-term memory, both implicit and explicit. Much of these investigations will examine memory function in those who have neurological disorders. Module 7.2 will also discuss the dementias and their specific impacts on memory and memory functions.

MODULE **7.2**
Disorders of Memory

With the exception of H.M., we have not really examined the neural bases of long-term memory, nor have we examined how a variety of experiences that alter brain function affect memory. The failure to encode, store, or retrieve a memory is known by the generic term *amnesia*. There are also everyday little amnesias, such as forgetting people's names or faces and where you put your keys. We also rapidly forget things we do not need to know, such as some telephone numbers. Many of these phenomena can be attributed to properties of the working memory system and not to problems in the long-term memory system. Certainly, we can agree that the type of amnesia experienced by H.M. is on a different scale than forgetting the name of the person who sits next to you in sociology class.

Amnesia: Retrograde and Anterograde

Although you might not know it, during your lifetime, you have already experienced at least one type of amnesia, which is known as **infantile amnesia.** Typically, we have no episodic memories of events that occurred before 2 years of age (although we have quite a number of implicit memories, such as being able to walk). Most people who have experienced a major event (e.g., the birth of a sibling, the death of a parent or grandparent) before the age of 2 cannot reliably recall the event. Some researchers suggest that although the nervous system is continuing to develop until at least 11 years of age, the largest changes in the nervous system are largely completed by 2 years of age. They suggest that infantile amnesia is a reflection of an inability of the immature nervous system to store episodic information. Other researchers suggest that infantile amnesia is related to language development. That is, they interpret infantile amnesia as being indicative of the tight relationship between consciousness and language (Chapter 11), in which they interpret the nonlinguistic child as being at best semiconscious and not able to process relevant events appropriately. Still others have suggested that until we are a certain age, we do not have enough experience to adequately tag events as being important and thus ensure their processing by episodic memory. (After all, when you are 18 months old, how do you know whether or not new siblings show up all the time?) It is likely that the phenomenon of infantile amnesia reflects the interaction between nervous system development, linguistic competence, and a growing repertoire of experiences. However, infantile amnesia also suggests that for most people, explicit memory begins at about the age of 2, whereas implicit memories might begin to be formed at birth.

Amnesia can also occur in adults, typically following some type of trauma to the central nervous system. **Dissociated amnesia,** in which there are no other cognitive deficits, is extremely rare, and memory loss is typically associated with other nonmemory

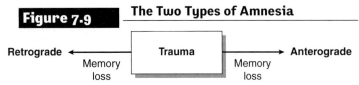

Figure 7.9   The Two Types of Amnesia

Retrograde ←——— | Trauma | ———→ Anterograde
Memory loss | | Memory loss

Retrograde and anterograde amnesia are distinguished by the time frame in which they disrupt memory. Retrograde amnesia disrupts memory for events that occurred before the trauma, whereas anterograde amnesia disrupts memory for events that occurred after the trauma.

problems, such as aphasia (see Chapter 8). Amnesia can be categorized into two general forms, which relate to the type of memory loss. **Retrograde amnesia** is the loss of memory for events that occurred before the trauma; **anterograde amnesia** is the loss of memory for events that occurred after the trauma (see Figure 7.9). Retrograde amnesia is quite common on soap operas, when characters are unable to recall their names or recognize their spouses and have lost other important information for the plot. (The actual incidence of retrograde amnesia in otherwise neurologically normal people is quite a bit lower than TV would suggest.) Conversely, H.M. primarily displays anterograde amnesia, although he also displayed mild retrograde amnesia for about two years before his surgery. However, rather than concluding that memories are stored in the temporal lobes for about two years before moving elsewhere, most people suspect that the retrograde amnesia displayed by H.M. is primarily due to the large doses of anticonvulsants and frequent seizures that occurred before the surgery.

A phenomenon similar to what is described on TV is **transient global amnesia,** in which people display no knowledge of their previous life but have intact skills and language. The onset is sudden, and although transient global amnesia has been associated with, among other conditions, migraines, epilepsy, cold showers, and stress hormones (e.g., Kessler, Markowitsch, Rudolf, & Heiss, 2001), there is often no apparent precipitating cause. Almost as abruptly as it begins, transient global amnesia is apparently resolved. We have used the word *apparently* because although there is improvement in the retrograde aspects of amnesia—and unlike what is depicted on TV—there is often an inability to form new memories. Often, the considerable memory loss is overlooked owing to the dramatic recovery (Kessler et al., 2001). Despite this "recovery," careful psychometric testing reveals that there are significant anterograde memory impairments that can persist, with reports for periods ranging from days to months after the initial incident (e.g., Jovin, Vitti, & McCluskey, 2000). A number of imaging studies have suggested that this amnesia results from decreased metabolism and blood flow to the mesial temporal lobes, which usually resolves spontaneously (e.g., Eustache, Desgranges, Aupee, Guillery, & Baron, 2000; Jovin et al., 2000; Masson, 2000).

AMNESIA RESULTING FROM CONCUSSION. Amnesia is commonly associated with concussion, which is defined as a nonpenetrating head injury (i.e., nothing sticking into or out of your skull) that results in unconsciousness. Concussions typically result in brief periods of unconsciousness, and people appear to recover quite quickly from concussions. Concussions are fairly common phenomena in a variety of sports (e.g., football, hockey). For instance, one study of the Canadian Football League suggested that over 40% of all players experienced at least one concussion (over 60% of these experienced more than one concussion) during the 1997 season (Delaney, Lacroix, Leclerc, & Johnston, 2000). One interesting study (Yarnell & Lynch, 1970) examined the memory functions of football players at a number of intervals following a concussion. Immediately after regaining consciousness, the participants were able to tell the researchers the play on which they had been injured. However, within minutes, this information had been lost, and the players were unable to provide the information about when their injury had occurred. This result suggests that these players had intact short-term or working memory and that the amnesia resulted from a failure of long-term memory to store the information.

Typically, it has been observed that concussion results in anterograde and retrograde amnesia for the period surrounding the head injury and that this amnesia is mild and resolves quickly (e.g., Lovell, Iverson, Collins, McKeag, & Maroon, 1999). In contrast, some researchers have observed that disruptions to memory function can be observed for periods of up to two months following the injury (e.g., Capruso & Levin, 1992). These previous studies have focused on athletes for whom head injury is not part of their sport. However, studies of boxers, who experience repeated blows to the head over long periods of time, have demonstrated that there are significant impairments of memory and other cognitive functions (e.g., Mendez, 1995; Heilbronner, Henry, & Carson-Brewer, 1991). Arguably, boxers represent the extreme end of a number of sports. Even when the player exhibits no obvious concussion and the repeated head impact is relatively mild, such as with heading a soccer ball, deficits in memory have been observed (Matser, Kessels, Lesak, Jordan, & Troost, 1999). On a final note, regardless of how long concussions affect memory after the injury, it must be noted that concussions are a risk factor for Alzheimer's disease (e.g., Emmerling, Morganti-Kossman, Kossman, Stahel, Watson, Evans, et al., 2000), which definitely results in memory deficits.

AMNESIA FOLLOWING ELECTROCONVULSIVE THERAPY. Electroconvulsive therapy (ECT) can be used for treatment of severe depression, especially when other therapies have failed to produce significant relief from the depression. ECT is a procedure in which a generalized convulsion is induced in an anaesthetized individual by briefly applying an electrical current (which can be applied either bilaterally or unilaterally). From our perspective, ECT is interesting because it produces mild anterograde and retrograde amnesia (Taylor, Tompkins, Demers, & Anderson, 1982). A number of studies have observed that bilateral ECT produces a greater effect on memory than does unilateral ECT and that these effects become greater with increased frequency of ECT (e.g., Lisanby, Maddox, Prudic, Devanand, & Sackelm, 2000; Taylor et al., 1982; Vakil, Grunhaus, Nagar, Ben-Chaim, Dolberg, & Dannon, 2000). These effects appear to be restricted to explicit memory functions, and the amnesia appears to affect memory for recent events rather than remote ones. Unlike what was observed in H.M., these effects on explicit memory are very mild and appear to be the greatest for ordinary events, as striking personal events are not impaired. As was the case with concussion, it appears that this effect is resolved over time (often within two months of the last treatment).

How ECT produces amnesia is unknown, as is the mechanism behind its effects on depression. Because ECT resulted in explicit memory loss but not in implicit memory loss, it seems likely that the amnesic effects of ECT are due to alterations in temporal lobe function. In fact, an EEG study following ECT observed that there were changes in temporal lobe activity that appeared to be related to the degree of memory impairment (Sackheim et al., 2000). Furthermore, although there were changes within the temporal lobes that were associated with ECT, it did not appear that there was evidence of cell death in the temporal lobes, which could have conceivably resulted in amnesia (Ende, Braus, Walter, Weber-Fahr, & Henn, 2000). However, there is a complication, as most of the people in these studies were depressed, and getting a baseline memory measure on depressed people may confound memory with depression. Furthermore, some research has found that some depressed people exhibit pathology in their temporal lobes and that the degree of pathology is related to the length of the depressive illness (Sheline, Sanghavi, Mintun, & Gado, 1999). As we cannot perform ECT on randomly chosen participants (who presumably would not be depressed and/or not have temporal lobe pathologies), we must interpret these results with caution, as they may not reflect the typical functioning of the temporal lobes.

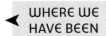 We have examined the separate memory systems in neurologically normal individuals. We have also defined two forms of amnesia: retrograde amnesia, in which there is an impairment of previously learned material, and anterograde amnesia, in which there is an inability to form new memories. We have also examined a number of conditions in which the amnesia produced is mild, such as concussion or following electroconvulsive therapy.

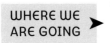 We are going to examine the dementias and their specific impacts on memory and memory functions. Finally, we will discuss current theories of how the brain encodes, stores, and retrieves memories.

The Dementias

Dementia is a general term that was introduced by Pinel (1809) and Esquirol (1814) to refer to a condition related to general loss of function. For the most part, the definition of dementia is quite loose and refers to a number of neurological conditions that result in the general decline of cognitive function. For the most part, dementia is a progressive, irreversible condition that eventually results in death. Although dementia is associated with a variety of cognitive deficits, memory deficits are a hallmark of the early stage of many of the dementias. Dementia can be divided into three common groups—cortical, subcortical, and mixed—which largely reflect the areas of the brain that are thought to undergo pathologic change.

Although dementia is correlated with aging, it does not appear to be a general consequence of aging itself. Instead, it appears to be associated with a number of changes in the nervous system that are also associated with advanced age. Dementia affects approximately 5–8% of the population over the age of 65; the prevalence jumps to between 25% and 50% in people who are more than 85 years of age (Monk & Brodaty, 2000). It is suggested that as our population ages and medical science increases life span, the incidence of dementia will continue to increase over the next twenty-five years, with estimates suggesting increases from a current prevalence of about 2 million people in the United States to over 12 million by 2025 (Marx, 1996).

CORTICAL DEMENTIAS. The common **cortical dementias** are Alzheimer's disease, and Pick's disease. Of all the dementias, Alzheimer's disease is the most common form and may account for as much as 50% of the diagnoses of dementia (Kay, 1994). The cortical dementias typically have an insidious onset, which may be marked by initial memory problems, such as word-finding problems or difficulty in remembering events, disorientation in familiar surroundings, and changes in personality and mood. This decline is steady and proceeds slowly. Associated with the deficits in memory, there is often a co-occurrence of other deficits such as aphasia, agnosia, and apraxia.

Although dementia was a recognized disorder in the 1800s, **Alzheimer's disease (AD)** was first described by Alois Alzheimer in 1906. In his paper, Alzheimer described a person who exhibited brain atrophy and senile dementia. Somewhat presciently, Alzheimer suggested that this disease was a function of slow deterioration of neurons and that the degree of dementia was related to the amount of brain deterioration.

AD is characterized by a progressive loss of function over a period of years, most notably in memory and memory function. New explicit learning is impaired, and it is the loss of recent memories that is often noticed first. Mild AD typically occurs during the first two years following diagnosis and is marked by impairments on a number of learning tasks, regardless of the modality (e.g., verbal, visual, tactile, gustatory). There also appears to be a large number of intrusions from nonrelated information. For example, if the task is to learn two lists, individuals with AD may have a difficult time keeping the two lists separate. Furthermore, it appears that the problem with memory is at all levels: encoding, storage, and retrieval. Therefore, many cues that often help people with non-AD-related memory loss, such as retrieval cues, do not help people with AD. As AD progresses to moderate severity (two to three years after diagnosis), there is a loss of more remote memories, along with parietal lobe dysfunction marked by dyspraxia and agnosia. As AD becomes severe, people with AD may fail to recognize their family members (or themselves in mirrors), and all higher cognitive functions and many basic motor functions are lost. Interestingly, there is relative sparing of short-term memory, working memory, and implicit memory tasks until the disease is quite advanced. Furthermore, many motor and sensory abilities (with the exception of olfaction, which is blunted very early) are relatively preserved through the course of the disease. Most people live for five to fifteen years from the time of diagnosis with AD until their death (Brinton, 2001).

Although AD can be characterized by changes in behavior, definitive diagnosis cannot be made until after death, when the brain can be autopsied. From a gross perspective, there is general atrophy of the brain, especially in the temporal and association cortices, and an increase in the size of the ventricles. When brain tissue is examined under the microscope, two observations are evident: There is a loss of medium and large cholinergic neurons, and large numbers of amyloid plaques and neurofibrillary tangles can be observed (Figure 7.10).

The amyloid plaques are an accumulation of **beta-amyloid protein,** and certain risk factors are associated with the formation of amyloid plaques. Individuals with trisomy 21 (Down syndrome) appear to contract AD much earlier than other people do, and on autopsy, they have brain changes similar to those with AD. People with Down syndrome have an extra copy of chromosome 21, so it seemed likely that the gene for AD might be found there. What was found was a gene for making the

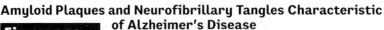

Amyloid Plaques and Neurofibrillary Tangles Characteristic of Alzheimer's Disease

Figure 7.10

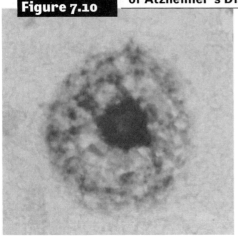
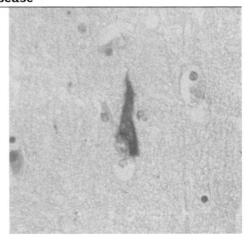

Source: Images courtesy of Mel Feany.

beta-amyloid precursor protein. However, most people with AD do not have a mutation in this gene. AD does appear to run in families, and genealogical studies indicated that familial AD appeared to result from an abnormal copy of a gene on chromosome 19, which makes a protein called apolipoprotein E (ApoE). There are four forms of the ApoE gene, of which ApoE 4 puts people at risk for developing AD. Although how ApoE 4 produces AD is unknown, it is thought that it may increase the production of beta-amyloid.

The severity of the dementia is correlated with the number of neurofibrillary tangles, which are characteristic of dead or dying neurons. These filaments are made up of the microtubule-associated protein tau. In normal brain tissue, tau acts as a bridge between microtubules in axons, ensuring that axons are healthy and have a stable structure. In AD, tau becomes detached from the microtubules and congregates in the soma, which causes the axons to shrink and die, thus becoming neurofibrillary tangles (Figure 7.10). No one knows for sure why tau changes in AD, although some researchers think that the abnormal amount of amyloid protein made by neurons in those who have AD may negatively impact the normal functioning of tau. It also appears that ApoE 4 is associated with abnormal tau formation and may facilitate tau regression to the soma.

There are four well-established risk factors for AD: age, the ApoE 4 gene, having family members with AD, and Down syndrome. As well, there are a number of other factors that may be related to increased risk of AD: being female, lower levels of education, head injury (which may interact with ApoE), and exposure to aluminum in drinking water (McDowell, 2001). Although there is no current treatment that can halt the progression of AD, many pharmacological treatments are aimed at restoring cholinergic function. (Recall that it is primarily cholinergic neurons that are damaged during the initial phase of the disease.) Much research is being conducted to examine whether estrogen replacement therapy, anti-inflammatory drugs (such as ibuprofen),

Current Controversy

Can Estrogen Replacement Therapy Help to Prevent Alzheimer's Disease in Women?

AD affects a large number of the elderly, and as our population ages, increasing numbers of people will be affected. Women appear to be two to three times more apt than men to develop AD, which is independent of their longer life span. Rather, some researchers have suggested that it is the lack of estrogen that women experience as a consequence of menopause (e.g., Carr, Goate, & Morris, 1997) that results in the increased incidence of AD. Furthermore, some researchers have observed a decreased prevalence of AD in women who take estrogen replacement therapy (ERT) following menopause than in those who did not take ERT (e.g., Paganini-Hill & Henderson, 1994). Furthermore, short-term ERT may improve cognitive function, especially memory in women who have undergone surgical removal of the ovaries. On the basis of these results (along with research that demonstrates benefits of ERT for osteoporosis), ERT has become the fastest-growing prescription in North America.

The cognitive research suggests that AD and memory decline associated with aging may be associated with decreased levels of estrogen following menopause. However, a number of other researchers have failed to observe this effect. In a meta-analysis of nineteen studies that looked at the effect of ERT and cognitive function, Haskell, Richardson, and Herwitz (1997) found that there was some support for the beneficial effects of ERT on cognitive function. They decided that they could not conclusively state their results, though, as most of the studies had important confounds in their methodology, including the failure to control for mood and other symptoms associated with ERT. Furthermore, most of these studies failed to use double-blind randomized trials and allowed their participants to self-select into groups. Self-selection is an important factor in studies of aging populations and cognitive function. For example, how likely would you be to volunteer for a study if you thought that you would be diagnosed with AD? Haskell and colleagues concluded that there is inadequate evidence to support the position that ERT improves cognitive function in menopausal women.

As a final comment, there is an ongoing study by Shumaker and colleagues (Shumaker, Reboussin, Espeland, Rapp, McBee, & Dailey, 1998) called the Women's Health Initiative Memory Study (WHIMS), which has as one of its goals to examine the relationship between ERT, cognitive function, and AD. Because this study is going to assign ERT randomly and follow women as they age, this should provide the kind of evidence that we will need to objectively determine the degree to which ERT can prevent or mediate the cognitive declines associated with AD.

---

and antioxidants (such as Vitamin E) can act to reduce or impair the progression of AD.

In 1892, Arnold Pick described an individual who had a severe language disorder. When an autopsy was conducted, it was observed that there was selective atrophy of the left temporal lobe (Pick, 1892). Interestingly, it was Alzheimer (1911) who described the histological features of the disease now known as **Pick's disease (PcD).** When PcD is compared to AD, there are a number of striking differences. First, PcD is extremely rare, occurring ten to twenty times less frequently than AD (Rossor, 2001). Furthermore, PcD tends to occur at an earlier age than AD and often appears before the age of 65. The onset of PcD is slower and more subtle than that of AD, although early in the disease, there are striking changes in social behaviors and personality, something that does not occur until late in AD. For instance, on tests of social function and examinations of daily living skills, individuals with early-stage AD outperform people with PcD (Brito-Marques, Mello, & Montenegro, 2001). There may also be hyperorality (increased exploration of objects with the mouth) and hyperphagia (excessive eating). Also quite unlike the case in AD, changes in memory do not occur until much later in the PcD disease process (Brito-Marques et al., 2001). Careful neuropsychological testing reveals that on tests of memory, individuals with early-stage PcD outperform people with early-stage AD.

PcD is also definitively diagnosed only after death. PcD is characterized by gross brain atrophy that is primarily limited to the temporal and frontal cortices (in contrast to AD in which the parietal lobe is also affected). Under the microscope, brain tissue of individuals with PcD typically shows no amyloid plaques or neurofibrillary tangles. Rather, PcD is characterized by swollen or ballooned neurons (in contrast to the atrophied neurons observed in AD) and by Pick bodies. Pick bodies, which are composed of tau, differ from neurofibrillary tangles in that they are straight (Armstrong, Cairns, & Lantos, 1999).

SUBCORTICAL DEMENTIAS. The **subcortical dementias** occur as a consequence of Huntington's chorea and Parkinson's disease. In contrast to the cortical dementias, the first symptoms of subcortical dementia are changes in personality, slowing of cognition, and difficulty with problem solving and attention. Of course, the hallmark features of these diseases is their motor symptoms (Chapter 5), and it is unclear whether or not subtle features of dementia precede the motor symptoms.

Parkinson's dementia (PD) is associated with specific dopaminergic cell loss in the substantia nigra, the main effect of which is a dramatic loss of the neurotransmitter dopamine throughout the brain. The loss of dopamine in the brain especially affects the functioning of the basal ganglia. Along with the motor symptoms associated with dopamine depletion, about 20–60% of people with Parkinson's disease also experience dementia.

PD is characterized by a slowness of thought (**bradyphenia**), difficulties with tasks requiring sustained attention, memory retrieval, and executive function (Spinnler, 1991). Bradyphenia is manifested by the slowness with which people arrive at solutions to problems, especially problems that require planning. Associated with bradyphenia are problems with vocabulary (particularly with naming items) and problems with articulation, which, because they are not global linguistic deficits, are distinguishable from aphasia. Memory problems are obvious in situations in which individuals must retrieve information in nonstructured settings, particularly when a structured search through memory stores must be performed. There are also problems with tasks of implicit memory and with judgments of recency or temporal order (Saint-Cyr, Taylor, & Lang, 1988). However, individuals with Parkinson's dementia typically exhibit intact long-term and visuospatial memory and respond normally to cued recall (e.g., "Which one of these pictures have you seen before?"). The difficulties with executive function appear to be related to difficulties with abstract reasoning, switching between strategies, and inhibition of competing information. Interestingly, although the motor symptoms of Parkinson's disease result from loss of dopamine, the cognitive symptoms appear to be largely unrelated to dopamine levels, as these symptoms are not improved by treatment aimed at augmenting dopamine levels.

Huntington's dementia (HD) is uncommon and results from a dominant mutation of the *huntingtin* gene on chromosome 4. (The mechanisms underlying the neural changes and the motor characteristics of Huntington's chorea are discussed in Chapter 5.) Early stages of dementia occur after the appearance of the motor symptoms of Huntington's chorea. HD is characterized by personality changes, depression, mania, and hallucinations. Anterograde amnesia often presents early in the disease process. In contrast with AD, HD is characterized by deficits in implicit memory, especially when the task requires motor planning (Folstein, 1991). It appears that HD results from atrophy of the basal ganglia, although the brains of HD individuals also show shrinking and thinning of the cortex.

MIXED-ETIOLOGY DEMENTIAS.   The **mixed-etiology dementias** are those that exhibit features of both cortical and subcortical dementia; they include multi-infarct dementia, Korsakoff's syndrome, Creutzfeldt-Jakob disease, and HIV-related dementia. As you might suspect, the pattern of deficits that is observed in these dementias is suggestive of both cortical and subcortical involvement.

The diagnosis of **multi-infarct dementia (MID)** is generally made when there is evidence of dementia that occurred along with the appearance of multiple small infarcts or lesions. MID is an umbrella term for any type of repeated vascular infarcts that result in cognitive impairment. It is significant to note that the risk of dementia is higher for vascular disease than is any other known risk factor (Tatemichi et al., 1993). MID typically has an acute onset and is characterized by progressive impairments in memory and other cognitive deficits, which eventually produce an inability to live independently. Typically, the onset of MID is sudden, and its progression is irregular. MID is usually associated with preserved personality and increased emotionality. As in AD, explicit memory deficits are observed early in the course of the disease, although there is relative sparing of remote memories. When compared to individuals with AD, people with MID often perform better on memory tasks, although eventually, the memory deficits associated with MID are undistinguishable from AD. Also, unlike the case in AD, motor coordination (including walking) is often affected quite early in MID.

Korsakoff's syndrome is sometimes referred to as Wernicke-Korsakoff's syndrome, in recognition of the early descriptions of the syndrome by both Wernicke (in 1881) and Korsakoff (in a series of papers from 1887 to 1891). Although rare, this disease is more frequent among alcoholics and in those with diseases of the gastrointestinal tract that inhibit the absorption of vitamins. Initially, it was thought that Korsakoff's syndrome resulted from the effects that chronic alcohol ingestion had on the nervous system, but it is now understood that the disease results from a deficiency of vitamin B1 or thiamine. Although any condition resulting in prolonged poor nutrition enhances the risk of Korsakoff's syndrome, alcoholics appear to have enhanced susceptibility to this disease. This is because alcoholics often have poor nutritional practices, because alcohol interferes with gastrointestinal absorption of vitamins, and because chronic liver disease (associated with alcoholism) reduces the ability of the liver to convert thiamine into its active metabolites. The mechanism by which thiamine deficiency results in Korsakoff's syndrome is unknown, although there is a known relationship between decreased thiamine concentration and decreased glucose metabolism in the brain.

Korsakoff's syndrome results in a pattern of global amnesia, with profound anterograde and retrograde amnesia. Specifically, individuals are unable to form new memories, and they have extensive impairments of remote memories (which may cover most of their adult life). One interesting feature of Korsakoff's syndrome is confabulation, the tendency to make up stories rather than admit that the person cannot remember. These confabulations are often plausible and tend to be based on previous experiences. Despite these confabulations, the content of the spontaneous speech is quite sparse, and these individuals appear to be quite apathetic about their condition. In fact, people who suffer from Korsakoff's syndrome appear to be almost unaware of their problems.

Although the pattern of brain pathology has been firmly established in Korsakoff's syndrome, how global amnesia is produced is still contentious. Korsakoff's syndrome results in diffuse brain damage and general cortical atrophy. It appears that there is damage to the medial thalamus and the mamillary bodies of the hypothalamus. In addition, over 80% of people with Korsakoff's syndrome exhibit gross atrophy of the frontal lobes. It has been suggested by Winocur and colleagues (Winocur, Kinsbourne, & Moscovitch, 1981) that the severity of the amnesia results from the combined damage to the diencephalon and the frontal lobes.

Prion diseases, which are also referred to as *slow viruses* (although they are not viruses), are neurodegenerative conditions related to the production and accumulation of a protein known as a **prion.** There are several forms of prion diseases, which are classified under the generic name of *spongiform encephalopathies.* Typically, symptoms of prion diseases may take many years to manifest. The most common form of the spongiform encephalopathies is **Creutzfeldt-Jakob disease (CJD),** of which there are a number of forms (e.g., Ironside, 2000).

CJD is easily distinguishable from AD and PcD in terms of both the clinical signs and the physiological effects of the disorder. CJD is diagnosed by spinal tap, because cerebrospinal fluid can be analyzed for the presence of the prion. Clinically, CJD results in dementia that is accompanied by changes in EEG and by involuntary movements. In addition the time course of the disease is much more rapid than that of either AD or PcD, in that death typically occurs within one year of diagnosis (and often within four months of diagnosis). Initially, CJD is characterized by fatigue, anxiety, and problems with concentration. Within weeks, these symptoms are accompanied by motor symptoms, which may include involuntary contractions of large muscle groups, ataxia (including difficulty walking), and blurred vision.

In CJD and the other spongiform encephalopathies, the brain undergoes widespread neuronal death, and there is a proliferation of glia, giving the brain a spongy look. Although some cases of CJD may have occurred from the ingestion of the protein or through contact with prion-infected tissue, there are also cases of familial CJD, and CJD may be overrepresented in people who have Parkinson's disease (Haltia, 2000). Currently, it is not known how CJD produces its effects, although some have suggested that, regardless of the type of CJD, neurons undergo prion-induced **apoptosis** (programmed cell death, discussed in detail in Chapter 14). A number of researchers have suggested that apoptosis in CJD may be mediated by changes in microglia function, free radicals, and changes in copper metabolism (Giese & Kretzschmar, 2001; Rezaie & Lantos, 2001).

AIDS is an infectious disease that is caused by the HIV virus. The primary feature of HIV is the severe impairment of the immune system. However, the HIV virus

the **Real** world

Mad Cow Disease

Bovine spongiform encephalopathy (BSE), widely known as "mad cow disease" was first noticed in the United Kingdom in 1986 and has affected over 200,000 cattle worldwide. BSE is a degenerative prion-based neuropathy that affects the central nervous systems of cattle. There are a number of prion diseases, including Creutzfeldt-Jakob disease (CJD) in humans and scrapie in sheep. Some researchers suggest that the outbreak of BSE in cattle was related to cattle feed that contained scrapie-infected sheep brains. Indeed, it has been shown that it is possible to infect a number of species with prions through ingestion of prion-infected materials. Although most of the affected cattle were found in Great Britain, cases of BSE have been confirmed in Belgium, Denmark, France, Ireland, Luxembourg, Liechtenstein, the Netherlands, Northern Ireland, Portugal, and Switzerland (Detwiler & Rubenstein, 2000).

Beginning in 1994, a number of people began to show signs of CJD in Great Britain (approximately ten to fifteen cases per year). Retrospective investigation revealed that these people may have consumed BSE-affected cattle, especially the brains of the affected cattle. Furthermore, molecular analyses of the prion protein in these people has confirmed that it is the same as was observed in BSE (Clarke, Jackson, & Collinge, 2001). Furthermore, because many infected people may not show symptoms of CJD, it may be that they are further spreading the disease through blood and other tissue donations. It remains to be seen how many people will be affected by CJD (Brown, Will, Bradley, Asher, & Detwiler, 2001).

Prions are not viruses, and unlike viruses, they appear to be difficult to get rid of. Standard methods of decontamination include washing with bleach or strong acids, treating with protein fixatives (such as ethanol or formalin), autoclaving with heat, and washing with strong acids or bases. Prions do not appear to be as susceptible as viruses and bacteria are to these standard decontamination procedures. This fact, along with the contagious nature of prions, has led to a widespread belief that prions are indestructible. This is not the case; strong solutions of sodium hypochlorite and/or hot solutions of sodium hydroxide do decontaminate objects that may have contacted prions.

Self-Test

1. Give an example of a type of memory loss that would characterize retrograde amnesia. Give an example of a type of memory loss that would characterize anterograde amnesia.

2. Why is it difficult to interpret the memory deficit associated with ECT? Are these reasons also applicable to interpreting H.M.'s memory deficit?

3. Define the cortical dementias. What memory deficits characterize the cortical dementias?

4. Define the subcortical dementias. What memory deficits characterize the subcortical dementias?

5. Why do alcoholics present with Korsakoff's syndrome more often than other people do? Where is the damage that is suspected to produce the memory deficits in Korsakoff's syndrome?

can affect any organ or tissue, including the brain. Although some cases of dementia in those who have HIV may be attributable to opportunistic infections, it appears that the HIV virus itself may also produce dementia. Some HIV-infected individuals exhibit **HIV-associated dementia,** which is distinguished by cognitive deterioration accompanied by motor difficulties and other behavioral disturbances. These disturbances may be mild or so severe that independent living is impossible. Neuropsychological testing demonstrates that these individuals have difficulties in concentrating and sustaining attention, that they have difficulty in performing tasks that require complex problem solving, and that they may also exhibit anterograde amnesia. Imaging studies show that the degree of cognitive impairment is related to the degree to which there is diffuse cerebral atrophy (e.g., Chang, 1995; Kramer & Sanger, 1990; Simpson, 1998).

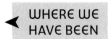 We have examined the separate memory systems in neurologically normal individuals and what happens to memories in a number of pathological disease states. Dementia can result from a number of different diseases and can produce various symptoms that appear to depend on the neural structures affected by the disease process.

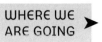 We are going to examine the data from these conditions and try to reconcile this information into a neural model of explicit and implicit memory.

MODULE **7.3**
Where Is Memory in the Brain?

To make some sense of what we have learned so far, let's look at the primary features of the material that has been presented (with the exception of the mixed-etiology dementias, which display a mixture of symptoms and neural deficits and therefore are difficult to interpret). Although Table 7.2 is a simplified, condensed summary of the material presented in Module 7.2, it is a good way to look for patterns.

In looking at the pattern of results, it appears that the temporal lobes subserve explicit memory, whereas the basal ganglia subserve implicit memory. Although this generality appears to have some basis in fact, is there further evidence that these assumptions are correct?

The Role of the Temporal Lobes in Explicit Memory

Much of the initial study of the role of the temporal lobes in explicit memory was pioneered in the studies of H.M. However, since H.M., a number of people with temporal lobe damage have had their memory studied. Hamann and Squire (1997) describe a case study, E.P., who sustained complete bilateral damage to the temporal lobes as a result of a viral infection. Zola-Morgan and colleagues (Zola-Morgan, Squire, & Amaral, 1986) describe a case study, R.B., and Rempel-Clower and colleagues (Rempel-Clower, Zola, Squire, & Amaral, 1996) describe a case study, G.D., both of whom had bilateral damage limited to the hippocampus. Interestingly, all of these individuals had severe anterograde amnesia for explicit memory, and all had intact implicit memory.

A number of imaging studies have investigated how episodic memories are encoded. Schacter (1996) suggests that the prefrontal cortex is involved in encoding of explicit information, although these changes in activity may reflect attentional and volitional aspects of episodic memory. If you recall, the prefrontal cortex was involved in tasks requiring the central executive component of working memory. It may be that accurate explicit memory (which may require prefrontal attention and strategy sys-

Table 7.2	**A Summary of the Treatments That Affect Memory and the Areas That Appear to Be Important in Producing These Effects**		
Person/Syndrome	**Primary Memory System Affected**	**Type of Amnesia**	**Areas Affected**
H.M.	Explicit	Anterograde	Bilateral removal of medial temporal lobes
Infantile amnesia	Explicit	Loss of explicit memory for first two years of life	??
Amnesia resulting from concussion	Explicit	Mild retrograde and anterograde	??
Amnesia resulting from electroconvulsive therapy	Explicit	Mild retrograde and anterograde	Temporal lobes
Transient global amnesia	Explicit	Retrograde and anterograde (mild)	Temporal lobes
Mild to moderate cortical dementia	Explicit	Mild anterograde	Temporal and association cortices
Severe cortical dementia	Generalized impairments	Anterograde and retrograde	Entire brain atrophy, enlarged ventricles
Mild to moderate subcortical dementia	Implicit	Anterograde	Basal ganglia
Severe subcortical dementia	Implicit and explicit	Anterograde and retrograde	Basal ganglia, atrophy of cortex

tems) may require interactions between the prefrontal and temporal memory systems. One puzzle is that many studies that have imaged the brain performing tasks of explicit memory tend not to observe temporal activation. This flies in the face of what has been observed in individuals with brain damage. However, careful analyses of the type of tasks that are given suggest that when cues are elicited that promote explicit memory formation, hippocampal activation is observed. Moscovitch (1994) suggests that for long-term explicit memory to be formed, both the prefrontal and hippocampal areas must be active.

The Role of the Temporal Lobes in Implicit Memory

Much of the initial information about the role of the basal ganglia in implicit memory comes from the study of individuals with PD. When people perform tasks of implicit memory, it becomes obvious that an intact explicit memory system is not required. For instance, one task of implicit memory requires participants to predict the weather on the basis of information given on a computer screen (Knowlton, Squire, & Gluck, 1994). Following each prediction, participants are given feedback about the accuracy of their answer. Neurologically normal participants often respond that they are guessing; however, an analysis of their performance demonstrates that they are performing well above chance (at about 70% correct). It seems that although the participants are unable to consciously articulate the rules of the game, they implicitly are able to perform the task. Individuals with temporal lobe damage behave similarly to the neurologically normal participants, although they could not answer questions about the task, as they did not remember ever playing the game. In contrast, people with PD were able to describe the task quite well, despite being unable to perform above chance levels on the task. This study suggests two things: Damage to the temporal lobes does not affect implicit memory tasks, and the basal ganglia are involved in performing implicit memory tasks. Knowlton and colleagues (Knowlton, Mangels, & Squire, 1996) review a number of studies that have replicated these effects and suggest that there is strong evidence that the normal functioning of the basal ganglia is to facilitate implicit learning.

Where Are Memories Stored in the Brain?

There is little information about where memories are stored in the brain. Evidence obtained from studying nonhuman animals suggests that successful encoding of information is associated with changes in synapses and dendritic spines. However, it is

Self-Test

1. Fill in the missing pieces of table.

Person/Syndrome	Primary Memory System Affected	Type of Amnesia	Areas Affected
_____	Explicit	Anterograde	Bilateral removal of medial temporal lobes
Severe cortical dementia	Generalized impairments	_____	Entire brain atrophy, enlarged ventricles
Amnesia resulting from concussion	Explicit	_____	??
Mild to moderate subcortical dementia	_____	Anterograde	_____
Transient global amnesia	Explicit	_____	Temporal lobes
Mild to moderate cortical dementia	Explicit	Mild anterograde	_____
Infantile amnesia	_____	Loss of explicit memory for first two years of life	??
Amnesia resulting from electroconvulsive therapy	Explicit	Mild retrograde and anterograde	_____

2. What neural areas appear to be responsible for explicit memory? How do they differ from those that are responsible for implicit memory?

3. In what ways are current ideas about memory storage in the brain similar to those proposed by Hebb?

widely assumed that information is stored throughout the cortex, especially in areas that were involved in the learning of the information. This hypothesis is interesting, as it returns us to the state of memory theory in the 1950s; it was Hebb who suggested that it was highly likely that sensory cortical areas involved in encoding were also involved in the storage of information. This hypothesis is supported by the retrograde amnesia that is observed after widespread loss of neurons in diseases such as AD and PcD. However, despite widespread interest and thousands of research articles about memory, the neural basis of memory is still unknown, and the details of how neurons encode and represent memories are still quite controversial.

◀ **WHERE WE HAVE BEEN** We have examined a variety of different memory systems in the brain and have examined a variety of diseases that affect memory. Furthermore, we have sifted through the evidence to suggest that there are two separable long-term memory systems: the explicit system that relies on the normal functioning of the temporal lobes and the implicit system that relies on the normal functioning of the basal ganglia.

WHERE WE ARE GOING ▶ We will investigate the neuroanatomical basis of memory storage and retrieval, asking "Where is the memory in the brain?" As you will discover, the various functions collectively referred to as "memory" are distributed widely throughout the brain.

Glossary

Alzheimer's disease (AD)—Cortical dementia characterized by a progressive loss of function over a period of years, most notably in memory and memory function; characterized by general atrophy of the brain, especially in temporal and association cortices, increase in the size of the ventricles, loss of medium and large cholinergic neurons, and a large number of amyloid plaque and neurofibrillary tangles.

Amnesia—A memory disorder characterized by the failure to encode, store, or retrieve a memory.

Anterograde amnesia—A form of amnesia in which the loss of memory is for events after the trauma.

Apoptosis—Programmed cell death; occurs in Creutzfeldt-Jakob disease and may be mediated by changes in microglia function, free radicals, and changes in copper metabolism.

Articulatory suppression—A form of the dual-task paradigm in which the primary task involves listening and the irrelevant task involves speaking; results in a disruption in the performance of the primary task.

Beta-amyloid protein—Accumulates to form amyloid plaques.

Bradyphenia—Slowness with which people arrive at solutions to problems, especially problems that require planning associated with Parkinson's dementia; characterized by problems with vocabulary and articulation.

Brixton test—A test consisting of a series of plates with ten dots on it, one of which is colored and moves from plate to plate over successive trials; participants must predict where the dot will be next.

Brown-Peterson design—An experimental design in which participants are given two sets of information to remember (e.g., a consonant trigram such as BFN and a three-digit numeral such as 235) followed by a distractor task (e.g., counting backward).

Central executive—Primary component of working memory responsible for controlling attention and supervising the phonological loop and the visuospatial sketchpad.

Chunking—Grouping pieces of information together in a way that reduces the load on short-term memory and improves the ability to hold larger sets of information in short-term memory (e.g., remembering eleven numbers as a phone number instead of as eleven individual numbers).

Consolidation—Storing information for later use.

Cortical dementias—Dementias typically having insidious onset, often marked by initial memory problems and changes in personality and mood (e.g., Alzheimer's disease, Pick's disease).

Creutzfeldt-Jakob disease—The most common form of the spongiform encephalopathies resulting in dementia that is accompanied by changes in EEG and by involuntary movements (e.g., involuntary contractions of large muscle groups, ataxia, including difficulty walking).

Dementia—Refers to a number of progressive, irreversible neurological conditions that result in the general decline of cognitive function; can be divided into three common groups (cortical, subcortical, and mixed), which largely reflect the areas of the brain that are thought to undergo pathological change.

Dissociated amnesia—An extremely rare form of amnesia in which there are no other cognitive deficits accompanying the memory loss.

Dual-task paradigm—A technique that is often used to investigate working memory wherein individuals perform one primary task (i.e., listening) and one irrelevant task (i.e., repeating the days of the week) at the same time.

Echoic memory—Sound-based sensory memory.

Encoding—Attending to information.

Engram—The cortical location of memory, the search for which was pioneered by Lashley.

Explicit memories—Memories for events (e.g., what you ate for breakfast) and facts (e.g., the capital of Arkansas).

Hayling test—A two-part test in which individuals are given a sentence with the last word missing. In the first part of the test, individuals are asked to provide a word that would finish the sentence in a meaningful way; in the second part of the test, individuals are required to finish the sentence with a word that makes no sense.

HIV-associated dementia—Dementia exhibited by HIV-infected individuals, distinguished by cognitive deterioration that is accompanied by motor difficulties and other behavioral disturbances (e.g., difficulties in concentrating and sustaining attention, difficulty in tasks requiring complex problem solving, anterograde amnesia); cognitive impairment is related to the degree to which there is diffuse cerebral atrophy.

Huntington's dementia—Subcortical dementia characterized by motor symptoms, personality changes, depression, mania, hallucinations, and deficits in implicit memory (especially when the task requires motor planning). Results from a dominant mutation of the *huntingtin* gene and from atrophy of the basal ganglia.

Iconic memory—Short-term visually based sensory memory.

Implicit memories—Memories for skills and habits (e.g., how to tie a bow in shoelaces).

Infantile amnesia—The term to describe the phenomenon in which we generally have no episodic memories of events that occurred before 2 years of age; likely a reflection of the interaction between nervous system development, linguistic competence, and a growing repertoire of experiences.

Korsakoff's syndrome—Dementia resulting from a deficiency of vitamin B1 or thiamine that results in damage to the medial thalamus and the mammillary bodies of the hypothalamus and atrophy of the frontal lobes. Results in a pattern of global amnesia, with profound anterograde and retrograde amnesia and confabulation.

Learning—A relatively permanent change in behavior as a function of experience; concerned with encoding and consolidating information.

Long-term memories—Memories that one can recall days, months, and even years after they were stored.

Memory—Concerned with retrieving information from where it is stored in the brain.

Mixed-etiology dementias—Dementias that exhibit features of both cortical and subcortical dementia (e.g., multi-infarct dementia, Korsakoff's syndrome, Creutzfeldt-Jakob disease, HIV-related dementia).

Multi-infarct dementia (MID)—The term for any type of repeated vascular infarcts that result in cognitive impairment; typically has an acute onset and is characterized by progressive impairments in memory, other cognitive deficits, and motor coordination and is usually associated with preserved personality and increased emotionality.

Parkinson's dementia (PD)—Subcortical dementia characterized by bradyphenia, difficulties with tasks requiring sustained attention, memory retrieval, and executive function.

Phonological loop—Component of the working memory responsible for manipulating linguistic information.

Pick's disease (PcD)—Cortical dementia similar to AD except that it is more rare, occurs at an earlier age, and has a more subtle and slower onset; characterized by gross brain atrophy that is primarily limited to the temporal and frontal cortices, swollen neurons, and Pick bodies.

Prion—A protein that is produced and accumulates in the brain and causes spongiform encephalopathies (e.g., Creutzfeldt-Jakob disease).

Proactive interference—Occurs when new learning is disrupted by previously learned material.

Retrieval—Retrieving information from where it is stored in the brain.

Retroactive interference—Occurs when the learning of new material interferes with the recall of previously learned material.

Retrograde amnesia—A form of amnesia in which the loss of memory is for events before the trauma.

Sensory memories—Memory for information that is directly encoded by the senses; although it has a relatively large scope, the duration of these memories is very short.

Short-term auditory memory—A form of auditory memory that differs from echoic memory and is responsible for holding relevant auditory information for slightly longer periods of time than echoic memory.

Short-term memory—Holds information for periods beyond what can be stored by sensory memory, although it does not hold information permanently; can be in either visual or auditory modalities.

Short-term visual memory—A form of visual memory that differs from iconic memory and is responsible for holding relevant visual information for slightly longer periods of time than iconic memory.

Subcortical dementias—Dementias in which the first symptoms involve changes in personality, slowing of cognition, difficulty with problem solving and attention, and motor symptoms (occur as a consequence of Huntington's disease and Parkinson's disease).

Trace discrimination theory—Suggests that short-term memories begin to degrade spontaneously over time and that retrieval of short-term memory requires that the information be distinct from other pieces of stored information.

Transient global amnesia—Memory loss with sudden onset and sudden resolution in which people display no knowledge of their previous life but have intact skills and language; often has no precipitating cause.

Visuospatial sketchpad—The component of the working memory that is responsible for manipulating visuospatial information, such as mental imagery and spatial locations.

Working memory—Contains information that is going to be acted on or used in some fashion; can manipulate information that is retrieved from long-term memory stores and does not require that the event be physically present.

Hearing and Language Processing

Language is beginning to submit to that uniquely satisfying kind of understanding that we call science.

—STEVEN PINKER

MODULE **8.1**
The Auditory System

Faced with an arbitrary choice between losing the use of one's eyes or one's ears, most people say that they would prefer to lose their sense of hearing. However, they may be underestimating the importance of audition. Although you are currently reading, most communication in which you engage is probably not strictly visual. Your eyes provide information about the objects and people that are in direct view, but your ears provide information about objects that are hidden from view (around corners, in the dark, etc.) as well as objects in plain sight. Localizing objects is often considered the domain of vision, but the auditory system is also exquisitely efficient at indicating object position in addition to object presence.

You have probably heard the classic conundrum: "If a tree falls in the forest and nobody hears it, does it make a sound?" This question often sparks considerable debate, but the answer is really quite simple: *No.* Sounds require a brain to perceive them. The physical stimuli that are perceived as sounds are simply vibrations of molecules of air. These vibrations produce waves that differ in terms of their frequency, amplitude, and complexity, and these dimensions determine the nature of the perceived sound. Although a falling tree undoubtedly produces vibrations in the surrounding air, unless there is a mechanism to sense these vibrations (such as an ear) and a system to perceive these changes as sound (such as a brain), the falling tree cannot create a sound. (Of course, there may be squirrel, bird, and rabbit ears and brains present, in which case the tree does make a sound.)

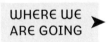 This module will describe the nature of auditory stimuli and describe the physiological system used to perceive them. This will involve descriptions of the outer and inner ear, auditory pathways, and auditory cortices.

The Properties of Sound

To understand how the brain creates the experience of sound, one must first understand the nature of the sound waves that are being perceived (see Figure 8.1). The first of these properties is the frequency of the sound. **Frequency** refers to the **rate of vibration** or the number of wave cycles completed per unit of time, and it is usually indicated in hertz (Hz), which is measured in cycles per second. Sounds waves can occur over a tremendous range of frequencies, but the human ear can only perceive vibrations between 20 and 20,000 Hz. Our sensitivity to sounds of different frequencies differs; humans are maximally sensitive to sounds between 1000 and 4000 Hz, corresponding roughly to the frequencies that the human voice can produce (Celine Dion excepted). The frequency of a sound should not be confused with its speed; sound travels at approximately 340 meters per second (depending on air temperature, etc.).

Perceptually, sounds of different frequencies have different **pitches.** The higher the frequency, the higher the perceived pitch. Some animals (such as dogs or deer)

The Relationship between the Physical and Perceptual Dimensions of Sound

Figure 8.1

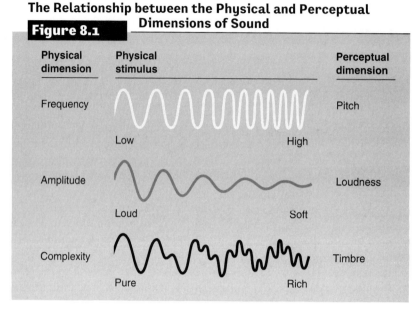

Physical dimension	Physical stimulus	Perceptual dimension
Frequency	Low High	Pitch
Amplitude	Loud Soft	Loudness
Complexity	Pure Rich	Timbre

Source: John P. J. Pinel, *Biopsychology,* 5e. Published by Allyn and Bacon, Boston, MA. Copyright © 2003 by Pearson Education. Reprinted by permission of the publisher.

can perceive sounds with frequencies higher than 20,000, which is why dog whistles are perceptually silent to humans. These whistles emit frequencies of 30,000–50,000 Hz—well outside humans' perceptual range. Other animals (such as many fish) can perceive only sounds with low (less than 2000 Hz) frequencies. The range of frequencies that an animal perceives also varies widely across species. Frogs and birds can generally perceive only a limited range of frequencies, whereas humans, whales, and dogs can detect a very wide range of frequencies.

Another perceptual property of sound is its **loudness.** Loudness corresponds to the amplitude of the sound wave. Waves of different amplitudes (or intensities) differ in the degree to which the high point (condensation of air) and the low point (rarefaction of air) of the wave differ from each other. Consider the example of playing the A note above middle C on a guitar. If you pluck the string lightly, the string will vibrate moderately, and the guitar will give off sound waves at a frequency of 440 Hz. If the string is plucked more strongly, it will vibrate back and forth over a larger area (producing waves of greater amplitude), but the frequency of those waves will still be 440 Hz. Of course, regardless of how strongly you pluck the string the note will still be an A.

The human ear is sensitive to a tremendous range of sound intensities, and typically sound **amplitude** is measured in decibels (dB), the sound pressure of a source when compared to a standard intensity of 10^{-12} watts. Depending on the frequency, someone with very good hearing can detect sounds as quiet as 1 dB. Conversational speech tends to occur at an average of 40–60 dB, whereas most alarm clocks emit sounds close to 80 dB. If you stand at the base of a pipe organ pipe at full blast (or in the front row of many concerts) you will be bombarded with 130 dB of sound, and sounds of this level typically produce painful sensations. Finally, standing one foot in front of a cannon when it fired would expose you to about 225 dB of sound, although that would be the least of your worries!

One final dimension on which sounds vary is their **complexity,** which is perceived as the sound's **timbre.** Some devices (such as tuning forks) are capable of producing relatively pure sounds, composed of a single frequency. However, most sounds are composed of a wide variety of frequencies—even the sounds produced by tuning forks. In addition to the intended frequency (or **fundamental frequency**), an instrument usually produces **overtones** that are at frequencies higher than (but mathematically related to) the fundamental frequency. To further complicate matters, these overtones also vary in their intensities.

Fortunately for the people who download music, complicated sounds can also be broken down into simple component waves in a mathematical process called **Fourier analysis.** Variants of this type of analysis are used to compress complex sounds on computers (in formats such as MPEG-1, Layer-3—a.k.a. MP3) because it is more efficient to represent a series of simple waveforms than it is to represent a single complicated waveform.

Although all sounds can be characterized in terms of their frequency, amplitude, and complexity, it is a gross oversimplification to state that the auditory system simply categorizes sounds resulting in auditory perception. We rarely listen to single, static, or unchanging tones. Most sounds in our environment are changing all the time. As an automobile accelerates past you, the pitch, intensity, and timbre of the sounds reaching each of your ears change. Furthermore, the sounds perceived by your left ear are not identical to those perceived by your right ear. Remarkably, all these changing factors are effortlessly integrated into the unitary percept of a moving car. In addition to identifying and monitoring its location, you can tell whether the car is accelerating or decelerating, and some of you might even be able to discern the make of the car.

Another factor in auditory perception that is often overlooked is the fact that people usually hear more than one thing at one time. As I sit at my desk writing this chapter, I can hear music, an overhead air exchange fan, someone walking down the hallway, the sound of my fingers hitting the keys, and the rather distracting racket of two pigeons on my windowsill. Thus, although I was only subjectively listening to the music, my auditory perceptual system detects a multitude of different parameters at the same time, including the implied tone of speech. Consider the example of hearing someone ask "Isn't that kind of underhanded?" In addition to perceiving each individual word, you can also tell this is a question because the pitch of the speaker's voice rises toward the end of the phrase. This type of cue in one's tone of voice is called **prosody,** which will be discussed in detail later in the chapter.

The Ear

The ear (see Figure 8.2) is a very efficient and robust mechanism that is capable of detecting and amplifying very subtle vibrations in the air and transforming these vibrations into neural signals, a process called *transduction* (which was also discussed in Chapter 5). Sound waves enter the funnellike outer ear, passing the **pinna** (the outermost,

| Figure 8.2 | Anatomy of the Inner and Outer Ear |

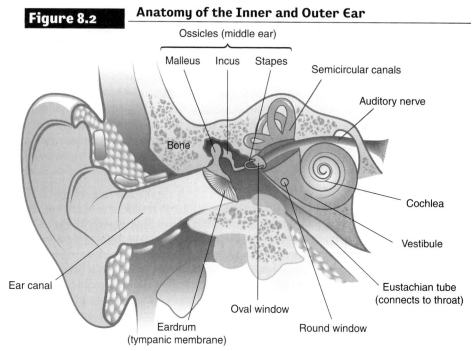

Source: Reprinted by permission of Paul Janzen.

visible portion of the ear) through the hole (called the **auditory meatus**) leading into the **external ear canal** that amplifies the vibrations and channels them onto the eardrum, or **tympanic membrane.** This membrane vibrates and passes the vibration along via three bones: the **malleus** ("hammer"), **incus** ("anvil"), and **stapes** ("stirrup"). Collectively, these bones are referred to as **ossicles,** and each successive bone further amplifies the vibration, transmitting the vibration through the **oval window.** The membrane covering the oval window transmits the vibrations into the cochlea through the **cochlear fluid.** The vibrations of this fluid cause a bending of both the **basilar membrane** and the **tectorial membrane,** which in turn elicits neural activity in the **hair cells.** These hair cells are the receptor cells of the auditory system (functionally similar to the rods and cones in the visual system), and they connect with the auditory nerve (see Figure 8.3).

All of the auditory system components described above can be grouped into three anatomical divisions. The **outer ear** comprises the pinna and external ear canal, and it serves to catch and amplify sound waves. The **middle ear** is the chamber (and its contents) between the tympanic membrane and the oval window. In the middle ear, sound waves are transduced from variations in air pressure (as they exist up to the tympanic membrane) into mechanical energy that is propagated and amplified along the ossicles to the oval window. In the **inner ear,** this mechanical energy is turned into neural activity.

The components of the inner ear are contained within the **cochlea,** which looks somewhat like a snail's shell (*cochlea* is Latin for "snail shell"). Within the cochlea

The Organ of Corti, Which Transduces Sound into Neural Impulses

Figure 8.3

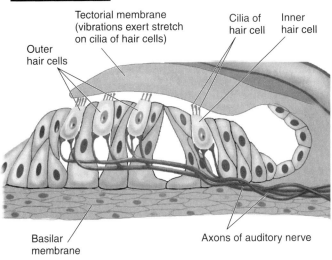

Organ of Corti

Source: Neil R. Carlson, *Physiology of Behavior,* 8e. Published by Allyn and Bacon, Boston, MA. Copyright © 2004 by Pearson Education. Reprinted by permission of the publisher.

are the inner hair cells and outer hair cells (outer hair cells outnumber inner hair cells by about 3 to 1), but it is the inner hair cells that serve as the receptors for the auditory system. Only 5% of the auditory nerve cells receive inputs from the outer cells, therefore an individual with intact outer hair cells but damaged inner hair cells is mostly deaf. This curious phenomenon leaves most students asking, "What are the outer hair cells for and why are there three times as many of them?" The outer hair cells appear to play a modulatory role, helping to "tune" the cochlea through contraction and relaxation. The mechanism that subserves the modulation is unclear, but it can be influenced by experience. Conditioning the cochlea over a long period of time can actually increase its sensitivity to similar sounds, presumably by modifying the outer hair cells and/or the mechanism that controls their contraction and relaxation (Kujawa & Liberman, 1999).

The inner hair cells (auditory receptors) have tiny filaments at their tips, called *cilia.* The cilia are arranged in order of height, and they are normally under a small amount of tension. When cilia move toward the direction containing the tallest cilium (singular of *cilia*), fibers within the cilia are stretched, resulting in increased firing in the axons of the cochlear nerve. If the cilia are forced in the opposite direction (toward the shortest cilium), firing in the cochlear nerve falls below the normal (resting) rate. The hair cells, their cilia, and the cells that support them are collectively referred to as the **organ of Corti** (see Figure 8.3).

Although we have described the receptor cells, we have not yet described how the mechanical energy from the middle ear influences them. What mechanism bends and applies force to the cilia? The hair cells (and their cilia) are located along the basilar membrane. There is a second membrane that runs parallel to the basilar membrane, called the tectorial membrane, located directly adjacent to the hair cells (see Figure 8.3). Although the movement of both membranes is critical to auditory perception, the tectorial membrane does not (normally) actually contact the cilia. Instead, the sound waves cause the two membranes to flex, and their relative movement causes cochlear fluid to flow past the cilia, causing them to bend.

Just as the retina is a highly organized system of rods and cones, the receptors of the auditory system are organized in a highly systematic way. Different sections of the cochlea respond maximally to different frequencies. The part of the basilar membrane closest to the oval window is quite stiff, and the receptors here are exposed to higher frequencies. Nearer to the **apex**, the basilar membrane is more flexible, and the receptors that are located here are exposed to vibrations of lower frequencies. This frequency-specific sensory organization is referred to as **tonotopic,** and as you will see later in this chapter, this tonotopic organization is preserved at higher levels in the auditory system.

As we have described the auditory system so far, it appears to be a relatively inflexible mechanical system for detecting changes in air pressure. However, it is not that simple. There is considerable evidence that the functioning of these components can be significantly influenced by cognition. One example we have already encountered involves the functioning of the outer hair cells. As we learned earlier, experience can significantly influence their efficiency.

However, even more transient and subtle changes occur in the auditory system. For instance, the efferent projections from the cochlea demonstrate differential activation under different attentional conditions (Ferber-Viart, Duclaux, Collet, & Guyonnard, 1995; Maison, Micheyl, & Collet, 2001). Other investigations found similar results for other relatively "low" brain areas, such as the brainstem (Hoorman, Falkenstein, & Hohnsbein, 2000). Although the mechanical nature of the outer and inner ear makes it seem extremely unlikely that any cognitive process could modulate their function, inner ear function can be affected by higher perceptual and attentional processes.

Auditory Pathways

Unfortunately for the student who is trying to memorize the auditory pathways, there is no auditory pathway that is analogous to the visual system's retino-geniculo-striate pathway. Audition is subserved by several functionally distinct and complex pathways. To make matters even more confusing, the pathways themselves may be interconnected. However, for the sake of clarity, only two of the pathways will be presented here (see Figure 8.4).

Axons from the cochlear nerve form a branch of the **eighth cranial nerve** (vestibulocochlear nerve), and they synapse on the ipsilateral

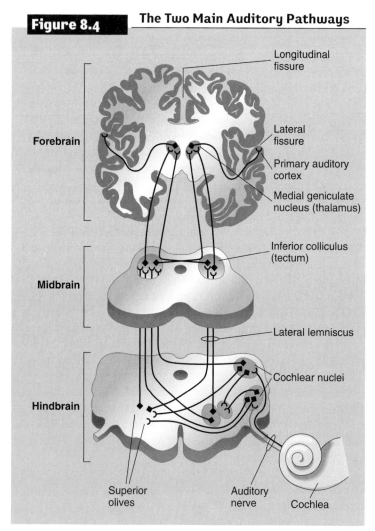

Figure 8.4   The Two Main Auditory Pathways

- Longitudinal fissure
- Lateral fissure
- Primary auditory cortex
- Medial geniculate nucleus (thalamus)
- Inferior colliculus (tectum)
- Lateral lemniscus
- Cochlear nuclei

Forebrain

Midbrain

Hindbrain

Superior olives   Auditory nerve   Cochlea

Source: John P. J. Pinel, *Biopsychology,* 5e. Published by Allyn and Bacon, Boston, MA. Copyright © 2003 by Pearson Education. Reprinted by permission of the publisher.

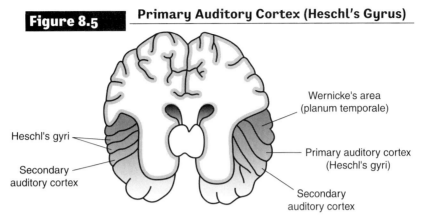

Figure 8.5 **Primary Auditory Cortex (Heschl's Gyrus)**

Wernicke's area
(planum temporale)

Heschl's gyri

Secondary
auditory cortex

Primary auditory cortex
(Heschl's gyri)

Secondary
auditory cortex

Source: Reprinted by permission of Paul Janzen.

cochlear nuclei. From here, most projections lead to the ipsilateral or contralateral **superior olives.** However, some lead directly to the **inferior colliculus** of the midbrain. From the olivary nuclei, projections travel to the (ipsilateral) inferior colliculus. After reaching the inferior colliculus, some projections cross to the contralateral side, whereas others project directly to the **medial geniculate nucleus of the thalamus** and then to the **primary auditory cortex** (also referred to as *Heschl's gyrus* or *BA41*). The subset of projections that cross to the contralateral side at the level of the inferior colliculus also eventually project to the medial geniculate nucleus of the thalamus (the ventral part) and then to the primary auditory cortex (see Figure 8.5). Therefore, unlike the visual system, auditory projections do not necessarily terminate in the cortex contralateral to their origin. There is some crossing at the level of the cochlear nuclei and some crossing at the level of the inferior colliculus, but a minority of all auditory projections are exclusively ipsilateral. Most fibers cross sides before the projections reach the cortex.

There is one way in which the auditory system pathways are analogous to the visual system pathways: Some pathways involve projections from receptors to the primary sensory cortex, and others appear to bypass the primary cortex, projecting directly to secondary or even tertiary cortical areas. The interconnected pathways described above all project to the primary auditory cortex. However, a second set of interconnected pathways does not. These pathways have the same destinations until they reach the inferior colliculus. At that point, the midbrain connections do not terminate in the ventral medial geniculate nucleus of the thalamus. Instead, they synapse on the dorsal medial geniculate nucleus of the thalamus, and then they project directly to the secondary and tertiary auditory cortices (corresponding to BA42 and 22).

Auditory Cortex

When we view the lateral surface of the brain, the primary auditory cortex is mostly hidden behind the secondary auditory cortex; it is located within the lateral fissure. The neurons within the primary auditory cortex are highly specialized to respond to certain frequencies of sound. The auditory cortex, like the cochlea, is organized in a tonotopic fashion (Wessinger, Buonocore, Kussmaul, & Mangun, 1997). Neurons within the auditory cortex are arranged in columns, and the columns in more anterior regions of the cortex respond maximally to higher frequencies, whereas neurons in posterior regions respond more to lower frequencies. However, these cortical neurons respond to a narrower range of frequencies than do the neurons located earlier in the processing stream. For example, a neuron in the cochlear nucleus might respond maximally to a tone at 10,000 Hz but also respond to tones between 6000 and 14,000 Hz. A comparable neuron in the primary auditory cortex might also respond maximally to 10,000-Hz tones but would be relatively uninfluenced by much higher (14,000-Hz) or lower (6000-Hz) tones.

As you learned in Chapter 4, the morphology of the primary auditory cortex differs between the right and left hemisphere. Most right-handers have a right Heschl's gyrus that is larger than the left. In fact, the right auditory cortex is often large enough to cover two gyri, collectively referred to as *Heschl's gyri*. Most left-handers also demonstrate this asymmetry, albeit to a lesser extent.

The areas immediately adjacent to the primary auditory cortex are referred to as the **secondary auditory cortex.** The secondary auditory cortex is located lateral and anterior to the primary auditory cortex (see Figure 8.5). Relatively little is known about the specific properties of the secondary auditory cortex, although the neurons in this region appear to be highly selective in the stimuli to which they respond. That is, these neurons are highly sensitive to specific frequencies of sound, and these cells are also sensitive to frequencies occurring in particular temporal patterns.

Self-Test

1. What are the three dimensions on which sound waves are described?

2. What is the difference between the tectorial membrane and the basilar membrane?

3. What do outer hair cells do?

4. Where does information cross from one side to the other in the two main auditory pathways?

5. Part of the compression used in MP3 music files takes advantage of a perceptual phenomenon. What is it, and how is it used to compress music files?

MODULE **8.2**
Language Systems in the Brain

As we learned in Chapter 1, a basic model of the functional neuroanatomy of language was formed by the end of the nineteenth century, long before other "higher functions" were mapped. However, this model was based solely on the study of individuals who had experienced focal brain injuries. Because the neuropsychologist's scientific toolkit is now considerably more diverse, we can study cases of acquired brain damage along with studying the normal and abnormal development of language in vivo. That is, we can now study language in the normal, intact brain.

Models of Spoken Language

There is no single, unitary language center that is responsible for auditory and visual language input and output. The neuropsychology of language is complicated, and understanding it requires the separate examination of the subtasks that occur during language processing. In the following sections, you will find separate discussions of auditory language (i.e., that which is spoken and heard) and visual language (i.e., that which is written and read). You will also be asked to consider the production of language (speaking and writing) separately from the reception of language (hearing and reading).

Language processing was initially viewed as a unitary function, all of which was subserved by a single module in the brain. This view was first advanced by Gall and Spurzheim but was later substantiated by clinical evidence provided by Paul Broca in 1861. According to both sets of evidence, language was subserved by the frontal lobe—the third gyrus of the left frontal lobe, according to Broca. This area is now referred to as **Broca's area** (see Figure 8.6). However, in 1874, Wernicke proposed a more complicated model. Instead of claiming that a single anatomical locus subserved all language processing, Wernicke suggested that one area was responsible for the output of spoken language (the same frontal lobe location described by Broca) and that another was responsible for mapping sounds to words. This second center was hypothetically located in the left temporal lobe, just posterior to the primary auditory cortex. This area is now referred to as **Wernicke's area.** Wernicke also proposed that these two centers would need to be connected to provide meaningful verbal output. This connection is now referred to as the **arcuate fasciculus.**

In 1885, Lichtheim proposed an alternative model—one that included an additional element, the **concept center** (Town, 1913). According to this model, Wernicke's area maps sounds to words, but its role in ascribing meaning to those sounds is minimal. Instead, the concept center, a center that is connected to both Wernicke's and Broca's areas, performs this role. Although this model could explain more of the language disorders than Wernicke's original model, it is still a gross oversimplification of language processing.

American neurologist Norman Geschwind updated the Wernicke-Lichtheim model in the 1960s, producing the **Wernicke-Lichtheim-Geschwind (WLG)** model (see Figure 8.7). Although the Wernicke-Lichtheim model could account for oral and aural language (that which is spoken and heard), it could not account for visual language (reading and writing). To expand the model, Geschwind included the **angular gyrus,** located at the junction between the temporal, parietal, and occipital lobes. The angular gyrus receives projections from primary and secondary visual areas and, according to Geschwind, provides a basis for **visual language.** The WLG

Figure 8.6   **Location of Broca's Area**

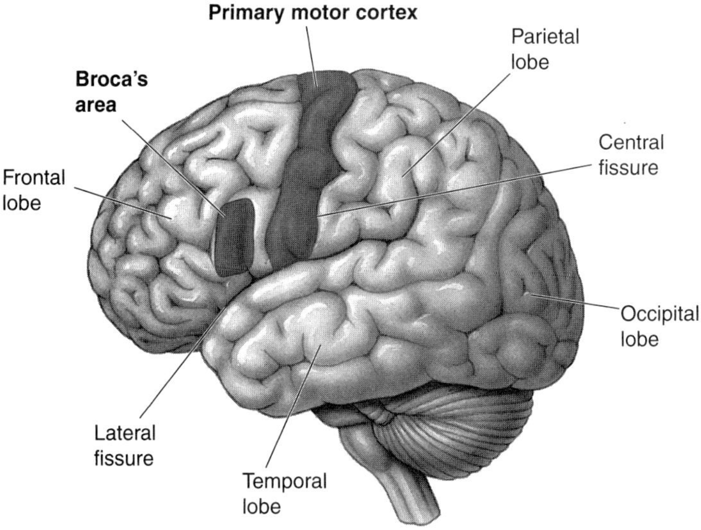

Source: John P. J. Pinel, *Biopsychology,* 5e. Published by Allyn and Bacon, Boston, MA. Copyright © 2003 by Pearson Education. Reprinted by permission of the publisher.

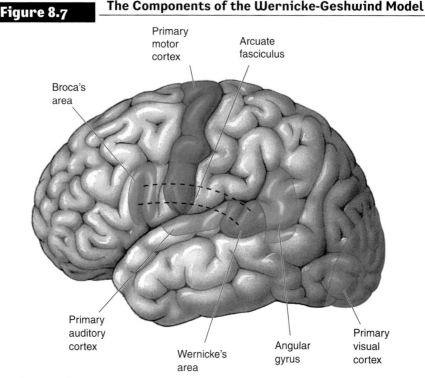

Figure 8.7   **The Components of the Wernicke-Geshwind Model**

Primary motor cortex

Arcuate fasciculus

Broca's area

Primary auditory cortex

Wernicke's area

Angular gyrus

Primary visual cortex

Source: John P. J. Pinel, *Biopsychology,* 5e. Published by Allyn and Bacon, Boston, MA. Copyright © 2003 by Pearson Education. Reprinted by permission of the publisher.

model incorporates considerably more detail about the roles of the primary sensory and motor cortices in the model, especially for the primary motor cortex and primary visual cortex.

The WLG model can account for many aspects of normal speech. According to the model, **spontaneous speech** is produced by accessing the mappings of sounds to meanings in Wernicke's area, projecting this information via the arcuate fasciculus to Broca's area, wherein the motor program is formulated and executed through the primary motor cortex that innervates the mouth, tongue, and so on. Repetition of speech occurs in much the same way. First, the person processes the auditory sounds that form the words to be repeated, but the sounds are not perceived as meaningful words until after they have been processed by Wernicke's area (receiving inputs from the primary auditory cortex). To initiate the repetition, the brain must then project these meaningful **sound images** to Broca's area through the arcuate fasciculus.

The WLG model can also account for some processing of visual language information (see Figure 8.8). For a person to silently read and understand written text, the text must be sensed and perceived by the visual system. After this information reaches the primary and secondary visual cortices, it is projected to the angular gyrus. At this point, the written words are "transcribed" into sound images, which can be interpreted and ascribed meaning by Wernicke's area (although this transformation is not

Figure 8.8   How the Wernicke-Geschwind Model Works

How the Wernicke-Geshwind model works

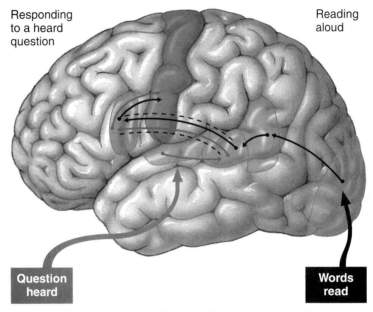

Source: John P. J. Pinel, *Biopsychology,* 5e. Published by Allyn and Bacon, Boston, MA. Copyright © 2003 by Pearson Education. Reprinted by permission of the publisher.

always necessary). The process of transcribing written words to sound images is presumably why you "hear a voice in your head" as you read. The model suggests that Wernicke's area is processing information in a similar way as when it is presented with "real" auditory stimulation.

There are numerous points of support for the WLG model. For instance, it provides a parsimonious account of many of the clinical speech disorders (described in the next module), largely because this is the type of evidence on which the work was based. Electrical stimulation and functional neuroimaging studies have also confirmed many of the model's claims. However, the WLG model has serious shortcomings. The most serious problem is one of oversimplification and omission. For example, if Wernicke's area subserves knowledge for mapping sound images to meanings, why does the mapping of spoken words to meaning depend on the meaning of the word in question? When individuals are asked to name people, this results in activation of anterior inferior temporal areas. When they name tools, the activation is more posterior along the inferior temporal lobe. If they are asked to name animals, the activation is in between these two areas. Additionally, the WLG model grossly oversimplifies the processing of visual language. More modern models of visual language are discussed in the following section. Despite these shortcomings, the WLG model can still explain the bulk of the clinical evidence regarding spoken language, which is why it is popular.

Figure 8.9

Summary of Language Models

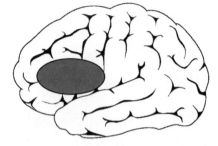

Single-center model
(Gall & Spurzheim,
Broca)

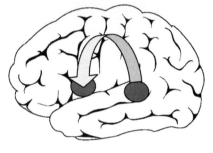

Wernicke's model

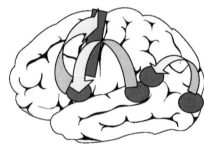

Wernicke-Lichtheim-
Geschwind model

Figure 8.9 summarizes the three language models we have discussed here.

Models of Visual Language

The differences between visual and auditory language are many; not only are different modalities employed, but auditory language abilities usually develop long before visual language does. Humans develop auditory language with relative ease, and it progresses well without formal instruction. Conversely, visual language is usually explicitly taught, and its acquisition is not effortless. It is also clear that humans used oral language long before systems of reading and writing were developed, but this does not necessarily mean that oral language developed before visual language. A number of researchers suggest that a system of communicating through gestures (a form of visual language) developed prior to the development of oral language (Diamond, 1959; Corballis, 2002).

Models of visual language emerged relatively recently. The WLG auditory language model made an attempt to include visual language functions, but simply attributing visual language processing to the angular gyrus oversimplifies the complexity of reading and writing. Most current visual language models are considerably more complicated. However, they can be divided into two general classes: **single-route** models and **dual-route** models. Both classes of models describe two ways in which words can be read: sounding out the words or reading the word as a whole.

Have you seen television commercials for the Hooked on Phonics® reading program? Or if you have ever watched *Sesame Street,* you undoubtedly have watched sketches in which a word is split in two pieces on the screen and the two pieces are sounded out separately as the pieces of the word get closer and closer together. (For example, the word *book* is split into *b* and *ook*, and the child hears, "Buh, . . . uck, Buh . . . uckk, Buh - uck, b-ook, book.) Both are examples of how English readers can use **phoneme–grapheme conversion rules** to read text. A **phoneme** is a small, pronounceable, and meaningful unit of sound in language. **Graphemes** are the smallest units of written language. In English, graphemes are letters. However, graphemes are not always simply letters. For example, in German *u* and *ü* are different graphemes that correspond to different phonemes. Although many languages (e.g., Spanish) have very regular, predictable phoneme–grapheme conversion rules, others (e.g., English) do not.

Using phoneme–grapheme conversion rules, we can read familiar words as well as words that we have never encountered before. Even if you have not seen *Mary Poppins*, you can probably read "Supercalifragilisticexpialidocious" using phoneme–grapheme correspondence rules. You can also probably decipher the sentence "Hukt awne foniks wurkt phore mee" despite the fact that none of the letter strings form real words. Instead, these letter strings form sounds that sound like real words. They are called **pseudo-homophones**. To further complicate matters, sometimes two words that sound the same have different meanings. Perhaps you have received a copy of the e-mail joke (author unknown) that goes like this:

I have a spelling chequer
It came with my pea sea
It plainly marques four my revue
Miss steaks eye cannot sea . . .

However, English is a complicated language, and being able to sound out words is not always helpful. Try sounding out the words *yacht*, *colonel*, and *epitome*. Compare the pronunciations of *goose* and *choose*, *heard* and *beard*, or *word* and *sword*.

. . . Beware of heard, a dreadful word,
That looks like beard and sounds like bird.
And dead—it's said like bed, not bead;
For goodness sake, don't call it deed!
Watch out for meat and great and threat.
(They rhyme with suite and straight and debt.)
A moth is not a moth in mother;
Nor both in bother, broth in brother.
    (author unknown)

As the poem makes clear, there are many situations in which the regular phoneme–grapheme correspondence rules are not very helpful. These irregular words appear to require memorization of the word as a whole. Although you might suspect that only a small subset of words are normally read this way, whole-word reading is probably the dominant manner in which people read. When words are unfamiliar, they must be pronounced by using phoneme–grapheme rules. Once they become familiar, their graphemic representation is "remembered" as a whole.

Given that words can be read either way, many have argued that there are two functionally distinct routes for receptive visual language (i.e., reading). These models are collectively referred to as *dual-route models* (Meyer, Schvaneveldt, & Ruddy, 1974). However, others have used computational models of word recognition to argue that both types of reading could be subserved by a single distributed network (Plaut, McClelland, & Seidenberg, 1995; Seidenberg & McClelland, 1989). These models are collectively referred to as *single-route models*. For a graphical rendering

Figure 8.10 ## The Dual-Route Model of Reading

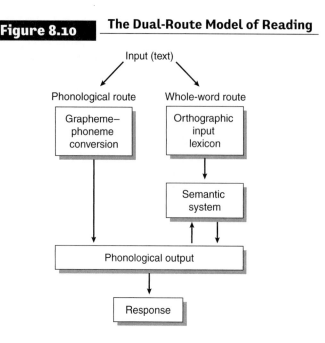

of a dual-route reading model, see Figure 8.10. The two routes are usually named the **phonological route** and the **whole-word route**. As you might expect, dual-route models of writing (analogous to the reading models) have also been proposed (see Figure 8.11).

In terms of the anatomical loci subserving these two routes, several candidate structures have been identified. Simos and colleagues (Simos, Breier, Wheless, Maggio, Fletcher, Castillo et al., 2000) used whole-head magnetic source imaging in patients undergoing electrocortical stimulation mapping. When reading using the whole-word route (or *assembled phonology*, to use these researchers' terminology), Simos and colleagues found activity in the posterior part of the left superior temporal gyrus. The evidence for an anatomically distinct phonological route is less clear. Although phonological processing appears to depend on structures other than the posterior left superior temporal gyrus, its localization is better informed by the clinical evidence that we discuss in the next module.

Figure 8.11 ## The Dual-Route Model of Writing

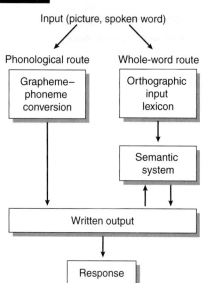

Prosody and the Role of the Right Hemisphere in Language Processing

Have you ever had an instructor who lectured in a flat, monotone manner? After listening to a lecture from a speaker with flat, invariant speech, students often complain that the lecture was boring and the speaker was difficult to understand. However, we are too quick to blame the difficulty in understanding on boredom. A speaker who does not vary his or her tone of voice while speaking is failing to use an important means for communication: prosody.

Prosody is the conveyance of meaning by varying the intonation in speech, including changes in pitch, tempo, intensity, and rhythm. These changes not only can augment the meaning of the words in a phrase, but also can reverse the meaning of words. Consider the case of sarcasm. Sometimes people say the opposite of what they really mean: "I just *love* reality television. There is nothing more entertaining than taking a bunch of average people off the street, forcing them to compete in silly, arbitrary competitions, and eavesdropping on their petty gossip during all hours of the day. I think it is a *brilliant* innovation in television programming that in *no* way resembles the perverse entertainment that was provided at the Roman Coliseum thousands of years ago."

What does the speaker *say* about reality television? What does the speaker *mean*? If you were listening to the passage above instead of reading it, you would have heard stresses on the words *love* and *no*, cueing you that the intended meaning was the opposite of what the words themselves indicate. (Aside: I actually enjoy watching reality television but am not proud of that fact.) Prosody can also cue the presence of a question, usually by a slight elevation in pitch toward the end of a phrase. Sometimes questions can be identified because of the words in the phrase (e.g., *who, what, where, why, how*), but some phrases question without the presence of such words. Consider the example of a person reaching into a dishwasher to retrieve a clean bowl and saying to his or her spouse, "You did the dishes." or "You did the dishes?" The first phrase is a statement (perhaps a veiled expression of gratitude); the second asks for confirmation that the retrieved bowl is actually clean.

These examples describe prosody influencing the meaning of phrases, but prosody can also convey the meaning of single words. A speaker's emotional state can be inferred from tone of voice alone, even if the word is emotionally neutral. For example, in one dichotic listening experiment the words *bower, dower, power,* and *tower* are spoken in angry, sad, happy, or neutral tones of voice. When participants were instructed to listen to the emotional tone of the voice, they exhibited a left ear/right hemisphere advantage on the task (Bryden & MacRae, 1988; Elias, Bryden, & Bulman-Fleming, 1998; Elias, Bulman-Fleming, & Guylee, 1999). However, when instructed to listen to the words, they exhibited a right ear/left hemisphere advantage on the task (Bryden & MacRae, 1988; Bulman-Fleming & Bryden, 1994). This demonstrates that the right hemisphere is specialized for the detection of prosody, a finding that has also been demonstrated with nonsense syllables (Erhan, Borod, Tenke, & Bruder, 1998) and short phrases (Herrero & Hillix, 1990). Functional neuroimaging has also confirmed the right hemisphere's specialization for the detection of prosody (Buchanan, Lutz, Mirzazade, Specht, Shah, Zilles et al., 2000).

There are large individual and cultural differences in the amount and type of prosody employed during conversation. Some speakers use extreme changes in intonation to convey meaning, whereas other speakers employ relatively monotone speech. Some recent evidence suggests that there are also sex differences in the production of prosody. According to Fitzsimons, Sheahan, and Staunton (2001), males employ higher rates of speech, more

Self-Test

1. How many language centers did Gall and Spurzheim claim were present?

2. What additional component did Lichtheim propose in addition to those described by Wernicke?

3. What is the difference between the single-route and dual-route models of visual language processing?

4. What is phoneme–grapheme conversion?

5. What is prosody?

narrow pitch ranges, but a greater pitch slope (rate of pitch change) than those of female speakers.

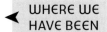
WHERE WE HAVE BEEN We have examined the structures and processes that subserve language perception and production. Visually processed language is related to auditory language, but the two systems are dissociable. Although the right hemisphere's contribution to the production and understanding of single words is minimal, it plays a vital role in processing the emotional content in language and encoding contextually relevant information.

the **Real** world

An Example of Whole-Word Reading Circulated on the Internet

I have lost count of how many times I have received the following e-mail:

"Aoccdrnig to a rscheearch at Cmabrigde Uinervtisy, it deosn't mttaer in waht oredr the ltteers in a wrod are, the olny iprmoetnt tihng is taht the frist and lsat ltteer be at the rghit pclae. The rset can be a toatl mses and you can sitll raed it wouthit porbelm. Tihs is bcuseae the huamn mnid deos not raed ervey lteter by istlef, but the wrod as a wlohe."

The passage first started circulating on the Internet in September of 2003, and like so many passages that get passed around online, it has mutated over time. Also, like many of these e-mails, there is a grain of truth, along with many falsehoods.

Falsehood #1: "Aoccdrnig to a rscheearch at Cmabrigde Uinervtisy . . . " (According to a researcher at Cambridge University). It is unclear which research paper sparked the original e-mail, but it does not appear to have come from Cambridge. Instead, a likely candidate is Graham Rawlinson's Ph.D. thesis, completed at Nottingham University in 1976.

Falsehood #2: "it deosn't mttaer in waht oredr the ltteers in a wrod are" (it doesn't matter in what order the letters in a word are). The only way to distinguish between many words is the order of the letters. Consider the following words: blamed, beldam, ambled, and bedlam.

Falsehood #3: "The olny iprmoetnt tihng is taht the frist and lsat ltteer be at the rghit pclae" (It doesn't matter in what order the letters in a word are, the only important thing is that the first and last letter be at the right place). Wrong. Try reading this sentence: A dootcr has aimttded the magltheuansr of a tageene ceacnr pintaet who deid aetfr a hatospil durg blendur. (A doctor has admitted the manslaughter of a teenage cancer patient who died after a hospital drug blunder; from the BBC News, September 22nd, 2003). You can probably read some of the words, but to decipher other ones, you need to use the context of the sentence, and maybe lots of processing time!

Falsehood #4: "the rset can be a toatl mses and you can sitll raed it wouthit porbelm" (the rest can be a total mess and you can still read it without problem). This is wrong for the same reasons described above.

Grain of Truth: "Tihs is bcuseae the huamn mnid deos not raed ervey lteter by istlef, but the wrod as a wlohe" (This is because the human mind does not read every letter by itself but the word as a whole). As you have learned in this module, a skilled reader is quite capable of whole-word reading. However, this does not imply that the letters in the middle of the word are irrelevant contributors to the "word shape."

An excellent review of the letter (along with examples in many other languages) can be found at a Cambridge University researcher's website: www.mrc-cbu.cam.ac.uk/personal/matt.davis/Cmabrigde.

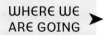

In the next module, we will investigate disorders of language processing and audition. As you will see, language disorders can be highly specific. These disorders have provided a wealth of information about the functional architecture of language systems in the brain.

MODULE **8.3**
Disorders of Language and Auditory Perception

As we mentioned previously, language production was one of the first cognitive abilities to be localized in the brain. Although many people contributed to this discovery (for a review, see Chapter 1), the patient described by Broca is widely known. Broca encountered an epileptic patient who had suffered brain damage some twenty years earlier that rendered him paralyzed on his right side (**right hemiparesis**) and virtually unable to speak (Broca, 1865). In the scientific literature that followed, Broca's patient (M. Leborgne) became known as "Tan" because it was one of the only words that the man could produce fluently (he also retained the ability to swear). Leborgne appeared to use the word *tan* as if it was in fact many different words and would speak "sentences" such as "Tan, tan tan, tan, tan tan tan. . . ." Despite this deficit, Leborgne did not exhibit difficulties comprehending language, and he otherwise seemed to possess normal intelligence. When Leborgne died, Broca performed an autopsy to investigate the claims made by others regarding the role of the left hemisphere and found that Leborgne had a softening of the tissue "the size of a hen's egg" along the third frontal convolution along the left hemisphere (see Figure 8.12). This area is now referred to as *Broca's area*. A CT scan of Leborgne's brain (conducted over 120 years later) confirmed Broca's conclusions about the location of the lesion (Signoret, Castaigne, Lhermitte, Abelanet, & Lavorel, 1984).

In the two years that followed, Broca encountered eight more cases with similar symptomology. The presentation of this evidence caught the attention of the medical and scientific community but not without encountering adversity (Marie, 1906; Souques, 1928; Town, 1913). Despite his detractors, it eventually became clear that Broca's position was correct. Although Broca is normally credited with the first description of aphasia, Broca himself readily acknowledged the claims made by Gall, Bouillaud, and Auburtin. He is also commonly credited as the first to describe language as a function that is dominated by the left hemisphere. As he put it, "Nous parlons avec l'hémisphère gauche" ("We speak with the left hemisphere").

Aphasia

The term **aphasia** is used too broadly in clinical and experimental neuropsychology, a mistake that we are about repeat here. Literally, *aphasia* means a "lack of language" or "no language." A deficit this severe is extremely rare. Most patients who are diagnosed with aphasia retain some (or even much) of their linguistic capacity. Therefore, the term **dysphasia,** referring to a partial loss of language, is usually more appropriate. However, use of the term *dysphasia* is so infrequent that we will use the more conventional term *aphasia*. When you read descriptions of the various types of

Figure 8.12   **Tan's Brain**

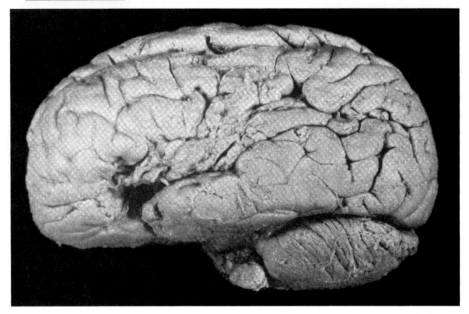

Source: Reprinted from *Brain and Language, 22,* J. L. Signoret, P. Castaigne, & F. Lhermite, "Rediscovery of Leborgne's brain: Anatomical description with CT scan," pp. 303–319, Copyright 1984, with permission from Elsevier.

aphasia, remember that these disorders vary considerably in their severity and that the deficits are almost never complete—some functionality of the impaired system or structure is virtually always retained.

BROCA'S APHASIA. The behavioral syndrome that results from damage to Broca's area is called **Broca's aphasia** (Broca, 1865). Its hallmark symptom is an inability to produce fluent speech, despite relatively intact speech comprehension and intact vocal mechanisms. However, Broca's aphasia can vary considerably from one individual to the next. Some individuals exhibit problems in producing speech fluently (often omitting function words, which are pronouns, conjunctions, prepositions, or articles such as *of, at,* or *and*) but still manage to produce some comprehensible sentences, albeit slowly. Others have such severe aphasia that they can produce only a few different words, and the production of these words appears to be quite difficult. The verbal problems that are evident in Broca's aphasia are not the result of a generalized inability to produce oral–facial movements. When asked to, an individual with severe Broca's aphasia can blow out a candle or clear his or her throat. Furthermore, individuals with Broca's aphasia do not exhibit generalized cognitive impairment; performance on nonverbal tasks (e.g., calculation, mental rotation, facial recognition) remains in the normal range, and the ability to understand and carry out verbal commands is preserved. Despite an ability to understand verbal commands, repetition of these commands is impaired.

Following is an example of Broca's aphasia described by Howard Gardner (1974). This is a partial transcript of a conversation between Gardner and David Ford, a 39-year-old radio operator who suffered a left hemisphere stroke. Ford could speak slowly but abruptly. The words transcribed below were usually vocalized quite harshly and quickly but with lengthy gaps between some of the words. Ford appeared to exert considerable effort when conversing.

Gardner: "Could you tell me Mr. Ford, what you've been doing in hospital?"
Ford: "Yes, sure. Me go, er, uh, P.T. nine o'cot, speech . . . two times . . . read . . . wr . . . ripe, er, rike, er, wite . . . practice . . . get-ting better."
Gardner: "And have you been going home on weekends?"
Ford: "Why, yes . . . Thursday, er, er, er, no, er, Friday . . . Bar-ba-ra . . . wife . . . and, oh, car . . . drive . . . purnpike . . . you know . . . rest and . . . tee-vee."
Gardner: "Are you able to understand everything on television?"
Ford: "Oh, yes, yes . . . well . . . almost." (Ford grinned a bit.) (Gardner, 1974, p. 61)

Ford appears to understand the questions asked of him, but he displays profound difficulty in articulating what he intends to communicate. He can often produce the appropriate nouns or verbs, but appears to have trouble finding words. The inability to find the correct word (usually nouns and verbs) is referred to as **anomia** (which means "no name"). People with Broca's aphasia often exhibit some degree of anomia, but most exclusions (words left out) are function words. This results in speech that is composed mostly of nouns, verbs, and some adjectives. Despite the missing words, these utterances can often carry the speaker's intended meaning. Because of its similarity to the type of communication that used to be common in telegrams (telegrams are normally priced per word, so small and unnecessary function words were often omitted to save money), speech by Broca's aphasics is sometimes referred to as *telegraphic speech*. In a more general sense, the inability to produce grammatically correct sentences is referred to as **agrammatism.** Broca's aphasics usually display agrammatism, but the types of errors are usually errors of omission.

Unfortunately, the agrammatism that is often displayed in Broca's aphasics is not limited to the production of speech. There is some evidence of comprehension problems, but these problems do not involve understanding the meanings of nouns or verbs. Instead, it appears as though the understanding of function words (the types of words often excluded) can be impaired. Therefore, when they encounter grammatically complicated sentences in which the meaning depends on word order and the meaning of the function words, individuals with agrammatism exhibit impairments. Consider the following string of words: "car, fast, screech, smash, ambulance, hospital, graveyard." What happened? Despite the complete lack of grammatical structure and function words, it should be clear to most readers that the example tells the story of a car crash that caused someone's death (possibly, but not necessarily, the driver).

Now consider following two sentences: "Dog bites man" and "Man bites dog." The nouns and verbs in the two sentences are identical, but the meanings of the two are very different. However, a Broca's aphasic demonstrating agrammatism might judge the two sentences to be equivalent in meaning. However, as the old saying goes, only the second sentence is news.

Fortunately for individuals with these deficits, the meaning of most sentences can be deduced using one's knowledge of semantics: the meanings of words. Consider the following sentence: "The deer was shot by the man." I have never encountered a story about a deer learning to shoot a rifle and successfully turning the tables on some unsuspecting hunter (well, maybe in a *Far Side* cartoon). Therefore, even in the absence of the grammatical information and function words in that sentence (i.e., deer, shot, man), one can reasonably guess what happened. Similarly, aphasics with agrammatism tend not to exhibit problems with the meanings of such sentences. Because they know that deer do not shoot people, the ordering of the words does not confuse them. Therefore, agrammatism compromises language comprehension only under certain circumstances.

The transcript of the conversation between Gardner and Ford also provides an example of another type of error common in Broca's aphasia. Note the spot where Ford mentions the "purnpike." Broca's aphasics often substitute similar sounds within a word, an error known as a **phonemic paraphasia.** Recall that a phoneme is a component sound that makes up a language. Therefore, a phonemic paraphasia is an aphasia in which the individual has difficulty producing the correct phoneme. In the example with Ford, he substituted a *p* sound for a *t* sound when intending to use the word *turnpike.* As you will discover in the next section, there is another type of paraphasic error, called a **semantic paraphasia,** in which individuals substitute words of similar meaning, such as substituting *leopard* for *tiger.* However, the paraphasic errors made by Broca's aphasics are normally of the phonemic type.

Phonemic paraphasic errors are not simply random substitutions of one letter for another. Instead, the errors that are made appear to vary systematically with the physical requirements of producing a particular sound. Making the sounds for various phonemes requires coordination of a number of motor processes. To help you learn about these processes, you are going to be asked to try making some nonsense sounds. To avoid disturbing others or becoming the butt of their jokes, you might want to find a quiet place where you can be alone for this next section.

One of these processes in articulating phonemes is the *voicing* of the phoneme, referring to the differences in the timing of the release of air and the vibration of your vocal cords. For example, **voiced consonants** involve almost identical timing between the release of air and vocal cord vibration. Try repeating the following sounds to yourself (quietly—you don't want people to think you are going crazy): *bah, dah, gah.* The *b, d,* and *g* are all voiced consonants—the release of air and vibration of vocal cords are simultaneous. In contrast, try repeating these sounds: *tah, kah, pah.* The *t, k,* and *p* in these examples are **unvoiced consonants.** There is a delay between the release of air and the onset of vocal cord vibration, resulting in a more airy feel. If you are not convinced of the difference, try alternating between voiced and unvoiced consonants: *bah–tah, dah–kah, gah–pah.* If this accomplishes nothing else, you should at least sound like a toddler.

One can also characterize the vocalizing of phonemes in terms of where they are articulated in the mouth, called the **place of articulation.** To use the same examples as above, some phonemes involve a complete constriction of air toward the front of the mouth. These are called **labial stops.** Try repeating the following sounds: *bah, pah.* If you noticed that the two sounds involved different voicing, you were quite correct.

However, both sounds involved the same *place* of articulation—could you feel the constriction of air right at your lips? In comparison, try repeating two examples of **alveolar stops,** in which the airflow is constricted a little farther back—against the alveolar ridge located behind your front teeth. Two such examples are *tah* and *dah.* Again, these examples involve differences in voicing, but they are articulated in the same place. You articulate phonemes even farther back in your mouth. These are referred to as **velar stops,** and these sounds involve placing your tongue toward the back of your mouth. Try repeating these examples: *kah, gah.* Just as in the previous examples, the voicing differed between the two examples but their place was the same. Could you feel the difference between the three places of articulation? If not, try the three in a row: *pah, dah, gah.*

So what does all of this have to do with Broca's aphasia? The phonemic substitution errors that occur in Broca's aphasia are not simply random intrusions. Instead, the errors tend to vary systematically according to the voicing or place of articulation for the phoneme. People with Broca's aphasia often make errors based on the place of articulation but rarely make errors based on the voicing of a phoneme (Baker, Blumstein, & Goodglass, 1981; Lecours & Lhermitte, 1969). Therefore, a typical error might be the substitution of *p* for *t* (e.g., *purnpike* for *turnpike*) or *b* for *d.* It is relatively more rare to substitute *b* for *p* or *d* for *t* (errors of voicing). Almost all errors occur across the place of articulation *or* voicing but not both. Therefore, it would be extremely rare to substitute *b* for *t* or *d* for *p,* because to do so would require getting both the place of articulation *and* the voicing wrong. The more similar the two phonemes (in terms of their place of articulation or voicing), the more likely they are to be substituted. See Table 8.1 for a clarification of these two dimensions.

Table 8.1	

Types of Errors in Broca's Aphasia

Voicing	Place of Articulation		
	Labial Stops	**Alveolar Stops**	**Velar Stops**
Voiced	B	D	G
Unvoiced	P	T	K

The lesions that give rise to Broca's aphasia are usually located at Brodmann's areas 44 and 45, although the depth of the lesion required is still a matter of debate. Some claim that lesions of the cortex alone are sufficient to give rise to the condition; others claim that some of the underlying subcortical tissue also needs to suffer damage for the syndrome to result.

Still others claim that the functions of Broca's area are broader than simply sequencing speech. Because individuals with Broca's aphasia also exhibit problems in solving nonverbal planning tasks, some have argued that the area serves the more fundamental problem of mental sequencing (Bartl-Storck & Mueeller, 1999). This function is necessary both for language production and for planning in a more general sense.

WERNICKE'S APHASIA. The aphasia described by Karl Wernicke (1848–1904) some twenty years after Broca's written description of "aphemia" is in many ways the opposite of Broca's aphasia. **Wernicke's aphasia** (sometimes called *sensory aphasia*) is characterized by fluent speech, but the meaning of the speech is severely compromised.

The term **word salad** is often used to described the seemingly random collection of words that form speech from an individual with Wernicke's aphasia, but this term probably underestimates the structure that underlies the nonsensical linguistic stream. A well-tossed salad is a truly random assortment of the ingredients (with the possible exception of well-placed garnishes on top of the salad after the tossing is complete). However, the speech produced by individuals with Wernicke's aphasia is not truly random. Instead of being composed of random function words, nouns, verbs, and adjectives, the speech includes many sensible orderings of the different parts of speech (e.g., subject, verb, object), but this alone does not make for successful communication.

When Wernicke first described this condition, he was making a number of claims that were inconsistent with those made by Broca. Broca claimed that there was one language area and that it was located in the frontal lobe. Others, including Wernicke and Theodore Meynert (1833–1892), suggested that damage to the temporal lobe produced linguistic deficits. In addition to resulting from damage to a different locus (the first temporal gyrus rather than the third frontal gyrus), the aphasia syndrome described by Wernicke (based on ten clinical cases) differed from that described by Broca in a number of respects. Broca's aphasia is normally comorbid with a right hemiplegia (paralysis of the right side), but Wernicke's aphasia can appear without any motor deficit. Individuals with Broca's aphasia exhibit great difficulty in producing speech, but an individual with Wernicke's aphasia produces speech effortlessly. Broca's aphasics understand speech reasonably well, but individuals with Wernicke's aphasia exhibit severe deficits in speech comprehension.

Consider the following example of Wernicke's aphasia. It is a partial transcript of a conversation between Philip Gorgan (a retired butcher who had spent the previous four weeks in the hospital) and Howard Gardner. Gorgan exhibited some difficulty speaking during his first few days in the hospital, but these difficulties were probably due to a more general weakness. In the days that followed, Gorgan spoke effortlessly—too effortlessly, in fact. It was nearly impossible to interrupt him once he started speaking.

Gardner: "What brings you to the hospital?"

Gorgan: "Boy, I'm sweating, I'm awful nervous, you know, once in a while I get caught up, I can't mention the tarripoi a month ago, quite a little, I've done a lot well, I impose a lot, while, on the other hand, you know what I mean, I have to run around, look it over, trebbin and all that sort of stuff."

Gardner: "Thank you, Mr. Gorgan. I want to ask you a few–"

Gorgan: "Oh sure, go ahead, any old think you want. If I could I would. Oh, I'm talking the word the wrong way to say, all of the barbers here whenever they stop you it's going around and around, if you know what I mean, that is tying and tying for repucer, repuceration, well, were trying the best that we could while another time it was with the beds over there the same thing. . . ." (Gardner, 1974, p. 68)

A number of features of Mr. Gorgan's speech are clearly pathological. Some are less clearly pathological and might even remind you of conversations with the stereotypical con artist, used-car salesman, or telemarketer—the inability to get a word in edgewise and the unpredictable appearance of meaningless jargon. What makes the verbal stream coming from a Wernicke's aphasic particularly special is its juxtaposition of effortless fluency with a lack of meaningful content. Unlike the extreme economy of words one encounters in Broca's aphasia, individuals with Wernicke's aphasia can produce great quantities of linguistic output, but the quality of the output is severely compromised. If a person in the relatively early stages of learning English were to attempt to converse with a Wernicke's aphasic, the person might not notice that there was anything amiss. The Wernicke's aphasic would provide them with a steady stream of nouns, function words, and even some correctly conjugated verbs. Even the prosody in the speech (the variations in tone, including pitch, volume, and tone) can sound quite normal.

Just as individuals with Broca's aphasia make paraphasic substitutions of letters or words, Wernicke's aphasia results in the same intrusions and substitutions. However, the severity of the paraphasia is more severe in Wernicke's aphasia. Not only do Wernicke's aphasics make more semantic paraphasic errors (substituting an incorrect word for the intended word), but they also make some phonemic paraphasic errors, just as Broca's aphasics do (Baker et al., 1981). In the example dialogue, Mr. Gorgan says, *tying* instead of *trying*, omitting the *r*.

At this point, you are probably gaining an appreciation for the degree to which speech is compromised in Wernicke's aphasia. Not only are individuals unable to correctly match linguistic sounds with their meanings, but when they attempt to converse, the words they produce might contain some of the wrong phonemes, or a different word entirely might be substituted in its place.

As if that alone were not enough, there is one more type of linguistic error that is commonplace in Wernicke's aphasia: the appearance of neologisms. A neologism is not a real word, but the sounds that it comprises are combined in ways that sound like words (e.g., *biznit, scrut, almod*). Therefore, neologisms follow the language-specific rules for combining sounds to produce a meaningless nonword. The sample dialogue between Dr. Gardner and Mr. Gorgan contains the neologism *tarripoi*. Differentiating between neologisms and paraphasic errors can be very difficult. In the dialogue between Dr. Gardner and Mr. Gorgan, *repuceration* is probably an attempt at the word *recuperation*—a paraphasic error rather than a neologism.

Despite the broad range of error types in Wernicke's aphasia and the frequency with which the errors are committed, one startling feature of the aphasia remains: Many people with Wernicke's aphasia seem completely unaware of their deficit. Not only do they fail to detect the errors in their own speech, but they also do not notice that they no longer understand the speech of others. This unawareness often makes individuals with Wernicke's aphasia appear much less impaired than they actually are. They will often "converse" in socially acceptable ways, taking turns speaking with their partner(s) and noting signs of bewilderment in their audience but not demonstrating these signs themselves. If asked a question, they will usually detect the presence of the question (despite their inability to understand the words that make up the question) by listening to their partner's tone of voice. If the phrase ends with a slight raise in pitch, this can serve as a cue for the aphasic individual to respond. The unawareness of deficit that is often found in Wernicke's aphasia is extremely rarely (if ever) present in Broca's aphasia.

After observing a number of individuals who had fluent but nonsensical speech after suffering left temporal damage, Wernicke formulated a model for how language functions are subserved in the normal brain. He claimed that the temporal lobe contained the memories for how sounds correspond to words and other objects (sometimes called *sound images*), whereas the frontal lobe served to help produce the necessary movements to create language sounds. Although this position appeared to contradict Broca's position (that there is one language area and it is located in the frontal lobe), it also supported his position that articulation deficits result from left frontal lesions and integrated this finding into a broader framework. Wernicke surmised that people with damage restricted to the left frontal language area should demonstrate difficulties producing speech, but their memories for sound images should be intact, and therefore their comprehension of speech should be unaffected. Conversely, individuals who suffer exclusively from temporal lesions should demonstrate impairments in comprehension and the meaningful production of speech despite preserved articulation.

CONDUCTION APHASIA. Wernicke also theorized that the two language areas would need to be connected (via the arcuate fasciculus, a band of subcortical white matter located between the areas; see Figure 8.8) and that damage to this connecting structure should result in a third, unique language disorder. He predicted that damage to the connection between what we now call Broca's area and Wernicke's area would disrupt the flow of information from one's knowledge of how sounds map onto words and one's knowledge about how to create such sounds. Therefore, an individual with such damage should not be able to repeat words or phrases. However, because both Wernicke's and Broca's areas are intact, comprehension and production would be spared. Wernicke called this (predicted) condition **Leitungsaphasia,** German for "conduction aphasia" (Wernicke, 1874).

Wernicke's prediction proved to be correct. If an individual suffers circumscribed damaged to the inferior parietal lobe and this damage is deep enough to penetrate the subcortical white matter connecting Wernicke's and Broca's areas, this results in an impairment in repetition despite fluent and meaningful spontaneous speech. However, the resultant speech is not completely flawless—it is marred by phonemic paraphasias, just as in Broca's and Wernicke's aphasia.

Consider the following example of an interview of Margolin and Walker's (1983) patient L.B. (a different person from the commissurotomy patient L.B. described in Chapter 4). Following are some of L.B.'s responses when he was asked to repeat words and nonwords:

Examiner: "hippopotamus"
L.B.: "hippopotamus"
Examiner: "blaynge"
L.B.: "I didn't get it."
Examiner: "Okay, some of these won't be real words, they'll just be sounds. Blaynge."
L.B.: "I'm not. . . . "
Examiner: "blanch"
L.B.: "blanch"

Examiner: "north"
L.B.: "north"
Examiner: "rilld"
L.B.: "Nope, I can't say." (Margolin & Walker, 1983)

Clearly, L.B. has trouble repeating nonwords but does not seem to have trouble repeating single real words. However, this does not mean that L.B. is unimpaired in repeating real words. Consider what happens when he is faced with combinations of words:

Examiner: "Up and down."
L.B.: "Up and down."
Examiner: "look, car, house."
L.B.: "I didn't get it."
Examiner: "Save your money."
L.B.: "Save your money."
Examiner: "yellow, big, south."
L.B.: "yellen. . . . Can't get it."
Examiner: "They ran away."
L.B.: "They ran away."
Examiner: "look, catch, sell."
L.B.: "like . . . [shakes head, laughs]. . . . That's the trouble!" (Margolin & Walker, 1983)

Word combinations did not appear to pose a problem for L.B., provided that the words could be grouped together in a meaningful fashion. When presented with a series of unrelated words, L.B. was profoundly impaired, a result that is also exhibited by others (McCarthy & Warrington, 1987). This effect complicates the interpretation of the syndrome. If it was simply a deficit in repetition, the type of repetition should not matter. However, given that repetition of single meaningful words or short meaningful phrases can be preserved, this suggests that a short-term memory component is also involved.

To further complicate matters, damage to a fairly wide variety of anatomical sites can give rise to conduction aphasia. Lesions to the arcuate fasciculus appear to produce the syndrome, but these lesions are extremely rare. Given the location of the arcuate fasciculus, this should come as no surprise to you. Take another look at Figure 8.8. The structure is not near the outside edge of the cortex, so any penetrating wound causing arcuate fasciculus damage would also injure other nearby structures. The same widespread damage usually follows damage to the blood supply around the arcuate. Highly local infections or tumors can cause damage that is selective enough to help solve scientific puzzles such as conduction aphasia, but these events are extremely rare. Some individuals who exhibit the symptoms of conduction aphasia have damage to the posterior sylvian region, which may or may not include damage to the supramarginal gyrus and underlying white matter. However, some appear to have damage only to Wernicke's area (Benson, Sheremata, Bouchard, Segarra, Price, & Geschwind, 1973) or the angular gyrus (Damasio, 1998; Damasio & Damasio, 1980). Given that the syndrome can result in the absence of damage to the arcuate fasciculus, the validity of the Wernicke-Geschwind model of language has been challenged.

Techniques beyond simple classification of the lesion site have also cast doubt on the simple disconnection hypothesis in conduction aphasia. PET imaging has failed to observe patterns of activation consistent with the hypothesis (Kempler, Metter, Jackson, Hanson, Riege, & Mazziotta, 1988). Further, conduction aphasia has been temporally induced following cortical (not subcortical) stimulation. Using a subdural stimulation technique (i.e., electrodes placed beneath the dura mater), Quigg and colleagues stimulated the posterior superior temporal gyrus in a woman undergoing evaluation for epilepsy surgery. The woman demonstrated temporary (reversible) conduction aphasia when current was applied to the cortex, a result suggesting that subcortical (white matter) need not be involved in the condition (Quigg & Fountain, 1999). Using similar methods, others have noted the same thing (Anderson, Gilmore, Roper, Crosson, Bauer, Nadeau et al., 1999). This has cast doubt on Wernicke's disconnection hypothesis. According to Brown, "This concept is deeply entrenched in neurological thinking, but is supported neither by clinical nor pathological evidence" (Brown, 1975, p. 37).

Modern models of conduction aphasia tend to include a store of learned phonological representations for familiar words (analogous to Wernicke's area of sound images), but this store is posited to contain both input and output components. If the output component is damaged, conduction aphasia results. If the input component is damaged, an individual's understanding of speech is compromised (Anderson et al., 1999). Some models also propose a more dynamic relationship between speech areas, rather than one in which the flow of information is unidirectional. The truth is probably somewhere in the middle. The original model proposed by Wernicke is an oversimplification of language processing in the human brain, and in light of recent evidence (both behavioral investigations and functional imaging), conduction aphasia can result from purely cortical damage. Further, it appears that interactions between Wernicke's and Broca's areas are more complex than was previously believed.

TRANSCORTICAL-MOTOR APHASIA. In a number of ways, transcortical aphasias are the opposite of conduction aphasia. In all transcortical aphasias, individuals retain their ability to repeat words and phrases (Berthier, 1999). **Transcortical-motor aphasia** is often mistakenly identified as Broca's aphasia because spontaneous speech is halting and laborious, and comprehension is intact. Unlike the case in Broca's aphasia, articulation is not impaired when the person is instructed to repeat words or phrases. However, the person often needs no such instruction. People with transcortical-motor aphasia often exhibit a compulsion to repeat whatever someone else just said, a phenomenon called **echolalia.** Simulating echolalia is a common childhood prank—probably because it is so successful at annoying the victim. Does the following conversation sound familiar?

Adult: "Hello."
Child: "Hello."
Adult: "What are you doing?"
Child: "What are you doing?"
Adult: "No, you first. What are you doing?"
Child: "No, you first. What are you doing?"

Adult: "Stop repeating everything I say."
Child: "Stop repeating everything I say!"
Adult: "STOP IT!"
Child: "STOP IT!!" [giggling]

Children (and the occasional adult) simulate echolalia as a prank, but people with transcortical-motor aphasia often exhibit it against their wishes. The reason for the symptom becomes quite clear when we consider the types of lesions that lead to it. Although damage to a variety of structures appears to result in transcortical-motor aphasia, one thing is common: These lesions involve a disruption to the connections between the dorsolateral prefrontal cortex and the anterior portion of Broca's area (Cappa & Vignolo, 1999). Effectively, this results in a disconnection between Broca's area and the supplementary motor area. Depending on the exact location of the lesion, other motor deficits can result. For example, if the damage includes the supplementary area (as is often the case after anterior cerebral artery damage), the transcortical motor aphasia would also be accompanied by deficits in sequencing complicated movements that do not involve the mouth (Cappa & Vignolo, 1999). In all of these cases, the connection between Wernicke's area and Broca's area (the arcuate fasciculus) remains intact, and this facilitates compulsive repetition.

TRANSCORTICAL-SENSORY APHASIA. Given that transcortical-motor aphasia is similar to Broca's aphasia but with the sparing of repetition, it should come as no surprise to you that **transcortical-sensory aphasia** is analogous to Wernicke's aphasia with spared repetition. The syndrome involves similar fluent but nonsensical speech, riddled with paraphasias and neologisms. Verbal comprehension is also severely compromised. However, oral naming of objects is sometimes preserved (Berthier, 1995). Despite these deficits, individuals with transcortical-sensory aphasia are relatively unimpaired at repetition. Just as is the case in transcortical-motor aphasia, this syndrome usually includes echolalia.

The condition usually follows lesions to the angular gyrus, but it has also occurred following frontal lesions (Berthier, 1999, 2001; Freedman, Alexander, & Naeser, 1984) or thalamic lesions (Maeshima, Komai, Kinoshita, Ueno, Nakai, Naka et al., 1992). The condition is also commonly observed during the latter stages of Alzheimer's disease (Appell, Kertesz, & Fisman, 1982; Murdoch, Chenery, Wilks, & Boyle, 1987). In all of these events, the arcuate fasciculus remains intact, presumably underlying the preserved repetition or even echolalia.

MIXED TRANSCORTICAL APHASIA. **Mixed transcortical aphasia** seems to result from the presence of two lesions: one in the frontal lobe that spares much of Broca's area and one that damages temporal structures (Grossi, Trojano, Chiacchio, Soricelli, Mansi, Postiglione, et al., 1991). Clinically, this rare condition shares the symptoms of both transcortical-motor aphasia and transcortical-sensory aphasia: It is characterized by halting, laborious, and meaningless speech; impaired auditory comprehension; but preserved repetition and echolalia (Cappa & Vignolo, 1999).

Some claim that the disorder appears only when the right hemisphere is capable of subserving some residual language functions (Grossi et al., 1991; Nagaratnam &

Nagaratnam, 2000). There are two lines of evidence that support this contention. First, the occurrence of a second lesion in the right hemisphere can eliminate the ability to repeat (Rapcsak, Krupp, Rubens, & Reim, 1990). Second, injecting amobarbital into the right hemisphere of a mixed transcortical aphasic can also (temporarily) impair repetition (Berthier, Starkstein, Leiguarda, Ruiz, Mayberg, Wagner et al., 1991).

GLOBAL APHASIA. The most severe of the aphasias, **global aphasia** involves a global impairment of language comprehension and production. Speech is meaningless and nonfluent (halting, laborious), comprehension is impaired, and repetition is not spared (unlike mixed transcortical aphasia). As is the case with Broca's aphasia, hemiparesis often accompanies the language deficits. The lesions that usually give rise to this condition are extensive, including Broca's area, Wernicke's area, and many of the cortical and subcortical structures in between. Lesions this widespread are often caused by damage to the middle cerebral artery. However, the lesions that give rise to global aphasia need not involve Wernicke's area or Broca's area. Even completely subcortical lesions can produce the disorder (Vignolo, Boccardi, & Caverni, 1986). Therefore, it appears as though the behavioral syndrome can result from different lesions, suggesting that there may be a number of subtypes.

ANOMIC APHASIA. Anomia is an impairment in word finding (the impairment is not restricted to naming). Anomia occurs in a number of language syndromes (some of which were already discussed) and in other neurological disorders, such as Alzheimer's disease (Chenery, Murdoch, & Ingram, 1996), or following head trauma (Cappa & Vignolo, 1999). However, anomia can also occur in isolation from other disorders, referred to as **anomic aphasia** (or *pure anomia*). Therefore, an individual with anomic aphasia will produce meaningful, fluent speech with preserved repetition but impaired word finding.

Consider the following example of a conversation between Richard MacArthur and Howard Gardner. The linguistic deficit exhibited by Mr. MacArthur is relatively subtle, and if the conversation were restricted entirely to small talk, one might not even notice it. When asked about his work, Mr. MacArthur replied:

MacArthur: "Well, let me tell you, Dr. Gardner. It's like this. I've been a supervisor for the Telephone Company up in Lawrence for all these years. About twenty years in fact. I was in charge of twenty-five men, the finest group of men you'll ever want to meet, I can assure you."
Gardner: "What specifically did you do, Mr. MacArthur?"
MacArthur: "Oh, specifically, why sure. Well, I would come in every morning about eight o'clock, check in, you know they have those big new time-clocks, and then I'd make the rounds checking up on all the fellows, like the electric lathes, and all that. Is that what you mean?"
Gardner: "But doesn't it have a specific name?"
MacArthur: "Why, of course it does. I just can't think of it. Let me look in my notebook." (Gardner, 1974, pp. 75–76)

Mr. MacArthur was a foreman in a factory, and the word *foreman* was very familiar to him at one time. However, when asked to come up with the name for his job, he could not, despite his ability to provide many other details about his work. Maintaining a conversation with someone with anomia can be quite trying; the person might talk in circles around what he or she is really trying to say (called **circumlocutions**), seemingly trying to trigger their memory for the word by talking about related matters. In this example, Mr. MacArthur mostly uses complete sentences in his attempts to find the word *foreman,* and he seems to demonstrate some difficulty focusing on the question at hand. In contrast, consider the following example of anomia in an individual who also demonstrated agrammatism. When the person was shown a picture of a girl giving flowers to her teacher and asked to describe the picture, this was the reply:

> "Girl . . . wants to . . . flowers . . . flowers and wants to . . . The woman . . . wants to . . . The girl wants to . . . the flowers and the woman." (Saffran, Schwartz, & Marin, 1980, p. 234)

Here, the fact that the girl is *giving* the flowers to the woman (her teacher) is missing from the answer, but the respondent focuses much more directly on the irretrievable word rather than talking in circles around it.

Anomic aphasia results from lesions to a variety of locations. If the lesion involves Wernicke's area, the resultant anomia can still be fluent. However, if the lesion includes Broca's area or more posterior areas, fluency is impaired, and agrammatism may occur (Foundas, Daniels, & Vasterling, 1998; Raymer, Foundas, Maher, Greenwald, Morris, Rothi, et al., 1997).

PURE WORD DEAFNESS. **Pure word deafness** is the inability to understand spoken language despite preserved speech, reading, and writing. These individuals can also correctly perceive other noises (i.e., a baby crying, an engine starting, etc.), including music. The disorder is extremely rare; according to Vignolo (1996), there are only six pure cases in the literature. Unlike cases of Wernicke's aphasia, individuals with pure word deafness are quite aware of their deficit, indicating that speech is incomprehensible and sounds as if it is a foreign language. Individuals might also complain that others are speaking too quietly or quickly. Speaking more slowly can aid comprehension, but speaking more loudly is not helpful (Vignolo, 1996). In most cases, the disorder appears to be caused by bilateral lesions to the posterior superior temporal lobe, close to (or including) its border with the parietal lobe (di Giovanni, D'Alessandro, Baldini, Cantalupi, & Bottacchi, 1992; Otsuki, Soma, Sato, Homma, & Tsuji, 1998; Vignolo, 1996).

AUDITORY SOUND AGNOSIA. **Auditory sound agnosia** resembles pure word deafness, but instead of impairments in the perception of words and preserved perception of other sounds, auditory sound agnosics display relatively little trouble perceiving words but have great difficulty in identifying environmental sounds. For example, the sound of a moving automobile might be mistaken for that of a train or applause, or the jingling of a bunch of keys might be mistaken for a doorbell (Vignolo, 1996). Most cases of auditory sound agnosia appear to have apperceptive rather than associative causes. Remember that apperceptive disorders result from perceptual problems, whereas associative disorders result from problems associating perceptions with meaning. Most

Table 8.2

Summary of Common Auditory and Language Disorders

Name of Disorder	Articulation	Comprehension	Repetition	Naming
Broca's aphasia	Poor	Good	Poor	Poor
Wernicke's aphasia	Good	Poor	Poor	Poor
Conduction aphasia	Good	Good	Poor	Poor
Transcortical motor aphasia	Poor	Good	Good	Poor
Transcortical sensory aphasia	Good	Poor	Good	Poor
Global aphasia	Poor	Poor	Poor	Poor
Pure Word Deafness	Good	Poor	Poor	Good
Auditory Sound Agnosia	Good	Good	Good	Poor

cases of auditory sound agnosia seem to be characterized by individuals confusing two perceptually similar sounds (both structurally and acoustically) rather than difficulty in associating sounds with meaning. Importantly, these individuals are relatively unimpaired at associating linguistic sounds with meaning (Vignolo, 1996).

Table 8.2 summarizes the aphasia disorders we have discussed.

Subtypes of Acquired Alexia

Acquired alexias are reading disorders that appear as a result of brain damage in people who previously demonstrated normal reading abilities. Just as the terms *aphasia* and *dysphasia* describe two severities of the same problem (a relative absence of language), **alexia** and **dyslexia** describe a lack of reading ability. This disorder is rarely pure, as often some reading ability is retained (making *dyslexia* the more appropriate term), but just as we used the term *aphasia* to be consistent with other writings on this topic, we will use the term *alexia* here. This also helps to avoid confusion between the acquired disorders that we discuss below and developmental reading problems that are referred to as *dyslexia*.

Alexia is a relatively recent problem. As one would expect, reading disorders became commonplace only after literacy became more widespread, starting in the twentieth century. Déjerine described the first two cases in 1891 and 1892 (Déjerine, 1891, 1892). Since then, alexia has been observed in many cultures, including Asian languages that use pictographic characters (Benson, 1984; Sakurai, Ichikawa, & Mannen, 2001). Many variants have been described, including one case in which the ability to read Chinese was retained but the ability to read Japanese was lost (Odani, 1935). At least eleven variants have been described (Benson, 1996; Lecours, 1999), but we will focus on a subset of these, interpreted in terms of dual-route models of reading.

There are three main linguistic types of alexia. The first is **phonological alexia** (sometimes called *letter alexia*), in which the reader is unable to attribute the correct sound (phoneme) to the graphemes in the written material. These individuals cannot sound out unfamiliar words, although they can recognize common words. For example, if a person with phonological alexia is asked to read a common word, such as *dog,* the person produces the appropriate response. When presented with an irregular (but familiar) word, such as *colonel,* the person can also produce the correct response. However, if asked to read a nonword, such as *glumpit,* the phonological alexic is unable to do so. Phonological alexics also make errors in the form of **visual paralexias:** They often substitute two similar looking words, such as *leaf* and *lead*.

This impairment is easily explained with the dual-route model of reading described in the previous module (see Figure 8.12). If an individual suffers damage to the phonological route, the intact, whole-word route can still subserve the reading of both regular and irregular words. Using nonwords to help diagnose the condition is particularly convenient because the examiner is virtually guaranteed that the individual will not have whole-word memories for them. The syndrome typically follows damage to the posterior inferior temporal lobe (Rapcsak, Gonzalez-Rothi, & Heilman, 1987; Sasanuma, Ito, Patterson, & Ito, 1996).

A second form of alexia is called **surface alexia;** it is characterized by an impairment in reading irregular words (e.g., *yacht, colonel*) but spared reading of regular words or even nonwords. Dual-route models of reading also easily characterize this impairment. If an individual suffers damage to the whole-word processing route, the intact phonological route can successfully process regular words and unfamiliar words, but it cannot produce the correct pronunciation of irregular words (see Figure 8.12). Relying exclusively on the phonological processing route causes surface alexics to confuse the meanings of written words that sound the same as other words with different meanings (called **homophones**). If asked what *peat* is, they might say it is a male name (i.e., Pete).

A third form of alexia, called **deep alexia,** shares many of the symptoms of phonological alexia. Reading regular and irregular words is relatively unimpaired, but reading nonwords is profoundly impaired. One symptom that differentiates the condition from phonological alexia is the substitution of words with semantically similar ones during reading. These substitutions are called **semantic paralexias.** As an example, in the phrase *the infant was crying,* a deep alexic might substitute the word *baby* for *infant*. Another symptom of deep alexia is the relative inability to read words that are not highly imageable. This includes words that describe abstract concepts (such as *justice*), but also includes very common function words, such as *on, it,* and *the*.

It is difficult to explain deep alexia in terms of dual-route models. Some have argued that it is a more severe version of phonological alexia, whereas others claim that it is the result of lesions in two locations: one along the phonological route and one disconnecting (or partially disconnecting) the whole-word route from the semantic center.

Alexia without Agraphia

Losing the ability to read is normally accompanied by a similar loss in the ability to write, a condition called **agraphia.** This disorder requires a definition of exclusion because there are many reasons why one might lose the ability to write (such as damaging one's writing hand or going blind). However, to be considered agraphia, the loss of ability to write must *not* be attributable to basic sensory or motor problems or a more generalized intellectual impairment. Both alexia and agraphia normally follow lesions to the angular gyrus at the posterior superior temporal and inferior parietal junction (Bradshaw & Mattingley, 1995). Counterintuitively, agraphia can occur in the absence of alexia and vice versa (Grossi, Fragassi, Orsini, DeFalco, & Sepe, 1984). Consider the following example:

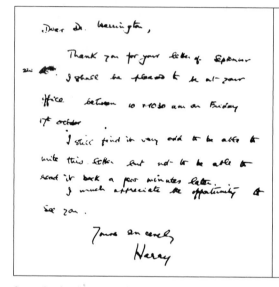

Dear Dr. Warrington,

Thank you for your letter of September the 16th. I shall be pleased to be at your office between 10 & 10:30 am on Friday 17th october.

I still find it very odd to be able to write this letter but not be able to read it back a few minutes later.

I much appreciate the opportunity to see you.

Yours sincerely,

Harry

Source: Reprinted from *Cognitive Neuropsychology,* R. A. McCarthy and E. K. Warrington, p. 261, Copyright 1990, with permission from Elsevier.

When individuals first experience alexia without agraphia, they often first complain of visual problems, attributing the reading problem to a visual disturbance (Kattouf, 1996). The underlying problem in alexia without agraphia seems to be a disconnection between visual perception and memory for orthographic representations of words. If words are spelled out loud or traced into their palm, affected individuals can often identify the words, indicating that their memories of the orthography of the words are intact (Bradshaw & Mattingley, 1995).

Agraphia without Alexia

Just as individuals can lose their ability to read while retaining their ability to write, the converse dissociation also occurs: the loss of ability to write despite retaining their ability to read. Exner first described this condition in 1881.

Subtypes of Acquired Agraphia

There are numerous classification schemes for the various forms of agraphia, and descriptions of almost thirty subtypes are reviewed by Hinkin and Cummings (1996).

We will review three linguistic categories of agraphia—the same three categories that we applied to alexia in the previous section: phonological, surface, and deep.

Phonological agraphia is the inability to write a word on the basis of "sounding it out," despite the ability to write both regular and irregular words. Therefore, the condition can be diagnosed by asking an individual to write nonwords. This disorder can be explained by using a dual-route model of writing in which the individual suffers damage along the phonological route, but the intact whole-word route is able to subserve the writing of words with preformed orthographic memories.

Surface agraphia is the inability to write irregular words (e.g., *yacht* or *colonel*) despite the ability to write regular words and nonwords by "sounding them out." This condition can also be interpreted using a dual-route model of reading. If the whole-word route is damaged (see Figure 8.13), the intact phonological route can subserve the writing of words or nonwords that follow phoneme–grapheme correspondence rules. As soon as these rules are broken, spelling errors occur. These errors tend to be phonetically correct representations of the irregular words. For example, *yacht* might be written as *yot*, whereas *colonel* could be written as *kernol*.

Deep agraphia is similar to phonological agraphia in that individuals cannot write words on the basis of phoneme–grapheme correspondence rules. However, it also involves **semantic paragraphias:** semantically related substitutions in writing. This condition can occur in the absence of such substitutions in reading. For example, when asked to read a sentence about a rose, an individual might read the word *rose* correctly. However, when asked to write out the sentence, the person might substitute the word *tulip* for *rose* (Hillis, Rapp, & Caramazza, 1999). As is the case with deep alexia, deep agraphia is a little more difficult to explain by using dual-route models of reading. It probably involves damage along the phonological route but might also involve lesions disconnecting (or partially disconnecting) the whole-word route from the semantic center (see Figure 8.13).

Aprosodias

Aprosodia is the loss of ability to produce or comprehend prosody in speech (changes in the intonation of speech), which usually follows right hemisphere damage. Some have proposed that its functional and anatomical organization mirrors that of speech in the left hemisphere (Gorelick & Ross, 1987; Ross, 1993). Anterior lesions tend to impair the production of prosody, generally termed **motor aprosodia,** which is analogous to Broca's aphasia. Posterior lesions selectively impair the comprehension of prosody, called **sensory aprosodia,** which is analogous to Wernicke's aphasia. In **conduction aprosodia,** both spontaneous production and comprehension are intact, but repetition is impaired (Gorelick & Ross, 1987). There are even reports of transcortical aprosodias that are analogous to the transcortical aphasias. For example, in **transcortical-motor aprosodia,** prosodic comprehension and repetition are intact, but spontaneous production is impaired (Stringer & Hodnett, 1991). In **transcortical-sensory aprosodia,** spontaneous production and repetition are intact, but comprehension is impaired (Gorelick & Ross, 1987; Ross, 1993).

Controversy

Current

How Is American Sign Language Represented in the Brain?

As we have seen, there are major differences between the production and comprehension of spoken language versus that of written language. However, studying the neural representation of American Sign Language (ASL) in native signers (i.e., individuals who essentially learned ASL as their first language) or congenitally deaf signers (individuals who have been deaf since birth) offers a unique chance to study language acquisition. If there are neural modules that are specialized for subserving language functions, regardless of the modality of the language, then ASL should not be represented differently from spoken language.

Both clinical and nonclinical evidence appears to confirm that prediction. The production of ASL appears to be dominated by the left frontal lobe. Functional neuroimaging studies find left frontal activation during the generation or imagined generation of ASL (Bavelier, Corina, Jezzard, Clark, Karni, Lalwani, et al., 1998; Neville & Mills, 1997). Injecting sodium amytal into the left hemisphere produces ASL motor aphasia (Damasio, Bellugi, Damasio, Poizner, & van Gelder, 1986), as does left frontal damage (Bradshaw, 1996; Kegl & Poizner, 1997; Poizner, Klima, & Bellugi, 1987). Right hemisphere damage appears to have minimal effects on ASL production or comprehension (Damasio et al., 1986). Examination of ASL comprehension yields similar results: The comprehension of ASL appears to be dominated by left temporal structures, as is indicated by both functional imaging (Bavelier et al., 1998) and studies of individuals with brain damage. After suffering posterior left hemisphere damage, one ASL signer exhibited symptoms that resembled Wernicke's aphasia, producing signs that were mostly properly executed (i.e., fluent), but the sequence of the signs was virtually meaningless (Poizner et al., 1987). Therefore, the neural representation of ASL appears to mirror that of spoken language.

These results alone are not terribly controversial. It is generally agreed that ASL and spoken language have similar neural representations. However, the interpretation of this evidence is extremely controversial. Some claim that the ability to acquire language evolved and is genetically determined, on the basis of evidence that humans are normally born with the cognitive/neural architecture necessary for language acquisition already in place. The exact nature of the language—whether verbal or visual—is irrelevant. Others claim that language acquisition is not determined by genetics and that it is simply a product of learning. The cases of Williams syndrome versus specific language impairment section are also relevant to this debate.

Self-Test

1. What is a semantic paraphasia?
2. What is the difference between transcortical-motor aphasia and transcortical-sensory aphasia?
3. Does conduction aphasia arise from cortical or subcortical lesions?
4. What are the symptoms of surface agraphia?
5. What is conduction aprosodia?
6. What are visual paralexias? When do they occur?
7. What is the difference between alexia and dyslexia?
8. Is it sometimes possible to write if you lose your ability to read?

◀ **WHERE WE HAVE BEEN**

This module described the various ways in which language and auditory processing can be altered following brain injuries or developmental disorders. These disorders have been very informative regarding the functional neuroanatomy of language.

Neuropsychological Celebrity

Crystal

After spending most of this module detailing the myriad of ways in which language can break down, we would like to end the chapter on language with a description of preservation of language function. Williams syndrome is a very rare (approximately 1 in 25,000) genetic disorder caused by the absence of some genetic material: there is a deletion of part of chromosome 7 (Ewart, Morris, Atkinson, Jin, Sternes, Spallone et al., 1993). Similar to Down syndrome, this genetic abnormality results in a characteristic appearance, usually described as "pixielike" or "elfin faced." Steven Pinker thinks they look more like Mick Jagger (Pinker, 1994).

Mental retardation caused by a genetic abnormality (or any other cause, for that matter) usually results in language deficits (Rondal, 1980). This is not the case in Williams syndrome—far from it. Despite I.Q.s in the forties or fifties and profound impairments on tasks such as way finding, and shoe tying, children with Williams syndrome display an impressive command of language. Coupled with their typ-ically gentle, courteous, and friendly manner, one might not detect the depth of their impairment through casual conversation. This dissociation between language and other abilities is one of the most remarkable features of the syndrome.

Compare the verbal and pictorial description (Figure 8.13) of an elephant provided by Crystal, an 18-year-old with Williams syndrome (Pinker, 1994, pp. 52–53).

There is a condition that virtually mirrors that of Williams syndrome and has the rather unspecific name of **specific language impairment (SLI).** Children with SLI exhibit severe deficits in the production and/or comprehension of language, and these deficits cannot be attributable to sensory problems (e.g., hearing loss), motor problems, or a more general intellectual impairment. The language deficits can include problems in articulation and almost always include impaired syntax. Because SLI also appears to have a genetic component (van der Lely & Stollwerk, 1996), many interpret the presence of both disorders as evidence that the neural architecture normally subserving language functions is genetically determined (Pinker, 1994). Others argue that Williams syndrome and SLI are not clear opposites (van der Lely & Stollwerk, 1996).

A Verbal Description and Diagram of an Elephant Provided by an 18-Year-Old with Williams Syndrome

Figure 8.13

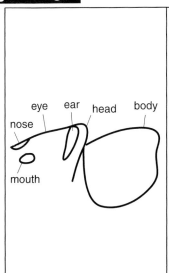

And what an elephant is, it is one of the animals. And what the elephant does, it lives in the jungle. It can also live in the zoo. And what it has, it has long gray ears, fan ears, ears that can blow in the wind. It has a long trunk that can pick up grass, or pick up hay. . . . If the elephant gets mad it could stomp; it could charge. Sometimes elephants can charge. They have big long tusks. They can damage a car. . . . It could be dangerous. When they're in a pinch, when they're in a bad mood it can be terrible. You don't want an elephant as a pet. You want a cat or a dog or a bird. . . .

Source: Copyright Ursula Bellugi, The Salk Institute for Biological Studies, La Jolla, California.

Glossary

Acquired alexias—Reading disorders that appear as a result of brain damage in people who have previously demonstrated normal reading abilities.

Agrammatism—The inability to produce grammatically correct sentences.

Agraphia—Loss in the ability to write.

Alexia—Describes a lack of reading ability; typically, the term *alexia* describes an acquired inability to read rather than a developmental problem.

Alveolar stops—Phonemes that are produced by constricting airflow against the alveolar ridge located behind your front teeth.

Amplitude—The size of the waveform; in sound, this corresponds to the loudness of the sound and measurement is usually indicated in decibels (dB).

Angular gyrus—Located at the junction between the temporal, parietal, and occipital lobes; receives projections from primary and secondary visual areas; subserves knowledge of visual language.

Anomia—Literally means "no name"; the inability to find the correct word (usually nouns and verbs).

Anomic aphasia (or pure anomia)—An impairment in word finding that occurs in isolation from other disorders; individuals may express circumlocutions (talking in circles) and are able to perceive environmental sounds.

Apex—Near this point, the basilar membrane is more flexible, and the receptors located here are exposed to vibrations of lower frequencies.

Aphasia—Literally means "a lack of language" or "no language"; a deficit this severe is extremely rare.

Aprosodia—The loss of ability to produce or comprehend prosody in speech that usually follows right hemisphere damage.

Arcuate fasciculus—A band of subcortical white matter located between Broca's area and Wernicke's area that connects Wernicke's area with Broca's area. Allows for the production of meaningful verbal output.

Auditory meatus—The hole in the ear.

Auditory sound agnosia—Individuals with this disorder display relatively little trouble in perceiving words but have great difficulty in identifying environmental sounds.

Basilar membrane—Bends in response to vibrations of the cochlear fluid; serves to elicit neural activity in the hair cells. The hair cells and their cilia are located along this structure.

Broca's aphasia—A behavioral syndrome that results from damage to Broca's area; typically Broca's aphasia is characterized by the inability to produce fluent speech, despite relatively intact speech comprehension and production mechanisms.

Broca's area—The third gyrus of the left frontal lobe.

Circumlocutions—Talking in circles around what one had intended to say.

Cochlea—Contains the components of the inner ear, including the inner and outer hair cells.

Cochlear fluid—The membrane covering the oval window transmits vibrations into the cochlea through this fluid; vibrations of this fluid cause a bending of the basilar membrane and the tectorial membrane.

Cochlear nuclei—Axons of the cochlear nerve synapse on the ipsilateral side of these.

Complexity—The number of different wave frequencies contained in a sound; in sound, this corresponds to timbre.

Concept center—An additional component of the alternative model of language proposed by Lichtheim; in essence, the concept center is involved in ascribing meaning to the sounds of language.

Conduction aprosodia—Both spontaneous production and comprehension of prosody are intact, but repetition is impaired.

Deep agraphia—Similar to phonological agraphia in that individuals cannot write words based on phoneme–grapheme correspondence rules; also involves semantic paragraphias, or substitutions that are semantically related.

Deep alexia—Reading regular words and irregular words is relatively unimpaired, but reading nonwords is profoundly impaired; shares many symptoms with phonological alexia.

Dual-route models—Models of visual language that rely on two networks to comprehend the phonemic and whole-word components of written language separately from each other; the two routes are usually named the *phonological route* and the *whole-word route.*

Dyslexia—Describes a lack of reading ability; typically, dyslexia describes a developmental problem with reading rather than an acquired deficit.

Dysphasia—A partial loss of language.

Echolalia—A compulsion to repeat whatever someone else has just said.

Eighth cranial nerve—A branch of this nerve is formed by axons from the cochlear nerve. Also called the vestibulocochlear nerve.

External ear canal—Part of the ear that amplifies the vibrations and channels.

Fourier analysis—A mathematical process in which complicated sounds are broken down into simple component waves.

Frequency—The number of wave cycles completed per unit of time; in sound, this corresponds to pitch and measurement is usually indicated in hertz (Hz), or cycles per second.

Fundamental frequency—The intended frequency of an instrument.

Global aphasia—Aphasia that is often a result of middle cerebral artery infarct, which results in widespread damage to the temporal and frontal lobes; speech is meaningless, halting, and laborious; comprehension is impaired, and repetition is *not* spared; hemiparesis often accompanies the language deficits.

Graphemes—The smallest units of written language; in English, graphemes are letters.

Hair cells—The receptor cells of the auditory system; they connect with the auditory nerve.

Homophones—Written words that sound the same as other words with different meanings (e.g., bark of a dog versus that of a tree).

Incus—Literally means "anvil." One of the three bones in the ear.

Inferior colliculus—Part of the midbrain that receives projections from the cochlear nuclei.

Inner ear—Part of the ear where mechanical energy is transduced into neural activity.

Labial stops—Phonemes that are produced by the complete constriction of air toward the front of the mouth.

Leitungsaphasia—The condition in which comprehension and production are intact, but repetition is impaired; results from damage to the arcuate fasciculus. German for *conduction aphasia.*

Loudness—Perception of the amplitude of the sound wave.

Malleus—Literally means "hammer." One of the three bones in the ear.

Medial geniculate nucleus of the thalamus—Receives projections from the olivary nuclei.

Middle ear—The chamber (and its contents) between the tympanic membrane and the oval window; sound waves are transduced here from variations in air pressure into mechanical energy propagated and amplified along the ossicles to the oval window.

Mixed transcortical aphasia—Aphasia that usually follows two lesions: one in the frontal lobe that spares much of Broca's area and one that damages temporal structures; sharing symptoms with both transcortical motor and transcortical sensory aphasia, speech is halting, laborious, and meaningless; repetition is intact, and echolalia is often present; auditory comprehension is impaired.

Motor aprosodia—The impairment in the comprehension of prosody resulting from anterior lesions of the right hemisphere; analogous to Broca's aphasia.

Organ of Corti—Collective name for the hair cells, the cilia, and the cells that support them.

Ossicles—The collective name for the malleus, incus, and stapes.

Outer ear—Comprises the pinna and external ear canal; this structure serves to catch and amplify sound waves.

Oval window—Vibration is transmitted through this structure.

Overtones—Frequencies that are higher than, but mathematically related to, the fundamental frequency.

Phoneme—A small, pronounceable, and meaningful unit of sound in a language.

Phoneme–grapheme conversion rules—The rules for converting written words into sounds.

Phonemic paraphasia—The substitution of similar sounds within a word; characteristic of Broca's aphasics.

Phonological agraphia—The inability to write a word based on its phonemes.

Phonological alexia—The inability to attribute the correct sound (phoneme) to the graphemes in the written material; this results in an inability to sound out unfamiliar words but a sparing of the recognition of common words. Also referred to as *letter alexia.*

Phonological route—Sounding out the words.

Pinna—The outmost and visible portion of the ear.

Pitch—Perception of frequencies of sounds; the higher the frequency, the higher the perceived pitch.

Place of articulation—The location in the mouth where phonemes are articulated.

Primary auditory cortex—Receives projections from the contralesional side of the infereior colliculi and projections from the medial geniculate nucleus of the thalamus. This area is also referred to as *Heschl's gyrus, Brodmann's area 41,* and *A-1.*

Prosody—The conveyance of meaning by varying the intonation in speech, including changes in pitch, tempo, intensity, and rhythm.

Pseudo-homophones—Letter strings that form sounds that sound like real words (e.g., *yot* instead of *yacht*).

Pure word deafness—The inability to understand spoken language, despite intact speech, reading, and writing.

Rate of vibration—Frequency.

Right hemiparesis—Paralysis of the right side.

Secondary auditory cortex—Areas immediately adjacent to the primary auditory cortex.

Semantic paragraphias—Semantically related substitutions in writing.

Semantic paralexias—Substitution of words with semantically similar ones during reading; these substitutions are characteristic of deep alexia but not phonological alexia.

Semantic paraphasia—Where individuals substitute words of similar meaning, such as substituting *leopard* for *tiger.*

Sensory aprosodia—The impairment in the comprehension of prosody resulting from posterior lesions of the right hemisphere; analogous to Wernicke's aphasia.

Single-route models—Models of visual language that rely on one distributed network to comprehend the phonemic and whole-word components of written language; there are multiple parallel processing streams within this network.

Sound images—Refers to how sounds correspond to words and other objects; the temporal lobe contains memories for these.

Specific language impairment (SLI)—A disorder marked by severe deficits in the production and/or comprehension of language; these deficits cannot be attributable to sensory problems, motor problems, or general intellectual impairment.

Spontaneous speech—According to the WLG model, this is produced by accessing the mappings of sounds to meanings in Wernicke's area and projecting this information via the arcuate fasciculus to Broca's area. Here the motor program is formulated and executed through the primary motor cortex.

Stapes—Literally means "stirrup." One of the three bones in the ear.

Superior olives—Receives projections from the cochlear nuclei.

Surface agraphia—The inability to write irregular words (e.g., *yacht* or *colonel*) despite the ability to write regular words and nonwords by phonological processing.

Surface alexia—Characterized by an impairment in the ability to read irregular words (e.g., *yacht, colonel*), but reading of irregular words or nonwords is spared.

Tectorial membrane—Bends in response to vibrations of the cochlear fluid; serves to elicit neural activity in the hair cells. This membrane runs parallel to the basilar membrane and is located directly adjacent to the hair cells.

Timbre—The perception of a sound's complexity, which differs from instrument to instrument. Timbre is how to describe how violins sound different from trumpets.

Tonotopic—A type of frequency-specific sensory organization; specifically, as the basilar membrane moves away from the apex, it becomes thinner and wider. This makes it more susceptible to vibrations at lower frequencies.

Transcortical-motor aphasia—Aphasia in which there is a disruption of the connections between the dorsolateral prefrontal cortex and the anterior portion of Broca's area. Similar to Broca's aphasia, spontaneous speech is halting and laborious, but comprehension is intact; however, unlike the case in Broca's aphasia, repetition is intact and echolalia is often present.

Transcortical-sensory aphasia—Aphasia that usually follows damage to the angular gyrus; speech is fluent but nonsensical and is often riddled with paraphasias and neologisms. Similar to Wernicke's aphasia, verbal comprehension is severely compromised; however, unlike the case in Wernicke's aphasia, repetition is intact, and echolalia is often present. Furthermore, oral naming of objects is sometimes preserved.

Transcortical-motor aprosodia—Prosodic comprehension and repetition are intact, but spontaneous production is impaired; analogous to transcortical aphasia.

Transcortical sensory aprosodia—A condition in which spontaneous production and repetition are intact but comprehension is impaired; analogous to transcortical aphasia.

Tympanic membrane—The eardrum.

Unvoiced consonants—Involves a delay between the release of air and the onset of vocal cord vibration; the *t*, *k*, and *p* in *tah*, *kah*, and *pah* are examples.

Velar stops—Phonemes that are produced by placing your tongue toward the back of your mouth.

Visual language—Language that relies on vision for communication; includes sign language and written text.

Visual paralexias—The substitution of two similar looking words, such as *leaf* and *lead*; phonological alexics make these types of errors.

Voiced consonants—Involve almost identical timing between the release of air and vocal cord vibration; the *b*, *d*, and *g* in *bah*, *dah*, and *gah* are all voiced consonants.

Wernicke-Lichtheim-Geschwind (WLG)—A model that accounts for oral, aural, and visual language processing.

Wernicke's aphasia (or *sensory aphasia*)—Characterized by fluent speech with the meaning of the speech severely compromised; word salad may also be present.

Wernicke's area—An area of the left temporal lobe, just posterior to the primary auditory cortex.

Whole-word route—Reading the word as a whole.

Word salad—The seemingly random collection of words that form speech from an individual with Wernicke's aphasia.

Emotion

*We know too much and feel too little. At least, we feel too little of those
creative emotions from which a good life springs.*
—BERTRAND RUSSELL

Star Trek (and the related series of *Star Trek* spin-offs) introduced us to Vulcans, a humanoid species who choose to live rationally and therefore must learn to ignore their illogical emotional side. The example of Vulcans provides us with the first important observation about emotion: that emotion is experienced privately, within the self, although the emotional state of an individual can be communicated to others. That is, humans have both the perception and experience of the emotional state in the self and the perception of the emotional state of others. However, humans also perceive that others cannot truly understand the nature or depth of a person's emotions, because they are subjective and personal.

To stretch the *Star Trek* analogy farther, the series contains a subtext that although the Vulcans and animate androids such as Data may have superior intellect, they are somehow deprived of the richness of life that is experienced by humans. The series also suggests that the Klingons, who are hyperemotional, tend to make foolish mistakes and can be goaded into making poor decisions by provoking their emotional nature (which makes humans similar to baby bear's porridge—"just right"). Contained within this subtext is the belief that higher cognitive function is the antithesis of emotionality. Is this the case? In the following module, we will discuss emotion: what it is, what emotion does for us as a species, how we perceive and experience emotions, and the roles of various neural structures in the expression and experience of emotion. Finally, we will come back to the question "Are decisions made without the presence of emotions better than those made in emotional states?" Are we more logical when we are not emotional?

WHERE WE ARE GOING ➤ In this chapter, we discuss emotions and disorders of emotion. The first module will begin with a definition of emotion and will examine how emotions are produced in neurologically normal individuals, including a definition of emotion and the neural substrates for the components of emotional states. The second module will explain the neuroanatomical and behavioral findings related to how the damaged brain understands and expresses emotions.

MODULE **9.1**
Emotion

When we describe our emotions to others, we tend to use words to do so. A quick look in the thesaurus suggests that there are numerous words that we use to describe emotional states. For instance, the word *happy* has more than fifty synonyms, including *joy, bliss, rapture, pleasure, contentment,* and *gladness.* Even the word *emotion* has a number of synonyms (e.g., *passion, desire, feelings*). However, when we examine the words, we see that the thesaurus, while correct, is describing only what most of us would call related emotions. That is, although joy is similar to happiness, it does not describe exactly the same emotion. Somehow words such as *bliss* seem to be more intense and happier than words such as *gladness*, revealing that emotions vary in intensity and in degree. Finally, it is my subjective experience that words such as *bliss* do not fully capture the emotional state that the word is attempting to describe because they cannot really describe the bodily sensations that accompany the cognitive state of bliss. So, then, what are emotions? What is their purpose? How does the brain produce emotions in ourselves and how does the brain perceive emotions in others?

Early views of emotions often localized emotions to various internal organs, such as the liver and heart (Finger, 1994). For instance, the Greek philosopher Plato suggested that the head was for reason, the liver was for desire, and the heart was for anger. Aristotle was of a similar opinion; he equated temperature changes of the heart with changes in emotional state. Aristotle also thought that the difference between passions and emotion explained the difference between humans and nonhuman animals. That is, Aristotle suggested that emotion occurred only when the intellect was engaged, whereas passions were more instinctive (Finger, 1994). As we will see, emotions are the product of the brain, and emotional states are the product of both conscious and unconscious processing.

What Is Emotion?

A DEFINITION OF EMOTION. Defining emotion is surprisingly difficult and complicated, when one considers that most of us intuitively know what emotions are. However, emotions are private events, and so our emotions must either be described to others or inferred by others, usually from observations of overt behaviors. When we are angry, we have the physical sensation of our heart pounding, a dry mouth, and an increase in blood pressure, and we have the feeling of anger. Therefore, **emotional states** have two components: the physical sensation of the **emotion** and the cognitive experience, or **feeling,** of the emotion itself. To perceive emotional states, humans have become adept at monitoring physiological change in their bodies and in the bodies of others. Changes in heart rate and blood pressure are frequently associated with specific emotions. Humans also self-monitor subjective cognitive states, which is why emotions that may result in increases in heart rate, such as anxiety and happiness, are rarely mistaken for each other.

Emotional states are the combination of the physical sensations of emotion and the cognitive experience of emotion (Figure 9.1). As you will see in subsequent sections, neurologically normal individuals process the cognitive and physical aspects of emotional states in distinct neural circuits. However, these circuits work in concert to produce the unified percept of an emotion.

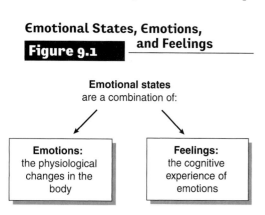

Figure 9.1 Emotional States, Emotions, and Feelings

Emotional states
are a combination of:

Emotions:
the physiological changes in the body

Feelings:
the cognitive experience of emotions

Emotional states produce behaviors, both internal and external. Emotional states produce internal changes associated with the autonomic nervous system, such as increases or decreases in heart rate, blood pressure, stomach motility (e.g., "butterflies"), and perspiration. Emotional states also produce external motor responses, including verbal statements (e.g., "I am absolutely furious"), facial expressions (e.g., smiling), and thoughts related to the experience (e.g., "Wow! That was fun!"). Finally, emotional states in others can provoke emotional states in ourselves (Wild, Erb, & Bartels, 2001), as we often react emotionally and experience feelings in response to emotional states in others.

BASIC EMOTIONAL STATES. One of the first individuals to recognize the significance of basic emotional states in humans was Charles Darwin (1872) in his book *The Expression of the Emotions in Man and Animals*. Darwin suggested that the emotional states occur innately in children and thus are not learned. He came to these conclusions on the basis of observations of his own children and those made by colleagues in other countries. Darwin suggested that there are universal emotional states that all humans express, primarily through invariant facial expressions. He theorized that these facial expressions evolved from similar expressions in nonhuman animals and served some adaptive purpose. Although Darwin's work influenced much in the scientific study of emotional states, there are two limitations to Darwin's theory: Darwin did not perform cross-cultural observations but instead relied on anecdotal reports, and he did not suggest that the emotional state was localized within the brain.

One of the first systematic cross-cultural studies of facial expressions was performed by studying the emotional expressions of the Fore tribe in a remote part of New Guinea (Ekman & Friesen, 1971). It is important to note that the members of the Fore tribe had never been exposed to Western culture, including such technology as videotape or photographs. Ekman and Friesen presented the Fore with photographs of European individuals making faces that were characteristic of specific emotional states. The Fore were asked to match the faces to stories that illustrated particular emotional states and to guess how the people in the photographs felt. Ekman and Friesen reasoned that if emotional displays are culturally mediated or learned, then among divergent groups of people, there should be significant variance in emotional facial displays and in the interpretation of these displays. However, they found that Fore participants were quite accurate in both matching faces with stories and attributing emotional states to the expressions in the photographs. In addition, the Fore participants made facial expressions similar to those of Europeans in response to emotional stimuli.

These effects have been replicated in a variety of cultures, in children, in individuals with brain damage, and even in nonsighted individuals (Izard, 1992). Even babies as young as 4 months old appear to evaluate the emotional expressions of others (Montague & Walker-Andrews, 2001). Although there are slight differences among groups, as a whole, individuals make the same facial expressions to express the same feelings (e.g., smile = happiness). Therefore, it appears that there are universal basic emotions that occur in all humans, which presumably are mediated by similar areas of the brain (Izard, 1992; but see Russell, 1995, for a different view). This view of basic emotional states is still quite controversial, and even agreement on what emotions constitute basic emotional states is far from complete. For instance, although many researchers suggest that happiness, sadness, fear, anger, surprise, and disgust are basic emotions (e.g., Izard, 1992), others do not consider surprise to be an emotion, suggesting instead that it is a reflex (Ekman, Friesen, & Simons, 1985).

Ekman (1998) suggests that for an emotional state to be considered as basic it must exhibit the following seven elements:

1. Distinctive facial expression.
2. Distinctive physiological state.

3. Facial expressions and physiological states that occur together and are relatively difficult to separate.
4. Almost instantaneous onset of the facial expression and physiological state, which lasts for only a brief duration.
5. Distinctive eliciting stimuli.
6. Automatic appraisal of the eliciting stimuli, not a result of deliberate cognitive appraisal. Furthermore, this appraisal is not desired or deliberate, as it is automatic.
7. Similar expressions of emotional states in the related primates.

Using these elements can be problematic, because there are some presumably valid emotions that have no corresponding unique facial expression (e.g., jealousy, greed, or lust). In addition, there is a scientific problem with attributing emotional states to nonverbal individuals (e.g., babies, other primates). Because emotional states are subjective and personal, it is difficult to be sure what an individual is experiencing without a corresponding linguistic confirmation. Even Ekman suggests that there might be an additional eight basic emotional states—awe, contempt, embarrassment, excitement, guilt, interest, shame, and surprise—that do not meet his criteria (Ekman, 1998). Thus, we can see that trying to define basic emotional states is difficult at best and that there is little agreement among researchers as to which emotions are basic and which ones are learned.

THE ADAPTIVE VALUE OF EMOTIONAL STATES. To understand the adaptive value of emotional states, we need first to consider what their function is. So what is the function of emotional states? What problems do they solve?

On the surface, emotional states may appear to have little relevance to our current lives. For instance, whenever I watch television and a snake appears, my palms get clammy, my stomach feels upset, and my pulse races. Even hearing about other people's encounters with snakes makes me unhappy. Why do we have these emotional reactions to situations and stimuli that we have never encountered?

Certainly, some emotional reactions to specific stimuli are learned responses to situations that the individual has encountered. However, other phobias appear to be innate. Take for instance, my snake phobia. I live in a region of Canada with relatively few snakes, and the snakes that could inhabit my backyard are definitely nonpoisonous. Furthermore, I have no experience with real snakes; I have only observed them behind glass at zoos (not for long!) and have certainly never touched one. So how could I have learned this fear? It is possible that I could have learned from others with greater experience with snakes that I should be afraid of them? However, snake and spider fears are extremely common cross-culturally. Ohman and Mineka (2001) suggest that common phobias and fears are elicited by stimuli that are relevant to survival. That is, they theorize that we have evolved mechanisms to produce fear of specific dangerous stimuli that were important in our evolutionary history. Thus, although I may live in a relatively snake-free zone, humans evolved in situations in which a fear of snakes, and therefore the avoidance of snakes, was adaptive.

Similarly, other emotions may motivate us to perform certain behaviors that may also be adaptive. For instance, Gilbert (2001) suggests that social anxiety (e.g., fear of speaking in a group) is not the fear of being attacked or fear of danger; rather, it is the consequence of the desire to be liked by other members of the group. The desire to be liked by the group is adaptive in that it may result in status and access to resources. Recall that status and access to resources contribute positively to the reproductive success of an individual, both individually and for their offspring. Gilbert (2001) hypothesizes that social anxiety allows an individual to monitor how others in the group are reacting and to act to ensure conformation to group norms. Because humans are a social species, our success depends on our social skills and on correct interpretations of social situations.

Emotional states act as signals to ensure that behaviors occur (or do not occur) appropriately, especially in social situations. Even secondary emotions or emotions that do not have characteristic facial expressions, such as shame or pride, have significant adaptive value (Gaulin & McBurney, 2001). Shame and pride both have significant social functions and often relate to status or loss of status within the group. According to Gaulin and McBurney (2001), it makes no sense to differentiate between basic and secondary emotional states, because both are evolved mechanisms that exist to solve or avoid previously encountered problems.

As signals, some emotional states are more salient than others. For instance, it is much easier to detect anger than happiness (Hansen & Hansen, 1988). If you think about it, anger may have greater immediate impact on well-being than happiness, because anger may predict that someone is going to do you harm, thus signaling the need for a quick reaction. Hansen and Hansen (1988) suggest that detecting emotional states in others and the self serves a predictive function, as emotional states help the organism to avoid negative situations and ensure that organisms take advantage of positive situations. An interesting study by Wild and colleagues (2001) observed that individuals who examine emotional faces tend to experience similar emotional states, and they tend to mimic the face that they are observing. These results are consistent with the view that emotional faces act as signals to the observer and that subsequent evoked emotional states act as a signal to the individual regarding future actions.

Finally, have you ever observed a happy dog or smiling cat? What about a bird, snake, or a spider? Which of the dogs in Figure 9.2 would you approach to pet? Why? Why do similar facial expressions accompany specific emotional states (e.g., smiling = happiness) in nonhuman animals? Darwin hypothesized that the constancy of facial expressions in nonhuman animals also served some adaptive purpose. As such, regardless of the species, facial expressions themselves serve as predictive signals. We are willing to attribute emotional states to other mammals because we evolved from a common ancestor and therefore most likely share many neural systems for the expression of emotional states. Thus, distinct facial expressions are adaptations to communicate emotional states to others to facilitate a solution to the problem that caused the initial emotional state (Gaulin & McBurney, 2001). Interestingly, Gaulin and McBurney (2001) suggest that some emotional states do not have characteristic facial expressions associated with them because some emotional states are better kept private (e.g., lust).

Figure 9.2 | **Which of These Dogs Looks Friendly?**

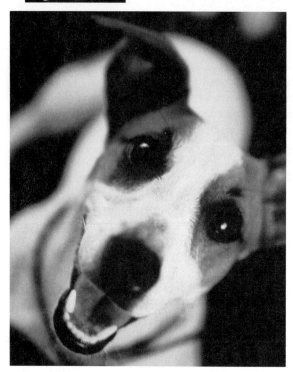 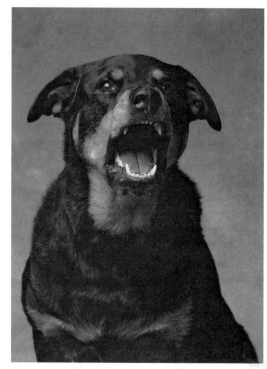

Source: © M. Meyer/Zefa/Corbis (left); GK Hart/Vikki Hart/Getty Images (right). Used with permission.

◀ **WHERE WE HAVE BEEN**

Emotional states are the combination of the physiological sensations and cognitive experiences of emotions. Although much of an emotional state is internal and subjective, emotional states produce externally observable events, including characteristic behaviors, such as facial expressions that do not vary cross-culturally. These expressions act as signals to others. As a species, we are very sensitive to the signals that others produce because this helps us to predict and react to events as they occur in our environment.

WHERE WE ARE GOING ▶

The following sections describe theories of how emotional states occur. The functional neuroanatomy of emotions and feelings in neurologically normal individuals will also be discussed. The second module will explain disorders of emotions and feelings that occur as a consequence of brain damage or brain dysfunction.

Theories of Emotional States

In some sense, the problem of understanding emotional states can be reduced to understanding how external stimuli produce emotional states. Contained within this question is an understanding of the relative contributions of the cognitive and phys-

Controversy

Current

Lie Detection: Do Autonomic Responses Give You Away When You Are Lying?

The story of Pinocchio is about a puppet whose nose grows whenever he tells a lie, making it obvious to others that he is not being truthful. Humans are slightly more accomplished at lying, which is why there are tests designed to detect lying. The best-known lie detection test, commonly referred to as a *polygraph test,* is designed to measure basic changes in physiological responses that occur when an individual is answering a series of questions. The polygraph test is often used in police investigations; it is also increasingly being used for job screening and the monitoring of employees within the government. For instance, the Department of Energy routinely investigates its employees this way.

In a procedure known as the control question test (CQT), changes in perspiration, respiration, blood pressure, and heart rate are recorded. Most polygraph examinations rely on the CQT technique, in which individuals are asked a series of control questions that the examiner knows to be true (e.g., name, date of birth) and a series of relevant questions that the examinee may lie about (e.g., "Do you know who killed John Doe?"). The questions are formulated to elicit either yes or no responses. Both the control questions and the relevant questions are expected to evoke emotional responses, although the relevant questions are anticipated to evoke emotional responses only when an individual is lying. The theory behind the polygraph test is that lying is a recognizable emotion that is accompanied by a stereotypic autonomic response. Which of the following questions would evoke a greater emotional response in you? "Is there anything in your background that you don't want the examiner to find out about?," which is a standard control question, or questions about your apparently suspicious behavior in a murder investigation. If the physiological changes that occur in the control questions are greater than those that occur in the relevant questions, then the exam-

iner assumes truthfulness on the part of the individual. If the physiological changes that occur in response to the relevant questions are greater or equal to those that occur in response to the control questions, then the examiner assumes either that the individual is lying or that the test is inconclusive. Thus, the accuracy of the polygraph test rests on assumptions about the autonomic responses that accompany fear, anxiety, and nervousness. Although fear, anxiety, and nervousness are likely to accompany interrogation, the presumption is that these emotional states can be accurately distinguished from lying.

Are the changes in the autonomic nervous system that accompany lying discriminable from those that are associated with negative emotional states? Although many people suggest that there are distinct physiological responses that are associated with specific emotional states, many individuals do not believe that a polygraph test can distinguish lies from the truth. One common criticism of polygraph tests is that they are based on deceptive practices and are conducted in highly emotional situations, such as a job interview or a police interrogation. Additionally, the literature on emotional states provides no evidence to suggest that lying produces consistent and reliable changes in breathing, perspiration, or blood pressure that are distinct from those that accompany other negative emotions such as fear.

Critics of the polygraph technique suggest that there are several easily learned tricks that can be employed to appear truthful when lying during a polygraph test. For instance, deliberately keeping your breathing shallow when asked the relevant questions and breathing more deeply or holding your breath when asked control questions can be an effective way to beat the polygraph. If you are tempted to try this, you must remember to keep your breathing at an even rate until you are disconnected from the polygraph (often, individuals stop monitoring their breathing when they think they are done but are still connected to the polygraph). Sudden changes in breathing rates are always thought to indicate lying, whenever they occur.

---

iological aspects of emotional states. That is, are the physical sensations that accompany emotional states responsible for the cognitive or affective experiences of emotional states, or is the converse true? Any attempt to understand emotional states must be able to account for the means by which external stimuli acquire the ability to induce emotional states and how emotions and feelings interact to produce an emotional state. From our perspective in neuropsychology, a valid theory should be able to describe the neural substrates of the cognitive, affective, and physiological components of the emotional state as well as describing how these areas of the brain interact to produce the emotional state.

There are a number of theories of how emotional states are produced, and although they all share a number of features, no one theory emphasizes the same relationships between emotions and feelings. Emotional states encompass many different behaviors and cognitions. A person who receives bad news ("Your daughter is dead") may respond by producing a verbal response ("Oh, no!"), an expressive behavior (crying), a physical response (striking the individual who brings the news), a physiological response mediated by the autonomic nervous system (trembling), or a combination of any or all these behaviors. It is therefore difficult for one theory to encompass all aspects of emotional states.

This section will describe the following prominent theories of emotional states: James–Lange theory, Cannon–Bard theory; Schachter–Singer theory, the somatic marker theory proposed by Damasio, and the appraisal theory proposed by Arnold. As you read the following theories, keep in mind the similarities among the theories as well as the differences. Although each of these theories is different, it is important to recognize that each of them has its strengths, in that it is able to describe or explain a particular facet of emotional states.

JAMES–LANGE THEORY. Working separately, the American psychologist William James and the Danish psychologist Carl Lange developed one of the first well-defined theories of emotional states. This theory, known as the **James–Lange theory,** suggests that the cognitive aspects of emotional states are secondary to the physiological response. Specifically, the James–Lange theory suggests that emotionally provocative stimuli automatically and unconsciously evoke physiological responses. The individual monitors the physiological changes associated with the emotional state, which then evoke specific conscious thoughts that are consistent with the experience (Figure 9.3). Thus, conscious experiences of emotional states are driven by unconscious physiological re-

Schematic Diagram of the James–Lange Theory of Emotions

Figure 9.3

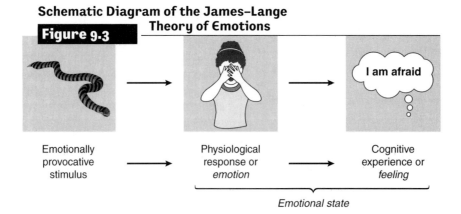

Emotionally provocative stimulus → Physiological response or *emotion* → Cognitive experience or *feeling*

I am afraid

Emotional state

sponses. For example, when we see a snake, we consciously feel afraid because our brains are interpreting the automatic and unconscious physiological changes associated with fear (racing heart, sweaty palms, trembling).

Although this theory may seem to be backward, there is some evidence to support it. For instance, some specific emotional states are associated with specific autonomic, endocrine, and behavioral responses (Kandel, Schwartz, & Jessell, 2000). Also, research has found that when participants make a particular emotional facial expression (e.g., smiling), they tend to interpret neutral events on the basis of their facial expressions (e.g., pleasant or happy event when smiling) (Izard, 1992; Levinson, Ekman, & Friesen, 1990). Even instructing participants to contract muscles of the arms or face results in changes in their affective experience (Schiff & Lamon, 1989, 1994). Consistent with the James–Lange theory, studies with individuals who can no longer consciously monitor their autonomic responses (e.g., quadriplegics) have found that these individuals experience a decrease in the intensity of their emotions (Jasnos & Hakmiller, 1975). However, the spinal cord is not the only way for information from the periphery to reach the central nervous system; the vagus nerve also sends this information to the brain, which makes the results of Jasnos and Hakmiller (1975) interesting but inconclusive.

CANNON–BARD THEORY. The James–Lange theory was the dominant theory from the time it was proposed, and the **Cannon–Bard theory** (1927) arose primarily as a response to the James–Lange theory. Walter Cannon, an American physiologist, and his student Philip Bard argued that the cognitive aspect of emotional states occurred too quickly to result from monitoring physiological responses. Instead, they suggested that cognitive aspects of affect could be experienced even when individuals could not sense any physiological changes (Figure 9.4). They based this conclusion on work that they performed with nonhuman animals in which the spinal cord was transected (severed), after which the nonhuman animal was placed in an emotion-provoking situation. Although these nonhuman animals could not experience the physiological changes in their periphery, they still produced emotional expressions with their faces and vocalizations (Kandel et al., 2000). Contrary to the findings of Jasnos and Hakmiller (1975), there are early reports of Cannon describing humans with spinal cord transections who reported that following paralysis, they experienced no change in their ability to sense feelings (Finger, 1994). Consistent with the Cannon–Bard theory is research by Keillor and colleagues (Keillor, Barrett, Crucian, Kortenkamp, & Heilman, 2002), who observed the emotional abilities of an individual with bilateral facial paralysis (known as F.P.). Although F.P. can no longer move or feel her face, she can recognize emotional states in others and reports that there has been no subjective change in her ability to experience emotions, and she continues to exhibit ordinary emotional responses, albeit with an absence of facial expression.

Cannon and Bard also suggested that the physiological states that accompanied emotional states also accompanied other physiological states. For instance, both fear and illness produce nausea and sweating, yet individuals with the flu do not interpret themselves as being afraid. Therefore, Cannon and Bard argued, the physiological states that accompany emotional states are not unique and so require some type of

Schematic Diagram of the Cannon–Bard Theory of Emotions

Figure 9.4

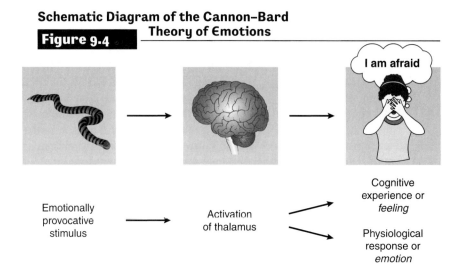

Emotionally provocative stimulus → Activation of thalamus → Cognitive experience or *feeling*

Physiological response or *emotion*

I am afraid

cognitive interpretation. The Cannon–Bard theory suggests that an emotion-inducing stimulus activates the thalamus, which then simultaneously activates the cortex (cognitions related to the emotional state) and the hypothalamus (responsible for releasing hormones that signal the autonomic physiological emotional response). Thus, the Cannon–Bard theory suggests that although the cognitive and physiological aspects of emotional states occur simultaneously in most individuals, it is possible for these components of emotional states to be dissociated.

SCHACHTER–SINGER THEORY. Critics of the Cannon–Bard theory included the American psychologists Stanley Schachter and Jerome Singer, who performed a classic experiment to test both the James–Lange and Cannon–Bard theories of emotional states. In the 1960s, Schachter began to develop a theory of emotional states based on cognitive interpretation of emotionally charged events. In this theory, the brain constructs emotion similarly to other experienced sensations. That is, the brain takes signals from the periphery and interprets and translates them into emotional states. Thus, similar emotions can produce different feelings depending on the context of the event. (Although the peripheral feelings when one is on a rollercoaster and when one is driving off a cliff are probably the same, presumably only one of these events is pleasurable.)

In a classic experiment, Schachter and Singer (1962) manipulated physiological arousal to determine whether or not the same state of arousal could be affected by situational variables (Table 9.1). Participants were told that the experimenters were going to test the effects of a vitamin on vision, when in fact half of the group received an injection of adrenaline and the other half of the group received a placebo injection (control group). As you may recall from Chapter 2, adrenaline is a hormone that is produced by the adrenal glands and has the effect of arousing the autonomic nervous system. Of those who received adrenaline injections, some participants were told that the vitamin had side effects that would result in a pounding heart and dry mouth (informed condition), some participants were told that the vitamin might make them

Table 9.1		
Predictions of the Three Major Theories of Emotion		
Group	**Euphoria Condition (cognitive signal = happy)**	**Anger Condition (cognitive signal = anger)**
Adrenaline + warning (explained physiological arousal)	**James–Lange predicted:** Should experience no emotion **Cannon–Bard predicted:** Should experience happiness **Schachter predicted:** No emotion	**James–Lange predicted:** Should experience no emotion **Cannon–Bard predicted:** Should experience anger **Schachter predicted:** No emotion
Adrenaline + no warning (unexplained physiological arousal)	**James–Lange predicted:** Should experience same emotion in both euphoria and anger **Cannon–Bard predicted:** Should experience happiness **Schachter predicted:** Happy	**James–Lange predicted:** Should experience same emotion in both euphoria and anger **Cannon–Bard predicted:** Should experience anger **Schachter predicted:** Anger
Adrenaline + false warning (unexplained physiological arousal)	**James–Lange predicted:** Should experience same emotion in both euphoria and anger **Cannon–Bard predicted:** Should experience happiness **Schachter predicted:** Happy	Not conducted.
Controls (placebo injection) (no physiological arousal)	**James–Lange predicted:** Should experience no emotion **Cannon–Bard predicted:** Should experience happiness **Schachter predicted:** No emotion	**James–Lange predicted:** Should experience no emotion **Cannon–Bard predicted:** Should experience anger **Schachter predicted:** No emotion

itch or give them a headache (misinformed condition), and some were told nothing about any side effect (uninformed condition). Participants were then placed into situations that were either happy (the participants played with toys) or angry (the participants had to complete insulting tasks while others in the room expressed anger).

Schachter and Singer predicted that if the James–Lange theory was correct, then participants in the uninformed and misinformed groups should experience similar feelings in both the anger and happy conditions (because physiological arousal was identical regardless of the situational events), whereas if the Cannon–Bard theory was correct, then participants in all conditions should experience the appropriate emotions for the conditions (euphoria or anger). However, Schachter and Singer (1962) had a third view of how the experiment would turn out: Schachter predicted that the physiological arousal in the misinformed and uninformed groups would be interpreted in light of the situation. That is, he predicted that physiological arousal in the happy condition would result in happiness and that physiological arousal in the anger condition would result in anger.

Schachter hypothesized that when an individual experienced arousal in a situation (emotion), the individual would label and experience the feeling to be congruent with the cognitive appraisal of the situation. Specifically, Schachter predicted that

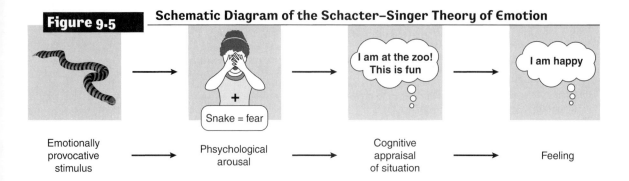

Figure 9.5

Schematic Diagram of the Schacter–Singer Theory of Emotion

exactly the same state of physiological arousal (what we have defined as emotions) would result in the attribution of different feelings depending on the cognitive appraisal of the situation. (In general, Schachter and Singer's experiment was thought to confirm the role of cognitive appraisal in the experience of feelings and emotions.) Thus, the **Schachter–Singer theory** suggests that cognitive processes are important in the production of emotional states and that the role of the periphery was to alert the organism to potential situations. Furthermore, the Schachter–Singer theory predicts that the degree of arousal is correlated with the degree to which an individual experiences an emotional state (Figure 9.5).

For a number of reasons, many researchers have suggested that the Schachter–Singer experiment is, at best, inconclusive. For instance, the control group (placebo injection) did not report that they experienced any less emotion than the aroused groups, a finding that was not predicted. Another criticism is that physiological arousal in the absence of any stimulus is a rare event. Therefore, the ability of Schachter and Singer (1962) to manipulate the feelings experienced by individuals in the two conditions is artificial and may represent only what individuals do in abnormal situations. Finally, studies that have attempted to replicate these effects have met with only limited success (e.g., Marshall & Zimbardo, 1979).

There was one other item of interest in the original study: The informed group (adrenaline injection + correct arousal information) that then experienced the anger manipulation tended to report feelings of happiness. Others have confirmed the relationship between physiological arousal and positive emotions. For instance, Dutton and Aron (1974) had a young women introduce herself to participants either when they were on a high, swinging suspension bridge (high arousal) or when they were on a low, stable bridge (low arousal). Participants later had to rate the attractiveness of the young woman. Participants in the high arousal condition rated the young woman as significantly more attractive than did the individuals who were in the low arousal condition. Dutton and Aron (1974) interpreted their results as support for the Schachter–Singer theory, in that individuals were using their heightened arousal in the one condition as a marker for heightened attraction.

THE SOMATIC MARKER THEORY. The **somatic marker theory** proposed by Portuguese-American neurologist Antonio Damasio differs from the Schachter–Singer theory in several ways. To begin with, Damasio formulated his initial theory on the basis of his observations of Elliot, an individual who had a large tumor in the meninges above his frontal lobes (Damasio, 1994). Surgery to remove the tumor was successful, but Elliot experienced a severe change in his personality. Before surgery, Elliot had been a good father and husband and was a successful businessman. After surgery, Elliot seemed fine. However, now he needed to be prompted to go to work. When he was at work, he would follow a task tirelessly, even when it was futile, rather than switching tasks to do something else relevant to the project. He also seemed to be unable to follow a schedule or to meet deadlines. In his personal life, he made a series of bad decisions leading to bankruptcy and divorces. Thus, although Elliot could still use language correctly and appeared to have intact cognitive skills, he no longer seemed to be able to reach decisions, to change activities once they were started, or to plan for the future (either hours or days ahead).

Many of Elliot's deficits should seem familiar, because they are very similar to those of Phineas Gage (see Chapter 3). In fact, research by Hanna Damasio and colleagues (Damasio et al., 1994) has demonstrated that Elliot and Phineas Gage suffered from very similar brain damage to the frontal lobes. However, unlike Phineas Gage, Elliot was given a full battery of neuropsychological tests. In all of the tests that Damasio could think of to give Elliot, including standardized personality tests and tasks that were designed to specifically test the functions of the frontal lobes, Elliot scored as well as neurologically intact individuals. So why had Elliot's personality undergone such a dramatic shift? Damasio suggests that much of Elliot's change can be attributed to the change in Elliot's ability to experience emotional states.

In a series of experiments, Damasio had Elliot try to solve ethical dilemmas. These dilemmas tested Elliot's awareness of consequences, social problem-solving ability, and moral reasoning ability. Again, Elliot scored as well as neurologically intact individuals on the ethical dilemmas and above average on the tasks that tested his awareness of consequences, social problem solving, and moral reasoning. Despite Elliot's good performance on these tasks, he was quite incapable of making rational choices in the real world. The only task on which Elliot's performance was unusual was one in which he was presented with pictures of emotional scenes (e.g., injured people, natural disasters). Although Elliot could describe how he should feel when he saw these pictures, he no longer had an autonomic arousal response to these pictures. That is, although he could describe feelings, he no longer could experience emotions. Further, Elliot described to Damasio this change in his ability to experience emotions: Although he could remember how he should feel, he no longer felt anything at all. Damasio suggests that although Elliot could distinguish several options for a given scenario, he could not decide which one was best because he could no longer rely on feelings to guide him.

In Damasio's somatic marker theory, emotion is represented by the brain similarly to how the senses are represented; that is, the brain synthesizes a wide variety of information that is obtained from the body to produce a unified percept (in this case, an emotional state). The association between emotional state and bodily change is the somatic marker. Somatic markers are means by which our brain evaluates novel situations on the basis of previous experience. In a sense, somatic marker theory suggests that the relationship between a stimulus and the emotional state produced by

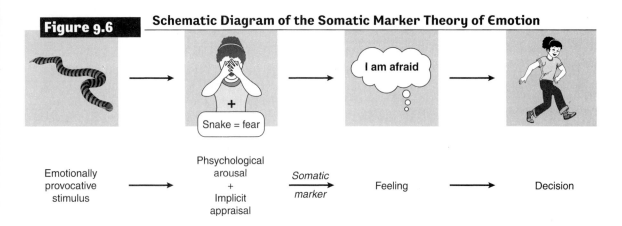

Figure 9.6	Schematic Diagram of the Somatic Marker Theory of Emotion

the stimulus can be a product of learning. However, Damasio states that the type of learning represented by the somatic marker theory is implicit rather than explicit. Thus, somatic markers are produced automatically by emotions and are not mediated directly by conscious recollection (Figure 9.6).

Damasio (1994) suggests that somatic markers are the basis on which we make decisions. In fact, Damasio suggests that the failure of patients such as Elliot to make rational decisions is the result of their inability to use somatic markers to assess possible outcomes. Thus, although Elliot can intellectually decide that there are a number of outcomes to a specific situation, he can no longer decide which outcome is best. Damasio does not resolve whether or not individuals with frontal damage similar to Elliot's are unable to access previously acquired somatic markers or are merely unable to use the information provided by these markers. Both are possibilities. If Elliot is no longer able to access somatic markers, then he would be unable to make decisions on the basis of previous experience, whereas if Elliot can no longer utilize the information provided by somatic markers, then he would be similarly unable to come to a decision. At this time, we do not know whether the frontal lobes are the site of storage for the somatic markers or whether they are the site at which these markers are interpreted.

THE APPRAISAL THEORY. The **appraisal theory** is one of the most dominant theories in the field of emotion, partly because it is one of the few theories that attempts to explain how emotional states are generated. The appraisal theory traces its roots to the work of Magda Arnold, an Austrian-Canadian psychologist. Arnold argues that emotional states are the process of cost–benefit analysis of situations. The physiological response is the product of unconscious evaluation of the situations that is based on the potential for the organism to either benefit or be damaged by the situation. The affective–cognitive portion of emotional states occurs when an individual consciously examines the unconscious appraisal. One important difference between the appraisal theory and other theories of emotion is that Arnold states that affective physiological responses also include the tendency to make specific responses to the stimulus. The appraisal theory suggests that emotional states differ from one another

Schematic Diagram of the Appraisal Theory of Emotion

Figure 9.7

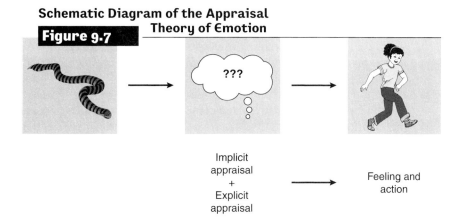

Implicit
appraisal
+
Explicit
appraisal

Feeling and
action

because they have different appraisals. That is, the appraisal theory suggests that emotional states are action tendencies, and that serve to alert the organism and to provide possibilities for action (Figure 9.7). Finally, Arnold suggests that emotional states may follow their own rules and that they most likely differ from the processes that are involved in either implicit or explicit learning.

One of the strengths of the appraisal theory is its ability to explain the relationship between the physiological and cognitive aspects of emotional states and to provide a framework for understanding why emotional states exist. The appraisal theory clearly explains how emotions are generated and the relationship between implicit and explicit affective evaluations. However, the appraisal theory has been criticized as being too cognitively heavy. For instance, some researchers have interpreted the appraisal theory as stating that an appraisal must be deliberate and conscious (e.g., LeDoux, 1996). As such, affective preferences for items that have not been consciously observed, such as stimuli that are presented too briefly to be identified are preferred over novel stimuli (e.g., Kunst-Wilson & Zajonc, 1980), are inconsistent with the theory. However, Arnold herself (1960) suggested that appraisals were "direct, immediate, nonreflective, nonintellectual [and] automatic" (p. 174). Therefore, affective preference based on unconscious or implicit processing of information does not necessarily pose a problem for the appraisal theory. Nonetheless, we are left wondering which of the two (implicit or explicit appraisal) leads to the action tendency and how they interact to produce an emotional state.

CONCLUSIONS AND SYNTHESIS. As you have read about these theories, you might have come to the conclusion that there is no conclusion. The failure to achieve consensus on which theory is correct should lead us to the conclusion that no single current theory can explain the variety of behaviors that exemplify emotional states. This is often the case when there is considerable research in an area; that is, the more we know about something, the more we realize that there is still much more that we do not know. Rather than trying to understand how stimuli acquire the ability to evoke emotions, many of the theories are an attempt to explain different classes of behaviors, including the nature of the relationship between the physiological and cognitive aspects of emotional states. It may be that many of the remaining questions surrounding emotional states cannot be answered by simply observing behavior. As we will see in the subsequent sections, functional imaging has provided important insights into explanations of how the brain understands and produces emotion.

Both the somatic marker theory and the appraisal theory are good at explaining the interaction between feelings, emotions, and conscious thought, because they both prominently emphasize the role of conscious and unconscious processing in producing emotions. Where the two theories differ is that the appraisal theory states that unconscious physiological responses automatically produce action plans that may be separate from consciously experienced cognitive appraisals of these states, whereas the somatic marker theory suggests that the physiological and cognitive aspects of emotion work together to play an important mutually beneficial role in decision making. Although the somatic marker theory is the only theory that is explicitly based on the brain, there appears to be growing consensus that the appraisal theory can also describe the relationship between the brain and emotional states (Kandel et al., 2000). Interestingly, neither theories address the unresolved question about the existence and definition of basic emotional states (Izard, 1992), though they both recognize the primacy of emotional states. Although the strength of both theories is that they provide a framework for understanding the role of emotional states and for potentially understanding their adaptive value, neither theory is currently capable of explaining precisely how the brain produces emotional states and how it perceives them in others.

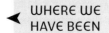

Emotional states combine the physiological responses and cognitive appraisals of emotion-provoking events or stimuli. There are numerous theories of emotional states, which tend to focus on different aspects of affective behavior. Two of the most prominent theories of emotional states are the somatic marker theory and the appraisal theory. Both theories emphasize the role of implicit/unconscious and explicit/conscious processing in producing emotional states, and both theories appear to be able to describe aspects of affective behaviors.

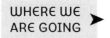

The following three sections will describe the laterality and functional neuroanatomy of emotions and feelings in neurologically normal individuals. As you are reading this section, keep in mind the somatic marker theory and the appraisal theory, and try to integrate the research that is described with the theory. The second module will explain disorders of emotions and feelings that occur as a consequence of brain damage or brain dysfunction.

Laterality of Emotion

In Chapter 4, you learned that laterality studies tend to use techniques that present material to only one hemisphere. For instance, information that is presented to only one visual field is initially sent to the contralateral visual cortex. Laterality studies interpret differences in the ability of the hemispheres to report presented stimuli to differences in the ability to translate and understand the information. For instance, if a participant tends to report correctly more of the stimuli that were presented to the right ear, we would conclude that the left hemisphere (the hemisphere contralateral to the right ear) is advantaged in processing the stimulus. Studies of the laterality of emotional states tend to focus either on the production of emotional behaviors (e.g., the ability to make facial expressions) or on the perception of emotional stimuli (e.g., the emotional content of speech).

PRODUCTION OF EMOTIONAL BEHAVIORS. One of the most common emotional stimuli available are the faces of individuals around us. Our faces are not perfectly symmetrical; that is, there are differences between the right side of the face and the left, such as the shape of mouth) (Figure 9.8). Interestingly, when we make facial expressions of emotions, our faces again exhibit asymmetries. Although differences in asymmetries of the face itself are most apparent when the face is relaxed, it does not appear that asymmetries of facial expressions of emotion can easily be attributed to these underlying structural features of the face itself. Rather, asymmetry in facial expressions of emotion is likely due to differences in the contraction of the muscles of one side of the face (van Gelder & Borod, 1990).

Contraction of the muscles of the face is dependent on the activity of the facial nerve (the seventh cranial nerve), which has two main pathways from the brain. Voluntary facial expressions are mediated by the precentral gyrus, which sends bilateral projections to the muscles of the upper face (e.g., eyebrows) and contralaterally to the muscles of the lower face (e.g., mouth). Involuntary facial expressions are most likely controlled by the thalamus, through bilateral projections. Thus, the right hemisphere is most likely to control and produce asymmetries involving the left side of the lower face, including the mouth, whereas the left hemisphere is most likely to be involved in asymmetries of the right lower side of the face (see Figure 9.9).

There are various ways in which facial asymmetry can be considered, for example, by having individuals make specific facial expressions or by observing individuals as they produce

Figure 9.8   An Example of Facial Asymmetry

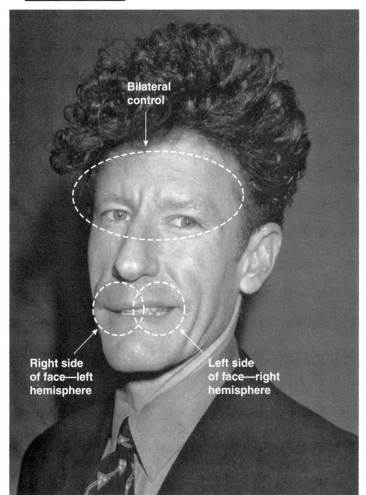

Source: Photo © Mitchell Gerber/Corbis. Used with permission.

spontaneous facial expressions. There are even a number of studies that suggest that photographs and paintings may be of use in examining facial asymmetries. For instance, one study of paintings and photographs of famous individuals found that the left side of their face was more likely to be prominent than the right (McManus & Humphrey, 1973). Although you could argue that this is some kind of an artifact, research by Nicholls suggests that the preference for exposing the left side of the face in portraits is determined by the person who is sitting for the portrait (Nicholls, Clode, Wood, & Wood, 1999). Furthermore, when participants are asked to make emotional facial expressions, they tend to have greater change in expression in the left hemiface, which is controlled by the right hemisphere (Borod & Caron, 1980; Borod, Caron, & Koff, 1981; Borod, Haywood, & Koff, 1997; Graves, Landis, & Simpson, 1985). When spontaneously emitted facial expressions were observed, it has also been noted that there is greater change in the expression of the left hemiface (Borod et al., 1997; Borod, Koff, & White, 1983; Borod, Koff, Yecker, Santschi, & Schmidt, 1998). Taken together, these indications of the dominance of the left side of the face for producing emotional displays is consistent with the conclusion that the right hemisphere is specialized for emotional expression. Consistent with other studies of laterality, most left-handed individuals exhibit a leftward bias in emotional facial expressions (Kim & Levine, 1991), and there are suggestions that women express less asymmetry than men, presumably reflecting increased bilateral involvement of the brain in producing emotional facial expressions (Borod et al., 1998).

There is also the suggestion that the valence of the emotion (i.e., whether it is a positive or negative emotion) can influence the asymmetry observed. For instance, Heller and Levy (1981) observed more leftward asymmetry when an individual was expressing happiness; Sackeim and Gur (1978) observed that negative emotions were displayed predominantly by the left hemiface; and Asthana and Mandal (2001) observed a leftward asymmetry for sadness and no asymmetry for happiness. However, because many researchers have consistently found leftward asymmetries for both positive and negative emotions (e.g., Moscovitch & Olds, 1982; Borod et al., 1983, 1997), we must conclude that there is currently no definitive evidence of asymmetrical facial expressions that relate to the type of emotion that an individual is trying to express.

This conclusion does not suggest that there is no relationship between facial asymmetry and emotional valence, as the relationship either may be subtle or may occur only in specific situations. For instance, Borod (1992) suggests that positive emotions may present with less lateralized expression because of their linguistic properties, whereas negative emotions are linked with survival and therefore are less likely to engage linguistic areas of the brain. According to Borod (1992), positive emotions are more likely to engage approach behaviors than are negative emotions (which engage avoidance behaviors). Therefore, negative behaviors may engage the right hemisphere more than positive emotions do, because the right hemisphere is specialized for automated movements. Conversely, approach behaviors may preferentially engage the left hemisphere, which is specialized for fine-motor control and sequencing of movements. Furthermore, Borod and colleagues (1998) suggest that valence effects are most likely to be observed when self-report measures of subjective experience are used, which reflect experimental demands that bias attention to facial musculature. Note that neither the approach–avoidance explanation nor the attentional biases explanation involves emotional states per se; rather, they suggest that the motor consequences of emotions may mediate facial expressions.

Facial expressions are not the only way in which individuals convey emotion to others. We routinely use speech to convey emotional state. Speech can convey emotional state directly ("I am happy!"), and it can convey emotional state indirectly. In fact, the term **prosody** was coined by Monrad-Krohn (1947) when he argued that communication through language required more than simply choosing the correct word and placing it in the appropriate grammatical context. There are components of verbal communication that direct meaning and inform the listener about emotional content (or state) that are *independent* of the words spoken. These components include the tone of voice (pitch, rhythm, duration, and stress). Therefore, prosody is the conveyance of meaning, often related to emotional tone, by varying the intonation in speech. These changes can fundamentally change the meanings of the spoken words and can even reverse their meaning.

Although it is difficult to convey prosody through written text, consider this example: "Todd is so smart" versus "Todd is *sooooo* smart!" Does the first statement seem to be sincere? How about the second statement? In the case of sarcasm, people say the opposite of what they really mean. The listener is informed of this intention from the speaker's tone of voice. Prosody can also cue the presence of a question, usually by a slight elevation in pitch toward the end of a phrase. Sometimes questions can be identified because of the words within the phrase (e.g., *who, what, where, why, how*), but some phrases question without the presence of such words. These two examples of prosody are cases of **propositional prosody,** wherein the semantic information that is being conveyed is qualified or augmented by the prosody that is employed. However, prosody can also convey emotional content. This type is termed **affective prosody.** A statement such as "The Lakers won again" might inform the listener about the outcome of the basketball game, but the manner in which the statement is spoken helps to indicate whether the speaker is a Laker fan or not. Thus, although the linguistic components of the phrase remain the same, the emotional tone of the words changes significantly from sincere to sarcastic.

Because the linguistic components that are required to directly convey emotional state may be confounded with the production of language (which typically is a function of the left hemisphere), we will consider only the indirect methods of indicating emotional state. Functional imaging studies of neurologically normal individuals have implicated right hemisphere activity in the production of both prosodic speech and prosodic singing (Dogil et al., 2002; Riecker, Ackermann, Wildgruber, Dogil, & Grodd, 2000). Consistent with this are the observations that individuals with right hemisphere damage exhibit profound difficulties in producing prosodic speech (e.g., Weintraub, Mesulam, & Kramer, 1981).

PERCEPTION OF EMOTIONAL STIMULI. Many more studies have been performed on the laterality of perceived emotional stimuli, in part because perception lends itself to experimentation more easily than expression does. Typical studies of perception of emotion have examined performance on the lateralized presentation of either auditory or visual stimuli. Auditory stimuli tend to take the form of dichotically presented words or sentences that are spoken in an emotional tone, such as the word *cat* said in a happy voice. Participants are asked to listen for the emotional tone of the speech and to indicate whenever they hear a specific emotion (e.g., sadness). Numerous studies have found that there is a left ear advantage (LEA) for reporting the emotional tone of either words or sentences (e.g., Bryden & MacRae, 1988; Haggard & Parkinson, 1971), which suggests that the perception of prosody is mediated by the right hemisphere. Interestingly, the LEA is obtained even when the stimuli are nonspeech sounds that have emotional tones, such as coughing, crying, and laughing (King & Kimura, 1972).

Although some researchers have argued that the observed LEA is a result of attentional asymmetries rather than processing, work by Bryden and MacRae (1988) demonstrates that the ear advantage depends on the target. Using the same stimuli, when participants in this study were told to detect specific words, a right ear advantage (REA) was obtained, and an LEA was obtained when participants were told to detect specific emotional tones. Using the exact same stimuli for emotions and words (e.g., the word *bower* spoken in an angry voice), Bulman-Fleming and Bryden (1994) observed the same pattern: Participants had an LEA for the affective part of the target and an REA for the linguistic part of the target. Taken together, there is strong evidence that the right hemisphere is dominant for both producing and expressing prosody.

Figure 9.9   **An Example of a Chimeric Face**

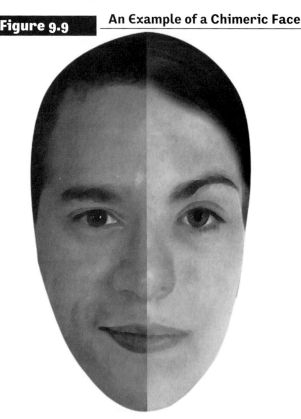

Studies of the perception of the emotional tone of visual stimuli tend to examine the responses of individuals to photographs of faces. Studies of this sort typically use either lateralized presentations of photos of faces or central presentations of chimeric faces. Recall from Chapter 3 that chimeric faces are composite faces that are split down the middle into a right hemiface and a left hemiface. Often, chimeric faces can be composed of two different hemifaces that are fused to make a novel face (e.g., Figure 9.9), although chimeric faces that are composed of one hemiface and its mirrored reflection are also common. Studies of tachistoscopically presented faces typically demonstrate that individuals are better at identifying the emotion portrayed by the face when the face is presented in the left visual field (LVF) (e.g., Strauss & Moscovitch, 1981). A series of studies conducted by Borod and others (e.g., Borod et al., 1997, 1998; Borod, St. Clair, Koff, & Alpert, 1990; Borod, Vingiano, & Cytryn, 1989; Heller & Levy, 1981) have demonstrated that an individual's assessment of the emotional content of chimeric faces is dependent primarily on the expression of the left hemiface. In addition, subsequent studies by Nicholls and colleagues demonstrated that individuals perceive portraits as being more emotional when the left side of the face is exposed to a greater degree than the right side of the face (Nicholls, Clode, et al., 1999; Nicholls, Wolfgang, Clode, & Lindell, 2002). Taken together, these results suggest that the right hemisphere is dominant for the perception and production of emotional facial expressions.

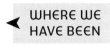 The perception and expression of emotional states are dominated by right hemispheric function. The right hemisphere is better than the left hemisphere at producing and recognizing both emotional faces and prosody.

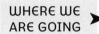 Although there is no unified theory of emotion that is based in the brain, much of the research presented suggests that there is both an autonomic or physiological component and a cognitive component to emotional states. As we will see in the next section, the autonomic components of an emotional response involve responses of the hypothalamus. The cognitive component of emotional states requires both implicit and explicit processing of emotion (LeDoux, 1996). The following section will examine the role of cortical structures in the perception and expression of emotional states. The second module will examine how brain damage or brain dysfunction can affect emotional states.

Role of Subcortical Structures in Emotional States

Although the brainstem is the site of many of the nuclei that regulate the autonomic nervous system, the hypothalamus exerts significant influence over these nuclei. For instance, stimulation of specific areas of the hypothalamus can elicit autonomic changes that include piloerection and changes in blood pressure and heart rate (Ranson, 1934). In the 1940s, Hess performed classic studies in awake and behaving cats in which he observed that stimulation of different areas of the hypothalamus produced behaviors that are characteristic of differing emotional states. For instance, stimulation of specific areas of the lateral hypothalamus resulted in autonomic responses that are consistent with anger: piloerection, increases in blood pressure and heart rate, constriction of the pupils, and a facial expression that was typical of an anger response in cats (Finger, 1994). Research suggests that the hypothalamus is responsible for integrating and coordinating the autonomic and somatic components of emotional states. In addition, the hypothalamus may play a role in ensuring the congruence between the autonomic and somatic responses.

Although the hypothalamus regulates the autonomic and somatic components of an emotional state, emotional states also contain the cognitive component, which must involve some recognition of the relevant stimulus by areas of the brain that are associated with higher-order cognition. One of the first attempts to understand how the physiological and cognitive components of emotional states were represented in the cortex was described by Papez (pronounced "Peeps") in 1937 (Finger, 1994). Papez hypothesized that the cortical areas for the cognitive components of emotional states

Figure 9.10 The Limbic System

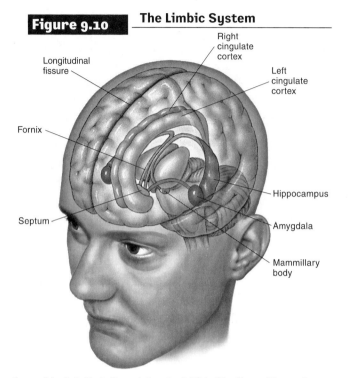

Right cingulate cortex
Left cingulate cortex
Longitudinal fissure
Fornix
Hippocampus
Septum
Amygdala
Mammillary body

Source: John P. J. Pinel, *Biopsychology*, 5e. Published by Allyn and Bacon, Boston, MA. Copyright © 2003 by Pearson Education. Reprinted by permission of the publisher.

involved activation of the limbic lobe, an area of the brain that includes the cingulate gyrus, the parahippocampal gyrus, and the hippocampal formation (Figure 9.10). Although areas such as the amygdala are cortical, they are definitely more primitive than other areas of the cortex are and therefore are often called the paleocortex and are often considered separately from the neocortex. Papez suggested that the ability of the hypothalamically mediated physiological responses and the cortically mediated cognitive components to influence each other could result from the reciprocal connections between the hypothalamus and areas of the limbic cortex. In addition, areas of the neocortex could influence both the limbic system and the hypothalamus through the cingulate and hippocampus, both of which are highly connected to neocortex. Thus, Papez suggested that emotional responses result from reciprocal interconnections between the limbic lobe, neocortex, and hypothalamus.

The role of the limbic lobe in emotional states was modified by MacLean, who theorized an entire limbic *system* (Finger, 1994). One of the biggest differences was that MacLean incorporated the original structures of the limbic lobe with the hypothalamus, septum, nucleus accumbens, and areas of the neocortex such as the orbitofrontal cortex. A number of studies have confirmed that there are extensive, direct, and reciprocal interconnections among the structures of the limbic system, especially the neocortex, hippocampal formation, and amygdala. MacLean suggested that it was the hippocampus that directed and organized the activity of the hypothalamus, partly on the basis of the research by Klüver and Bucy (1939), who demonstrated that bilateral removal of the temporal lobes of monkeys resulted in major changes in affective behaviors (Finger, 1994). However, subsequent research suggests that this role is accomplished by the amygdala, not the hippocampus (for a review, see Ohman, Flykt, & Esteves, 2001). Important for both the appraisal and somatic marker theory, the amygdala appears to be involved in both implicit and explicit emotional states. For instance, stimulation of the amygdala in humans results in feelings of fear, and activation of the amygdala is observed in learned fear responses (Ohman & Mineka, 2001). Bilateral amygdala lesions have also been associated with impaired ability to recognize emotional faces (Adolphs et al., 1999) and emotional speech (Scott, Young, Calder, Hellawell, Aggleton, & Johnson, 1997). However, because many of these studies relied on individuals who had widespread damage to the limbic system, it is not possible to determine which single structure was primarily responsible for the results.

Neuropsychological Celebrity

S.M.

How do you decide whom to trust? Is it the way a person looks? Is it their facial expression? Is it their tone of voice? Is it the way they dress? Do you sometimes get the feeling that someone is not very trustworthy, but you do not know *why* you are suspicious? We make judgments of trustworthiness all the time. Some more obvious examples include choosing a car salesperson, a babysitter, or a dating partner. If you have allergies to foods such as nuts and you ask the server at a restaurant what ingredients a certain dish contains, how do you decide whether you believe the answer? Imagine *not* being able to make accurate judgments in these situations. Wouldn't that be scary? Not if you cannot feel fear!

S.M. has complete lesions of both the left and right amygdalae (plural of *amygdala*) as a result of Urbach–Wiethe disease. This extremely rare lesion pattern has resulted in a unique behavioral pattern. S.M. does not appear to exhibit fear (at least not the autonomic responses that are associated with fear), nor can she perceive fear in the facial expressions of others. This is particularly remarkable in light of her apparent ability to recognize faces (Adolphs, Tranel, Damasio, & Damasio, 1995) and even recognize other emotions (such as happiness) on the basis of facial expressions (Adolphs et al., 1999). Therefore, it appears that the human amygdala plays an important role in both experiencing and perceiving fear.

Is the amygdala also involved in other real-world social judgments such as those about trustworthiness or approachability? Adolphs and colleagues investigated this question by presenting S.M. with pictures of unfamiliar people and asking her to rate the trustworthiness and approachability of 100 faces that control participants had rated as either highly trustworthy and approachable or very untrustworthy and unapproachable. During the testing session, S.M. commented that "in real life, she would not know how to judge if a person were trustworthy, consistent with her tendency to approach and engage in physical contact with other people rather indiscriminately" (Adolphs, Tranel, & Damsio, 1998, p. 471). Her prediction proved to be correct. She gave relatively positive ratings to faces that the control participants had deemed untrustworthy or unapproachable, indicating that she could not make these judgments.

To test whether S.M.'s impairment was specific to judgments of faces, Adolphs and colleagues read short verbal biographies of fictitious people to her and asked her to make similar judgments. Quite unlike the case with facial stimuli, S.M. could perform that task normally, giving answers that were comparable to the responses of the control participants. Collectively, these studies suggest that the human amygdala plays an important role in triggering socially and emotionally relevant responses when presented with visual stimuli. The extent to which this function is innate versus acquired has yet to be determined.

Because of the location of the amygdala within the brain, lesions of the amygdala are rare in humans. However, Urbach–Wiethe disease results in the progressive calcification of the limbic areas, including the amygdala. Individuals with this disease may experience emotional lability, often expressed as periods of rage (e.g., Kleinert, Cerros-Navarro, Kleinert, Walter, & Steiner, 1987). Individuals who are affected by Urbach–Wiethe disease often fail to correctly discriminate among facial expressions, though their ability to recognize the identity of the faces is unimpaired. Nevertheless, this effect is not always observed, especially when damage is restricted to limbic areas such as the hippocampus (e.g., Ghika-Schmid et al., 1997). Given that the discrimination of facial expressions of emotion relies on implicit memory, results from studying individuals with Urbach–Wiethe disease suggest that there are links between the function of the amygdala and the implicit processing that goes with processing of emotional stimuli (Markowitsch et al., 1994; Newton, Rosenberg, Lampert, & O'Brien, 1971).

Functional imaging of neurologically intact individuals suggests that the recognition of emotional facial expressions results in activity of the amygdala. Curiously, the left amygdala was preferentially activated for negative emotions, and the degree of activation was positively correlated with the degree to which the facial expression was intense (Morris et al., 1998; Morris et al., 1996, 1998; Phillips et al., 1997). That is, extremely unhappy faces resulted in greater activation than did mildly unhappy faces. This result is inconsistent with the valence theory of facial expressions, which suggests that the negative emotional states should exhibit greater lateralized activity in the right hemisphere. However, similar results have been obtained with negative auditory stimuli (Phillips et al., 1998), suggesting that the left amygdala plays a central role in the perception of negative emotional states. Interestingly, Tabert and colleagues (Tabert et al., 2001) reported that the right amygdala was active when emotional long-term memory consolidation was required. It may be that the left amygdala is involved in immediate, implicit processing of a stimulus and the right amygdala is involved in the explicit processing of a stimulus (Tabert et al., 2001).

Role of the Cortex in Emotional States

Although the amygdala plays a critical role in affective perception and expression, neuroimaging studies of neurologically intact individuals also consistently observe extra-amygdalar cortical activation. Studies of conditioned fear typically involve pairing specific facial expressions with unpleasant consequences (e.g., pairing the viewing of a happy face with a very loud noise). Using these paradigms, these studies tend to observe significant cortical activation associated with conditioned fear responses. Specifically, evoked fear responses were associated with increased activation of the right orbital frontal area (BA10) and superior frontal cortex (BA46) (Morris, Friston, & Dolan, 1997), along with significant activation of the amygdala, thalamus, and pulvinar. These changes in activity were interpreted as being indicative of both the implicit (subcortical) and explicit (cortical) expression of fear by the participants. If the amygdala is the site at which cross-modal sensory integration of emotional stimuli is achieved and cortical areas are responsible for mediating and recognizing the emotional state (Dolan, Morris, & de Gelder, 2001), then lesions of either cortical areas or the amygdala would result in deficits of affective responsiveness.

When participants observed emotional faces, fearful faces appear to be associated with increased activation in the left anterior insula and bilateral activation of the anterior cingulate (Morris et al., 1998). Conversely, happy faces were associated with more posterior activation in the right superior temporal gyrus and bilateral activations of the striate cortex and the lingual and fusiform gyri (Morris et al., 1998). A series of studies performed by Phillips and colleagues observed that there was significant activation of the anterior insula in the perception of visual and auditory displays of disgust (Phillips et al., 1997, 1998).

It has been suggested that the sensitivity of anterior cingulate to fearful stimuli reflects the role that the cingulate plays in responding to pain and its role in mediating social behavior (e.g., Morris et al., 1998; Phillips et al., 1997, 1998). These researchers hypothesize that the responsiveness of the anterior insula to the intensity of fearful stimuli reflects the role of the anterior insula in mediating responses to noxious stimuli and in the learning of avoidance behaviors. It is interesting to note that the insula has been implicated in phobias, specifically in the experience of phobic symptoms (Rauch et al., 1995). Others have suggested that the insula coordinates sensorimotor information on the basis of overall activity in the limbic system (e.g., Augustine, 1996). When trying to understand these results, it is important to keep in mind that all of the areas of the limbic system are extensively interconnected.

Before you begin to think that neuropsychologists study only unpleasant things, there are a number of studies that have examined the neural basis of positive emotions, such as happiness and love. Both the viewing of a happy experience on film and autobiographical recall of happy events result in activation of the frontal and temporal cortices, especially the medial prefrontal cortex (BA9), which is an area that is hypothesized to play a critical role in the somatic marker theory of emotion (Lane, Reiman, Ahern, Schwartz, & Davidson, 1997). Others have observed that viewing happy faces resulted in bilateral activation of the areas in which the occipital and temporal lobes meet (Gorno-Tempini et al., 2001). Significant activation of subcortical areas (including the amygdala) was also observed, suggesting that subcortical areas are also important in the processing of positive affect.

Neuroimaging studies have compared the neural activation of participants who viewed pictures of friends (whom they reported as liking) and their life partners (whom they reported as loving). Bartels and Zeki (2000) reported that when participants viewed pictures of their loved ones, there was significant activation of the left medial insula and bilateral activation of the anterior cingulate. When participants viewed pictures of their friends, there was significant activation of the right prefrontal, parietal, and middle temporal cortex and the posterior cingulate and medial prefrontal cortex. Thus, it appears that positively viewed stimuli (either happy faces, films, or friends) resulted in the activation of the medial prefrontal and middle temporal areas, whereas love has a separate neural substrate in the insula and cingulate.

Finally, studies of individuals who had undergone a prefrontal lobotomy have observed significant changes in emotional output (among other significant changes). That is, these individuals appeared to be less anxious, and they engaged in significantly fewer emotional behaviors of any sort. In primates, lesions of the orbitofrontal cortex reduced aggression and anger responses, whereas stimulation of the orbitofrontal cortex resulted in autonomic responses involved in arousal. It is suggested that the reciprocal connections between the amygdala and neocortex provide the ability for affective experience to result in learning. Cortical aspects of emotional states allow an individual to use affective information to affect cognitive processing. However, it must be recognized that cognitive processing mediated by the cortex is most likely responsible for the ability to suppress emotional responses. Research suggests that the ventromedial frontal cortex is one area that exerts such control, allowing either somatic markers or cognitive appraisals to affect emotional states and/or decision making (e.g., Damasio, 1994).

1. What are the criteria for basic emotional states? What are the problems with these criteria?

2. Are emotional states adaptive? Why would facial expressions of emotion be adaptive? On the basis of adaptation, when would you predict that the absence of stereotypic facial expressions of emotion would occur?

3. Describe the research that supports the Cannon–Bard theory of emotion. Describe the research that supports the James–Lange theory of emotion. Why is the experiment performed by Schachter and Singer inconsistent with either theory of emotion?

4. What research supports the role of implicit processing in emotional states? What research supports the role of explicit processing in emotional states? What neuroimaging evidence suggests whether implicit or explicit processes are more important in emotions? What neuroimaging evidence suggests whether implicit or explicit processes are more important in feelings?

5. What are the candidate structures in the brain that are responsible for feelings? What are the candidate structures in the brain that are responsible for emotions? What are the candidate structures in the brain that are responsible for the integration of feelings and emotions?

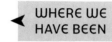

◀ **WHERE WE HAVE BEEN**

The limbic system, especially the amygdala, plays a major role in the perception and expression of emotional states. Although the amygdala plays a larger role in the perception and expression of negative emotions, the amygdala is also involved in positive emotional states. Cortical structures such as the insula and cingulate also play a role in emotional states. Consistent with other types of functions, it appears that emotional states are functionally localized in the cortex.

WHERE WE ARE GOING ▶

The following sections detail the functional and neuroanatomical changes that accompany a disturbance in affective processing. As you will see, subcortical or cortical brain damage can impair one's ability to process emotion. It can also spark the release of abnormal emotional responses. We also discuss the anatomical and neurochemical characteristics of relatively common mood disorders, such as depression. Finally, we take a look into the brains of psychopaths to investigate what underlies this rare but important emotional disorder.

MODULE **9.2**
Disorders of Emotion

In previous chapters of this book, we described a variety of cases of abnormal affect. In Chapter 3, you learned about Phineas Gage and the results of his frontal lobe injury. In Chapter 4, you learned about abnormalities in affective processing in people with lateralized lesions or corpus callosum lesions. In Chapter 7, you learned about the role of the right hemisphere in varying one's tone of voice and the consequences of right hemisphere damage. In some of these cases, brain damage resulted in a major reduction in emotional experience, be it the spontaneous production of emotion or the perception of emotion in others. However, this is not always the case. Brain damage can also result in increases in the experience of emotion. The same can be said for neurochemical changes. Some agents can cause heightened sensation of emotion (e.g., many drugs that are commonly abused), whereas others (such as lithium carbonate) appear to dull emotional states. The following sections detail some of these changes, starting with a discussion of reductions in emotional experience following brain injury.

Brain Damage and Lack of Affect

As we learned in the previous section, **prosody** is often used to convey meaning by varying the intonation in speech. Prosody can be used to cue both semantic information (propositional prosody) and emotional content (affective prosody). Recall from Chapter 4 that when participants are instructed to listen to the emotional tone of a speaker during a dichotic listening task, they exhibit a left ear/right hemisphere advantage (Bryden & MacRae, 1988; Bulman-Fleming & Bryden, 1994; Elias et al., 1998). Functional neuroimaging has also confirmed that the right hemisphere is specialized for the detection of prosody (Buchanan et al., 2000). Therefore, it should come as no surprise that people who suffer right hemisphere damage often display deficits in prosodic processing (called **aprosodia**).

Aprosodia is particularly pronounced when areas analogous to the language areas of the left hemisphere (such as Broca's area and Wernicke's area) are damaged. As you might imagine, assessing aprosodia can be quite difficult. How would you assess the degree to which a person's speech is monotone? One strategy has been to ask individuals with brain damage to repeat sentences or words in different emotional tones (such as happy, sad, or angry) and then judge the appropriateness of their affect (Tucker, Watson, & Heilman, 1977). This procedure can be more formalized with the use of a device (an **audio spectrogram**) that measures the amount of pitch variance in the person's speech. This method is somewhat problematic because there are large individual and cultural differences in the amount and type of prosody that are used during conversation. Some speakers use extreme changes in intonation to convey meaning; other speakers employ relatively monotone speech. Some recent evidence suggests that there are also sex differences in the production of prosody. According to Fitzsimons and colleagues (Fitzsimons, Sheahan, & Staunton, 2001), males employ higher rates of speech, more narrow pitch ranges, but a greater pitch slope (rate of pitch change) than those of female speakers.

Linguistic expression has dissociable expressive and receptive components. A person can be impaired in his or her ability to produce speech (Broca's aphasia) but retain the ability to understand it. Similarly, production can be spared, but comprehension can be impaired (Wernicke's aphasia). The same dissociation appears to be present for aprosodia. In some cases (especially following damage to the middle cerebral artery of the right hemisphere), people lose their ability to produce prosody normally, resulting in monotone speech. However, they retain the ability to recognize affective prosody and propositional prosody in others. This deficit has been termed **motor aprosodia.** Conversely, the inability to understand the prosody of others coupled with the retained ability to produce it is called **sensory aprosodia** (Ross, 1993, 2000). It is possible that other aprosodias exist that are analogous to the other aphasias, including global, conduction, transcortical-motor, and transcortical-sensory aprosodia. However, we must caution that the evidence is not clear on this point, and the topic remains controversial

Brain damage also produces emotional-processing deficits in the visual modality. In the previous module, you learned about the universality of emotional facial expression. Following right hemisphere damage, both the expression and recognition of these expressions are impaired. Curiously, the inability to distinguish between *facial expressions* is dissociable from the ability to recognize *faces*. Two examples of this were provided by Bornstein (1963). He described two people who made partial recoveries from prosopagnosia but complained of a difficulty in recognizing facial expressions. According to one of the patients, "It is clear that I have lost the ability to read a person's facial expression. This is apparent in situations such as seeing a film in which everyone can easily understand what is taking place from the facial expression" (Bornstein, 1963). One strategy that is typically adopted by such patients is to adopt a feature-searching strategy. When people smile, they typically show their teeth, or perhaps dimples are present. This strategy is helpful for identifying some emotions (such as happiness), but it not does reliably discriminate among other emotions (Etkoff, 1984).

Klüver–Bucy Syndrome

We previously described a behavioral syndrome that is evident in rhesus monkeys following anterior temporal lobe damage. Named after the scientists who described it in 1939, Klüver–Bucy syndrome was characterized by "psychic blindness" (the inability to recognize familiar objects), the tendency to examine objects orally, emotional unresponsiveness, an increase in sexual activity, **hypermetamorphosis** (a strong tendency to react to every visual stimulus), and a lack of fear (possibly related to the psychic blindness). Rhesus monkeys that were fierce and not amenable to being handled before the surgery became docile and tame afterward.

The first report of Klüver–Bucy syndrome in a human came in 1955, sixteen years after the original report. Terzian and Dalle-Ore (1955) described an adult male who had undergone a temporal lobectomy to treat his otherwise intractable seizures. Following the surgery, he displayed all of the classic symptoms of Klüver–Bucy syndrome except the tendency to place objects in one's mouth. Twenty years later, the first account of a "complete" case of Klüver–Bucy syndrome in a human was reported. Marlowe and colleagues (Marlow, Mancall, & Thomas, 1975) described a twenty-year-old male who had suffered brain damage as a result of viral meningoencephalitis:

> He exhibited a flat affect, and although originally restless, ultimately became remarkably placid. He appeared indifferent to people or situations. He spent much time gazing at the television, but never learned to turn it on; when the set was off, he tended to watch reflections of others in the room on the glass screen. On occasion he became facetious, smiling inappropriately and mimicking the gestures and actions of other. Once initiating an imitative series, he would perseverate copying all movements made by another for extended periods of time. . . . He engaged in oral exploration of all objects within his grasp, appearing unable to gain information via tactile or visual means alone. All objects that he could lift were placed in his mouth and sucked or chewed. . . .
>
> Although vigorously heterosexual prior to his illness, he was observed in hospital to make advances towards male patients. . . . [H]e never made advances toward women, and, in fact, his apparent reversal of sexual polarity prompted his fiancée to sever their relationship. (Marlowe et al., 1975, pp. 55–56, as quoted in Pinel, 1997)

In primates, the symptoms of the syndrome appear to result from bilateral amygdala damage. It is difficult to generalize about the type of brain damage that produces the syndrome in humans, given the rarity of the syndrome and lack of neuroradiological or postmortem examinations of the cases that exist. However, it appears as though damage that extends beyond the amygdala is necessary to produce the syndrome in humans. There are several well-studied cases of individuals with bilateral amygdala damage (such as H.M., who was featured in Chapter 8, and S.M., who is featured in this chapter) who do *not* exhibit the symptoms of the syndrome. It is entirely possible that the cortex surrounding the amygdala and other limbic structures needs to be damaged before humans will exhibit Klüver–Bucy syndrome.

Mood Disorders

Mood disorder is a diagnostic term that refers to a class of disorders characterized by long-term disruptions in mood. The diagnostic manual referred to as the DSM-IV (American Psychological Association, 1994) includes within this category major depressive disorder and bipolar disorder. Both of these diseases are serious and common and are often associated with significant impairments in the ability to work and have relationships with others. These diseases have no known cause, although there are theories that relate the illness to abnormal neurotransmission and genetic factors.

MAJOR DEPRESSIVE DISORDER. Major depressive disorder is characterized by long-lasting periods of depressed mood (persisting sadness), lack of interest, and/or the lack of ability to feel pleasure. The lifetime risk for depression is 7–12% for men and 20–25% for women, which translates to about 17 million Americans per year (American Psychological Association, 1994). Depression can be distinguished from simple sadness by its duration. Although most of us may feel sad or low for a few days, without treatment, depressed individuals feel this way for long periods of time, even years. Associated with depression are changes in sleep patterns, weight, energy levels, and the ability to concentrate. Theories regarding the biological basis of depression typically focus on the neurotransmitter serotonin and on genetic factors.

Drugs that increase monoamine neurotransmission are often effective in reducing depression. Recall from Chapter 2 that the monoamine neurotransmitters are the catecholamines (dopamine, epinephrine, and norepinephrine) and the indoleamine (serotonin). Conversely, drugs that reduce monoamine levels in the brain induce depression. Some researchers therefore suggest that depression is a result of lower than normal levels of monoamines (most likely serotonin) in the brain. In fact, the popular antidepressant Prozac (fluoxetine) works by inhibiting the reabsorption of serotonin from the synapse. Depression also seems to run in families, suggesting that there may also be a genetic component. There is evidence to suggest that genes that code for the serotonin receptor and genes that regulate serotonin metabolism may be related to depressive illness (Du, Faludi, Palkovits, Bakish, & Hrdina, 2001).

It has been reported that individuals with major depressive disorder also demonstrate cognitive impairments. As in individuals with schizophrenia, the impairments associated with depression relate to motor speed, memory (long-term and working memory), executive function, and attention. However, unlike the case in schizophrenia, it appears that these deficits are quite minor and occur only when the individual is experiencing a depressive episode. Furthermore, not all researchers have observed all of the deficits in cognitive function (e.g., Sweeney, Kmiec, & Kupfer, 2000), suggesting that the severity of the depression may also be related to the degree of cognitive impairment.

Neuropsychologists must be aware of the prevalence of depression in the elderly, because depression in the elderly may result in cognitive impairments that are similar to those associated with dementia. Unlike the case in dementia, these cognitive deficits appear to be reversible when the depression is treated (Sweeney et al., 2000). Therefore, neuropsychologists who suspect dementia in elderly clients should be sensitive to their clients' moods to rule out depression as a possible confounding factor.

Imaging studies of depressed individuals suggest that there are abnormally high levels of activity in the limbic system, especially the amygdala (Drevets, Price, Bardgett, Relch, Todd, & Raichler, 2002). It may be that abnormal levels of activity in the amygdala relate to the depressed emotional state. Depressed individuals also appear to have abnormal activity in the dorsal prefrontal cortex and anterior cingulate, which may account for the cognitive deficits that are associated with depression, because these areas are thought to be involved in attention and memory (Drevets et al., 2002).

BIPOLAR DISORDER. **Bipolar disorder** is also known as *manic-depressive disorder,* although the correct term is *bipolar disorder.* Bipolar disorder is characterized by periods of depressed mood (persisting sadness) followed by periods of mania (elevated mood and activity). The lifetime risk for bipolar disorder is 1% for severe cases and 2–3% for milder cases, which translates to about 5–7 million Americans who are affected with this disorder (American Psychological Association, 1994). Bipolar disorder can be distinguished from depression by the presence of mania, which may persist for durations ranging from hours to months. Associated with mania are changes in mood (excessively elevated or irritated moods), increased distractibility, high levels of risk taking, an increased tendency to talk, and a decreased need for sleep. Theories regarding the biological basis of bipolar disorder focus on abnormalities in neurotransmitters and on genetic factors. However, it is clear that bipolar disorder and major depressive disorder are separate syndromes that have different patterns of inheritance.

Unlike the case with depression, an examination of the drugs that alleviate the symptoms of bipolar disorder does not provide clear-cut insights into the neurotransmitter systems that may cause this disorder. Lithium is historically the drug of choice for treating the manic portion of bipolar disorder. Although the means by which lithium works is unknown, it is thought that lithium's antidepressive effects may relate to its ability to block presynaptic serotonin receptors (Shaldubina, Agam, & Belmaker, 2001). Furthermore, it appears that bipolar disorder may relate to abnormalities in a number of neurotransmitters, including GABA and serotonin (Benes & Berretta, 2001; Craddock, Dave, & Greening, 2001; Shaldubina et al., 2001; Shiah & Yatham, 2000). There may be inherited differences in the receptors for these neurotransmitters, which may account for the observation that bipolar disorder is familial (Craddock et al., 2001; Jones & Craddock, 2001).

Imaging studies of individuals with bipolar disorder suggest that there may be abnormalities in the frontal and temporal lobes, cingulate cortex, and basal ganglia (Blumberg et al., 2000). For instance, when affected individuals are asked to distinguish emotions in others, there is abnormally high activity in the limbic system, especially the amygdala, and abnormally low activity in the prefrontal cortex (Yurgelun-Todd, Gruber, Kanayama, Killgore, Baird, & Young, 2000). It may be that these differences in activity levels relate to the abnormal emotional state and cognitive deficits that are associated with bipolar disorder. Others have reported that there are abnormalities in the axonal connections between the frontal lobes and basal ganglia, decreases in cerebellar size, and microscopic anatomical abnormalities in the midbrain and brainstem (Baumann & Bogerts, 2001; Stoll, Renshaw, Yurgelun-Todd, & Cohen, 2000; Strakowski, DelBello, Adler, Cecil, & Sax, 2000). Needless to say, much more research needs to be done before a clear picture of the neural changes associated with bipolar disorder are known.

Not surprisingly, there are conflicting reports as to whether or not bipolar disorder is associated with cognitive deficits. Some have reported that bipolar disorder is associated with deficits in executive function, motor skills, and memory. For instance, Sweeney and colleagues (2000) reported cognitive declines in individuals with either major depression or bipolar disorder. However, the decline in cognitive function was more severe in individuals with bipolar disorder than was observed in individuals with major depression. These researchers suggest that this pattern of cognitive deficits is consistent with dysfunction in the frontal and temporal lobes. However, others have failed to find significant cognitive impairments associated with bipolar disorder, suggesting that the severity of the disease may be related to the degree of cognitive impairment (Bearden, Hoffman, & Cannon, 2001).

ANXIETY DISORDERS. Experiencing bouts of anxiety (even severe anxiety) is normal, provided that the episode is provoked by some sort of stimulus. In fact, *not* experiencing instances of anxiety is abnormal. However, there are a number of anxiety disorders in which the experience of anxiety is more intense and/or longer lasting than normal. One such disorder, called **generalized anxiety disorder,** is the subjective experience of anxiety coupled with the somatic markers for anxiety in the absence of an identifiable anxiety-provoking stimulus.

Other anxiety disorders, such as **phobias,** are characterized by very similar symptoms except that the anxiety is provoked by a specific stimulus. The stimulus itself might not provoke severe anxiety in most people, but phobic individuals experience extreme emotional responses to these stimuli. For example, an agoraphobic person usually becomes anxious when in a crowd, and the anxiety might be accompanied by a panic attack or fear of fainting or losing control (Martin, 1998).

Obsessive-compulsive disorder is characterized by unwanted obsessions and recurrent behaviors accompanied by an urge to do something to relieve the discomfort caused by the obsession. Although people with obsessive-compulsive disorder realize that their obsessions are excessive and/or unreasonable, the symptoms can be overwhelming and may result in severe impairment and dysfunction.

In **posttraumatic stress disorder** (PTSD), a person who has been exposed to a traumatic event suffers from persistent reexperiencing of the event. These individuals typically take steps to avoid exposure to stimuli that remind them of the event. As with the other anxiety disorders, these symptoms can be very debilitating and can result in severe impairment and dysfunction.

It is important to remember that all of these disorders are anxiety disorders, but they are characterized by different symptoms and often appear to have different causes. According to PET and SPECT (single photon emission computed tomography) studies, the changes in brain metabolism associated with these disorders also vary with the condition. In generalized anxiety disorder, increases in frontal and temporal activation have been found. Anxiety disorders appear to be characterized by decreases in activation for these same regions, along with decreases in occipital activity compared to individuals without panic disorder. In obsessive-compulsive disorder, there is decreased metabolism in the orbitofrontal cortex, caudate nucleus and anterior cingulate gyrus, thalamus, parietal cortex, and basal ganglia.

Recently, a number of imaging studies (PET, fMRI, MRI) examining the neural bases of individuals who are experiencing PTSD have appeared in the literature. Studies of individuals with PTSD have reported that affected individuals may have reduced hippocampal volumes, increased activity in the amygdala, and decreased activity in Broca's area (e.g., Hull, 2002; Villarreal, Hamilton, et al., 2002; Villarreal, Petropoulos, 2002). Other researchers have observed that the induction of a dissociative state, a hallmark symptom of PTSD, was associated with increased limbic and prefrontal activation (Lanius et al., 2002). For people who experience flashbacks as a result of PTSD, changes in cortical/subcortical and right caudate nucleus, limbic, paralimbic, and visual area rCBF ratios have been reported (Kugu & Bolayir, 2001). Finally, an interesting study by Lanius and colleagues has found that the brains of individuals who were abused as children but did not develop PTSD differed from individuals who were abused as children and developed PTSD (Lanius et al., 2003). Specifically, when participants were exposed to emotionally provocative stimuli, participants who had PTSD exhibited significantly less cingulate and thalamic activity than did the participants who did not have PTSD. This study suggests that PTSD may be responsible for the changes in neural functions observed in these studies, rather than the person's experiences leading to PTSD (Lanius et al., 2003). Because this study is quasi-experimental, it is possible that individuals with lower thalamic or cingulate activity are at greater risk for developing PTSD.

Most anxiety disorders are treated with antianxiety drugs called **anxiolytics.** The most commonly prescribed anxiolytics are benzodiazepines, such as diazepam (Valium) or chlordiazepoxide (Librium) (Hood, Argyropoulos, & Nutt, 2000). These drugs are relatively effective in alleviating the symptoms of many anxiety disorders, and they have few side effects. Unfortunately, the brain becomes tolerant to these drugs relatively quickly (in about four weeks), so the compounds can be used to help manage symptoms over short periods of time, but they are less useful for long-term management of anxiety disorders (Hood et al., 2000; Isojaervi & Tokola, 1998). Other compounds such as antidepressant drugs (which are less vulnerable to tolerance) have proven effective in treating some specific anxiety disorders, such as generalized anxiety disorder or various phobias (Bourin, Chue, & Guillon, 2001; van der Linden, Stein, & van Balkom, 2000). In addition to medications that are normally prescribed, there is one extremely commonly used anxiolytic that is available without a prescription: alcohol. It is the most used and abused psychoactive substance in the world, in part because of its anxiolytic effect, in part because it is vulnerable to the development of tolerance, and in part because it is addictive. All of these anxiolytics can be effective in treating

1. What are the two types of prosody? How do they differ?

2. How is aprosodia like aphasia?

3. What are the symptoms of Klüver–Bucy syndrome? What sort of brain damage is necessary to produce the syndrome in monkeys? What sort of brain damage is necessary to produce the syndrome in humans?

4. What are the clinical features of major depression? How is the condition treated?

5. What is generalized anxiety disorder? What metabolic changes in the brain are associated with the disorder?

the symptoms of anxiety disorders, at least in the short run, but they tend to be devoid of long-term benefits. These disorders are best treated by combining pharmacotherapy with other therapeutic techniques.

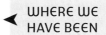 **WHERE WE HAVE BEEN**

In this module, we examined disturbances in emotional processing. Following right hemisphere damage, both the perception and production of emotion in language (prosody) and facial expressions can be impaired. Klüver–Bucy syndrome has been

the **Real** world

The Brain of a Psychopath

A **psychopath** is an individual whose behavioral patterns—specifically, the level of compassion, empathy, and guilt—appear to differ significantly from those of the general population (Bartol, 1999). This disorder is estimated to affect one out of 100 people in the general population and 15–25% of people in prison (Hare, 1991; Kiehl et al., 2001). The device that is used to measure psychopathy is called the Psychopathy Checklist–Revised (PCL-R), which was developed by University of British Columbia researcher Robert Hare. Hare's PCL-R is conducted through a highly structured interview process that is carried out by a highly trained examiner. Some of the key characteristics that are marked by the PCL-R include shallow affect, impulsivity, and glibness/superficial charm (Hare, 1991).

Because of recent advances in neuroimaging techniques, it is now possible to attain a greater understanding of the mind of individuals who exhibit psychopathy. In fact, there is evidence to suggest that physiologically, people with psychopathy have neurological differences compared to neurologically normal controls. In a structural MRI study, for example, individuals with antisocial personality disorder, a much broader term that includes psychopathy (Alison, 2001), have reduced prefrontal gray matter volume and reduced autonomic activity (Raine, Lencz, Bihrle, LaCasse, & Colletti, 2000). This deficit in the prefrontal cortex may be the mechanism that causes many of the marked behavioral features of psychopathy, such as lack of conscience and poor fear conditioning (Raine et al., 2000).

Blair and colleagues (Blair, Morris, Frith, Pervett, & Dolan, 1999) found that increasing the intensity of sad facial expressions resulted in greater activity in the left amygdala. Because previous research had shown that there is a reduced level of responsiveness to sad expressions in psychopaths, whereby amygdala dysfunction has been demonstrated, this study draws support for abnormal amygdala functioning in the psychopath population.

Kiehl and colleagues (2001) found that criminal psychopaths showed abnormal functioning in limbic and frontal cortex regions while viewing affective stimuli when compared to criminal nonpsychopaths and controls. Specifically, Kiehl and colleagues (2001) found that there was less activity of the amygdala/hippocampal formation, parahippocampal gyrus, ventral striatum, and anterior and posterior cingulate gyri and overactivation of the frontal temporal cortex. This evidence suggests that when viewing emotive stimuli, psychopaths demonstrate abnormal and even nonlimbic strategies to process emotional information.

This piece was contributed by Brent M. Robinson.

studied in detail in monkeys; there have been a couple of cases of humans who exhibit a similar syndrome. Unlike the case for lower primates, bilateral amygdala damage alone does not appear to produce these symptoms in humans. Mood disorders such as major depressive disorder, biopolar disorder, and generalized anxiety disorder are associated with a variety of subcortical and cortical abnormalities in metabolism. Currently, the best treatment for these disorders appears to be pharmacotherapy coupled with other forms of therapy.

Glossary

Affective prosody—Prosody that is related to the emotional content of the words (e.g., "I really like carrots" can mean that you enjoy them or you hate them, depending on how you emphasize the word *like*).

Anxiolytics—Antianxiety drugs. The most commonly prescribed anxiolytics are benzodiazepines.

Appraisal theory—Emotional states are the process of cost–benefit analysis of situations. Physiological reactions (emotions) are the product of unconscious evaluation of the situations that is based on the potential for the organism to either benefit from or be damaged by the situation. Cognitive components of the emotional state (feelings) are produced when an individual consciously examines the unconscious appraisal.

Aprosodia—People who suffer right hemisphere damage often display deficits in prosodic processing.

Audio spectrogram—A device that measures the amount of pitch variance in the person's speech.

Bipolar disorder—A disorder that is characterized by periods of mania (elevated mood and activity) followed by periods of depressed mood (persisting sadness).

Cannon–Bard theory—Emotionally provocative stimuli evoke both physiological and cognitive aspects of emotion simultaneously. Although the cognitive and physiological aspects of emotional states occur simultaneously in most individuals, it is possible for these components of emotional states to be dissociated.

Emotional state—Refers to the combination of emotions with feelings.

Emotions—The physical sensations of emotion.

Feelings—The cognitive experience of emotion.

Generalized anxiety disorder—The subjective experience of anxiety coupled with the somatic markers for anxiety in the absence of an identifiable anxiety-provoking stimulus.

Hypermetamorphosis—The strong tendency to react to every visual stimulus, characteristic of individuals with Klüver–Bucy syndrome.

James–Lange theory—Emotionally provocative stimuli automatically and unconsciously evoke physiological responses, which are monitored by the individual. The conscious experience of the emotional state is secondary to the unconscious response to the stimulus, which then evoke a specific feeling.

Major depressive disorder—A disorder that is characterized by long-lasting periods of depressed mood (persisting sadness), lack of interest, and the lack of ability to feel pleasure.

Motor aprosodia—Aprosodia occurring following damage to the middle cerebral artery of the right hemisphere in which people lose their ability to produce prosodic speech despite being able to recognize affective prosody and propositional prosody in others.

Obsessive-compulsive disorder—An anxiety disorder that is characterized by unwanted obsessions and recurrent behaviors accompanied by an urge to do something to relieve the discomfort caused by the obsession.

Phobias—An anxiety disorder that is characterized by symptoms similar to those of generalized anxiety disorder except that in a phobia, the anxiety is provoked by a specific stimulus.

Posttraumatic stress disorder—An anxiety disorder in which a person who has been exposed to a traumatic event suffers from persistent reexperiencing of the event and typically takes steps to avoid exposure to stimuli that remind the person of the event.

Propositional prosody—Prosody related to the meaning of the words (e.g., "Is that so?" said with an elevation of tone at the end is indicative of a question).

Prosody—Components of verbal communication (pitch, rhythm/duration, and stress of the speech) that affect meaning and inform the listener about the meaning of speech independent of the words spoken.

Psychopath—An individual whose levels of compassion, empathy, and guilt appear to be significantly lower those of the general population.

Schachter–Singer theory—When an individual experiences physiological arousal in a situation (emotion),

the cognitive components (feelings) of the emotional state are congruent with the cognitive appraisal of the situation.

Sensory aprosodia—The inability to understand the prosody of others coupled with the retained ability to produce it.

Somatic marker theory—Somatic marker theory suggests that the relationship between a stimulus and the emotional state produced by the stimulus can be a product of implicit learning. The association between emotional state and bodily change is the somatic marker, which provides us with a means by which our brain evaluates novel situations on the basis of previous experience.

10 Spatial Ability

Space, the final frontier.
—CAPTAIN JAMES T. KIRK

MODULE **10.1**
Spatial Ability

As you are sitting here reading this chapter, take notice of your surroundings. Maybe you are reading this book in your room. If so, perhaps you have a soft drink, a high-lighter, and some paper within reach. If you expand your awareness of your surroundings beyond what you can pick up easily, you might notice that the room also contains a television or a stereo, along with your bed or a chair, and some pictures on the wall. Now expand your awareness of your environment farther. Can you imagine where you are on your street or in your city or town? Now reach out and pick up your pen or highlighter. Did you have to think about where your pen was, or did you simply make the correct computation? These exercises all require your brain to process spatial information, and this chapter deals with how your brain accomplishes this task.

What Is Spatial Ability?

Put simply, all objects occupy space. When we process the position, direction, or movement of objects or points in space, we are using some form of **spatial ability.** When we notice the orientation of an object—for example, whether the handle of a mug is facing toward us or away from us—we are using spatial ability. When we look at a shoe and decide whether it is for the right or the left foot, we are using spatial ability. You may have noticed that many of these tasks incorporate other functions that were discussed in other chapters. In fact, many functions that are included in this chapter also appear in the chapters about memory, motor function, and sensory abilities.

Space is a multifaceted construct that includes both *real* space (what you can sense right now) and *imagined* space (space that you can think about even though you cannot directly experience it right now). Many people have tried to define spatial ability, and at last count, it was thought to have at least six discrete basic components. When a statistical technique known as factor analysis is used, it appears that spatial ability is made up of a number of individual skills that correspond quite nicely to the variety of ways in which we interact with space (Linn & Petersen, 1985). These six skills are *targeting,* or how well you can throw an object at a target; *spatial orientation,* or how well you can recognize items even when they are placed in different orientations, or directions; *spatial location memory,* or how well you can remember the location of objects; *spatial visualization,* or how well you can imagine how well pieces of an object would go together; *disembedding,* or how well you can find figures that are hidden within other pictures; and *spatial perception,* or how well you can determine where horizontal or vertical is in the real world even if you are given distracting information. However, as you will discover later in this chapter, spatial ability can also be more complex and can involve both real and imagined features.

Hemispheric Representation of Space

The commonly held belief that the left hemisphere of the brain is specialized for language processing and the right hemisphere is specialized for spatial processing has its roots in a paper published by Hughlings-Jackson in 1874, entitled "On the Nature of the Duality of the Brain" (Jackson, 1931). As we will see, although there is much evidence that supports this position, there are certainly exceptions, in which lesions to the left hemisphere or bilateral damage results in difficulties with spatial perception.

Perhaps the most basic spatial ability is the ability to localize a point in space (Figure 10.1). To localize a point in space, we need to know where the point is absolutely and the relative position of that point. That is, to know whether the point occupies the same location as another point requires depth perception. Research has found that neurologically normal people can identify the location of a dot more readily when it occurs in the left visual field (Kimura, 1969). Recall that for vision, information that is presented to the left visual field is projected to the right hemisphere. Researchers interpret the left visual field advantage for dot location as being indicative of superiority of the right hemisphere for processing spatial location. Studies using PET imaging have also found that the right hemisphere (especially the right prefrontal cortex) appears to be involved with the recall of spatial location information (Jonides, Smith, Koeppe, Awh, Minorhima, & Mintun, 1993).

The ability to determine relative position of an object, or **depth perception,** is another very basic spatial ability. Typically, depth perception is divided into two types: local and global. **Local depth perception** is the ability to use detailed features of objects point by point to assess relative position. For instance, in looking at this page, you might look at the relative position of these words with the corners of the book to determine which corner of the book was closer to you. In contrast, **global depth perception** is the ability to use the difference between the information reaching each

Figure 10.1   Test of One's Ability to Localize a Point in Space

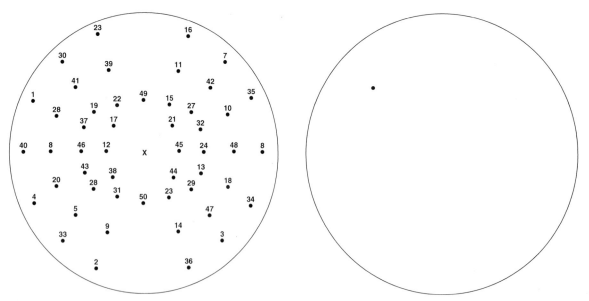

Which number corresponds to the point located within the circle on the right?

eye to compute the entire visual scene. If you have ever tried Magic Eye pictures (random dot stereograms), then you have performed a task that requires global depth perception (Figure 10.2). A very simplified explanation of how these pictures produce what appear to be three-dimensional images is that your brain computes the differences in the images presented to the two eyes and fuses these images to produce depth. Because there are no obvious features in these pictures, local depth perception cues cannot be responsible for this effect. As was the case with dot location, the right hemisphere is also better at determining global depth perception (Carmon & Bechtoldt, 1969). However, local depth perception is not as simple; the determination of which object is in front of another shows a left visual field advantage in normals (Durnford & Kimura, 1971), whereas both right and left hemisphere lesions disrupt local depth perception (Danta, Hiton, & O'Boyle, 1978).

Related to localizing points is the ability to localize a line and to identify its orientation. Many tasks in our daily lives require that we accurately identify **line orientation** (e.g., being able to differentiate between the letters *d* and *p*). Researchers have found that there is a right hemisphere advantage for both tactile and visual assessment of line orientation (Deutsch, Bourbon, Papanicolaou, & Eisenberg, 1988; Zoccolotti, Passafiume, & Pizzamiglio, 1979). However, if the lines can be described verbally, such as "the horizontal line" or "the vertical line," then often a left hemisphere advantage emerges. This illustrates an important point in testing all types of

Figure 10.2   **Random Dot Stereogram**

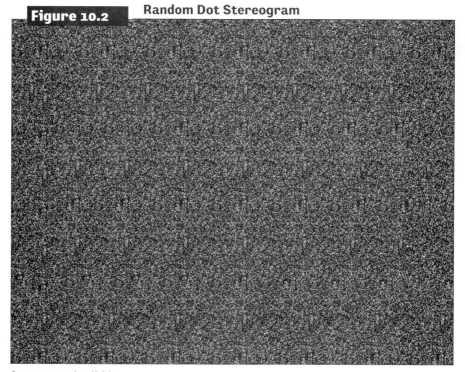

Can you see the disk?

cognitive abilities. Often a task that is supposed to be measuring only one type of ability may actually be measuring other different abilities as well.

However, most of what we do in the world is more complex than simply judging the relative position of a line or its orientation. Often, we have to determine the spatial relationship between the points on the line, lines, or objects. Determinations of the spatial relationships between objects may rely on the ability to determine whether or not an item shares spatial properties with another (the **object geometry**), but it also relies on the ability to reconstruct previously viewed items. Investigations of the spatial properties of items have tended to focus on judgments of similarity between curved lines (e.g., Franco & Sperry, 1977; Longden, Ellis, & Iversen, 1976) and have found that there is a right hemisphere advantage for these types of judgments when using either visual or tactile modalities. The ability to reconstruct previously viewed items tends to rely on having people reconstruct complex, novel figures from memory. A number of researchers have found that decisions regarding whether or not a complex novel figure had been viewed previously were more accurate when the figure was presented in the left visual field. This suggests that as in other spatial abilities, the right hemisphere is superior at this task (e.g., Fontenot, 1973; Umilta, Bagnara, & Simion, 1978).

What happens when objects move? Our world is far from the static types of comparisons that we considered in the previous paragraphs. When objects move, some parts of the object that were visible are obscured whereas some parts of the object that were obscured are now visible. We routinely and rapidly track and identify moving objects. Thus, our ability to identify a moving object must relate to our ability to track an object and to identify that object when it is rotated. Tracking an object also relates to our ability to determine where an object is currently and where it will be momentarily. As such, motion detection and prediction of trajectory are fundamental and complex spatial abilities. Much of what is known about motion detection comes from experiments with monkeys, although recent studies using fMRI techniques have been able to confirm that similar areas are involved in humans. Specifically, it appears that in humans, the detection of motion is related to increased activity in the right hemisphere, particularly in occipital, temporal, and parietal areas associated with the processing of visual information (Cornette et al., 1998; Grossman et al., 2000; Shulman et al., 1999).

Position your hand with your palm facing you, and rotate it slowly so that your palm is facing away from you. Notice how the image of your hand that your brain is processing is changing but that you never fail to recognize your hand. Although the rotation of your hand is a simple demonstration of the factors that are involved in rotation, the same event occurs in many of our daily lives; for example, most of us leave home every day by driving or walking in one direction and return home by traveling in the opposite direction. We are rarely startled on the return trip by viewing the street in a different orientation (although it is only ourselves that have been rotated, not our neighborhood). Rotation that does not occur overtly (such as the rotation of your hand in front of you) is often referred to as **mental rotation**. In these tasks, participants are often required to look at two items and decide if they are the same or if they are different (see Figure 7.6 in the chapter on memory to refresh your own memory about this task). A number of researchers have found that mental rotation abilities rely on the right hemisphere (e.g., Ratcliff, 1979), as measured by enhanced accuracy in the left visual field (Burton, Wagner, Lim, & Levy, 1992) or tasks of mental rotation that result in greater activation of the right hemisphere (Deutsch et al., 1988).

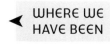

The preceding paragraphs dealt with definitions of spatial ability, the basic components of spatial ability, and evidence that supports the notion that the right hemisphere is specialized for utilizing spatial information.

The following sections will examine the specific areas of the brain that appear to be involved in processing spatial information, with respect to more complex spatial tasks, and with what happens when parts of the brain that mediate spatial ability are damaged.

Parietal Lobes

As you learned in Chapter 6, the brain processes visual information in a very systematic fashion. Visual information is received in the primary visual area of the brain (area V1 of the occipital lobe or striate cortex) and is transferred to other areas of the occipital lobe (over twenty-five different extrastriate areas at last count). As you recall from Chapter 6, the visual system is hierarchically organized, with each of the extrastriate areas performing a specific function, such as analyzing the spatial frequency or retinal disparity of the visual information. Remember that most of the information passes up the hierarchy for further analysis and that most systems in the brain communicate extensively with other, related parts of the brain. It is important to remember that most functions in the brain are integrative and that they rely on the performance of multiple areas.

Beyond the occipital lobes, the information appears to be divided into the complementary dorsal and ventral streams. If the **ventral visual stream** is considered the "what" pathway useful for identifying objects, then the **dorsal visual stream** can be considered the "how" pathway. One role of the dorsal stream is to know how motor acts must be performed to manipulate an object (Goodale et al., 1991). To use our example from the beginning of the chapter, when you pick up a pen, you must know how to position your hand and fingers and how fast to move your hand toward the object as well as the location of the pen. It is the dorsal stream that supports spatial processing of information, and projects from the primary visual areas to parietal regions (Figure 10.3).

Figure 10.3 ——— **Visual Information Pathways**

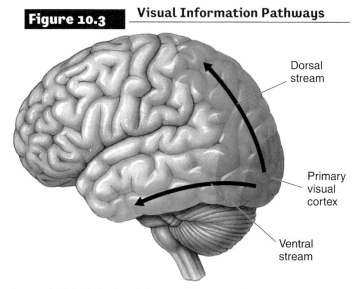

Source: John P. J. Pinel, *Biopsychology,* 5e. Published by Allyn and Bacon, Boston, MA. Copyright © 2003 by Pearson Education. Reprinted by permission of the publisher.

The dorsal stream receives information that makes it well suited to process this type of spatial information. The properties of the cells within parietal areas 5 and 7 are sensitive to certain attributes that allow stable cognitive maps to be made. Importantly, the cells within areas 5 and 7 do not receive much information about the color of the object or the fine details of the object, which would be needed to identify the object. Rather, cells in areas 5 and 7 seem to respond to movements that occur in specific directions, allowing objects to be tracked in space. The speed of the movement is also critical, and areas 5 and 7 respond the best to movements that are similar in speed to either walking or running (e.g., Motter & Mountcastle, 1981). Sensitivity to movement and speed allows area 7 to analyze space, and update positions of objects in space. When these two factors are combined with the ability of areas 5 and 7 to integrate large areas of ipsilateral and contralateral space, we can see that areas 5 and 7 are able to generate a stable spatial map of the world (Motter & Mountcastle, 1981). That is, the cells in the inferior parietal region are sensitive to retinotopic representations of space as well as head position, movement, and the speed of the movement. Areas 5 and 7 integrate quite a number of the pieces of information that are required for you to pick up your pen!

The role that these regions play in spatial processing has been studied by using the lesion method. When these parietal regions are lesioned in monkeys, there are some striking deficits in spatial ability. Monkeys with parietal lobe lesions appear to be quite impaired at computing spatial relations among objects. That is, if monkeys are required to pick an object (a cup) according to whether or not it is closer to another object (a tower), monkeys with parietal lobe lesions cannot learn this rule very well (Mishkin, Ungerleider, & Macko, 1983), although they can learn to pick an object consistently. Studies in humans confirm that our brains work similarly (Haxby, Horowitz, Underleider, Maisog, Pietrini, & Grady, 1994; Mellet, Tzourio, Crivello, Joliot, Denis, & Mazoyer, 1996). It appears that when we are asked to discriminate either form or spatial location, different parts of our brains are active. Discrimination of form involves the ventral stream, whereas discrimination of spatial location involves the dorsal stream. Consistent with the laterality experiments, Haxby and colleagues (1994) observed that there was greater activation in the right parietal lobes when participants were asked to perform tasks that required the processing of spatial location.

It appears that some cells in the parietal lobe are sensitive to the visual qualities of the object, such as texture, and further influence how the hands manipulate an object. Think about how you would pick up a real apple versus a similarly shaped object that was made of Jell-O. The difference in how you would shape your hands to pick up these two objects is most likely mediated by these cells in the parietal lobe.

Thus, it appears that the properties of the dorsal stream of the parietal lobe are well suited to processing information about how to interact with objects and where they are in space. Although we have some convincing evidence to suggest that the parietal lobes are involved with processing the spatial locations of the object, how does the dorsal stream direct movement to an object? As we will discuss in the next section, it is the reciprocal connections of the parietal lobes with the frontal lobes that make the dorsal stream important for coordinating movements with the spatial locations of objects.

Frontal Lobes

There is also a system of parietal cells that project to areas of the frontal lobes, to both the premotor and prefrontal cortex. These frontal areas receive massive inputs from somatosensory, auditory, and visual association areas of the parietal lobes. The function of this system is somewhat unclear, although the associative nature of the inputs to this system suggests that one of the functions is to provide an accurate coordinate system of visual space and to locate objects in space. Neurons in the posterior parietal cortex respond to stimuli within grasping space and project to the frontal motor system to guide movements. Within the frontal lobes, there are also nuclei that are responsible for directing head and eye movements toward stimuli in grasping space. These nuclei communicate extensively with the parietal lobes, further enhancing our ability to program motor movements aimed at reaching and grasping objects in space.

In one study, participants were asked to think about constructing a three-dimensional object (e.g., think about a red block, on the left side of the red block put a blue block, on top of the blue block put a green block, etc.) while they were undergoing an fMRI scan. This resulted in predictable activation of the dorsal stream in the parietal lobe (Mellet et al., 1996). However, activation of the dorsal premotor cortex in the frontal lobe was also observed. This task relies on short-term visuospatial memory, also known as visuospatial working memory. A number of studies have suggested that it is visuospatial working memory that is reflected by the activation of the dorsal premotor cortex. This type of research was performed primarily on monkeys (Watanabe, 1996, 1998), although recently some studies using fMRI on human patients with lesions to the dorsolateral prefrontal cortex have confirmed a role for the dorsal premotor cortex in visuospatial working memory (Carlson, Martinkauppi, Rama, Salli, Korvenoja, & Aronen, 1998; Ferreira, Verin, Pillon, Levy, Dubois, & Agid, 1998; Garavan, Kelley, Rosen, Rao, & Stein, 2000; Owen, 2000; Pollmann & von Cramon, 2000). All of these studies also found parietal lobe activation, along with activation in other, more lateral frontal areas, including the inferior, middle, and precentral gyri and the superior frontal sulcus. Again, it is important to emphasize that there was also activation within the motor areas of the frontal lobes, particularly those that are involved in moving the head, such as the frontal eye fields and the presupplementary motor area. This appears to reflect potential planning of motor movements that would be required if the imagined task were real. This is particularly evident in the patients with dorsolateral prefrontal lesions, who were the most impaired when visuospatial working memory was required to guide their motor responses. Thus, it appears that the performance of visuospatial working memory tasks engage the dorsal stream, along with its connections to the frontal lobe.

Temporal Lobes

As we mentioned earlier, visual information appears to be segregated into the complementary dorsal and ventral streams. There is a lot of evidence to suggest that the dorsal stream is involved with identifying where an object is in space and guiding motor movements. Conversely, there is evidence to suggest that the ventral stream is involved in the identifying of the object, that is, in deciding what the object is. As the ventral stream radiates from the occipital lobes to the temporal lobes, you might be tempted to conclude that the ventral stream is not very important in spatial ability. This conclusion, as we are going to learn, is incorrect.

A number of the studies that implicated the parietal and frontal lobes as playing a role in spatial localization of objects have also found that these tasks resulted in an increase in activity in the temporal lobes. Because much of this research was performed on normal human participants, some of this activation can be attributed to the role that the ventral stream and the temporal lobes play in the naming of objects. As you can imagine, it is very difficult to look at an object and decide on its position without naming it as well. However, not all of the activation within the temporal lobes can be attributed to its facility with naming objects. It appears that the temporal lobes, specifically the hippocampal formation, are also involved in tasks that require spatial learning.

As we saw in Chapter 7, the hippocampal formation plays a major role in tasks of explicit memory. The hippocampal formation is located within the temporal lobes and includes the dentate gyrus, the specific areas of the hippocampus itself, and the subiculum. The hippocampus receives information from the entorhinal cortex, which in turn receives major inputs from the various cortical association areas. Therefore, the hippocampus is well placed to integrate information from a variety of cortical and subcortical areas.

The hippocampus appears to engage in processing memory for places, such as how to get to your home or the location of your next class. We know this because studies with nonhuman animals and studies with humans have all shown that damage to the hippocampal formation results in an inability to form new memories for places. (However, memories for places that were formed before the damage appear to be unaffected.) A number of studies using rats have shown that rats with hippocampal lesions are unable to remember important locations (e.g., Morris, Gertrud, Rawlins, & O'Keefe, 1982). Similarly, people with hippocampal lesions have great difficulty in utilizing spatial information to produce memories about location (Squire, 1992). O'Keefe and Dostrovsky (1971), along with other researchers, have observed that cells within the hippocampus respond when the rat is moving through space. These cells, called place cells, respond in a very precise fashion, in that some cells respond only to certain locations and other cells respond only to other locations. For example, when a rat is placed in an unfamiliar environment, none of the place cells responds. As the rat becomes more familiar with the environment, a place cell will begin to respond preferentially to specific locations within the environment. Thus, it appears that cells within the hippocampus respond preferentially and selectively to spatial locations, and it may be that these cells form the basis of the hippocampus to form memories about space.

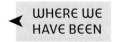

◄ WHERE WE HAVE BEEN The previous sections examined the specific areas of the brain that are important for the processing of spatial information.

WHERE WE ARE GOING ► Tasks that are performed in different parts of space appear to involve different brain areas. Using evidence involving both the normally functioning brain and injured brains, we will discuss these dissociations in the following sections.

When we interact with the spatial locations of objects, we can utilize three types of information about the object, typically referred to as position, cue, and place responses. **Position responses** are those that are made with movements using the body as a referent. Position responses do not need any cues that are external to the body, and they are relatively automatic. **Cued responses** are the types of movements that are guided by a cue. For instance, move your face toward the book, stopping just before you touch the book with your nose. As your face approaches the book, the image that the book presents on your retina becomes larger. The speed with which the image grows (optic flow) guides your movement and stops you just before your nose touches this page. Cued responses are also guided by changes in how we perceive the stimulus. Thus, cued responses rely on the perception of information that is external to your body. **Place responses** are the responses that you make toward a particular location or object. An example of a place response is if you were to point toward the nearest store. It is likely that you cannot see a store from where you are reading this book. Thus, an important feature of place responses is that they can be made when the stimulus is not currently present. Another important feature of place responses is that they tend to be relational. Notice that you were asked to point to the nearest store, not just any store. For you to do this accurately, you needed to compute your present location and determine which store was the closest.

When examining position, cue, and place responses, you can differentiate among them with respect to how your body is used. Position responses require only information about your body, cue responses require information that compares your body with another object, and place responses may use knowledge that you gained about the environment previously. Many people classify these types of space as either intrapersonal or extrapersonal. Typically, **intrapersonal space** is the space immediately around your body, including your body, whereas **extrapersonal space** is the space more than 5 feet away from you (Figure 10.4).

Personal Representations of Space

In the first paragraph of the chapter, we asked you to reach for your pen. When you did so, your brain computed the distance between your hand and the location of the pen. It also computed how to shape your hand so that you would be able to grasp the pen. Most likely, you did not bang your hand into the table, miss the pen, or find out that the pen was much larger or smaller than you thought it was. Most of the computations that your brain performed while you were picking up the pen relied on your brain's knowledge of your intrapersonal space. That is, the space that your body occupies and/or is within arm's reach of your body. As we have discussed, it appears that the dorsal stream, collaborating the activity of the parietal and frontal lobes, performs controlling movements directed at personal space.

Some examples of spatial abilities that can be performed in intrapersonal space include position responses. Position responses are performed in intrapersonal space, because they require the monitoring of space with respect to body position. One test of spatial ability that can rely on knowledge of intrapersonal space is known as the Acredolo test (Acredolo, 1976). In this test, a participant is seated at a chair in a room with a table, a window, and a door. The participant is blindfolded and then walks

Figure 10.4 | Difference between Intrapersonal and Extrapersonal Space

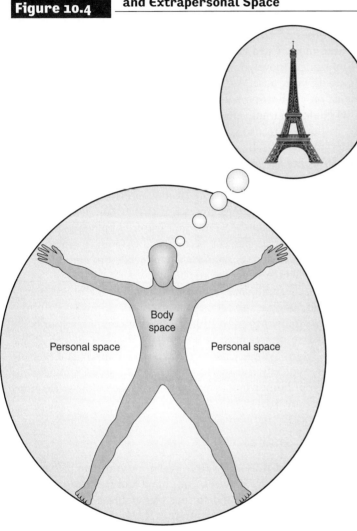

Extrapersonal space

Personal space includes the space that your body occupies and the space that is easily reached. Extrapersonal space is the space that extends five feet or more past your body.

Source: Reprinted by permission of Paul Janzen.

around the room. Without the participant's knowledge, the desk and chair are moved across the room while the participant is navigating blindfolded. When the blindfold is removed, the participant is asked to return to his or her original position. A position location would be one in which the participant used the information received from his or her body while the participant was navigating blindly. For example, if the person had turned right, walked 3 meters, and then turned left and walked 3 meters, a person making a position response to return to the original position would turn completely around, walk 3 meters, turn right, and walk 3 meters and turn left (Figure 10.5). As you can see, a position response is made only by monitoring the information that the participant received from his or her body.

Extrapersonal Space

In the first paragraph of the chapter, we asked you to imagine your location in your city or town. When you did so, your brain placed your current position within its knowledge of your city. These computations relied on your brain's knowledge of extrapersonal space, that is, the space that extends beyond what you could easily reach with your arms. Many people define extrapersonal space as the area beyond arm's reach or more than five feet from your body. Many of the basic spatial abilities that were discussed at the beginning of the chapter are performed in extrapersonal space. These abilities can include targeting, spatial orientation, spatial location memory, and navigational tasks including both place and cued responses.

To extend the example of the Acredolo test, a participant making a cued response would walk toward the desk and the chair (and in this case would be incorrect be-

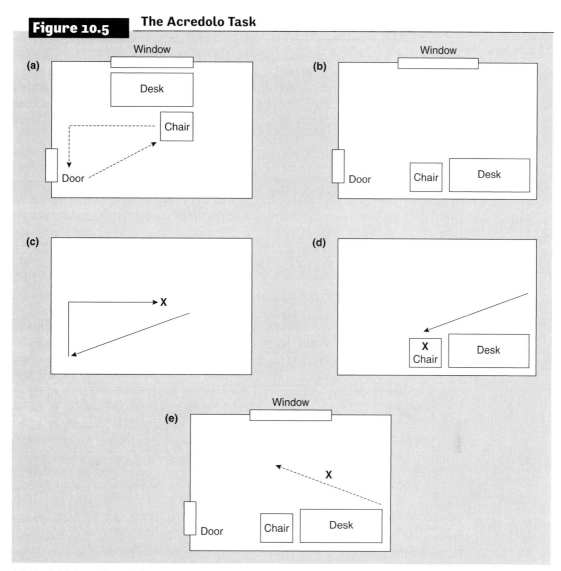

| **Figure 10.5** | **The Acredolo Task** |

(A) The initial position of objects within the room. The dotted lines indicate the path taken by the participant when blindfolded. (B) The final position of the objects within the room. (Note the desk and chair have changed locations, although the door and the window have remained constant.) (C) A position response, with the final position marked by an X. (D) A cued response, with the final position marked by an X. (E) A place response, with the final position marked by an X.

cause both the desk and the chair had been moved). Depending on the size of the room, a cued response could take place in either intrapersonal space or extrapersonal space. (How many times have you set something down on your desk, only to realize that you cannot find it minutes later?) In the same test, a participant making a place response would study the position of the desk with respect to the position of the door and the window (which did not move). A person making a place response would be able to notice the movement of the desk and the chair, compensate for these changes in the environment, and return to the correct original position.

Most studies of extrapersonal spatial abilities require the participant to navigate through the environment, often through mazes of some sort. There are a number of types of mazes that are used to study spatial abilities in nonhuman animals. One of the most common is the water maze, which is a circular pool that is filled with milky water, with a platform submerged just below the surface of the water (Morris et al., 1982). There are typically no identifying features within the pool or the water (both are white). Consequently, to find the hidden platform and get out of the pool, the animal must learn the spatial relationship between objects in the room that are outside of the pool. Unlesioned rats can learn this task very quickly and tend to swim directly toward the hidden platform. However, rats with hippocampal lesions do not learn where the hidden platform is located. Notice that if the platform were placed above the level of the water, solution of the water maze task would rely on a cued response. Both unlesioned and hippocampally lesioned rats can solve the cued version of the water maze task.

A series of intriguing and inventive studies have been performed to examine the role of the hippocampus in spatial cognition in humans. For instance, one study examined how people performed in a virtual water maze (Astur, Ortiz, & Sutherland, 1998). The researchers found that people, like rats, quickly learned how to find the hidden platform. Using a different type of virtual maze (a virtual-reality computer game), Maguire and colleagues (Maguire, Frith, Burgess, Donnell, & O'Keefe, 1998) observed that people navigating in this environment had enhanced activity in the right hippocampus. In fact, greater activation of the right hippocampus was associated with better learning of the maze (fewer mistakes). Using MRI and PET scanning techniques, taxi drivers were studied while they were imagining driving a variety of routes (Maguire, Frackowiak, & Frith, 1997; Maguire et al., 2000). To do their jobs efficiently, taxi drivers must have larger cognitive maps of cities than the average person, and they must use these maps routinely. When the taxi drivers were performing imagined navigation, there was enhanced activity in the right hippocampus. Furthermore, the posterior portion of the hippocampal formation was significantly larger in the taxi drivers than those of the control group. Interestingly, the volume of the hippocampus appeared to be related to how long the participant had been a taxi driver; that is, the longer the person had been a taxi driver, the larger the person's hippocampus was. The authors suggest that this increase in hippocampal size reflects the brain's ability to change in response to the daily demands that a person places on his or her brain. Alternatively, these results could reflect that only people who have large hippocampi stay employed as taxi drivers.

Using a slightly different maze task, Whishaw and Gorny (1999) found that the hippocampal formation is implicated in a related form of spatial learning. Rats in this task were placed in the dark and were required to follow a scented string to obtain a piece of food. Once the food had been retrieved, unlesioned rats turned around and went directly to their cage, using a short cut. These short cuts are also known as **dead reckoning**, the ability to use dead reckoning demonstrates a place response, which indicates very good knowledge of the spatial configuration of the environment. Rats with lesions to the fornix, which disrupts the functioning of the hippocampus, also retrieved the food. However, they did not dead reckon; rather they followed the string back to their cages, which is a cued response. Thus, it seems that the hippocampus is essential for learning the spatial configuration of the environment or creating a map of space. The results of the experiment with the scented string also illustrate that visual information in the environment is not required for the development of the map. Because the rats navigated in the dark, they had to create their mental map using scent cues and information about the movements of their body in space.

Humans may also be able to dead reckon (Bovet, 1994; Gould, 1981; Pick & Rieser, 1982; Westby & Partridge, 1986), although this ability is somewhat controversial. For instance, it has been reported that Pulawat Islanders in Micronesia are able to undertake long ocean voyages using a cognitive map of their environment. Accounts of their navigation ability suggest that Pulawat Islanders imagine a hypothetical island just over the horizon that is off to one side from their final destination (Pick & Rieser, 1982). By keeping track of their current position, the imaginary island, stars, and the time that has passed, the Pulawat Islanders are able to successfully navigate large distances over the ocean. A number of studies investigating the ability to monitor space in undergraduate students have found conflicting results. Typically, these studies measure the participants' ability to orient toward home following a long and circuitous path. Although some studies have found that participants can accurately point toward a previously occupied space, a number of other studies have failed to replicate these results. Certainly, as is demonstrated by the Acredolo task, humans can return to the origin of very short paths. Therefore, it may be that humans can dead reckon but that dead reckoning in complex paths may be a skill that must be learned over a number of trials.

Complex navigational abilities are not restricted to mammals; a number of avian species can navigate large distances and/or perform complex spatial navigation tasks that require place responses. For instance, some bird species use the night sky and/or the position of the sun to determine their location in space. The ability to learn how to use the relational positions of the stars or to use the sun as a compass appears to rely on the hippocampal formation. Homing pigeons and chickadees have been studied extensively, and hippocampal lesions in these species severely impair these species' ability to perform navigation tasks and maze tasks and to use spatial information to guide their behavior. Even though a number of these species use visual cues to perform these tasks, as is the case with rats, other senses are important for the creation of these maps. For instance, homing pigeons can integrate odors and magnetic information within their maps. Thus, as is the case with humans and other mammals, it appears that the hippocampus is responsible for the creation of cognitive maps and for the performance of novel complex spatial tasks.

The converging evidence regarding the involvement of the hippocampus in spatial navigation tasks across species suggests that these types of behaviors may have evolved as a response to the demands of the environment. The research with avian species is particularly illustrative of this point. A number of avian species (e.g., chickadees) hide food and retrieve it later, a behavior called **caching**. Although they may live in similar environments, some other avian species (e.g., sparrows) do not cache food. When we look at the hippocampi of the birds that cache and compare them to

the **Real** world

Navigation Descriptions as Clues to Cognitive Maps

How would you describe how to get to the bookstore on your campus? By examining the descriptions of people's cognitive maps, researchers can get a glimpse of what features are important in cognitive maps (Lawton, 1994). Typically, when giving directions to unseen locations, people rely on cardinal directions (north, south, west, east); relative turns (turn right or left); distances (1 meter, 10 miles); and landmarks (the old church). However, some research suggests that men and women do not attend to the same features in the environment. That is, it appears that when men give directions, they tend to rely more on cardinal directions and distances and less on landmarks and relative turns. When women give directions, they tend to rely more on relative turns and landmarks. There is also evidence to suggest that these preferences for types of directions may relate to the strategies that men and women prefer to use when navigating. When women were asked to evaluate how they would find a place that they had never been to before, they tended to report that they were more likely to ask for directions that told them about landmarks and whether to turn right or left at certain landmarks. Men, on the other hand, reported that they preferred to keep track of cardinal directions and mileage. Next time you are navigating around your town, keep track of how you encode the environment.

the hippocampi of birds that do not cache, we see striking differences. The hippocampi of birds that cache are much larger than those of birds that do not cache (Sherry, 1997). However, chickadees tend to cache their food much more in some seasons than in others, typically increasing their hoarding as the weather becomes colder (Smulders, Sasson, & DeVoogd, 1995; Smulders, Shiflett, Sperling, & DeVoogd, 2000). When we look at the hippocampus of chickadees in the summer, we can see that the hippocampus is smaller than those of the chickadees that were studied in the winter. Thus, it appears that two factors are involved. The first is that species who perform complex spatial tasks, such as caching, tend to have larger hippocampi; the second is that the brains of these species appear to be quite plastic, reducing the volume of the hippocampus when it is not in constant use.

These effects are also observed in mammals, such as voles. Some species of voles (e.g., pine voles) do not navigate long distances from their nest site, whereas some species of voles (e.g., meadow voles) travel long distances from their nest site to breed. The hippocampal volume of meadow voles is larger than that of pine voles, and the hippocampal volume in meadow voles fluctuates with the breeding season. That is, the hippocampal volumes in meadow voles increase during breeding seasons, when they also perform

Self-Test

1. What are the types of basic spatial abilities?

2. Which hemisphere is better at processing spatial information?

3. How does the dorsal stream process spatial information?

4. How do interactions between the frontal and parietal lobes produce what is known as the "how" pathway?

5. What role does the temporal lobe play in spatial learning?

6. How would you test place, cue, and position responses?

7. What evidence is there that birds and mammals process space similarly?

navigation tasks, and decrease during nonbreeding seasons, when they tend to stay closer to home (Jacobs, Gaulin, Sherry, & Hoffman, 1990). Hormones control these changes in hippocampal volumes (Galea & McEwen, 1999). It is currently unknown whether hormonal fluctuations in humans (such as those that occur across the menstrual cycle in women or the seasons in men) also result in modifications to the hippocampus. However, spatial ability does vary across the menstrual cycle in women and across the seasons in men (Kimura, 1996).

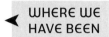

The previous section examined what spatial ability is, how the brain processes spatial information, and research investigating complex spatial tasks, including navigation and dead reckoning.

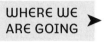

The following sections will deal with research about what happens when parts of the brain that mediate spatial ability are damaged.

MODULE **10.2**
Disorders of Spatial Ability

Our discussion of disturbances in spatial ability starts with a section on disturbances in intrapersonal space, in which individuals exhibit problems processing space that is within reach. This includes disorders of body schema (an inability to accurately represent the spatial relationships among the parts of one's body). This section is followed by a description of disturbances in extrapersonal space, in which individuals have difficulty perceiving or processing events or objects outside of their reach yet are relatively unimpaired at processing intrapersonal space. This distinction might appear to be an arbitrary one, but as we saw earlier in this chapter, the neural mechanisms that are involved in processing personal space are dissociable from those that are involved in processing extrapersonal space. Therefore, it should not be surprising that focal brain damage can selectively impair one's ability to process these two types of spatial information.

However, some disorders of spatial cognition impair processing of both types of spatial information. An example of this is Bálint–Holmes syndrome, which we will discuss in Chapter 11. Although the spatial disorders that are detailed below are discussed in isolation, this does not imply that the disorders usually *appear* in isolation. Brain damage often produces constellations of deficits, and some disorders have a tendency to appear along with certain other disorders. For example, left–right confusion often occurs along with finger agnosia.

Disturbances in Intrapersonal Space

MICROSOMATOGNOSIA AND MACROSOMATOGNOSIA. Neurological disorders can be accompanied by strange secondary behavioral symptoms. In some cases of epilepsy, individuals experience the erroneous perception that parts of their body are much larger or smaller than normal. The body parts that are usually implicated in this rare disorder are the hands and feet, and the symptoms are usually transient, occurring along with seizure activity. In **macrosomatognosia,** an individual believes that part of his or her body is much larger than normal. For example, an individual might perceive his or her hands to be quite large and cumbersome during seizure activity, but at other times the person's perceptions of his or her limbs are quite normal. **Microsomatognosia** is the opposite condition: the perception of parts of the body (or the body as a whole) being smaller than is actually the case. Macrosomatognosia is more common than microsomatognosia, and it is usually applied to single parts of the body, whereas microsomatognosia often affects the entire body.

Microsomatognosia and macrosomatognosia can also occur in the absence of epileptic activity. Some migraine sufferers experience these conditions as aura symptoms (Podoll & Robinson, 2000). The conditions have also been associated with schizophrenia, drug-induced psychosis, and sleep disorders such as sleep paralysis (Schneck, 1977). Although it is not yet clear which neural systems are producing these strange sensations, the temporal lobes are prime candidates. Temporal lobe dysfunction has been associated with epilepsy, schizophrenia, and sleep disorders. Furthermore, the anatomical projections that are received by the temporal lobe make it a prime candidate for subserving one's body image (Trimble, 1988).

AUTOTOPAGNOSIA. **Autotopagnosia** is a loss of spatial knowledge about one's own body (Denes, 1999). People with this disorder can recognize and name body parts but have difficulty pointing to the correct body part on command (regardless of side). In addition to manifesting the disorder when questioned about their own body, individuals with autotopagnosia cannot correctly point to body parts on the individual who is doing the examination, nor can they indicate the parts on a model or doll. Despite this inability, people with autotopagnosia appear to retain their knowledge of the *function* of body parts (Denes, Cappelletti, Zilli, Porta, & Gallana, 2000). Furthermore, if they are asked to point to specific items of clothing or jewelry that are associated with specific body parts (e.g., socks, earrings), autotopagnosics perform much better than they do when they are simply asked to point to feet or ears. Fortunately for autotopagnosics, their deficits rarely impinge on their everyday activities. Although the deficits are clearly identifiable in a clinical situation, autotopagnosics do not usually demonstrate a disability to perform tasks that draw on one's knowledge of body parts, such as dressing oneself (Denes, 1999).

LEFT–RIGHT CONFUSION. Do you have trouble keeping your rights and lefts straight? Have you ever held up both your hands with your palms downward and thumbs pointing at one another to see which hand makes the L shape to remind you which hand is your left one? If so, you are not alone. Many people exhibit left–right confusion at a subclinical level. Women generally report more problems with left–right confusion, and they tend to make left–right distinctions more slowly than men do, but they generally do not make more errors on such tasks (Snyder, 1991). Subjective reports of problems confusing right and left are particularly common among left-handed females (Harris & Gitterman, 1978).

However, a more severe manifestation of confusing left and right results in **left–right confusion,** a condition that co-occurs with a great variety of other disorders (such as topographical amnesia). One can test for left–right confusion in two ways

(Semmes, Weinstein, Ghent, & Teuber, 1960). The first way involves a series of verbal instructions, such as "Touch your left knee with your right hand" or "Touch my right hand with your left hand." The verbal instructions can also take the form of asking "show me" questions, such as "Show me your left eye" or "Show me my right hand" (Lezak, 1995).

Another method involves presenting line drawings of body parts and asking people to judge whether the parts are from the body's right or left side. Culver (1969) developed one such test consisting of drawings of sixteen hands, eight feet, four eyes, and four ears, each of which is presented on a card. After having been shown an image, the individual is asked to identify whether the body part belongs to the right or left side of the body. Damage to the left parietal lobe or the left frontal lobe leads to deficits on both types of tests. However, one must be careful to eliminate aphasia as a possible cause of the deficits. When a random sample of brain-damaged individuals are tested, more than two thirds will fail at left–right orientation tests, but many of these individuals will fail because of language deficits or a more generalized intellectual impairment (Denes, 1999).

FINGER AGNOSIA. Finger agnosia is, in many ways, a more specific manifestation of autotopagnosia. In **finger agnosia,** a person selectively loses the ability to recognize, name, or identify fingers. In addition to being unable to name or recognize their own fingers, finger agnosics cannot identify fingers from others' hands. As one might expect, the disorder can also be expressed with regards to one's toes (Tucha, Steup, Smely, & Lange, 1997). Although finger agnosia can occur in the absence of other deficits, it is often accompanied by left–right confusion. When an individual demonstrates finger agnosia, left–right confusion, dyscalculia (deficits in calculation), and dysgraphia (deficits in writing, discussed in Chapter 8), this constellation of deficits is called **Gerstmann syndrome** (Gerstmann, 1924, 1930). Although Gerstmann is often credited with the first description of this tetrad of symptoms, Jules Badal, a French ophthalmologist, described the syndrome earlier, in 1888 (Benton & Meyers, 1956).

ANOSOGNOSIA. One of the most striking disorders of body schema is **anosognosia.** Here, an individual with hemiparesis or other unilateral neurological disorders denies that the disorder exists, both verbally and through his or her motor behavior. Explicit denial of a physical disability or other illness can be caused by any number of factors (e.g., confusion, reduced arousal, memory difficulties), but anosognosia is a rather specific manifestation of this denial. An anosognosic individual is unaware of his or her hemiplegia, hemianopia, or hemianaesthesia. The condition is usually temporary, lasting for just days or even hours after its sudden appearance.

Although anosognosics often do not display conscious awareness of their deficits, they can display tacit knowledge. For example, when given a choice between performing a task that requires both hands (e.g., tying one's shoes) or a task that requires only one hand (e.g., threading a bolt), they choose the unimanual task far more often (Ramachandran, 1995). The same is not the case for neurologically normal controls. This demonstrates that anosognosics do not attempt to behave as though they are neurologically normal, despite their conscious claims to the contrary.

Neuropsychological Celebrity

Anosognosic Woman Examined by P.H. Sandifer

In July 1945, a 66-year-old woman was admitted to a hospital in England for stomach problems. She had a large gastric ulcer, and during the course of her treatment, she received a blood transfusion. Ten hours after the transfusion, she became comatose. Two days later, she exhibited left hemiparesis and exhibited some disorientation. In addition to incorrectly naming the current day or month, she also stated that the current king and queen were George V and Mary. (George V had died of influenza on January 20, 1936, some ten years earlier.) She demonstrated agnosia for the left side of her body and an apparent unawareness that there was anything wrong with the left side of her body. The following is an excerpt from her conversation with an examiner (Sandifer, 1946, pp. 122–123):

Examiner: "Give me your right hand."
(Patient presented the right hand.)

Examiner: "Now give me your left hand."
(Patient presented the right hand again.)
The right hand was then held. (by the examiner)
Examiner: "Give me your left hand."
(Patient looked puzzled and moved neither arm.)
Examiner: "Is anything wrong with your left hand?"
Patient: "No doctor."
Examiner: "Why don't you move it then?"
Patient: "I don't know."

The left hand was then held before her eyes.

Examiner: "Is this your hand?"
Patient: "Not mine doctor."
Examiner: "Whose hand is it then?"
Patient: "I suppose it is yours doctor."
Examiner: "No it is not; look at it carefully."
Patient: "It is not mine doctor."
Examiner: "Look at it—it is your hand."
Patient: "Oh, no doctor."
Examiner: "Where is your left hand then?"
Patient: "Somewhere here, I think."

(Patient made groping movements near her left shoulder.)

In most cases of anosognosia, the person suffers from left hemiparesis (following right hemisphere injury). This general finding is complicated by the fact that left hemisphere lesions often lead to severe language disorders, making anosognosia much more difficult to detect. Even though the disorder might be underdiagnosed following left hemisphere injury, most researchers agree that the condition is far more commonly the result of left hemisphere injury. However, a single lesion does not appear to be sufficient to cause anosognosia. Instead, it appears to follow the co-occurrence of two lesions: one that causes the hemiplegia, hemianaesthesia, or hemianopia and one that causes the lack of awareness of deficit. The second lesion is usually in the parietal lobe, and the thalamus and internal capsule can also be involved (Bisiach, 1999).

Disturbances of Extrapersonal Space

REDUPLICATIVE PARAMNESIA. Reduplicative paramnesia for places is an example of a *misidentification syndrome,* in which individuals incorrectly identify and reduplicate persons, places, objects, or events (Feinberg & Roane, 2000). The same disorder is also called *environmental reduplication* (Leiguarda, 1983; Ruff & Volpe, 1981).

For example, in a case involving the "duplication" of a person, a 16-year-old boy had the delusion that a double of himself (one year younger and without his physical impairments) was occupying the same space and time. There is also a more purely spatial manifestation of the disorder in which a place in space that is familiar to the individual is "duplicated and relocated from one site to another" (Nichelli, 1999). For example, Benson and colleagues (Benson, Gardner, & Meadows, 1976) describe three males who suffered severe head trauma and "relocated" their hospital to another geographical site despite compelling evidence to the contrary. This delusion can appear in two different forms. In one form, the reduplicated world appears to exist in parallel with the present one. In another form, the previously familiar world (often from a time and place that were known well earlier in the individual's life) is displaced from one place to another (see Luzzatti & Verga, 1996). When exhibiting the latter type, the individual often displays temporal disorientation as well.

The lesion locations that are associated with reduplicative paramnesia are quite varied, but the right hemisphere (particularly right frontal and limbic regions) is often affected (Hakim, Verma, & Greiffenstein, 1988; Moser, Cohen, Malloy, Stone, & Rogg, 1998; Murai, Toichi, Sengoku, Miyoshi, & Morimune, 1997). However, lower brain areas such as the brainstem and cerebellum have also been implicated (Joseph, O'Leary, Kurland, & Ellis, 1999).

TOPOGRAPHICAL AMNESIA. **Topographical amnesia** is the loss of ability to navigate in environments that were previously familiar and navigable. Hughlings-Jackson (1931) was the first to describe this rare condition (only a few dozen cases have been reported since). After a tumor formed in her right temporal lobe, a woman had trouble navigating through a park near her home. Förster (1890) reported on a similar case of a male postal clerk who lost the ability to learn the location of objects, even in a space as small as a room. In addition to the anterograde components (the loss of ability to remember new information), his topographical amnesia also had retrograde components. Locations of objects that were previously familiar (such as famous landmarks in his city or the spatial arrangement of his home) could not be recalled. Despite his training and experience as a postal clerk, he could no longer draw accurate maps of his local environment or the world.

The deficits that these individuals exhibit in navigation are not simply due to their failure to recognize landmarks. Instead, they often identify landmarks correctly (such as an individual building), but they fail to recall whether the landmark is to the left, right, front, or back of another recognized landmark. This leaves the individuals unable to place the landmarks on maps or give landmark-based directions verbally (DeRenzi, Faglioni, & Villa, 1977).

In addition to deficits in real-world navigation, individuals with topographical amnesia can demonstrate impairments on a much smaller scale. Using a stylus maze (in which people must use a stylus to indicate the correct path out of the maze), DeRenzi and colleagues (1977) tested fifty-one patients with right hemisphere damage, fifty-four patients with left hemisphere damage, fifty non-brain-damaged controls, and one topographical amnesic patient. Although both brain-damaged groups showed impairments on the task, the group with right hemisphere damage (particularly if the damage was posterior) had the most difficulty learning the task. The individual with topographical amnesia had great difficulty with the task, requiring 275 trials to learn the maze.

Although right hemisphere damage appears to impair one's ability to navigate (see also Barrash, 1998), damaging some more central brain structures can produce the same symptoms. Bottini and colleagues (Bottini, Cappa, Geminiani, & Sterzi, 1990) reported the case of a 72-year-old man who acquired topographical amnesia (both retrograde and anterograde) after a tumor formed in the splenium of his corpus callosum. There are also cases of transient topographical amnesia (i.e., the condition comes and goes), particularly in individuals with epilepsy (Cammalleri et al., 1996; Mazzoni, Del-Torto, Vista, & Moretti, 1993; Stracciari, 1992; Stracciari, Lorusso, & Pazzaglia, 1994). In at least one case, the transient disorder appears to have been caused by a reduction in blood flow to the cingulate cortex (Cammalleri et al., 1996). In this case, a 53-year-old man suffered transient attacks of both transient topographical amnesia and rigidity in his left arm and leg, again implicating the role of the right hemisphere in this rare condition.

TOPOGRAPHICAL AGNOSIA. Paterson and Zangwill (1944) proposed that disorders in navigation could be divided into two dissociable impairments: Topographical amnesia and topographical agnosia. In the case of topographical amnesia, the deficit appears to be caused by a memory problem. In **topographical agnosia** (sometimes called *environmental agnosia;* see Benson, 1994), the individual exhibits deficits in identifying features of landmarks (buildings or other objects) with their orienting value but retains the ability to identify classes of similar objects (e.g., high-rise buildings, churches, drive-through restaurants, hills). Because of this specificity, some people refer to the disorder as *landmark agnosia* (Aguirre & D'Esposito, 1999).

Individuals with topographical agnosia erroneously claim that all locations and routes are novel. Unlike the case in topographical amnesia, these agnosics can often retain their ability to give appropriate directions (particularly when using cardinal directions) or draw simple maps. One such patient even retained his ability to play chess (Pallis, 1955). In a group of sixteen people with a loss of ability to recognize familiar surroundings, all had right medial temporo-occipital lesions, although three of the individuals also had left side lesions (Landis, Cummings, Benson, & Palmer, 1986).

More recently, other researchers have argued that the amnesia/agnosia dichotomy is an oversimplification of topographical dysfunction. The two deficits are difficult to tease apart, and they often co-occur (Barrash, 1998). Instead, the retrograde and anterograde aspects of the disorders can be examined separately. The anterograde components of the disorder are associated with medial occipitotemporal lesions in either hemisphere (especially posterior parahippocampal gyrus), whereas the retrograde components are often attributable to right medial occipitotemporal lesions.

Self-Test

1. Microsomatognosia and macrosomatognosia are probably the result of dysfunction in which lobe of the brain? Why?

2. Do anosognosics display any awareness of their deficits? If so, how?

3. What is the difference between topographical amnesia and topographical agnosia?

◀ **WHERE WE HAVE BEEN** This chapter was divided into two modules. The first dealt with how the brain processes space, and the second dealt with damage to these areas and resulting behaviors. Spatial abilities can be as simple as perceiving the location of a single point in space and as complex as navigation through a large city. The evidence from both human and nonhuman animal research and from research using participants with brain damage all points to the dominance of the right hemisphere for most spatial tasks. There appears to be relevant differences in how people process intrapersonal space and extrapersonal space, especially when we examine the behaviors of people who have suffered brain damage.

Glossary

Anosognosia—Occurs when an individual with hemiparesis (or other unilateral neurological disorders, e.g., hemiplegia, hemianaesthesia, hemianopia) denies that the disorder exists, both verbally and through the person's motor behavior. It appears to be the result of two lesions: one that causes the unilateral neurological disorder and one that causes the lack of awareness of the deficit (usually in the parietal lobe, though, the thalamus and internal capsule can also be involved).

Autopagnosia—A loss of spatial knowledge about one's own body. People with this disorder can recognize and name body parts but have difficulty pointing to the correct body part on command (regardless of side) of themselves, the examiner, or a model or doll.

Caching—A behavior that is characterized by hiding food and retrieving it later. Species that demonstrate this behavior tend to have a larger volume of hippocampi.

Cued responses—Responses to the spatial location of an object, in which movements are guided by a cue. Cued responses are also guided by changes in how we perceive the stimulus and thus rely on the perception of information that is external to your body.

Dead reckoning—A short cut that is adapted through spatial learning. The ability to use dead reckoning demonstrates a place response, which indicates very good knowledge of the spatial configuration of the environment.

Depth perception—A very basic ability that is used to determine the relative position of an object. Depth perception is divided into local and global depth perception.

Dorsal visual stream—The visual stream extending from the primary visual cortex to parietal regions; considered the "how" pathway, responsible for identifying where an object is in space and guiding motor movements.

Extrapersonal space—The space more than five feet away from one's body.

Finger agnosia—A disorder in which a person selectively loses the ability to recognize, name, or identify fingers of both themselves and others; often accompanied by left–right confusion.

Gerstmann syndrome—A disorder in which an individual demonstrates finger agnosia, left–right confusion, dyscalculia (deficits in calculation), and dysgraphia (deficits in writing).

Global depth perception—The ability to use the difference between the information reaching one eye and the information reaching the other to compute the entire visual scene.

Intrapersonal space—The space immediately around your body including your body.

Left–right confusion—A severe manifestation of confusing left and right that co-occurs with a great variety of other disorders.

Line orientation—The position in which a line is oriented in space; many tasks require accurate identification of line orientation, such as being able to differentiate between the letters *d* and *p*.

Local depth perception—The ability to use detailed features of objects point by point to assess relative position.

Macrosomatognosia—A neurological disorder of personal space in which an individual believes that part of his or her body is much larger than normal. It is most likely due to temporal lobe dysfunction.

Mental rotation—Rotation of an object that does not occur overtly. In many mental rotation tasks, participants are often presented with two or more items that are rotated in different positions and asked to determine whether they are the same or different objects.

Microsomatognosia—A neurological disorder of personal space in which an individual believes that part of his or her body (or the body as a whole) is much smaller than is actually the case; most likely due to temporal lobe dysfunction.

Object geometry—The spatial properties of an object that are used to determine whether or not an item shares similar spatial properties with another.

Place responses—The responses that a person makes toward a particular location or object. An important feature of place responses is that they can be made even when the stimulus is not present. Place responses also tend to be relational.

Position responses—Responses to the spatial location of an object, in which movements are made using the body as a referent; do not need any cues that are external to the body and are relatively automatic.

Reduplicative paramnesia—A disorder in which an individual incorrectly identifies and reduplicates people, places, objects, or even events. This disorder is usually the result of damage to the right hemisphere, particularly the right frontal and limbic regions. The brainstem and cerebellum have also been found to be implicated however.

Spatial ability—The ability to understand space and process spatial information. This general term is used to describe the six individual spatial skills of targeting, spatial orientation, spatial location memory, spatial visualization, disembedding, and spatial perception.

Topographical agnosia—A disorder in which an individual exhibits deficits in identifying features of landmarks (buildings or other objects) with their orienting value but retains the ability to identify classes of similar objects (high-rise buildings, churches, drive-through restaurants, hills, etc.). Individuals with this disorder claim that all locations and routes are novel.

Topographical amnesia—The loss of ability to navigate in environments that were previously familiar and navigable.

Ventral visual stream—The visual stream extending from the primary visual cortex into the temporal lobe; considered the "what" pathway, used for the identification of objects.

11

Attention and Consciousness

The moment we try to fix our attention upon consciousness and to see what, distinctly, it is, it seems to vanish: it seems as if we had before us a mere emptiness.

—GEORGE EDWARD MOORE

A student of mine asked an insightful question when reviewing the table of contents for this chapter: "Why is the study of attention grouped with the study of consciousness? Can't consciousness also be grouped together with memory, visual object recognition, spatial ability, or emotion?" She was (and still is) quite right. There are clearly conscious and unconscious aspects of all of the functions that you have studied in this book so far. Visual object recognition involves both conscious and unconscious components, and some impairments (such as the visual form agnosia exhibited by D.F. in Chapter 6) seem to affect these components separately. Similarly, memory has conscious and unconscious components. In the case of H.M., conscious recollection of experiences after his surgery was terrible, but he retained the ability to form unconscious memories.

These examples might be interesting, but they do not answer the student's question: Why are attention and consciousness often studied together in neuropsychology? My answer was that attention can mediate conscious experience. For example, consider all of the tactile sensations that you are experiencing right now. If you are seated, you should be able to feel the back and bottom of your chair, your feet on the ground, and perhaps both hands on this book. Could you feel those things a moment ago? Well, you *could* have felt them, but you probably did not. Instead, chances are that your attention was focused elsewhere (ideally, on your reading), and these sensations did not reach conscious awareness. Therefore, your conscious experience of the world is modulated or even gated by attention. Personally, I am quite thankful for this. The world would be a completely overwhelming place if we were unable to selectively attend to things. As expressed by Mesulam (1981), "If the brain had infinite capacity for information processing, there would be little need for attentional mechanisms."

WHERE WE ARE GOING ➤ The following sections discuss the various ways in which attention can be defined. Then we discuss three current issues in the neuropsychology of attention. The first issue is the debate over when attention exerts its effect during perception. The second issue is the difference between voluntary and involuntary control of attention. The third issue is the question of where the neural substrate(s) of attention might be in the brain.

MODULE **11.1**
Studying Attention

Typically, these modules start with definitions of important terms. However, according to the founder of modern psychology, William James (1842–1910), attention needs no definition:

> Everyone knows what attention is. It is the taking possession by the mind, in clear vivid form, of one out of what seem several simultaneously possible objects or trains of thought. Focalization, concentration of consciousness are of its essence. It implies withdrawal from some things in order to deal effectively with others, and is a condition which has a real opposite in the confused, dazed, scatterbrain state.

Are you clear on what attention is now? Neither am I. *Attention* is a word that most people are quite comfortable using in everyday conversation, but it is notoriously difficult to define. As you will discover in Module 11.2, defining consciousness is even more difficult. However, what makes the quote from William James so interesting and relevant to current studies of attention is the fact that he clearly identifies two basic features of attention. The first is the selection of sensory information from several simultaneously available inputs. These inputs can be sensory, but they need not be. As James mentions, attention can also be directed to internal mental processes. This type of attention is now referred to as **selective attention,** the process that allows the selection of inputs, thoughts, or actions while other ones are ignored. Note that this process can be a covert one. The shifting of attention from one input to another can occur without adjusting sensory structures, such as moving one's eyes.

The second feature of attention is the selection of a mental state, allowing either an internal or external flow of information (Marzi, 1999). In a broad sense, attention can be described as either **voluntary attention,** in which one intentionally shifts attention from one input to another, or **reflexive attention,** in which the shift occurs in response to some external event. Your decision to read and attend to this passage is a result of voluntary attention, but if you were to take this book and drop in on the floor, the attention that the sudden noise would garner from the people around you would be reflexive. Because attention covers all of these phenomena, James's definition is more commonly used in psychology than any other definition. Unfortunately for James, although he correctly identified many of the most fundamental features of attention, he missed most of the subsequent scientific enquiry on the subject. At the time of James and for many subsequent years, the topic was not really regarded as worthy of rigorous investigation by most psychologists and philosophers. Thus, during James's lifetime, theories about the processes mediating behavior rarely included attention.

Notably, Hermann von Helmholtz did discuss attention in his studies of visual perception (published in the year of his death, 1894). Helmholtz was interested in studying the visual perception of briefly presented stimuli. Such studies are now relatively easy to perform using computers or tachistoscopes, but these technologies were not available to Helmholtz. Instead, he had to go to considerable trouble to be able to present his stimuli rapidly. Helmholtz made a room in his laboratory almost completely dark and then constructed a large screen on one of the walls and covered the wall with letters. To control the duration of a participant's exposure to the letters, Helmholtz used a brief flash of light (like that of a camera flash). This design suited his needs quite nicely, but the size of the screen led to an interesting perceptual phenomenon. That is, when Helmholtz focused his eyes in the center of the screen but paid attention to a region of the screen other than where his eyes focused, he could correctly identify the letters outside of the region where his eyes were focused (see Figure 11.1). Helmholtz noted this effect only when he directed his attention to another region in advance, although subsequent studies demonstrated that the effect can occur even when one directs attention after the sensory event. (These studies are described in Chapter 7). On the basis of his results, Helmholtz concluded that

These experiments demonstrated, so it seems to me, that by a voluntary kind of intention, even without eye movements, and without changes of accommodation, one can concentrate

Figure 11.1	**Effects of Attention in Vision**

F 3 L 8 T 1 C 7 W 9 G 2 D 4 U 6 Z 0 C 8 L 3 X 9 B 2 M 7 J 5 S 2 Q 6 Y 4 P 6 F 1 W 8 H 3 A	F 3 L 8 T 1 C 7 W 9 G 2 D 4 U 6 Z 0 C 8 L 3 X 9 B 2 M 7 J 5 S 2 Q 6 Y 4 P 6 F 1 W 8 H 3 A	F 3 L 8 T 1 C 7 W 9 G 2 D 4 U 6 Z 0 C 8 L 3 X 9 B 2 M 7 J 5 S 2 Q 6 Y 4 P 6 F 1 W 8 H 3 A
1. A screen of characters was placed on the wall, and Helmholtz gazed in the middle of the screen. The room was too dark to read the characters.	2. The screen was briefly illuminated by a flash of light. Helmholtz focused his gaze at the middle of the screen (at the *X*), but directed his attention to another region (top right).	3. After the flash, Helmholtz could recall characters from the region where his attention (but not his gaze) was focused.

attention on the sensation from a particular part of our peripheral nervous system and at the same time exclude attention from all other parts.

The next important study of attention came over fifty years later, but this time it was an investigation of selective *hearing*. E.C. Cherry (1953) published the first technical work on what is now called the **cocktail party effect.** Simply put, this effect is the ability to focus one's listening attention on a single speaker among a cacophony of conversations and background noises. However, most of the early experimental work in this area was not motivated by a wish to understand party behavior. The goal of this research was to facilitate the work of air traffic controllers in the early 1950s. At that time, air traffic controllers received messages from pilots over a loudspeaker, and when there were many pilots close by, hearing the intermixed voices of many pilots over a single central loudspeaker made the job very difficult.

Cherry conducted a number of experiments that involved the presentation of simultaneous auditory stimuli. In one such experiment, words were presented through headphones, but the two speakers provided competing inputs. (As you learned in Chapter 4, this technique later became known as dichotic listening.) Cherry asked his participants to selectively attend to the information that was presented to one ear (and verbally "shadow," or repeat, that information) while ignoring the information presented to the other ear. Cherry found that people could successfully extract the information from the attended ear and could not recall information that was presented to the other.

Since Cherry's original work, a great number of experiments have been conducted to investigate the cocktail party effect. The vast majority of these studies have employed only two sources of auditory information, although some have used more sources, and others have even found evidence for the phenomenon in vision (Shapiro, Caldwell, & Sorensen, 1997; Yost, 1997). Cherry suggested that "spatial hearing" was the main mechanism for segregating auditory inputs. In an attempt to make the tasks of air traffic controllers a little easier, Cherry proposed some tactics that could ease the task of filtering different voices, including having the voices come from different directions; using voices with different pitch, speeds, or tones; and using speakers who have different accents.

Most recent experimental work indicates that spatial hearing is not the major cue for segregating sound inputs, although it certainly can help. The neural substrates of selective auditory attention are beginning to be uncovered, in part through investigations of individuals with surgical lesions of the temporal lobes. Efron and colleagues (Efron, Crandall, Koss, DiVenyi, & Yund, 1983) compared a group of neurologically normal volunteers with a group that had anterior temporal lobectomies in terms of their ability to selectively attend to spatially separated audio channels. The anterior temporal lobectomy patients were impaired on the task, but only when the attended channel was on the side opposite to their lesion. On the basis of this result, it appears that auditory selective attention is mediated by the contralateral anterior temporal lobe. Several laboratories are currently investigating this possibility using neuroimaging.

One important issue raised by the early cocktail party experiments was the question of *when* conscious perception can be influenced by attentional processes. This issue is still being vigorously debated today. There are two other major issues that dominate most neuropsychological investigations of attention. One is the question of how attention shifts from one thing to another. This question must be addressed by studying the difference between consciously mediated attentional processes and those that are controlled by more automatic processes. The other major issue is whether attention is subserved by a mechanism that is distinct from sensorimotor systems. The subsequent sections will investigate these issues.

Early versus Late Selection

If we are attending to one sensory event while ignoring another, where is the "gate" that blocks out the unattended stimulus? William James (1890) suggested that the gate was actually very early in the sensory processing chain. He described the "accommodation and adjustment of sensory organs" and "anticipatory preparation of the ideational centers concerned with the object to which attention is paid." The early experiments of Helmholtz also seem to suggest that attentional selection is quite early. When Helmholtz attended to a particular region on his screen *before* the flash of light, he could report which letter was located there. However, the same effect was not present when attention was allocated *after* the flash. The central idea behind **early selection** is that the encoding and perceptual analysis (e.g., categorizing or naming) of an input need not be complete before it is selected or rejected from further processing. If selection is this early, attention could modulate our perceptions by influencing which sensory events are processed at very early points in sensation and perception (Treisman & Gelade, 1980; Umilta, 2001).

James suggested one possible mechanism for early selection: the accommodation or adjustment of sensory organs. Some animals clearly orient their sensory organs when they shift attention, such as the shifting of position or orientation of the ears. However, there is also evidence for covert changes that are relatively "low" or "early" in our sensory systems. Recall from Chapter 8 that the efferent projections from the cochlea demonstrate differential activation under different attentional conditions but identical stimulus conditions (Ferber-Viart et al., 1995; Maison et al., 2001). Although it seems extremely unlikely that any cognitive process could modulate the function of the outer or middle ear, it appears that inner ear function is vulnerable to higher perceptual and attentional processes.

Most of the evidence favoring early selection comes from basic psychophysical experiments. In tasks that require basic detection or even identification, performance is enhanced (both accuracy and reaction time) when attention is focused on the relevant dimension. Unfortunately, interpreting the results of these experiments is not straightforward. It is possible that the accuracy and reaction time benefits provided by focusing one's attention appropriately are due to attentional influences on postperceptual processes, such as categorization or even response selection. Therefore, attention could be exerting its effect relatively late in the perceptual process. One way of dealing with this problem is to refrain from using accuracy or reaction time measures in these experiments. Tsal and colleagues (Tsal, Shaler, Zakay, & Lubow, 1994) had participants make judgments about the brightness of briefly presented small gray squares. In one experiment, participants matched the brightness of two peripheral squares while attending to only one of the squares. When the stimulus appeared on a white background, it was judged as being brighter but only when attention was directed to its location. When the same stimulus appeared on a dark background, the opposite effect was observed. Because the attentional manipulation resulted in a difference in perceived brightness (rather than an improvement in accuracy or reaction time), it appears as though the manipulation had an impact on fairly basic perceptual processing.

There is also a considerable body of event-related potential (ERP) research that supports the early selection account of attention. One famous example is an ERP experiment published in the journal *Science* by Hillyard and colleagues (Hillyard, Hink, Schwent, & Picton, 1973). A rapid sequence of tones was presented to both ears, and the participants were instructed to selectively attend to one ear during some of the blocks of trials and to attend to the other ear during other blocks. Whenever their target (a high-pitched tone) was presented to the attended ear, they had to press a button. Sometimes the target was presented to the attended ear, and sometimes it was presented to the unattended ear. When the target was presented to the attended ear, it was accompanied by a larger negative waveform (N1) than was the case for unattended tones. Presentations to the attended ear were accompanied by a smaller positive waveform (P1). Because the P1 waveform emerged 20–50 milliseconds after presentation of the stimulus and the N1 waveform emerged after 60–70 milliseconds, one could reasonably assume that the effect of attention was quite early. Indeed, these results suggest that attention is possibly even as early in perceptual processing as the processing in the primary auditory cortex. Similar procedures have been used to study visual attention. Here, too, attention appears to be capable of operating at very early stages of processing. However, most studies have indicated that the changes in ERPs take place at the level of the extrastriate visual cortex rather than the primary visual cortex (Mangun & Hillyard, 1988; Mangun, Hillyard, & Luck, 1993; Rugg, Milner, Lines, & Phalp, 1987; Umilta, 2001). Therefore, attention might operate later in the visual system than it does in the auditory system. Similar studies using tactile stimuli have not produced consistent results. According to Desmedt and colleagues (Desmedt, Robertson, Brunko, & Debecker, 1977), attention modulates both early and later components of the ERP for tactile sensations.

The central idea behind **late selection** is that attention operates after the sensory information has been perceived, identified, and/or categorized (Banich, 1997; Deutsch & Deutsch, 1963). Many of the early studies of attention (those of Helmholtz, Cherry, and Broadbent) seemed to support the early selection view, but what might be the most famous psychological experiment ever performed actually provides support for late selection. In the Stroop effect, unattended semantic information influences the processing of attended information (Stroop, 1935). When color words (such as *green*) are presented in colored ink that does not match the word (such as *green* printed in red ink), people are slower to name the color of the print. This effect can happen only if the word is recognized at a semantic level, despite the fact that the individuals were told *not* to read the word. Evidence gathered in the 1970s also demonstrated that nonattended stimuli can have semantic effects (Corteen & Wood, 1972; Lewis, 1970). For example, back when psychologists still routinely gave human participants shocks as part of their research programs, Corteen and Wood (1972) classically conditioned people to associate certain city names with an electrical shock. Once the conditioning was complete, Corteen and Wood presented words dichotically and instructed their participants to attend to a particular channel. When the words associated with shock were presented to the unattended ear, the participants could not consciously recall or identify the word. However, the words still produced autonomic responses that are consistent with their being correctly recognized and associated with shock. Studies of individuals with deficits in selective attention also provide evidence consistent with late selection. As you will discover later in this chapter, individuals with contralateral neglect (in which stimuli in the contralesional field are ignored, or neglected) display evidence of semantic knowledge of information presented in the neglected field, yet they fail to explicitly attend to these stimuli.

Of course, the debate between early selection theorists and late selection theorists might be resolved if there were concrete evidence of two distinct attentional mechanisms. It is quite possible that both positions are correct but the position that there is a single attentional mechanism is incorrect. Currently, it appears that there may be one attentional mechanism that could operate at an early level of selection and another that may operate later.

How Does Attention Shift?: Voluntary versus Reflexive Orienting

In the 1970s, experimental psychologists started to selectively study automatic versus controlled processes. It became clear that automatic processes had significant influence on controlled ones, and early studies attempted to examine these two types of processes in isolation. It also became clear that shifts in attention could be overt (such as moving the eyes when shifting visual attention) or covert (such as in Helmholtz's experiment in which visual attention did not correspond to the location of visual fixation). The following sections detail the difference between voluntary and reflexive attention.

VOLUNTARY SHIFTS IN ATTENTION. Voluntary shifts in attention are the changes that you intentionally initiate, changing the focus of your attention from one thing, such as a point in space or object, to another. Currently, you are trying to focus your attention on the words in front of you, although you undoubtedly have several other distracting options available. In attention experiments, one common paradigm for studying voluntary attention to space is to employ a cueing task. Participants are instructed to respond as quickly as possible to targets presented on a computer screen, and they are told that the target will most likely appear in a location that is cued before the presentation of the target. When trials are consistent with the cued location, we call them valid trials. However, sometimes the target appears in a location other than the one that was cued (see Figure 11.2). These trials are termed invalid trials, because the cue was misleading. In still other trials, the cue did not yield any information about the possible location of the target; these are referred to as neutral trials. Ironically, the results of the invalid trials are often more interesting than those obtained with valid cues.

When there are many more valid trials than invalid ones (e.g., 80% valid versus 20% invalid), participants learn to use the cue to help anticipate the location of the target. This results in a reduction in their average reaction time, which is called a benefit in this paradigm. However, under the same circumstances, invalid cues *increase* average reaction time, resulting in a **cost**. Both benefits and costs are traditionally

Examples of Valid, Invalid, and Neutral Trials Used in Spatial Cueing Experiments

Figure 11.2

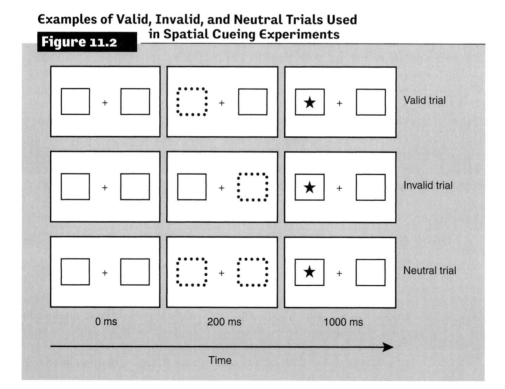

attributed to the influence of attention. Most of the time, users of this paradigm require their participants to keep their eyes focused on a central point. Therefore, the participants cannot directly look at the cued point, although they pay more attention to it. This type of paradigm can be used to study the effects of covert attention to a point in space. Unfortunately, interpreting the results of these experiments can be quite complicated. Consider the early versus late selection debate that we discussed a few paragraphs earlier. As we saw, the costs and benefits that are observed can be attributed to either early or late selection. For instance, early selection theorists might claim that the shift in covert attention influenced perceptual processing. Alternatively, late selection theorists might argue that the response required in the task was influenced by attention at a later (i.e., postperceptual) stage of processing. Although voluntary shifts in attention clearly have an effect, the level at which this effect is occurring is not clear.

REFLEXIVE SHIFTS IN ATTENTION. Many shifts in attention are not the result of a conscious decision about where to focus. If someone sneaks up behind you and drops a large book on the floor, the sudden, loud noise will seize your attention. In fact, for it to *not* seize your attention, you would need to either anticipate the noise and consciously avoid orienting to it (in effect, overriding a reflexive shift in attention with a voluntary one) or have a relatively large right frontal lobe lesion. Reflexive (or involuntary) changes in attention are usually adaptive. When a potentially threatening event happens, a failure to orient to the event and react appropriately might mean that one will be killed and therefore one's genes will not be passed along to subsequent generations. However, involuntary shifts in attention are not always useful or adaptive. Individuals with attention deficit disorder (which is discussed in more detail in Chapter 13) exhibit more attentional shifts from stimulus to stimulus than is typically observed, which can result in rather abnormal behavior.

Reflexive shifts in attention can be manipulated similarly to voluntary ones. Reconsider the cueing paradigm described in the previous section. If the participant's task is the same but the cues are presented randomly and the participant is instructed to ignore them, should this influence the speed of response? It does, but not always in the manner that you might predict. This method, called **exogenous cueing**, also produces costs and benefits, but both effects are possible for valid cues, depending on the timing. If a valid flash precedes the target by a short amount of time, such as 50–200 milliseconds, this results in a reaction time benefit. However, if the valid flash appears farther in advance of the target, such as 300+ milliseconds, this results in a cost (Gazzaniga, Ivry, & Mangun, 2002; Klein & Dick, 2002). This cost has been called an **inhibitory aftereffect** or **inhibition of return.**

The debate about what causes this effect has not been resolved, but there are two leading possibilities. One is that reflexive orienting responses are normally very short, on the order of 200 or fewer milliseconds. Much longer durations (such as multiple seconds) could potentially result in a life-threatening situation. For instance, what if reflexive changes in attention lasted a long time and while you were driving a car, your passenger suddenly sneezed? During the time that you reflexively oriented to the sudden noise and movement, your car could drift into opposing traffic. Obviously, benefits are observed when reflexive changes in attention are short rather than when attentional changes must be maintained for longer periods of time.

A second possibility is that when the cues tend not to provide valid information, there is a reluctance to respond to changes on that side, assuming (at first) that the visual changes that are detected are *not* the appearance of the target. This position assumes that it takes much of the 200–300 milliseconds after the presentation of a cue for people to recognize it as something other than the target and decide not to act on its presentation. Both positions have some supporters, but as with many topics in attention research, the debate is not over yet (Gazzaniga et al., 2002; Klein & Dick, 2002).

Neural System(s) Subserving Attention

Is attention subserved by a component of the sensorimotor system, or is it the product of one or more relatively independent systems? More simply put, where in the brain is attention? According to some phrenologists, it is at the back. As convenient as that might be to learn, current evidence paints a more complicated picture. Recordings taken from single cells in nonhuman primates over the past thirty years have clearly demonstrated that practically every cortical cell (with the exception of some primary visual and motor areas) can have its activity influenced by attention (Marzi, 1999). One interpretation of this finding is that attention is an extremely diffusely represented system, although a single attentional system could possibly have wide-reaching effects. Recordings taken from subcortical sites (e.g., the pulvinar nucleus of the thalamus, superior colliculus, inferior colliculus, and basal ganglia) suggest that attention is not strictly controlled by cortical structures. Rather than discussing the roles of these structures separately, we will discuss the neural correlates of attention in terms of their functional role within a diffusely represented attentional system.

In Chapter 7, you were presented with Baddeley's model of working memory. He suggests that working memory can be thought of as having three components, with the primary component (or **central executive**) responsible for controlling attention and supervising the two "slave" subsystems. Recall that the two slave subsystems are known as the **phonological loop** and the **visuospatial sketchpad,** which are separate and responsible for manipulating different types of information. In this view, attention is controlled by a single system, the central executive. However, there has been far less research on the central executive than on either of the two slave systems. One reason for this is that it is very difficult to study the central executive without involving either of the slave systems.

A related challenge is defining the central executive itself. As was the case with the two slave subsystems, the central executive is defined by what it does. That is, when performing a task, the central executive is involved with the allocation of attention, strategy selection, and the integration of information received from the two slave systems. It is rather difficult to study all of these facets of the central executive at one time. Additionally, although components such as strategy selection or allocation of attention appear to be rather concrete, trying to pin an operational definition on them can be rather challenging. Thus, although Baddeley's working memory model explains behavioral data quite well and is a well-accepted model in cognition, the central executive as a model of attention has not received much direct study.

Of those who have attempted to study the central executive, most functional imaging studies have reported that tasks that are demanding of the central executive result in activation of the dorsolateral prefrontal cortex (e.g., D'Esposito, Detre, Alsop, Shin, Atlas, & Grossman, 1995). Consistent with the observations of diffuse representation of attention in the brains of nonhuman primates, these tasks also result in activation of subcortical structures and more posterior regions of the brain, including the parietal cortex (e.g., Collette, van der Linden, Delfiore, Degueldre, Luxon, & Salmon, 2001; van der Linden et al., 2000).

Beyond the central executive is the widely studied model of attention proposed by Posner and Peterson, which involves three visual attentional mechanisms (Posner & Peterson, 1990). Although their theory describes only visual attention, as we will see in the following paragraphs, the model is consistent with the position that a single, anatomically distinct region of the brain does not mediate attention. Posner and Peterson hypothesize that three functionally and anatomically distinct attentional systems are involved in visual attention. Two are named after their location, and one is named after its function: a posterior attentional system (PAS), an anterior attentional system (AAS), and a vigilance system (VS).

According to functional imaging (mostly PET) and lesion studies, the PAS is functionally distinct from the other two systems in that it is primarily involved in orienting spatial attention, including object search and inspection of the object once it is found. When describing the PAS, people often suggest that it is like a zoom lens on a swiveling tripod. Given what you learned in Chapter 6, it should not surprise you that one of the main inputs of the PAS is the dorsal (i.e., "how?" and "where?") visual pathway. In fact, one could even think of the role of the PAS as one of ensuring that the ventral (i.e., "what?") visual pathway is actually activated by the objects of interest. Other anatomical sites within this system include the pulvinar nucleus of the thalamus, superior colliculus, secondary visual areas, inferior temporal lobe, and posterior parietal lobe. As we discussed in previous chapters, these structures are involved in the localization and identification of visual stimuli.

Functionally, the AAS is responsible for both the working memory and the executive control system that subserves the conscious control of attention. Therefore, the components of such a system would need to be involved in memory, semantics, and control of motor behavior. Anatomically, the AAS includes the cingulate gyrus (involved in response selection during various visual and motor tasks) and frontal cortex and contains many connections to structures with mnemonic functions, such as the hippocampus, amygdala, and medial temporal cortex. The control of the movements themselves appears to be mediated through the premotor cortex.

A successful attentional system must be able to prepare and sustain alertness toward signals that demand high priority. This is the function of the VS. Anatomically, the VS appears to be functionally lateralized. Right frontal damage compromises the ability to develop and maintain an alert state or perform vigilance tasks (Coslett, Bowers, & Heilman, 1987; Heilman, Bowers, Coslett, Whelan, & Watson, 1985), but similar left hemisphere damage does not produce the same behavioral deficits. The VS also appears to be selectively dependent on norepinephrine (NE)-containing neurons arising in the locus coeruleus. For example, depleting right (but not left) hemispheric NE in rats produces changes in arousal and vigilance (Robinson, 1985).

The neuropsychological community has not universally accepted Posner and Peterson's model of visual attention, and other models (which are beyond the scope of our discussion here) have been proposed (LaBerge, 1990; Mesulam, 1981). However, Posner and Peterson's model has certainly received support from other investigators, and it has even provided a plausible account of the deficits exhibited by people with focal brain injuries (Leon-Carrion et al., 1996). However, the model is mostly limited to the visual modality; it has yet to be seen whether auditory or tactile attention is mediated in a similar way.

◀ **WHERE WE HAVE BEEN** We examined three current debates about the neuropsychology of attention. One of these debates concerns when attention exerts its effect during perception. There is considerable evidence for both early and late selection, suggesting that there could be more than a single attentional mechanism. We also differentiated between voluntary shifts in attention, which have mostly been studied by using valid/invalid cueing paradigms, and reflexive shifts in attention, which is often studied by using exogenous cueing. We also considered some neural systems that could subserve attentional processing, including Baddeley's model and that of Posner and Peterson.

WHERE WE ARE GOING ▶ In the following sections, we focus on the state and trait of consciousness. Following a discussion of various definitions of consciousness, we outline some of the methods that are used to study it and the potential neural substrates of conscious and unconscious processing.

MODULE **11.2**
Studying Consciousness

What is consciousness? Is it being awake or alert? Is it being able to form explicit memories and recall them at a later time? Is it being self-aware? Is it being able to carry on an inner dialogue? Is it all of these things in combination? As you discovered in the previous module, people are generally quite comfortable using the word *attention* in everyday conversation, yet the term is notoriously difficult to define. The same can be said for the term *consciousness*. Here too, there is no generally accepted definition in the neuropsychological community, yet it is an issue that is central to many avenues of investigation in the field. Consciousness is a deceptively simple term, one that we tend to characterize in a dichotomy: One is either conscious or not. Is it really that simple?

Consider the example of sleep. When people are sleeping, are they conscious? Before you answer "no," think of all the things that are possible during sleep. You can dream and remember the dream when you wake up (sometimes). You can incorporate elements of the environment around you in your dream, such as the ringing of a telephone. You can also be aware of yourself during the dream or even realize that you are dreaming (called **lucid dreaming** by Frederik van Eeden in 1913) and perhaps take control of the dream. Is a person conscious during a lucid dream? People are even capable of learning during normal sleep or when under anaesthetic. Does that mean that they are conscious?

Consider another example. How about a person who is too drunk to be able to control his or her actions and will not remember those actions the next day. This person is still walking (badly), talking (also badly), somewhat alert, and presumably self-aware, but is he or she conscious? The answer has major implications for experimental neuropsychology—but also for our legal system. Similarly, what about a primate that demonstrates alertness, explicit memory, some rudimentary language skills (including the ability to use syntax), and even some evidence of self-awareness? Does that mean that the animal is conscious? If language and self-awareness are the keys to consciousness, are human infants conscious? How about hypnotized people? How about *self*-hypnotized people? What would it take for a machine to reach consciousness?

Defining Consciousness

The string of unanswered questions in the preceding section is not simply meant to annoy you. Instead, it is an attempt to demonstrate that the simple conscious/unconscious dichotomy is an oversimplification. We might be better off if we considered consciousness along a continuum. These examples also identify some of the problems in defining consciousness. What criteria must be satisfied before consciousness is demonstrated? Some of these might include selective attention, explicit memory, language, and self-awareness. However, these criteria alone might not be enough. The computer on which I am writing this has its own language, memory, and selective attention (what the Windows® operating system terms *task priority*), and it regularly makes self-referential statements (especially when something has gone catastrophically wrong); for these reasons, it could possibly meet the criteria for self-awareness! Faced with these problems, some have claimed that consciousness, like jazz, cannot be defined (Perry, 1904). Others have at least tried to define the phenomenon (Tassi & Muzet, 2001), although no consensus has been reached.

Of those who have defined consciousness, Bisiach (1988) proposed that there are three different senses of consciousness. The first includes nonphysical entities, such as the soul or immaterial mind. The second is the experience of sensation, thought, or action. The third is the monitoring of internal representations. However, Coslett (1997) points out that this definition fails to address the component of consciousness that most people mention first when asked to define the phenomenon: awareness. Niedermeyer (1994) identifies some of the same components of consciousness, including selective attentiveness, changes in mental states, and vigilance. Damasio (1999) approaches the problem quite differently, drawing a distinction between two kinds of consciousness: core consciousness and extended consciousness. Core consciousness is described as the transient process that is generated as an organism interacts with an object. This does not require working memory or language; short-term memory will suffice. However, extended consciousness is more complicated. It is generated out of the gradual buildup of "autobiographical self," requiring long-term memory. It can be enhanced by language, but language is not necessary (although testing autobiographical memory without using language is quite a task).

These are some of the ways in which consciousness has been described for the purposes of neuropsychological inquiry, although there are other characterizations that are even less useful (though not necessarily wrong) for guiding scientific inquiry. For example, Eccles described consciousness as "the process of knowing what one knows" (Kolb & Whishaw, 1990). From a neuropsychological perspective, the goal in studying consciousness is to understand the neural basis of the phenomenon and how brain damage produces disruptions in consciousness. This goal is obviously quite difficult when neuropsychologists cannot agree on a definition for the phenomenon. One helpful (but seldom used) distinction is to consider consciousness as either a state or a trait. A human being can exhibit the trait of consciousness but not always be in a conscious state. Other organisms, such as bacteria, presumably cannot exhibit the

Current Controversy

To What Extent Are Nonhuman Primates Conscious?

Although a generally accepted definition of consciousness has yet to be proposed, this has not stopped some researchers from studying the extent to which nonhuman animals might be conscious. Much of this research has focused on whether or not nonhuman primates have the most complex level of conscious awareness, that is, a theory of mind (TOM). Most of these researchers define TOM as an understanding that others can have beliefs and thoughts that are different from their own (Budiansky, 1998; O'Connell, 1995).

One assumption of TOM is that people or animals that have TOM understand the relationship between seeing and knowing (that is, they understand that an individual who sees an event has knowledge of that event). To test this in nonhuman primates, guesser–knower (GK) experiments have been performed. These experiments involve human confederates: one who leaves the room or covers his or her head with a paper bag (the guesser) and one who shows a chimpanzee a piece of food and then hides it under one of several opaque cups (the knower). After the food has been hidden, both the guesser and the knower point to the cups (the knower always points to the correct cup), and the chimpanzee must decide who is pointing to the cup with the food hidden under it. It is expected that if chimpanzees can make inferences about others' mental states, they would be more likely to choose the cup to which the knower points, which is what was found with many (but not all)

chimpanzees that were tested (Povinelli, Nelson, & Boysen, 1990).

So on the basis of this evidence, can we conclude that chimpanzees have TOM? Not exactly. One critique of experiments like this is that the chimpanzees could have simply relied on behavioral cues to figure out how to get the reward. In other words, the successful chimpanzees could have easily learned that they would receive rewards by trusting the person who stayed in the room or who did not do anything abnormal (such as putting a paper bag over his or her head), which does not require an understanding of the relationship between seeing and knowing (Roberts, 1998).

Given these problems in interpreting the results of GK experiments, you might conclude that studying TOM in nonhuman animals is fruitless. However, consider the behavior of rhesus monkeys in GK paradigms. Unlike chimpanzees, rhesus monkeys do not consistently choose the cup to which the knower is pointing (Povinelli, Parks, & Novak, 1991). This dissociation between the two species suggests that simple behavioral clues alone (available to either species during both experiments) do not mediate performance on the task. The dissociation also suggests that rhesus monkeys and chimpanzees differ in their cognitive capacity for such tasks. However, it is unclear whether chimpanzees have better-developed TOM or whether they are simply more sensitive to behavioral clues. There is much more work to be done in this area, and carefully designed experiments should help to answer many of our questions about TOM and primate consciousness.

This piece was contributed by Marla Pender.

state of consciousness and therefore cannot exhibit the trait either. However, imposing a strict dichotomy between the trait and state of conscious or unconscious is probably not as useful as it could be, because it appears that these states (and possibly traits) are graded rather than all-or-none phenomena (Delacour, 1996).

The Neural Basis of Consciousness

Given the many difficulties in defining consciousness, Farah (2001) proposes three general theoretical positions (and subsequent lines of inquiry) that neuropsychologists can adopt when studying consciousness. She states that we should (1) consider consciousness as the privileged role of particular neural structures, (2) consider consciousness as a state of integration between otherwise distinct brain systems, and (3) consider consciousness as a graded property of neural information processing in general. We will consider these three positions separately.

CONSCIOUSNESS AS THE PRIVILEGED ROLE OF PARTICULAR NEURAL STRUCTURES. This view might have originated with Descartes, who hypothesized that activity influencing the pineal gland was experienced consciously, whereas other patterns of activity were not. In many ways, this approach is the simplest conceptualization of consciousness, and the central idea behind it remains popular today. This is not to claim that the pineal gland is still the prime candidate structure. Other parts of the brain, including the right frontal lobe and the cingulate cortex are now burdened with this responsibility. Several investigators have proposed models of how an anatomically and functionally distinct "consciousness module" could interact with other brain systems. Perhaps the most influential of these models is that of Schacter, McAndrews, and Moscovitch (1998). In their Dissociated Interactions and Conscious Experience (DICE) model (see Figure 11.3), the conscious awareness system (CAS) is not part of the brain systems responsible for memory, perception, or action. This model is quite simple,

Figure 11.3   **Schematic Diagram of the DICE Model of Attention**

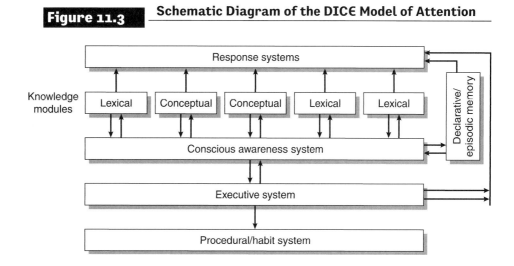

and it provides a convenient account of many disorders. For example, in the case of blindsight, the disorder can be conceptualized as a disconnection between the CAS and the visual system.

CONSCIOUSNESS AS A STATE OF INTEGRATION BETWEEN OTHERWISE DISTINCT BRAIN SYSTEMS. A somewhat more complicated (but popular) position is that consciousness is an emergent property resulting from the interaction among several otherwise distinct neural systems. According to this view, consciousness is not subserved by a single functionally and anatomically distinct system, and diagrams of such models do not include a separate consciousness module. Some examples of these modules include Crick and Koch's (1990) theory of visual awareness, in which the conscious percept of an object is the result of the binding together of the different visual properties of the object, including factors such as shape, size, color, and motion. Damasio's (1989) theory of awareness is similar but extends beyond the visual modality. These and other integration theories of consciousness are just as capable as the privileged role theories of accounting for disturbances in conscious awareness following brain damage (Crick & Koch, 1990; Damasio, 1989; Kinsbourne, 1988). The major difference between this position and that of a dedicated consciousness center is that they assert that anatomical disconnection among centers is to blame for the lack of awareness in individuals with brain damage.

CONSCIOUSNESS AS A GRADED PROPERTY OF NEURAL INFORMATION PROCESSING IN GENERAL. This position is a less modular view than the first two options that we presented. In the privileged role accounts, there is a consciousness module. In the state of integration accounts, modules that are responsible for different functions (e.g., identifying visual form or subserving language comprehension) interact to collectively produce consciousness. The graded property theories, in contrast, posit that perception (regardless of modality) is not an all-or-none phenomenon. Instead, the perception of an object can be incomplete, depending on the stimulus conditions or the integrity of the perceptual system. The quality of the perceptual representation is related to the probability that it will be available to conscious awareness. One could easily argue that all neuropsychological impairments that appear to be disorders of conscious awareness are simply perceptual disorders (Farah, Monheit, & Wallace, 1991).

Of course, these three perspectives on consciousness are not necessarily mutually exclusive. For example, if one part of the brain subserved conscious awareness and required activation from a number of other areas to become active, both the first and second perspectives would be correct. It is also possible that a degradation of the perceptual representation by one brain region could lead to a diminished role in a more integrated state of awareness, in which case both the second and third perspectives would be accurate accounts of the deficit.

Methods of Studying Consciousness

Although many neuropsychologists have difficulty in defining consciousness, many still choose to study the state (and, to a much lesser extent, the trait) of consciousness. Some of the methods focus on relatively normal or even everyday variations in consciousness, such as studying the differences between sleep and wakefulness. Other methods involve less common experiences, such as undergoing hypnosis.

SLEEP AND WAKEFULNESS. People rest, but brains do not. The nervous system is always spontaneously active, and sleep is a very active process indeed. Sleep can be differentiated from similar-appearing states, such as coma or anaesthesia, in that **sleep** "is a readily reversible state of reduced responsiveness to and interaction with the environment" (Bear, 2001, p. 614). Although we tend to think of only two different states of consciousness, sleep and wakefulness, this is a gross oversimplification of both states. Sleep takes many different forms, and so does wakefulness.

When I was in my first year of graduate school, I (L.E.) traveled with my classmates to a nearby university to tour a neuropsychology professor's ERP laboratory. To demonstrate some of the equipment and tasks, the local professor asked for a volunteer. Foolishly, I offered my own brain. Electrodes were pasted to my scalp, and a research assistant familiarized me with the task I was about to perform. I won't belabor you with the details of the task; I will simply describe it with one sentence: It was repetitive and boring—really boring. Once things were set up, I started doing the task as others watched the electrical activity of my brain in real time. The task went on and on and on. I was getting bored. Suddenly, the professor burst out laughing and called others (including my supervisor) to look at the output from my brain. "He's sleeping," the professor remarked. "He is taking naps between trials." It turns out that during the couple of seconds between trials, I had enough of a chance to relax that my brain could give off small bursts of **alpha waves,** a pattern consistent with resting with one's eyes closed or being in a trance. Some of the onlookers seemed quite impressed with my behavior, though my supervisor was not one of them. Had you been watching me perform the task, would you have said that I was awake or asleep? As we will learn, wakefulness is not a single state; neither is sleep.

Most experimental work on sleep has employed electrophysiological (EEG) measures. There are a number of reasons for this: They are noninvasive and readily available, they are fairly inexpensive, and they are much quieter than other brain-imaging techniques. fMRI is a fabulous imaging technique, but it is terribly loud, which is not an environment that is usually conducive to sleep. According to the EEG data, there are four different stages of sleep, each of which is characterized by unique brain activity. Stage 1 sleep is a transitional state characterized by **theta waves** (4–8 Hz). Stage 2 is similar, except that it also contains an occasional 8 to 14-Hz oscillation called a **sleep spindle,** which originates in the thalamus (Velasco et al., 1997). Stage 3 is characterized by slower waves, including **delta waves** (< 4 Hz). Stage 4 is the deepest stage of sleep and is also characterized by delta waves, but they are even slower on average than those during stage 3, often occurring at frequencies of less than 2 Hz.

A typical night's sleep is not a simple linear progression through these stages of sleep. Instead, the pattern is considerably more variable (see Figure 11.4). Furthermore, a state of sleep that was discovered in 1953, called **rapid eye movement (REM)** sleep, is an important part of the cycle, yet the electrical activity that characterizes REM sleep seems to resemble wakefulness more than rest (which is why REM sleep is sometimes called *paradoxical sleep*). REM sleep is accompanied by low-voltage, fast changes in EEG that are often accompanied by highly detailed and vivid illusions called *dreams*.

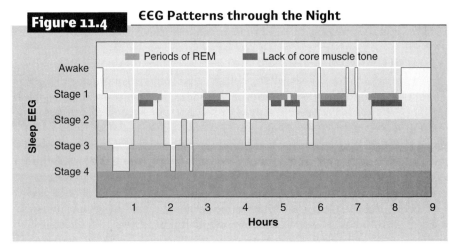

Figure 11.4

EEG Patterns through the Night

Source: John P. J. Pinel, *Biopsychology*, 5e. Published by Allyn and Bacon, Boston, MA. Copyright © 2003 by Pearson Education. Reprinted by permission of the publisher.

In contrast to other types of sleep, your body cannot move during REM sleep. Instead, you are paralyzed with the exception of the muscles that control eye movements, the muscles within the inner ear, and the muscles that are required to sustain vegetative functions such as breathing.

Although the electrical activity of the brain during REM sleep resembles wakefulness, the metabolic activity of the brain appears to be quite different. Because PET imaging can be considerably quieter than fMRI, there have been quite a number of PET studies of sleep. A study by Braun and colleagues (1998) compared brain activation during REM sleep to that during other stages of sleep or wakefulness. REM sleep was associated with the selective activation of extrastriate visual cortices (which is probably why those dreams seem so vivid) and a decrease in activity of the primary visual cortex. Consistent with these findings are the few studies that have been performed in the fMRI, in which similar patterns of activation were observed (e.g., Maquet et al., 1996; Maquet, 2005). This pattern of activity suggests that REM sleep is supported by higher cortical areas but operates independently of the primary sensory cortex.

Interestingly, although REM sleep is most often associated with dreaming, dreaming can be observed in other stages of sleep. Kjaer and colleagues (Kjaer, Law, Wiltschiotz, Paulson, & Madsen, 2002) have observed that the patterns of brain activation that are observed during REM sleep are quite different from those that are observed when participants are in stage 1 sleep and report that they were dreaming. In contrast to REM sleep, the pattern of brain activation during stage 1 dreaming was more like patterns that are observed when people meditate (Kjaer et al., 2002). Interestingly, recent research suggests that sleep may play an important role in the consolidation of memories (e.g., Nofzinger et al., 2002), because many structures associated with the consolidation of memories show increases in activity during sleep. Furthermore, when participants were trained on a particular task, imaging studies revealed that during sleep, there was selective activation of neural areas associated with the performance of these tasks (e.g., Maquet, 2005). Thus, it may be that beyond restorative body functions, sleep also plays an important role in maintenance of higher-level cognitive function.

PRESENTING STIMULI WITHOUT AWARENESS. Perhaps the most famous example of the influence of subliminal perception was actually a hoax. In 1957, a market researcher named James Vicary claimed that over a six-week period, 45,699 patrons at a movie theater in Fort Lee, New Jersey, were exposed to two subliminal advertising messages: "Eat Popcorn" and "Drink Coca-Cola." The message was supposedly presented for only 3/1000 of a second once every five seconds, a duration so short that the messages could not be consciously perceived. Vicary claimed that as a result of these messages, the sales of popcorn rose 57.7% and the sales of Coca-Cola rose 18.1% over the six-week period. Although these claims have often been accepted as established facts, Vicary admitted in 1962 that the results were a fabrication (Merikle, 2000).

Despite this early hoax and other subsequent hoaxes, recent studies have done an excellent job of illustrating the conscious influences of information that is presented without awareness. Marcel pioneered one often-employed paradigm in the 1970s and 1980s, in which either a blank screen or a word was presented and then was quickly covered up by a **masking stimulus,** a series of crosshatches or letters meant to occupy the participant's sensory memory of the event. (Recall the discussion of sensory memory in Chapter 7.) Following this presentation, the participants had to do one of two things: either indicate whether a word had been presented or not (which they could not do above chance levels of performance) or look at a string of letters presented after the mask and make a judgment about whether the letters formed a legitimate word (a task called **lexical decision**). Despite being unable to report whether a word had preceded the masking stimulus, the presentation of these words had significant effects on subsequent behavior. If the subliminally presented word had a meaning similar to that of the word presented after the mask (e.g., the word *doctor* followed by the word *nurse*), this resulted in faster lexical decisions (i.e., judging whether the letters *n-u-r-s-e* form a real word). If the two words were unrelated (e.g., the word *doctor* followed by the word *sandwich*), the lexical decision was not facilitated. These results have been replicated numerous times with other stimuli, such as spoken words and faces.

Kunst-Wilson and Zajonc (1980) provided another excellent example of unconsciously perceived stimuli influencing subsequent reactions. In this study, participants were briefly exposed (for 1 millisecond) to ten meaningless, irregular, geometric shapes, five times each (see Figure 11.5). At durations this short, none of the participants reported seeing *any* of the shapes. After these fifty presentations, the participants completed two tasks. Each of the tasks involved the presentation of a pair of shapes in which one old (i.e., previously exposed) shape and one new shape were presented. In the recognition task, the participants were instructed to select the member of each pair that had been previously presented. The participants performed the recognition task no better than if they were guessing. However, when the participants were instructed to indicate which shape they *preferred,* the participants tended to select the previously presented object despite their inability to recognize the object. This experiment has been successfully replicated dozens of times, and some recent studies have

| **Figure 11.5** | **Geometric Shapes Used for Tests of Memory without Awareness** |

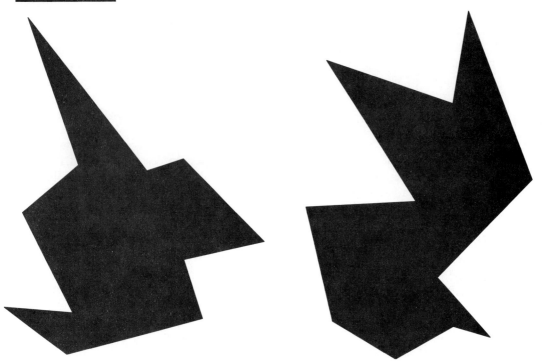

Although participants could not consciously recollect which of the shapes like these they had seen before, they preferred the one that had been previously presented.

provided neuroimaging of the phenomenon. When participants are performing the task, the right lateral prefrontal cortex appears to be most active during preference judgments of unfamiliar stimuli, whereas the right hippocampus is most active during the recognition task.

One common interpretation of this phenomenon is that people tend to report liking something more if they are exposed to it more often. This interpretation of Kunst-Wilson and Zajonc's mere exposure effect is not correct. When the experiment is repeated with the variation of asking people to identify which object they *dislike*, they again tend to choose the previously presented object. Furthermore, if the instructions are changed to ask people to identify which object looks brighter or darker (the pairs are identical in size and brightness), they tend to choose the previously presented object. Therefore, it appears that the mere exposure effect has enough of an consequence to make people think that there is something different about the previously presented object, but this difference is not necessarily positive.

HYPNOSIS. The neural mechanisms that underlie hypnotic states are only starting to be uncovered. Research in this area has been complicated by the wide variety of hypnotic states and phenomena to choose from. Hypnosis can be used to help people re-

1. List two pieces of evidence in favor of early selection and two pieces that favor late selection.

2. Describe the cueing paradigm that is often employed to study voluntary orienting. What are costs and benefits within this paradigm?

3. According to Farah (2001), what are the three general theoretical positions that a neuroscientist can adopt when studying consciousness?

4. According to PET imaging, what neural activity is different under hypnosis when a person's hand is placed in painfully hot water?

member events in their distant past, alter perceptions, quit smoking, or control pain. The efficacy of hypnosis at controlling pain has been objectively (and positively) evaluated (Faymonville, Fissette, Mambourg, Roediger, Joris, & Lamy, 1995), whereas the utility of hypnosis for other manipulations such as memory recall is questionable. Therefore, we will focus on the neural correlates of hypnotic pain control.

A classic example of the ability of hypnosis to modify the experience of pain is the "ice water experiment." In the 1950s, Hilgard had three groups of participants place their hands in ice water and repeatedly rate the painfulness of this experience. Normally, the cold is not terribly uncomfortable at first, but it becomes worse and worse until it is almost unbearable. Hilgard's three groups included participants who were highly hypnotizable, those who were moderately hypnotizable, and those who were hardly hypnotizable at all. Following the hypnotic suggestion that the ice water would not provide discomfort, the "highs" reported very low levels of discomfort, the "mediums" reported moderate levels of discomfort, and the "lows" reported discomfort that was comparable to that experienced during their waking state.

A variation of this classic experiment (using hot water and a single experimental group) was performed during PET imaging. Without the hypnotic suggestion that the water would be painfully hot, the sensation of dunking a hand into painfully hot water produced activation in the primary somatosensory cortex, as well as some secondary cortices and the anterior cingulate cortex, a structure that is known to be active during the sensation of pain. However, following the hypnotic suggestion that the water would only be mildly unpleasant, the primary and secondary somatosensory cortex was just as active, but the cingulate cortex was not. Therefore, the effect that hypnosis was having on the conscious experience of pain appeared to result in differential anterior cingulate activation.

◄ **WHERE WE HAVE BEEN**

After considering some definitions of consciousness, we outlined three theoretical positions that neuroscientists can adopt when studying consciousness: Considering consciousness as the privileged role of particular neural structures, considering consciousness as a state of integration between otherwise distinct brain systems, and consider consciousness as a graded property of neural information processing in general. Variations in consciousness can be studied by examining sleep/wakefulness cycles, presenting stimuli without awareness, using hypnosis to vary one's state of consciousness, or studying alterations in consciousness arising from focal brain damage.

WHERE WE ARE GOING ►

The following sections focus on disturbances in conscious processing of stimuli as a result of focal brain damage. We will examine three conditions in detail. Blindsight is a condition in which visual stimuli

the **Real** world

Are Human Infants Conscious?

"What Is an Infant but a Human in Lower Form?"[1]
The Development of Consciousness in the Infant

Before a month is up cells migrate together (the process of gastrulation)[2]
Fold into a groove and roll into a tube (the process of neuralation)[2]

The structure swells into three parts:
The forebrain, midbrain, hindbrain (while synapses dart)[2]

At birth: abound dendritic spines, glial cells and myelin
The organism is less primitive now, and more like kin

No longer thought to be merely sensorimotor,[3]
The being can approach and avoid[4] and experience the sense of another[5]

When did you become conscious?
Were you looking at insects on your haunches?

Or opening a gift at a favorite party?
(Probably not before age 3 or 4, after that memories are hardy)[6]

Were you using the words "I" and "you"?[7]
When you looked in the mirror did you know what to do?[8]

Strategizing, decision-making, understanding what you said
If they had a seat, it'd be the front of the head

The frontal lobe undergoes lengthy development
Growing bit by bit, but during infancy? A mere dent

Into the faculties it will eventually hold
Such as planning, self-monitoring, and resisting the impulse to be bold

The frontal lobe develops functions of complexity and broadness
Thus subserving the quintessence of consciousness.

[1]Refers to the development of the brain in the first month of gestation.

[2]Refers to the historical belief that infants are relatively unsophisticated organisms.

[3]Refers to the classification of "minimal consciousness" that has been proposed for human infants. This includes approach and avoidance behavior, and "being-like-something," which corresponds roughly to the experience of a first-person perspective.

[4]Refers to the notion of intersubjectivity, awareness of self and others.

[5]Refers to the finding that people's earliest memories are not before age 3 or 4, at which time they are also able to report verbally on personal events that have occurred in their lives (autobiographical memory).

[6]Refers to the first verifiable (i.e., verbal) identification of self, which occurs in approximately the second year of life.

[7]Refers to the rouge test, in which a red spot is placed on an infant's forehead, and the infant is placed in front of the mirror. At approximately age 2, the infant is able to identify and remove the spot, which is taken to be evidence of self-concept. Similarly, at this age, infants will self-reference (i.e., point to self) and demonstrate self-consciousness (i.e., embarrassment) when placed in front of a mirror.

Source: Reprinted by permission of Marianne Hrabok.

are not processed consciously but unconscious perception of visual information guides conscious decision making. In spatial neglect, an individual does not normally consciously perceive or respond to stimuli in a given spatial location, despite relatively intact sensation. Finally, Bálint–Holmes syndrome is a disorder of covert visual attention in which attention to multiple objects is severely impaired but the perception of single objects can be accomplished relatively normally.

MODULE **11.3**
Disorders of Attention and Consciousness

Blindsight

As you learned in Chapter 6, blindsight is a phenomenon that follows damage to the visual cortex. As you know, damage to the visual cortex results in blindness for specific areas of the visual field, called a *scotoma*. Objects that are presented in the scotoma cannot be consciously perceived. However, what is interesting is that some people appear to be able to "see" in their scotoma, which is referred to as *blindsight*. Some people with blindsight are able discriminate among stimuli, or identify objects presented in their scotomas, although they state that they do not see the stimuli. G.Y., a famous man with blindsight, suggested that describing his deficit was the same as "trying to tell a blind man what it is like to see" (Weiskrantz, 1995).

To some extent, being in a blindsight experiment is something like being in an ESP experiment. That is, the researcher deliberately puts a stimulus, such as an X, in the participant's scotoma. The participant is then asked to describe the visual properties of the stimulus. Because the stimulus is in the participant's scotoma, the participant quite correctly says that he or she cannot see anything. Experimenters often ask the participants to make a yes or no response to questions such as "Is it a flower?" Participants often give correct responses, sometimes as much as 90% of the time. As you may imagine, some participants simply refuse to respond, repeatedly stating that they cannot see. To increase the frustration quotient, when participants go along with the experimenter and guess, they get to perform another trial. People with blindsight often state that their abilities are based on feelings rather than seeing. For instance, when participants have to discriminate between Xs and Os, they may say that the Xs felt spiky, and the Os were smooth.

Individuals with blindsight may be able to perform even more complicated visual functions than discrimination among simple forms and position. For instance, words presented in the scotoma can sometimes influence behavior. When Marcel (1998) asked individuals with blindsight to define ambiguous words (e.g., *bank*), he found that if he had previously presented the word *river* in their scotoma that the participants were more likely to define *bank* as the edge of a stream or river. This is an intriguing result, because the most common definition of the word bank refers to a financial institution. Thus, Marcel (1998) has some evidence that the visual perception that occurs in blindsight may be far more complicated than previously thought.

So what is the neural basis of blindsight? Although some researchers have suggested that blindsight might be due to islands of preserved primary visual cortex that performed these rudimentary visual functions, this hypothesis is not widely believed today. One major problem with this idea is that when G.Y. was studied with functional neuroimaging, there was no evidence of activity within the primary visual cortex. Thus, at least in G.Y.'s case, islands of activity in V1 cannot account for his correct responses. Other investigations have also failed to confirm the islands hypothesis (Barbur, Weiskrantz, & Harlow, 1999).

Recall from Chapter 6 that not all projections from the LGN go directly to V1 (some go directly to visual association areas) and that there are direct projections from the retina that go directly to the superior colliculus (which projects to the pulvinar nucleus and visual association areas). It may be that these projections are intact in individuals with blindsight and they provide residual visual function (Stoerig & Cowey, 1997). Cowey and others suggest that the ability to perform explicit judgments about stimuli depends on the visual association cortex. These projections may perform the nonconscious visual functions that occur in blindsight (Cowey & Wilkinson, 1991; Rafal et al.,1990). If you remember the study on G.Y. from Chapter 6, you know that although there was no activity in V1 during blindsight; activity was detected in visual association areas and other brain regions, which is consistent with Cowey's hypothesis.

Interestingly, similar phenomena occur in other senses, although it is rare. There have been reports of "deaf hearing" in audition and numbsense/blindtouch in somesthesis (Garde & Cowey, 2000; Halligan, Hunt, Marshall, & Wade, 1995). Some suggest that these phenomena may rely on similar systems in both subcortical and secondary cortical systems. This hypothesis would be consistent with a common organizational structure being evident in all sensory systems.

Spatial Neglect

Another disorder of attention goes by many names; we use the term **spatial neglect** here; others are *unilateral spatial neglect, hemi-inattention, spatial hemineglect,* and simply *neglect.* As the names suggest, the disorder is a failure to report, respond to, or attend to stimuli or events in one hemifield when the impairment is not caused by sensory or motor deficits (Heilman, Watson, & Valenstein, 2000). The neglected side is always opposite the site of the lesion (contralesional), although the disorder is much more common following right hemisphere damage, resulting in neglect of the left side of space (McCarthy & Warringtron, 1990). In the rare cases in which right spatial neglect (following left hemisphere damage) is observed, the symptoms are typically much less severe.

Accompanying the lack of awareness for information in one hemifield is a lack of knowledge of the deficit. That is, individuals with spatial neglect behave as though they are unaware that they are attending to only one side of space. For this reason, individuals with spatial neglect often seek help for complaints other than their primary deficit. For example, an elderly man may visit his physician to complain of injuries to his left arm and leg. Although the bruises to his left limbs are quite real, their underlying cause is the unilateral spatial neglect, which causes him to walk into furniture and other obstacles located toward the left side of space. Other common be-

Sample of a Clock Drawn by a Patient with Left Spatial Neglect

Figure 11.6

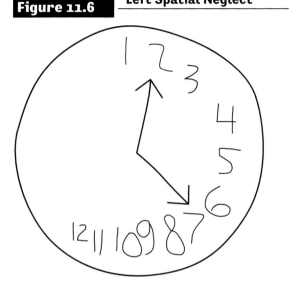

havioral symptoms include eating the food from one half of the plate, shaving half of one's face, dressing one half of one's body, or difficulty telling the time. Not only do individuals with spatial neglect cease to perceive events in one hemifield, but also they often cannot even conceive the existence of the contralesional hemifield (Bisiach, 1999).

One common bedside test for spatial neglect is the clock-drawing test. In this test, an individual will often draw a complete circle, but all the elements of the clock are transposed to one side (usually the right) of the clock. Despite this distortion, the drawing often contains all of the numbers from 1 to 12, but the 1 and the 12 are often quite distant from one another (see Figure 11.6). Another common test of spatial neglect is line bisection. Here, a person is presented with a horizontal line on a piece of paper and asked to draw a mark where he or she perceives the midpoint of the line to be. Most patients who demonstrate spatial neglect bisect to the right of center, and the degree of their errors increases as line length increases. There are also a variety of cancellation tasks that have been employed (Albert, 1973), in which an array of items (short lines, stars, O's, etc.) covering a piece of paper is presented to the person and they are instructed to cross out (cancel) all occurrences of those items (see Figure 11.7).

Figure 11.7   **Sample of a Line Cancellation Task from a Patient with Left Spatial Neglect**

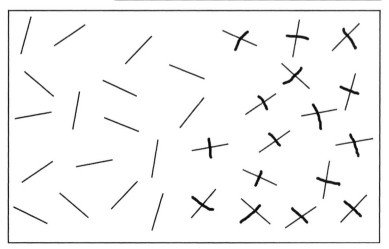

Spatial neglect is not simply a memory or perceptual problem. Instead, there is some very convincing evidence that the disorder results from a failure to construct representations of one's spatial environment. Bisiach and Luzzatti (1978) provided one of the most compelling arguments for this phenomenon. Two people with hemispatial neglect who were both familiar with the same Italian square (the Piazza del Duomo in Milan, shown in Figure 11.8) were asked to describe the square. However, Bisiach and Luzzatti controlled their perspective on the problem by instructing the participants to imagine the scene from two different vantage points. When asked to imagine and describe the visual scene when facing the cathedral, they correctly recalled many of the features and landmarks on the right side of what would be visible from that point but very few points from the left side of space. When their imaginary perspective was reversed, and they were asked to describe what the visual scene would look like from the front of the cathedral, they reported landmarks on the right side of their new imagined perspective but neglected those on the left. Notably, these individuals now failed to report landmarks that they had previously described. Using this strategy, Bisiach and Luzzotti demonstrated that the patients with spatial neglect could construct relatively complete visual scenes—but only one half at a time!

Spatial neglect was not discussed in Chapter 10 along with disorders of personal space and disorders of extrapersonal space because it can occur in either realm or

Figure 11.8 **The Piazza del Duomo in Milan**

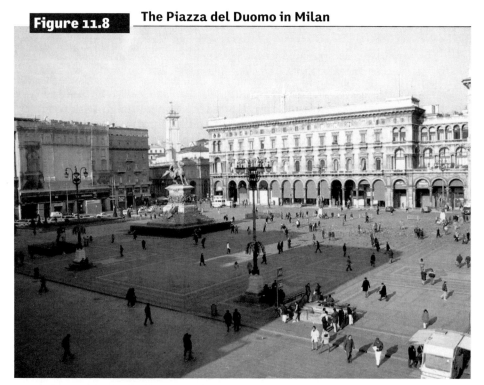

Source: Photo courtesy of Howard Lu.

even in both. Although perception of personal space, or space that is within your reach, can be selectively impaired in spatial neglect, this disorder can also affect perception of extrapersonal space—space that is beyond your reach. For example, Barrett and colleagues (Barrett, Schwartz, Crucian, Kim, & Heilman, 2000) reported the case of a woman who suffered a thalamic infarction and subsequently complained that she was consistently veering toward one side of the road when driving. They administered two line bisection tasks, in both of which she was instructed to respond by using a laser pointer. In the near condition (personal space), she bisected lines that were placed 30 centimeters away. In the far condition (extrapersonal space), she bisected lines that were placed 5 meters farther away. She performed similarly to the control participants when bisecting lines in personal space. However, in extrapersonal space, unlike controls, she made consistent and large errors away from the midline. Therefore, she was demonstrating neglect for extrapersonal space (making her a most hazardous driver) but perceived personal space relatively normally.

Spatial neglect can be manifested in a variety of other ways (each of which could actually be a unique disorder, replete with its own etiology); one such variant deserves special attention here. In some cases, the spatial neglect is not strictly bound by the hemifield in which the stimuli are presented. Instead, the spatial neglect can be "object centered," in which the person neglects one half of an object, word, or letter string, regardless of where these stimuli are presented in the person's visual field (Driver & Halligan, 1991; Hills & Caramazza, 1995; Subbiah & Caramazza, 2000). Although one can devise clever experiments to demonstrate object-centered neglect (see Driver & Halligan, 1991), it can sometimes be demonstrated in simple figure copying or spontaneous drawing (see Figure 11.9).

Figure 11.9   **Object-Centered Neglect**

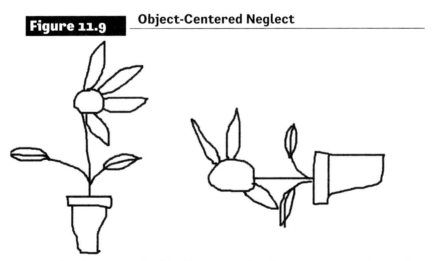

When copying objects, people with object-centered neglect cannot accurately reproduce the left side of an object. In this picture, an upright and rotated flower were copied. Note that the left side of the flower is missing petals in both drawings, even though it does not appear in the left side of space in the rotated image. Therefore it is the side of the object that matters most in object-centered neglect, not the side of space.

Spatial neglect is a lateralized disorder in that its symptoms are contralesional, but as was previously stated, the disorder is much more common following right hemisphere damage. In those cases in which spatial neglect arises from left hemisphere damage, the behavioral manifestations of the disorder are usually much less severe. However, the differences do not end there. The anatomical areas that are implicated in spatial neglect after left hemisphere damage are not the same as those that are implicated in right hemisphere damaged individuals. After damage to the left hemisphere, spatial neglect is associated with lesions anterior to the central sulcus. Conversely, after damage to the right hemisphere, spatial neglect is associated with lesions posterior to the central sulcus (Bradshaw & Mattingley, 1995). Taken together, these findings suggest that the anatomical structures that subserve our representation of space are localized to different regions in the two hemispheres. However, this generalization is complicated by the fact that spatial neglect can also arise after subcortical damage to structures such as the internal capsule, caudate nucleus, or thalamus (Heilman, Watson, & Rothi, 2000).

Bálint–Holmes Syndrome

As originally described by Bálint (Bálint, 1909; Harvey & Milner, 1995), there are three cardinal symptoms of the syndrome: (1) optic ataxia, (2) impaired visual attention, and (3) defective estimation of distance. Bálint's original case study reported an individual who had suffered a stroke and exhibited marked deficits in visually guided reaching and distance estimation, despite an intact ability to recognize and name objects. Holmes (1919) later described individuals with penetrating wounds who exhibited similar symptoms, but he also described an additional symptom: an oculomotor disturbance called *optic apraxia*. Much of the time, these four symptoms occur together in what we now call **Bálint–Holmes syndrome** (DeRenzi, 1985). However, not all four symptoms are always present. Despite these visuospatial deficits, people with Bálint–Holmes syndrome do not typically exhibit other cognitive or visual impairments.

OPTIC ATAXIA. Optic ataxia is a difficulty with visually guided reaching that is not related to motor, somatosensory, visual acuity, or other visual field defects (Nichelli, 1999). It occurs with varying degrees of severity. In its most severe form, individuals demonstrate great difficulty in accurately reaching for objects using either arm, even if they are fixating directly on the object. However, the reaching problem can also be more specific. In the case originally described by Bálint (1909), the individual demonstrated difficulty reaching with the right hand but virtually no impairment in reaching with the left hand. The fact that the reaching problems can be specific to one limb is quite important in explaining the cause of the optic ataxia. If the symptom were caused exclusively by a problem localizing an object in space, individuals would exhibit problems reaching with either arm. However, if the optic ataxia is caused by a problem integrating visual information with the movement (which appears to be the case), the symptom would be exhibited unilaterally.

IMPAIRED VISUAL ATTENTION. The impairment of visual attention in Bálint–Holmes syndrome is usually characterized by an extreme narrowing of attention. The narrow-

Visual Attention Problems in Bálint–Holmes Syndrome

Figure 11.10

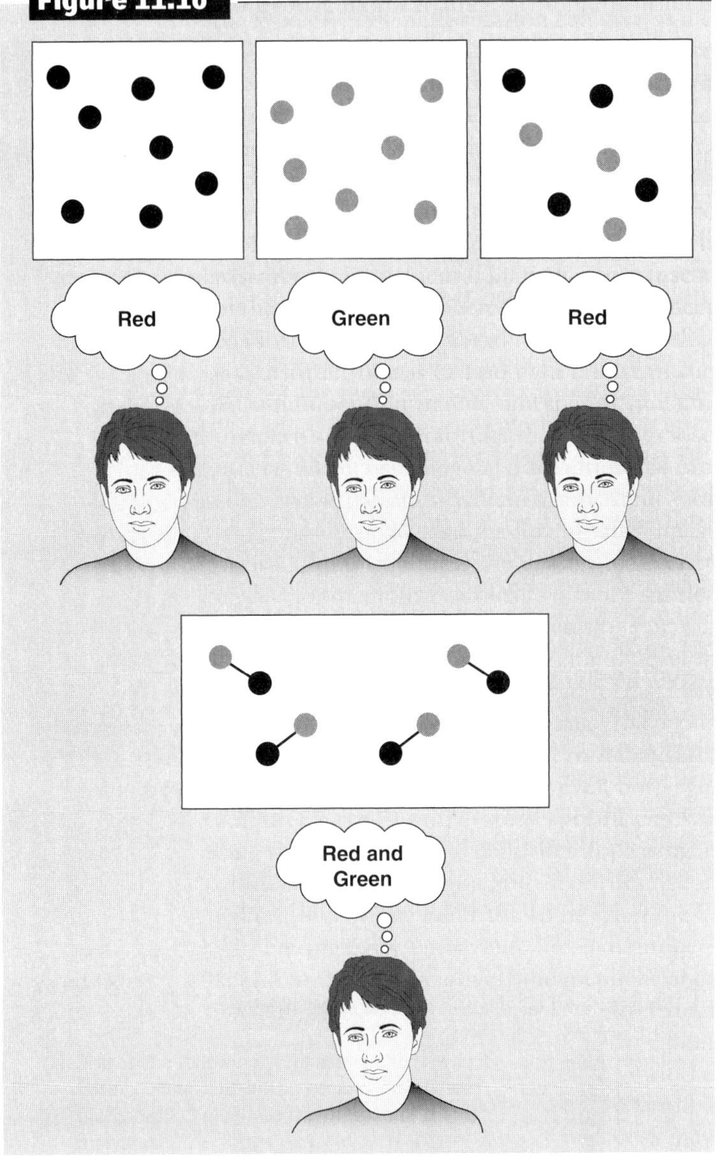

Source: Adapted from Humphreys & Riddoch (1993). Reprinted by permission of Paul Janzen.

ing of attention is so extreme that the person can usually attend to only one object at a time. Although the visual fields are usually intact, objects that are not attended to cannot be seen. (To contrast this with your own perception, place two pens a few inches apart on a desk in front of you such that they are not touching each other. Focus your attention on one of the pens. Can you still see the other pen? An individual with Bálint–Holmes syndrome could not.) When two objects are very close together or even touch each other, people with Bálint–Holmes syndrome might be able to perceive them both simultaneously. Some individuals with this syndrome retain (or regain) their ability to read, but only if the words are small and the letters are close together. When reading a newspaper, an individual with Bálint–Holmes syndrome might be able to read the articles at a relatively normal speed but exhibit severe difficulties reading the headlines (Nichelli, 1999).

Humphreys and Riddoch (1993) devised a very clever study of the visual attentive problems exhibited in Bálint–Holmes syndrome (Figure 11.10). They created visual arrays of thirty-two circles. The arrays were composed entirely of green circles, red circles, or a mixture of sixteen red and sixteen green circles. They presented these arrays to their patients and asked the patients to report whether the displays contained one or two colors. When the display was composed of all red or all green circles, the patients correctly identified that one color was present. However, when the arrays were mixed, the patients typically reported seeing either red or green (but not both). When Humphreys and Riddoch connected the red and green circles with a line (forming a single dumbbell-shaped object), a couple of the patients were much better at identifying that two

the **Real** world

Is Neglect Normal?

Line bisection is a useful task for detecting spatial neglect. Following right hemisphere damage, individuals often bisect lines to the right of center (neglecting the left side of space). One might expect that neurologically normal people should be able to bisect lines accurately. However, most people make small errors, consistently bisecting lines to the *left* of center. Bowers and Heilman (1980) named this phenomenon *pseudoneglect*. A recent meta-analysis (in which the results from a number of studies were combined and analyzed together) by Jewell and McCourt (2000) confirmed that the leftward bias occurs frequently in neurologically normal individuals. However, this study also identified a number of factors that influence these errors. For example, males appear to make larger leftward errors than females do, and right-handers make larger leftward errors than left-handers do (see Figure 11.11). The direction in which the lines were scanned also appears to affect these errors. When instructed to scan the line from left to right, people bisect the line to the left of center. When instructed to scan the line from right to left, people bisect the line slightly to the right of center. Some have claimed that the leftward bias that most people exhibit is simply an artifact of the left–right scanning that is required in reading English and many other languages.

However, line bisection is not the only task that demonstrates free-viewing perceptual asymmetries. If people view chimeric faces (discussed and illustrated in Chapters 4 and 9), in which the two halves of the face display different emotional expressions, people tend to base their judgments of the emotions on the expressions on the left side of the face (Moreno, Borod, Welkowitz, & Alpert, 1990).

A task that exhibits exceptionally strong and reliable free-viewing asymmetries is one developed by Mattingley and colleagues (Mattingly, Bradshaw, Nettleton, & Bradshaw, 1994). In this study, patients with right hemisphere lesions and normal controls viewed two shaded rectangles that were darker on one side. The participants were asked to indicate which rectangle was darker, but unbeknownst to them, the two rectangles were equal in brightness—in fact, they were mirror images of each other. As was expected, the people with right hemisphere lesions tended to choose the rectangle with the darkest edge on the right side. Surprisingly, the normal controls were much more likely to choose the rectangle with the darkest edge on the left side.

This finding was extended in a study by Nicholls and colleagues

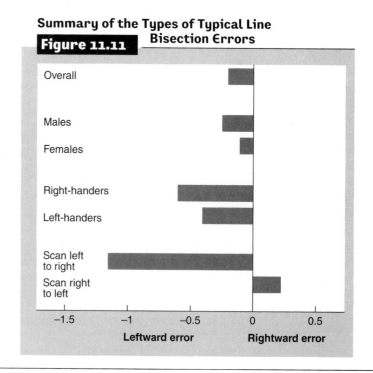

Summary of the Types of Typical Line Bisection Errors

Figure 11.11

Samples of Stimuli That Lead to Perceptual Asymmetries

Figure 11.12

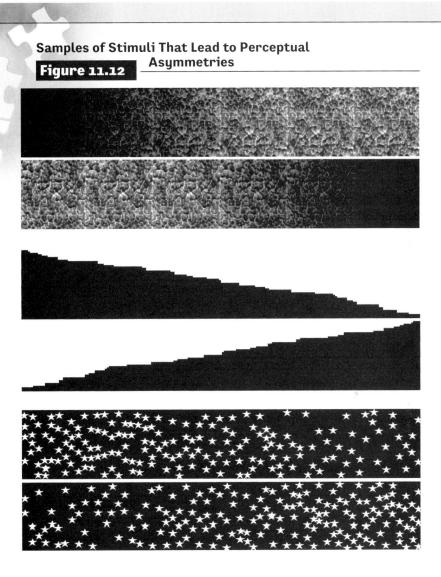

(Nicholls, Bradshaw, et al., 1999), who employed a number of similar tasks that demonstrated the same effect. When neurologically normal participants viewed two mirror images of stimuli whose features changed from left to right (see Figure 11.12) and were asked to make judgments about brightness, size, or quantity, people chose the object with the salient feature on the left over two-thirds of the time. Whether this finding is related to the leftward errors that people normally make in line bisection has yet to be determined.

colors were present. Therefore, when the mixed array of unconnected green and red circles was presented, only one of the objects could be attended to at any given time. However, when lines connected two circles of different colors, they were perceived as one object, and the presence of two different colors was detected.

DEFECTIVE ESTIMATION OF DISTANCE. Bálint's original report described the problems his patients had with a task in which they were presented with two objects and were asked to identify which object was closer to them. After observing marked deficits in this task, Bálint concluded that the cause of the impairment was an inability to perceive both objects at the same time. Although problems with visual attention probably contribute to the impairments on this task, people with Bálint–Holmes syndrome also have more general problems evaluating the spatial characteristics of single stimuli. For example, Holmes (1919) presented his patients with objects (one at a time) that they recognized and then asked the patients to describe the object's distance or size. The patients exhibited severe deficits on these tasks that cannot be attributed to impairments in visual attention.

GAZE APRAXIA. As we discussed in Chapter 5, apraxia is a disorder of purposeful movement that "is not caused by weakness, deafferentation, abnormal tone/posture or movement disorder" (Heilman, Watson, & Valentine, 2000). **Gaze apraxia** (also called *ocular apraxia*) is apraxia specific to eye movements. People with Bálint–Holmes syndrome can move their eyes in any direction but cannot shift their gaze intentionally to fixate on an object or point in space. When given instructions to look at a specific location, they might make random eye movements or even look in the wrong direction. If they eventually manage to fixate on the object, the fixation is very difficult to maintain and can be lost quickly. Because of this inability to voluntarily direct gaze, individuals with Bálint–Holmes syndrome also have trouble pursuing moving objects with their eyes.

PROBABLE CAUSES OF BÁLINT–HOLMES SYNDROME. Bilateral lesions to the parieto-occipital junction (posterior parietal lobe and lateral occipital lobe) typically cause Bálint–Holmes syndrome. These lesions are often caused by ischemia, but individuals in the early stages of Alzheimer's dementia can also exhibit Bálint–Holmes syndrome. When people in the early stages of dementia exhibit the syndrome, functional imaging shows a selective bilateral reduction in metabolism by parietal and occipital cortical regions (Pietrini et al., 1996).

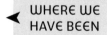 **◄ WHERE WE HAVE BEEN** The preceding sections focused on disturbances in the conscious processing of stimuli as a result of focal brain damage. We examined three conditions in detail. Blindsight, the condition in which visual stimuli are not processed consciously but unconscious perception of visual information guides conscious decision making. In spatial neglect, an individual does not normally consciously perceive or respond to stimuli in a given spatial location, despite relatively intact sensation. Finally, Bálint–Holmes syndrome is a disorder of covert visual attention in which attention to multiple objects is severely impaired but the perception of single objects can be accomplished relatively normally.

Glossary

Alpha waves—Brain activity with a pattern that appears when individuals have their eyes closed or are in a trance. Waves range from 8 to 12 Hz.

Bálint–Holmes syndrome—A syndrome following bilateral damage to the parieto-occipital junction. It is categorized by the presence of one to four cardinal symptoms: optic ataxia, impaired visual attention, defective estimation of distance, and optic apraxia.

Central executive—Primary component of Baddeley's model of working memory that is responsible for controlling attention and supervising the phonological loop and the visuospatial sketchpad.

Cocktail party effect—The ability to focus attention on one speaker in the midst of a number of speakers.

Cost—When cueing results in a slower or more erroneous response.

Delta waves—Brain activity that characterizes sleep stages 3 and 4; waves range from 1 to 2 Hz.

Early selection—Attention to an input and the decision to further encode and analyze it (e.g., categorizing, naming) occurs very early in the perceptual process. The stimulus does not need to be completely encoded or perceived prior to selection or rejection from further processing.

Exogenous cueing—A paradigm in which reaction times to targets can be influenced by the time between the presentation of the cue and the presentation of the target.

Gaze apraxia—A disorder resulting in an inability to voluntarily direct gaze.

Inhibitory aftereffect (inhibition of return)—In an exogenous cueing paradigm, the cost associated with a cue that occurs more than 300 milliseconds before the presentation of the target.

Invalid trials—Trials in which cues mislead the participant as to the location of a target.

Late selection—The idea that attention operates after the sensory information has been perceived, identified, and/or categorized.

Lexical decision tasks—Tasks that require an individual to decide whether a letter string was a word.

Lucid dreaming—Dreaming while knowing that one is dreaming.

Masking stimulus—A stimulus that rapidly replaces, or masks, a target stimulus that is developed to occupy a participant's sensory memory of an event during experiments.

Optic ataxia—A disorder that results in difficulty with visually guided reaching that is not related to motor, somatosensory, visual acuity, or other visual field defects.

Phonological loop—The component of the working memory that is responsible for manipulating linguistic information.

Rapid eye movement (REM)—A stage of sleep that involves electrical activity that resembles wakefulness more than rest; accompanied by dreams and paralysis of all muscles except the muscles controlling eye movements, the muscles within the inner ear, and the muscles that are required to sustain vegetative functions such as breathing.

Reflexive attention—A shift in attention that occurs in response to some external event.

Scotoma—An area of partial or complete loss of vision that can occur following damage to the primary visual cortex. When it is a result of cortical damage, the scotoma appears in the visual field opposite to the side of the brain in which the damage has occurred.

Selective attention—The process that allows the selection of inputs, thoughts, or actions while ignoring other ones.

Sleep—A readily reversible state of reduced responsiveness to and interaction with the environment.

Sleep spindle—Occurs occasionally during stage 2 sleep; an 8- to 14-Hz oscillation that originates in the thalamus.

Spatial neglect—A disorder that results in the failure to report, respond to, or attend to stimuli or events in one hemifield in which the impairment is not caused by sensory or motor deficits.

Theta waves—Brain activity that characterizes stage 1 sleep. Waves range from 4 to 8 Hz.

Visuospatial sketchpad—The component of the working memory that is responsible for manipulating visuospatial information, such as mental imagery and spatial locations.

Voluntary attention—An intentional shift of attention from one input to another.

12

Humans, Human Brains, and Evolution

Evolution is cleverer than you are.

—FRANCIS CRICK

MODULE **12.1**
Evolution of Humans

In November 1859, Charles Darwin published *On the Origin of Species* and fundamentally changed our understanding of biology, if not society as well. Darwin's theories tell us that all living creatures have been and continue to be subject to selection. These theories represent a fundamental paradigm shift in the natural sciences that have allowed us to understand speciation. Furthermore, these principles apply to more than just physical changes; evolutionary theory provides important insights into behaviors that also have been subject to selection pressures (e.g., the mating preferences of birds).

Despite the long history of research into the evolution of the physical structures of humans, few researchers applied the principles of evolution to human behavior, and many would agree that only now is such research beginning. This new research is very controversial—even more controversial than early research on the evolution of species. There are still controversies in the study of physical evolution; however, the disagreements within the scientific community typically revolve around the mechanisms of evolution or the placement of a specific artifact within a time frame. There is very little doubt among scientists that humans have been and continue to be subjected to evolutionary forces.

This level of acceptance has yet not been achieved for **evolutionary psychology**, which attempts to apply the principles of adaptation and selection to human behavior. Although evolutionary psychology has increased in popularity, a lack of acceptance of evolutionary psychology can be largely attributed to its relative newness and to the difficulties that are inherent whenever a new theory challenges accepted social and scientific views (for review, see Pinker, 2002). As a species, we have difficulty applying the principles of evolution to ourselves. It appears that we do not like thinking of ourselves as animals and as being subject to the laws of nature (although we also have a multitude of examples of evolutionary theory being used to promulgate racist views about people of certain ethnicities). However, the evolutionary perspective on brain and behavior provides us with important insights into how our environment has affected the development of our species as well as the specific demands and subsequent adaptations that evolved to deal with these challenges. Thus, evolutionary psychology provides us with a means by which we can integrate our behavior with our prehistory and gain profound insights into what it means to be human (and what it doesn't).

This chapter will take the perspective that we are animals and that our brains and therefore our behaviors have been shaped by the principles of evolution, just as it has shaped the bodies and behaviors of other animals.

WHERE WE ARE GOING ➤ This module will discuss the development of evolutionary theory and the evolution of hominid brains. This module will also discuss the inferences that we are entitled to make (and those that we are not) on the basis of the evolution of the human species. The second module will discuss how the principles of evolution can be used to understand brain function and behavior.

Evolutionary Theory

The discovery of evolutionary theory is generally credited to both Charles Darwin and Alfred Russel Wallace, who on July 1, 1858, presented the theory of evolution to the Linnean Society of London (Wallace was in absentia). The development of this theory was made independently by these two researchers, both of whom were naturalists with interests in geology.

Darwin sailed on the *H.M.S Beagle* in December 1831, traveling to such places as the Galapagos Islands. His voyage lasted five years, and during this time, he became intrigued with understanding how species emerged and how geographic isolation on islands produced such a variety of features in what he presumed were the same species. Wallace explored the Amazon River basin and parts of Indonesia for eleven years, becoming intrigued with the relationships between the geography of a particular location and its effects on specific characteristics of the species that inhabited that niche. During this time, Wallace wrote the essay "On the Tendency of Varieties to Depart Indefinitely from the Original Type" and sent it to Darwin for comment. It was this essay that confirmed Darwin's theories of evolution and pushed him to publish the book *On the Origin of Species* in 1859.

Although Darwin and Wallace are generally credited with discovering the principles of natural selection, they credited others with providing important insights that allowed them to produce the theory of evolution. In fact, some would argue that their true genius was their ability to synthesize a wide variety of diverse ideas. The ideas on which Darwin and Wallace drew include the following:

1. The classification of organisms based on structure by Carolus Linnaeus. Linnaeus observed that there were commonalities in structure among related species. This commonality is now thought to support the principles of evolution (although Linnaeus did not recognize this at the time).

2. Work by the geologists Charles Lyell and William Smith supported the notion that the earth was far older than was previously thought. Smith studied fossils and observed that some species of animals had changed very little, whereas others were now extinct. Furthermore, when changes occurred, they occurred in a predictable manner in the strata of the earth, with more primitive forms occurring in the oldest strata of the earth. Lyell studied geological processes, including erosion and volcanism, and argued that the length of time required for these events to occur suggested that the earth was much older than had previously been thought. Lyell's work also suggested the idea that the processes that shaped the earth were still in effect. That is, the forces that were active in shaping the earth as we know it are still active and will continue to produce changes in the future.

3. Thomas Malthus, a philosopher, wrote about the effects of poverty on the population during the industrial revolution. Simply put, Malthus observed that food supplies affect populations. Similar to what would become the staple of evolutionary theory (survival of the fittest), Malthus suggested that populations grow exponentially until they surpass their food supply, which leads to a struggle for existence.

HISTORICAL THEORY OF EVOLUTION. The historical theory of evolution can be summarized by three terms: **variation, inheritance,** and **differential reproduction.** That is, all individuals vary, which results in differences in morphology. These differences in morphology can be passed from one generation to the next. Finally, these individual differences in morphology result in variations in success in the environment, in terms of survival and reproduction. For example, we all vary in height (variation), although our heights are similar to that of our parents (inheritance). If the environment suddenly changed such that all tall individuals had a much harder time surviving, then shorter people would have an advantage, and they should have an easier time surviving longer to produce a greater number of infants (differential reproduction). Evolutionary theory predicts that over time, this scenario would result in more short people than tall ones.

Darwin suggested that the mechanism underlying these changes was **natural selection.** Natural selection requires that all individuals are unique and that characteristics that give an animal a reproductive advantage will result in the magnification of these traits in the population. When a trait results in a reproductive advantage and is selected for, it is called an **adaptation.** For a trait to be an adaptation, it must be inherited from one generation to the next. However, because the animals are adapted to specific environments, different environments may result in the selection of different traits, often in geographically distinct populations of related species. Because the environment is not static and variation never truly goes away, natural selection must be continually occurring (suggesting that existing and new species are being shaped currently).

However, this "survivalist" account of evolution cannot explain all of the physical and behavioral traits that influence a gene's success (i.e., survival). For example, why does a male (but not female) peacock have such an incredibly large and colorful tail? Certainly not to help avoid being eaten by predators! Darwin himself was puzzled by some of the physical traits observed in species such as peacocks and eventually became dissatisfied with natural selection as the only possible cause (or force) of evolution. In Darwin's second book on evolution, *The Descent of Man*, he proposed another type of selection: **sexual selection.** In natural selection, it is competition among individuals for survival to reproduce that determines which genes remain in the gene pool and which genes disappear from the face of the planet. In sexual selection, it is competition among individuals for reproduction that determine a gene's fate. There are two types of sexual selection:

1. In **intersexual selection,** one sex chooses a mate from among members of the other sex on the basis of specific traits. For human men, the choice appears to be most influenced by factors such as attractiveness and youth. For human women, the choice is also influenced by physical factors such as height and muscularity, but the man's resources also come into play.

2. In **intrasexual selection,** members of the same sex compete for partners of the opposite sex. Males might compete with each other by becoming more muscular or acquiring and displaying resources (such as wealth), whereas females might compete with each other by enhancing their appearance and youthfulness.

We refer to the original theory of evolution as the **historical theory of evolution** because of the changes to the theory that have occurred since its inception. For instance, although Darwin and Wallace formulated the theory of natural selection, they did not know why variation occurred, nor did they know the means by which traits were passed from generation to generation. We now know that traits are passed on by **genes** and that the original source of variation is the random **mutation** of these genes. The current version of evolutionary theory is referred to as the **modern synthetic theory of evolution** or the *modern synthesis*.

MODERN SYNTHESIS. The modern synthesis combines information from such diverse areas as molecular biology and paleontology. It is based on what is known about genes, **DNA** (deoxyribonucleic acid), **chromosomes,** and population biology. Before we discuss the principles of the modern synthesis, a basic knowledge of genetics will help.

Genes, made of DNA, assort in pairs and are located on chromosomes, which are simply strings of genes. Humans have twenty-three pairs of chromosomes, and it is estimated that we have between 26,000 and 40,000 genes (making us more like a short story than an epic novel), which are located on these chromosomes. When an egg is fertilized, the sperm contributes its twenty-three chromosomes to the egg's twenty-three chromosomes, resulting in twenty-three pairs of chromosomes. This allows for a large variation in genetic material that is passed from parents to offspring. It is important to remember that although there is a large variation among individuals, genetically speaking, there is more the same in the genetic makeup of individuals than there is different. These similarities allow for there to be common features, such as eyes and **bipedal gait** (walking upright on two legs), among members of our species. The differences among individuals allows for unique features, such as the subtle differences in the shape or color of the eyes, to occur. When someone undergoes a DNA test in a legal proceeding, it is the person's unique differences that are being examined.

Your genotype is the entirety of your genetic composition, and barring exposure to certain chemicals or radiation, your genotype is invariant during your lifetime. Your phenotype is the interaction of your genotype with the environment in which you develop. For example, your genotype may say that your maximum height should be six feet. However, if you live in an environment in which you are starved of nutrients, you may grow to be only five feet tall. Regardless of your phenotype, only your genotype will be passed on to your children. In essence, it can be said that while natural selection operates on phenotypes, only genotypes are transmitted from generation to generation.

Although we frequently use the shorthand phrase "the gene for some trait or other," this does not really represent the truth about the function of genes. Genes do not make traits or diseases, they make proteins. In addition, there is often more than one form of a given gene; these different forms are called **alleles.** When we say that there is a gene for blue eyes and one for brown, what we really mean is that there is an allele for eye color that in one form makes a protein (melanin) in the iris that looks brown and another allele that does not produce this protein, resulting in an iris that looks blue. Therefore, when we say that we have found the gene for Alzheimer's disease, what we mean is that we have found one allele of a gene that, in interaction with the environment, produces some of the symptoms associated with Alzheimer's disease. However, it is also possible that this same allele of the gene or a different one altogether produces some type of protein that is associated with the ordinary function of the brain.

The inheritance patterns of genes often follow very simple rules of expression. Although the composition of genes (DNA) was not known at the time, these rules of expression were first expressed by Gregor Mendel in *Experiments in Plant Hybridization,* written in 1885. The inheritance of eye color is a common example that illustrates simple, Mendelian genetics (Table 12.1). In this example, the gene for brown eyes (B) is **dominant,** and the gene for blue eyes (b) is **recessive.** As genes assort in pairs, dominant genes are always expressed whenever they are present. In contrast, recessive genes are expressed only when there are no dominant genes present. When both alleles are the same, we say that an individual is **homozygous** for that trait. When the two alleles are different, we say that an individual is **heterozygous** for that trait. In Table 12.1, both parents express the phenotype of brown eyes, and 75% of their offspring will have the phenotype for brown eyes and 25% will have the phenotype for blue eyes.

However, this view of genes is too simplistic, as very few traits are completely determined by a single gene. When multiple genes (often on different chromosomes) affect a trait, we say that the trait is **polygenic.** In fact, the example in Table 12.1 is not correct, as eye color is affected by at least three different genes on two different chromosomes. Chromosome 19 contains two genes for eye color: *bey2,* which has a brown and a blue allele, and *bey1,* which is associated with a central brown ring on the iris (Eiberg & Mohr, 1987). Chromosome 15 contains one gene for eye color, *gey,* which has a blue and a green allele. Table 12.2 presents a simplified polygenic model of eye color inheritance. As you can see, the polygenic model of eye color inheritance (Table 12.2) is more complex than the simple one presented in Table 12.1. Notice that this model does not explained eye colors such as hazel or gray, or the different shades within each color (light or dark brown), suggesting that there may be even more genes that are involved with the production of eye color.

It is also important to remember that many polygenic traits associate; that is, they behave like best friends, and although they are individual genes, they go everywhere

Table 12.1
Two Parents with Brown €yes and Their Possible Offspring

Parent 1 (phenotype: brown eyes; genotype Bb) & Parent 2 (phenotype: brown eyes; genotype Bb).

	Mom B		**b**	
Dad B	Genotype: BB	Phenotype: brown	Genotype: Bb	Phenotype: brown
b	Genotype: Bb	Phenotype: brown	Genotype: bb	Phenotype: blue

Table 12.2				
A Polygenic Model of the Inheritance of Eye Color				
Gene	**Allele**	**Mode of Inheritance**	**Genotype**	**Phenotype**
bey2	Brown (b-B)	Dominant	b-B/b-B (*gey* absent)	Brown
gey	Blue (b-b)	Recessive	b-b/b-b (*gey* absent)	Blue
			b-b/b-B (*gey* absent)	Brown
bey2 + *gey*	Green (g-G)	Dominant	g-B/g-B (*bey2* absent)	Brown
	Blue (g-b)	Recessive	g-b/g-b (*bey2* absent)	Blue
			g-B/g-b (*bey2* absent)	Brown
	b-B	Dominant	b-B + any other 3 alleles, including g-G	Brown
	g-G	Recessive to b-B dominant to b-b, g-b	g-G + any other 3 alleles except b-B	Green
	b-b	Recessive	b-b/b-b; g-b/g-b; b-b/g-b	Blue
	g-b	Recessive	b-b/b-b; g-b/g-b; b-b/g-b	Blue

together. This explains the observation that people with brown hair tend to have brown eyes and that people with blond hair tend to have blue eyes. The genes for hair color and eye color are associated and tend to pass from one generation to the next together. Furthermore, many polygenic traits are additive and do not follow the simple dominant/recessive pattern; that is, each allele has a small effect in determining the final phenotype. It is especially likely that inherited behaviors, such as bipedal gait, are most likely polygenic traits.

In any population, there is genetic variation. These variations may come about by random mutation and/or recombination of DNA. Mutation occurs when there is a change in the genotype due to an error in the replication of DNA. (DNA makes copies of itself; this process is known as **replication.**) Typically, the rate of mutation is slow, and most mutations are harmful to the organism, resulting in reduced ability to survive. This variation, whatever the cause, mutation or recombination, results in differing ability to adapt to the environment. Evolution works by selecting individuals who are better able to survive and reproduce, thus passing their genes on to their offspring.

The following list summarizes the modern synthesis.

1. *The central tenet of the modern synthesis is that certain environments select certain* **phenotypes,** *and phenotypes are an expression of the* **genotype** *interacting with the environment.* It is critical to remember that natural selection can not directly "see" the genotype, only the phenotype, and that although the environment can change the phenotype (e.g., colored contact lenses), the environment cannot typically change the genotype (with the exception of exposure to radiation). Although environmental factors may affect rates of mutation, they do not provide a direction for the mutation to occur. That is, the environment does not

Neuropsychological Celebrity

Children with PKU

Phenylketonuria (PKU) is a relatively rare inherited (autosomal, or nonsex chromosome, recessive) disease in metabolism that results from a deficiency of the phenylalanine hydroxylase enzyme. It is characterized by mental retardation. However, the extent of the retardation is dependent on two things. First, it depends on how early the condition is detected. Most hospitals in the developed world screen for PKU at birth using a blood test. The condition is also detectable without a blood test because it leads to light skin, light hair, and the development of a musty odor (created by the excess phenylalanine in the skin). Left untreated, PKU results in abnormally high levels of phenylalanine that damage the brain and other organs. However, when it is detected early, levels of phenylalanine can be kept low through dietary management, and the brain damage that it causes can be kept to a minimum. The second factor in the degree of brain damage produced by PKU is diet.

Phenylalanine can be kept from building up in the body by adhering to a diet with very low levels of protein.

The example of PKU demonstrates two important things about genetics and behavior. First, it is an example of the way in which an individual's genes interact with his or her environment. The genetic abnormality that causes PKU can be controlled as long as the individual's environment (in this case, the person's diet) can also be controlled. Second, it is an example of how some disease-causing genetic mutations manage to survive the selection pressures of evolution. If having a certain gene compromises one's ability to survive and reproduce, shouldn't the gene be selected out of the population? Woolf (1986) has suggested that there may be a heterozygous (adaptive) advantage in PKU. More specifically, an individual who has only one copy of the recessive gene is relatively well protected against the toxic effects of ochratoxin A, a mycotoxin that appears in stored grains and other foods. However, when an individual inherits two copies of the recessive gene, this results in the (maladaptive) condition of PKU.

produce adaptations; rather, mutations result in characteristics that in a specific environment are either adaptive, neutral, or deleterious (adverse) for the organism. Different environments may result in the same mutation being either adaptive, neutral, or deleterious.

2. *Although genes occur at the level of the individual, evolutionary change occurs at the level of populations.* Populations evolve by changes in gene frequency that are brought about by natural selection, random genetic drift, and gene flow. Natural selection can produce evolutionary change if a gene or genes provides a slight fitness, or reproductive, advantage (e.g., increases in the number of offspring that survive to reproduce). Small differences in genes can result in large changes in the genetic makeup of a population in a relatively short period of time if they provide tangible survival and/or reproductive advantages for those who possess the gene. **Genetic drift**, the tendency for isolated populations to depart from the original genetic composition of the population, also can produce evolutionary change. This drift away from the original genetic composition of the population is most likely the result of extensive **inbreeding** (offspring resulting from related parents) and adaptation to the isolated environment. **Gene flow** is the movement of genes through a population that results from mating. Gene flow can be profound when

there is extensive inbreeding. Finally, as was mentioned in point 1, because environments change over time, genes that were once adaptive may become maladaptive and result in a decreased frequency of occurrence in a population.

3. *Species represent different gene pools, rather than fundamentally unique groups.* Species are judged as such by their genotype, not their phenotype. When we judge speciation on the basis of phenotype, we can often be misled, because there is often great variation in phenotype among individuals of a population. For example, although both chihuahuas and Great Danes are quite phenotypically distinct, they are both phenotypes of dog (and theoretically could successfully mate). There is often considerable genetic overlap among different species. For instance, there is a 98.4% overlap between chimpanzees and human beings. This overlap provides support for the view that evolution is a gradual process that tends to make small changes over time in existing species rather than new species developing from nothing. However, there are those who point out that the fossil record also indicates rapid morphological changes and relatively long periods of stasis in populations.

There are three major differences between the modern synthetic theory of evolution and the historical evolutionary theory. The first and perhaps most important difference is that the modern theory recognizes that traits are the result of genes that are inherited from one's parents and interact with the environment. The second difference is the recognition that there are mechanisms other than natural selection that can effect evolutionary change. Finally, there is the recognition that what we call *species* are only differences in gene pools of a population, not totally distinct or new organisms that arrived fully formed from nowhere.

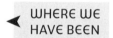 We have discussed the history of evolution, the historical theory of evolution, and the modern synthetic theory of evolution. A number of important physical modifications can be observed by studying our history. For example, evolution has resulted in fundamental changes to the shape of our hands, our faces, and, most important, the size of our brains.

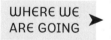 We will now trace the evolution of the nervous system. The second module will discuss how the principles of evolution can be used to understand brain function and behavior.

Evolution of the Nervous System

Unlike bones, the brain tissue is soft and quickly deteriorates under natural conditions, thus leaving no fossilized remains. Instead of looking directly at fossilized brain, researchers examine fossilized skulls to obtain clues regarding the brains of our ancestors. From direct observation of the skulls of our fossil ancestors, we can see an increase in skull size and in the size of the brain. However, we must be cautious about directly implicating brain size with increased intelligence or "humanness." Figure 12.1 demonstrates that although humans do not have the largest brains in the animal kingdom, we tend to have one of the larger brains for the size of our body. Even when we

Differences in Relative Size between the Cortex and Brainstem in Several Species
Figure 12.1

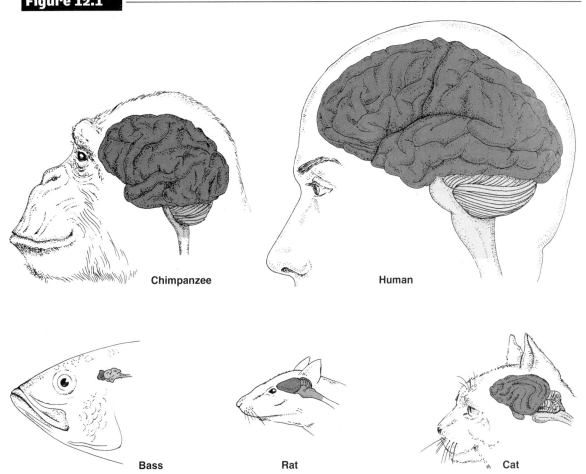

Chimpanzee

Human

Bass

Rat

Cat

Note the relatively higher proportion of cortex as evolutionary age increases.

Source: John P. J. Pinel, *Biopsychology,* 5e. Published by Allyn and Bacon, MA. Copyright © 2003 by Pearson Education. Reprinted by permission of the publisher.

take into account our body size (Jerison, 1990), we do not have the largest brains. Our brains are only 2.33% of our body weight, but the tree shrew has a brain that is 3.33% of its body weight. It is only when we examine how much of the brain is cortex that humans are startling: The human brain has almost 3.2 times the amount of cortex than other species. Thus, although over our evolutionary history, an increase in brain size is associated with an increased ability to perform complex behaviors, we must remember that absolute brain size can be misleading.

Another way to examine the skull of animals is to make an **endocast,** or a mold of the inside of the skull. In mammals, the endocasts look much like the brain when it is covered with the meninges, allowing for the inspection of the major sulci and gyri of the brain. From studying endocasts, we can see that the brain has undergone significant changes in organization. For instance, human brains are asymmetrical, and the degree of asymmetry is not as pronounced in endocasts from australopithecines, a very early ancestor who lived from four million on to as recently as one million years ago, suggesting that this asymmetry has evolved over time (Holloway, 1982).

Many scientists believe that changes in the placement of sulci on the endocasts is associated with changes in brain organization (Wilkins & Wakefield, 1995). Another area that is intriguing is the development of the frontal lobe area associated with language in humans. Although there is some debate, at least one endocast from *Homo erectus* appears to demonstrate a more humanlike frontal area. Since *Homo erectus* lived from 1.6 million years ago to as recently as 400,000 years ago, this is a relatively recent change. Unfortunately, the endocasts from australopithecines and other *Homo* species do not preserve this feature well, which makes it difficult to determine when this change occurred. However, the possibility that the features of the brain associated with language appear in *H. erectus* is suggestive of some rudimentary forms of speech. Furthermore, for the frontal language areas, there are no significant differences between endocasts obtained from Neanderthals and from humans, suggesting that Neanderthals could have used language (Johanson & Edgar, 1996). Neanderthals are a species related to humans that lived from 250,000 years ago and disappeared from Europe approximately 30,000 years ago. Again, caution must be used in the interpretation of this information; there are relatively few endocasts of fossil hominids, which makes it difficult to know whether a change in sulcal position reflects actual evolutionary change for the entire species or just some type of individual variation in brain organization. However, many researchers suggest that the study of endocasts, although flawed, is the best way that we currently have to study the evolution of the brain.

It seems reasonably safe to say that the observed increases in the size of the frontal lobe occur in australopithecines and all subsequent hominid brains. The switch from olfactory areas of the brain to frontal regions suggests that there may have been changes in behavior from olfactory analysis to more complex reasoning tasks. However, the largest changes in the modern human brain are in the parietal lobe, which is very flattened in ancient primates and quite rounded in modern humans. The increase in the size of the parietal lobe is associated with tool-making and hunting. Interestingly, early species of australopithecines appear to have enhanced frontal lobes, whereas later species have enlarged parietal lobes, suggesting an independent evolution of these structures (Deacon, 1997).

Other researchers suggest that brain evolution can be studied by comparing brains of humans with those of other primates. DNA evidence can tell us approximately when we had common ancestors with living primates, so studying the neuroanatomy of related species may also provide important insights into the evolution of the brain. Consistent with the observations from the endocasts, the brain of the common chimpanzee, *Pan trogolodytes*, also shows a lesser degree of hemispheric asymmetry, reduced frontal linguistic areas, and smaller parietal lobes. Other comparisons among species tend to focus on the relative size of the brainstem (regulating reflexive activities such as blood pressure and heart rate) and the cortex (regulating more complex

Current Controversy

What Caused Selection Pressure for Encephalization?

For the most part, bigger brains are better brains. However, there are several exceptions to the rule. For example, a whale brain is much larger than a human brain, and yet our planet is not run by whales. Human males enjoy larger brains than human females, although the intellectual benefits of this difference in size are not clear, if there are any benefits at all. When comparing across species though, it is usually pretty clear that bigger brains are more capable than smaller ones. The increases in brain size from our primate relatives to early hominids were dramatic, but what caused these increases? What made bigger brains so much better? The most common answer you will find is that bigger brains provided better support for language development. Others have argued that consciousness is only possible with larger brains. Still others have argued that the answer lies in one's capacity for social skills (especially the ability to predict and manipulate the behavior of others). The University of Washington's William Calvin (2002) has a very different idea. He blames the weather.

We appear to be experiencing a worldwide global warming trend right now, and many would have you believe that this is a unique event in the earth's history, caused solely by negligent environmental practices worldwide. However, several paleoclimate and oceanography researchers claim that the current warming trend is just one part of a repetitive cycle of warming and cooling, and that every few thousand years the Earth's weather does a large flip-flop, going from an ice-age to a period of rapid warming. These rapid changes in temperature would have huge impacts on many species, often resulting in dramatic population crashes. A cycle of repetitive population crashes (often referred to as "bottlenecks") dramatically increases selection pressure for adaptive traits, effectively increasing the rate of evolution.

Calvin (2002) argues that the large human brain evolved to be "a brain for all seasons," one that was (and hopefully still is) capable of adapting to these large climate changes, even if the change happens within a single generation. This is because our distant ancestors had to live through hundreds of these cycles, each of which produced a bottleneck in the primate (not just human) population, driving the intense selection pressure toward big brains. Most of our ancestors did not survive these periods of change, but the ones who did found ways to adapt. Those with big brains were capable of finding food, making shelter, and reproducing in a wide range of climates, enjoying "a brain for all seasons." Calvin's theory is not the most popular one at the moment, but it sure is one of the most interesting accounts of encephalization!

---

behaviors, including language and learning). Comparisons of the brainstem with the cortex tend to focus on three major points of difference among the species:

1. Newer species (defined as species that have evolved relatively recently) have larger brains.
2. The increase in size that is observed in newer species is primarily in cortical areas.
3. Newer species have an increasingly complex cortex, as defined by the number of layers of cells and the number of cortical convolutions (wrinkles).

Increases in convolutions allow greater cortical surface area in the same size skull.

In summary, the brain of humans has undergone significant change over the course of evolution, becoming more complex and larger in a fairly short period of time. It is important to remember that large brains may not, in themselves, be adaptive. Large brains are more difficult to cool than small brains, and large brains require more energy to function, both of which require dedicated metabolic resources. Our large brains

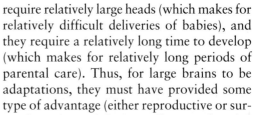

Self-Test

1. What are the three main characteristics of the modern synthetic theory of evolution?

2. How does sexual selection differ from natural selection?

3. What aspects of the human brain make it so unique?

require relatively large heads (which makes for relatively difficult deliveries of babies), and they require a relatively long time to develop (which makes for relatively long periods of parental care). Thus, for large brains to be adaptations, they must have provided some type of advantage (either reproductive or survival) that has ensured their selection. In the next module, we will argue that this advantage is behavioral.

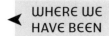

◀ **WHERE WE HAVE BEEN**

We have traced the evolution of the human brain, which provides important insights into behavior. We must remember that large brains are likely to provide an evolutionary advantage (perhaps behavioral) because they are very costly to maintain and would not have evolved if they did not offer something of value.

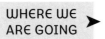

WHERE WE ARE GOING ▶

The next module will examine the statement that the changes in our brains allow us the tremendous flexibility in behavior that our species exhibits. It will focus on how the principles of evolution can be used to understand brain function and behavior.

MODULE **12.2**
Evolution and Behavior

As we stated at the beginning of this chapter, many people are quite comfortable with thinking about evolution in terms of its influence on the physical structure of many species. Species survive, thrive, or go extinct depending on their ability to feed and shelter themselves or their relatives and to cope with their environment and competitors. A glance through a children's book on animals gives the reader a quick tour of some physical adaptations: the long neck of the giraffe for eating food that is unreachable by other species, the large ears of the rabbit for detecting predators, the sharp teeth and claws of the crocodile for catching and consuming prey. These physical adaptations and their functions are obvious to the naked eye. However, what might be less obvious is the adaptive *behavior* exhibited by all animals, including humans.

The origin of adaptive behavior can be even less obvious. How much of your behavior do you attribute to learning? Try to imagine how you would act in your present situation if you were acting without the benefit of experience. What would your behavior be like? You certainly would not be able to read this book—in fact, you would not even be able to hold the book. So much of our behavior is made possible by the learning experiences that constitute our personal past. However, some behaviors are not exclusively dependent on learning. Instead, they appear to be dependent on our *evolutionary* past. Are you afraid of spiders? How about snakes? How about heights? Most humans are easily scared by all three, although most of us have never been bitten by a spider or snake, nor have we fallen from a great height. Are these fears the result of experience? Not entirely. They certainly can be modified by experience (mak-

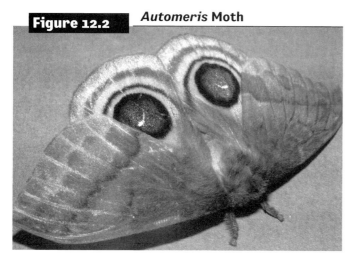

Figure 12.2   *Automeris* **Moth**

Source: Photo courtesy of Roger Chalkley.

ing one more or less frightened depending on the experience), but the origins of the fears tend not to be the result of personal experience.

Applying Evolutionary Theory to Behavior

The *Automeris* moth of Costa Rica has a very distinctive set of wings (see Figure 12.2). When the moth is in resting position, its forewings cover its hindwings, resulting in a relatively normal-looking yellowish moth. However, when the forewings are pulled forward, this reveals two large circular patches that resemble eyes on the hindwings. If the moth is antagonized, instead of flying away, it typically reveals these "eyes." It even looks as though the moth is looking back at you through these huge "eyes," in effect making itself even more noticeable. How and why does the moth exhibit this behavior? Should it not try to fly away? Questions about the cause of a given behavior can be addressed on many different levels of analysis. Consider these examples. One can describe the physiology that allows the moth to move its wings, the chemistry and genetics behind the formation of the colored patches, the neural processes that signal for the movement, or the past experiences of the moth in situations in which the patches were revealed versus when they were not.

PROXIMATE VERSUS ULTIMATE CAUSE. All of these types of explanations can provide valid accounts of the cause of the behavior, but the approaches can generally be divided into two types of questions. "How" questions address the **proximate cause** of a behavior. Proximate causes describe the internal mechanisms that underlie a behavior. They can also be characterized as the immediate cause of the behavior. "Why" questions are fundamentally different in that they address the **ultimate cause** of a behavior. Ultimate causes describe the evolutionary basis behind a behavior, including a description of what makes a given behavior adaptive. If we apply this distinction to the example of the *Automeris* moth, the proximate causes of the "eye"-bearing behavior can be described in terms such as the genetic coding for the formation of the circular patterns, the mechanisms for the sensation of a threat, or the physiology of the wing movement itself. The ultimate cause of the behavior must be described in terms of the adaptive value of the behavior. How did it increase the likelihood of survival and reproduction? According to British scientist David Blest, this behavior probably frightened off some of the moth's predators (such as smaller birds) because the "eyes" on the wings were mistaken for the eyes of their own predators, such as owls (Alcock, 2001; Blest, 1957).

Consider the examples of common fears that we provided a few paragraphs ago. Most people are scared of things such as spiders, snakes, heights, or even darkness, even in the absence of negative experiences with these stimuli. What causes this behavior? Descriptions of the proximate causes of the behavior might include an account of how the amygdala, a component of the limbic system (see more about the amygdala and fear in Chapter 10), is primarily responsible for the expression of fear or perhaps a description of how the visual system detects and recognizes creepy-crawly things. Although these are perfectly valid accounts of *how* the behavior is produced, they fail to address *why* people behave in this way. Presumably, the development of these fears in so many humans was ultimately caused by their facilitation of survival and reproduction in human ancestral environments. Consider the behaviors that arise as a consequence of fear. As a large spider moves in close to your bare hand, this produces arousal accompanied by a wide range of physiological responses, such as pupil dilation and increased rate of heartbeat. As the spider gets closer and closer, a whole host of behavioral options become available to you. Do you stomp on it? Run away? Scream? All three? These behaviors would presumably lower the odds of receiving a poisonous spider bite in our human ancestral environments. Therefore, the result of a fear of spiders is increased reproductive fitness. Some people have argued that an examination of human fears provides us with a glimpse into some of the survival hazards faced by our common ancestors (Buss, 1999; Marks, 1987).

ADAPTATIONS ARE NOT ALWAYS ADAPTIVE FOREVER. Until this point, we have considered some rather distressing examples of how our evolutionary past influences present-day behavior. However, in addition to human aversions, human preferences can also result from evolutionary mechanisms. Most studies of preference focus on how humans differ from one another. Do you remember discussing your favorite color with your friends when you were a child? How about your favorite food? Did all of you agree? Probably not. The preferences that humans exhibit vary considerably. Some people's preferences may seem completely baffling. Why would anyone ever ingest black licorice or listen to David Hasselhoff sing? (If you like these things, you can probably think of examples of preferences that make no sense to you.) Despite these differences in preference, there are some preferences that all humans appear to exhibit. One such example is our preference for fatty, salty, or sweet foods. When our early ancestors lived on the African savanna, sweet foods (such as fruits) would have been hard to come by but would provide nutrients such as vitamins. Individuals with a "sweet tooth" would be more likely to seek sweet foods and obtain vitamins necessary for survival and reproduction. Today, we are a species that generally loves sweets, but the sweets that are readily available now come in the form of junk food (which is practically devoid of the nutrients provided in the natural sweets of the savanna), and this preference is no longer adaptive. A preference that helped humans to stay healthy in ancestral environments now compromises our genetic and physical fitness (Buss, 1999).

The problem with evolution is that it tends to be quite slow. It takes generations for a random mutation to be selected by natural selection if it provides an advantage in terms of reproductive fitness. Unfortunately, the environment in which we currently live is changing at a furious pace. The vast majority of adaptations (physical or behavioral) are with us because they solved survival problems in our past, but they are not necessarily adaptive today.

Consider the example of automobile exhaust. It is not surprising that the lungs of humans (and other animals) have not adapted to the ever-present threat of automobile exhaust because this threat has been present for only a few human generations. In addition to living without adaptations that would be helpful in our present environment, we carry around adaptations that no longer help us. An example of a physical adaptation that no longer serves a function is the human appendix. This vestigial organ is part of the colon, and it is probably most famous for its penchant for perforating or rupturing, either of which can be fatal if not treated surgically. In addition to these examples of physical adaptations, some of our behavioral adaptations also appear to be out of date. Our love of junk food is certainly one damaging example, but our physiological reactions to stress are similarly damaging (Gaulin & McBurney, 2001).

This point is illustrated clearly by Ted Kaczinski (better known as the Unabomber) in his manifesto, "Industrial Society and its Future":

> [I] attribute the social and psychological problems of modern society to the fact that society requires people to live under conditions radically different from those under which the human race evolved and to behave in ways that conflict with the patterns of behavior that the human race developed while living under the earlier conditions. (quoted by Wright, 1995, p. 50)

There is considerable research to bolster Kaczinski's claim. Stress-related diseases such as high blood pressure are extremely rare among traditional, tribal cultures in Africa, South America, and the Pacific Islands. However, when people migrate from rural to urban areas, stress-related diseases become much more prevalent:

> Consistent and persuasive evidence links coronary and hypertensive disease with prolonged emotional stress, behavioral patterns, sociocultural mobility and changing life events. These disease states appear to be the major epidemic afflictions of industrialized communities in the twentieth century. Indeed the prevalence of coronary heart disease and hypertension parallel the increasing complexity of social system and social order. (Eliot & Buell, 1981, p. 25)

Modern life has provided us with many luxuries and advances compared to the lifestyle experienced by our ancestors on the African savanna. By comparison to them, we enjoy an abundance of food, shelter, and freedom from disease. Infant mortality is low, death from starvation is rare, and we can traverse the globe in a matter of days. However, along with these changes, modern life has become stressful, and we are regularly in contact with strangers (something that would have been relatively rare but stressful on the savanna). Our physiological adaptations to the *acute* stresses found in the environment of our ancestors are not adaptive in response to the *chronic* stresses that modern life delivers.

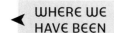

WHERE WE HAVE BEEN We have discussed the influence that evolutionary processes have on behavior as well as physical structure. The cause of a given behavior can be described in terms of the proximate events that make a behavior possible (such as the physiological changes that underlie a muscle movement) or the ultimate reason why individuals or species demonstrating a certain behavior would be more likely to survive and/or reproduce.

WHERE WE
ARE GOING ➤ The next section outlines some of the assumptions made by evolutionary psychologists as well as some of the prominent views of human behavior that are contradicted by this perspective. We will argue
that evolutionary psychology can be used to help guide neuropsychological investigations
of the relationship between brain activity and behavior.

Evolutionary Psychology

Imagine a researcher who specializes in studying evolution. How does he or she collect data? What sort of evidence is used to make inferences about evolutionary
processes? When most people are asked these questions, they describe an archeolo-
gist digging for fossils, searching for extinct species or perhaps rare "intermediate
forms" that bridge the gaps between present-day species. This answer is certainly a
good one; much of research into evolutionary processes takes this general form.
However, studying fossils tells the investigator only about the structure of an organism but not its behavior. Or does it? Is the researcher who is interested in ancient behavior out of luck because behaviors do not leave fossils the same way that structures
do? Consider the following vignette:

> As the archeologist dusted off the dirt and debris from the skeleton, she noticed some-
> thing strange: the left side of the skull had a large dent, apparently from a ferocious blow,
> and the rib cage—also on the left side—had the head of a spear lodged in it. Back in the
> laboratory scientists determined that the skeleton was that of a Neanderthal man who had
> died roughly 50,000 years ago, the earliest known homicide victim. His killer, judging
> from the damage to the skull and rib cage, bore the lethal weapon in his right hand. (Buss,
> 1999, p. 3)

The fossil record informs us about more than structural changes during evolution. It also provides clues about ancient behavior. It is difficult to make general inferences about human behavior on the basis of a single case, but this is no less true
in studying present-day individuals than it is in studying fossils from thousands of
years ago. However, in studying data from a group, many more inferences are possible in both instances. The fossil record certainly reveals some important themes that
are relevant to human behavior. The skeletons of males tend to contain far more dents
and fractures than do the skeletons of females, suggesting that males were much more
likely to die during combat. Furthermore, these injuries tend to be located on the left
front side of the skeletons and skulls, suggesting that most attacks (at least successful ones) were delivered by using the right hand (Trinkaus & Zimmerman, 1982).

Fortunately, old bones are not the only source of data for the evolutionary psychologist. In fact, studying present-day people often suffices. Testing a clearly formulated evolutionary hypothesis can be accomplished by comparing different species,
comparing males and females, comparing individuals within a species, studying the
behavior of the same individuals in different contexts, or using a variety of experimental methods. Surprisingly, one can compare animals from different species to gain
some understanding of the behavior of a species other than the ones being studied.
For example, if a researcher suspected that sex differences in spatial ability were related to polygamy in humans during ancestral times, one could test this hypothesis

by studying the sex differences in spatial ability for two species that are very similar in every respect except for their mating practices—polygamy versus monogamy. One can also compare males and females within the same species because the adaptive problems faced by the two human sexes can be quite different. In addition to comparing two sexes within a species, individuals can be grouped according to a different criterion, such as age. A teenage human female has many more years of potential reproduction ahead of her than does a middle-aged female; therefore, one could compare rates of abortion, miscarriage, or even infanticide between these two groups to investigate hypotheses about issues such as parental investment. There are also experimental methods that can be used to investigate evolutionary hypotheses. Given how slow evolutionary processes are (i.e., changes occurring over many generations), you might think that such methods would require the use of a time machine. A time machine would be nice, but until we have one, we must rely on methods such as subjecting different groups of people to different conditions and studying their reactions. Specific hypotheses, such as "group cohesion will increase in response to threat" can be tested in this way over a relatively short period of time. Curiously, such experiments are no longer being performed exclusively by the scientific community. Under the guise of "reality television," the entertainment industry appears to be conducting these experiments in many areas of behavior.

THE TABULA RASA. Long before Darwin's publication of *On the Origin of Species* in 1859, there was a commonly held belief that the human brain resembles a blank slate (**tabula rasa**) at birth and that all knowledge must be acquired through experience. This position was clearly articulated by John Locke (1632–1704), who claimed that no person's knowledge can go beyond his or her experience and that there are no such things as innate ideas. Beginning as a blank slate, the human brain must acquire knowledge through the use of the five senses and a process of reflection. This position was quite popular, though at odds with some other prominent views, such as the writings of Socrates that describe "innate knowledge." The tabula rasa view was also adopted by some of the founders of modern psychology, including behaviorist John Watson (1878–1958), who said,

> "Give me a dozen healthy infants, well-formed and my own specified world to bring them up in and I'll guarantee to take any one at random and train him to become any type of specialist I might select—doctor, lawyer, artist, merchant, chief and yes even beggarman and thief, regardless of the talents, penchants, tendencies abilities, vocations, and race of his ancestors." (Watson, 1924, p. 104)

Over the years, the tabula rasa metaphor has been updated to reflect current technologies. For example, the human brain at birth can be described as a general-purpose computer that has not yet been programmed. This general view has been termed the Standard Social Science Model (SSSM) by Tooby and Cosmides (1992), and it is still widely believed today.

INNATE HUMAN CHARACTERISTICS. The SSSM is not consistent with modern evolutionary psychology. Just as other animals are born with instincts, so too are humans. I adopted a very young and sickly kitten a few years ago. She was the runt of the litter and was not being fed very well by her mother. After she was separated from her littermates and bottle-fed by humans in a previously cat-free environment, her eyes opened, and she began to grow into a more and more healthy kitten. Eventually, she became extremely playful, stalking and pouncing on any moving thing that was smaller than she was. Where did she learn this behavior? She was separated from other cats for all of her sighted life, and I certainly didn't run around the house pouncing on things to demonstrate proper kitten behavior to her. Instead, these behaviors were instinctive. Most humans have very little difficulty accepting the fact that the behavior of "lower" animals can be determined without the benefit of experience, but we are generally quite reluctant to accept that possibility regarding our own behavior.

There are clearly some human behaviors that are "universal" in that they are exhibited by all cultures and ethnicities. Some behaviors are relatively simple and obvious ones, such as the presence of reflexes or the ability to learn simple motor tasks. However, others are very complex and influenced by socialization, such as the selection of a mate. Among the many examples are such disparate phenomena as infant reflexes, a love for rough-and-tumble play early in development, the imposition of grammatical structure on systems of communication, the use of tools, the telling of myths and legends, the formation of social groups, the development of aggression between individuals and social groups, the use of gestures during communication, the drive to have sex, and perhaps even the development of psychological defense mechanisms.

Many of these behaviors (if not all) appear to be adaptations. An adaptation is a system of properties or mechanisms molded by natural selection because it helped to solve a specific adaptive problem posed by the physical, chemical, developmental, ecological, demographic, social, or informational environment (Tooby & Cosmides, 1990). Adaptations have a number of properties:

1. They recur across generations.
2. They appear reliably over the developmental life of the organism.
3. Their appearance is influenced by genetic specifications.
4. They interact with features of the environment that are normally present.
5. They help to solve an "adaptive problem" that the organism's ancestors would have faced.
6. They were propagated during a period of selection because they enhanced the survival and/or reproduction of the individual (Tooby & Cosmides, 1990).

HOW DOES EVOLUTIONARY PSYCHOLOGY INFORM NEUROPSYCHOLOGY? As you will notice, the majority of this book is dedicated to providing proximate explanations of behavior. Describing the neural structures that subserve a given function answers "how" questions about behavior but not "why" questions. Consider the example of language processing. Following left hemisphere temporal lobe damage, people often have difficulty discerning the meaning of spoken words. This deficit is usually the result of damage to Wernicke's area, a region of the brain that is specialized for linking sounds with linguistic labels and meanings. However, this explanation is only a proximate one. Why does Wernicke's area perform this function? This question about the ultimate cause of the behavior is an evolutionary one, and it is currently fodder for debate.

the **Real** world

Are Allergies Adaptive?

Our planet is increasingly replete with toxins that are poisonous to humans and other animals. The presence of some of these toxins is clearly attributable to human environmental policy (or lack thereof), but there is also an impressive array of naturally occurring toxins present in fruits and vegetables such as bananas, broccoli, nuts, and potatoes. These plants produce toxins to protect themselves from herbivores and omnivores that eat them for their own survival. Margie Profet (1991) has argued that allergies evolved as a way to counteract the potentially deadly effects of these toxins. According to her toxin hypothesis, the bodily mechanisms triggered by allergies are adaptations. The manner in which mild allergic reactions manifest themselves through sneezing, coughing, or watering eyes would certainly help to purge toxins from the body. Even a reaction such as scratching in response to an itch could help to extrude toxins from the skin. The benefits of more extreme allergic reactions are less obvious. One common reaction is a sharp drop in blood pressure. Under normal circumstances, this is a very bad thing. However, if the bloodstream is carrying toxic substances, this can help to limit the body's exposure.

Allergies are becoming more and more common, and we probably experience them more than our ancestors did (Buss, 1999; Profet, 1991). Respiratory allergies alone afflict as many as 27% of people in the industrialized world. According to Buss (1999), we are particularly vulnerable to allergies in the modern world for the following reasons:

1. Hunter-gatherers could identify which substance is producing an allergic reaction and avoid it. In modern society, we are usually not fully aware of the substances we are ingesting, making them much harder to identify and avoid.
2. Modern humans are regularly exposed to harsh chemicals in forms such as soaps, preservatives, and pesticides.
3. Modern humans are less likely to breastfeed than was previously the case. Infants who are breastfed for at least six months are much less likely to develop allergies as adults, although the mechanism for this effect is not well understood.

Profet's position that allergies developed to solve an adaptive problem has not been met with unconditional acceptance, but her theory has the ability to explain a large number of previously puzzling facts about the nature of allergies.

Given that the brain was shaped by evolutionary processes, how does this help to guide our exploration of this incredibly complex structure? Much of neuropsychology and cognitive neuroscience proceeds without much influence from evolutionary theory. However, evolutionary psychology can simplify our explorations of the brain in a number of ways. First of all, it can help us to define which functions we should attempt to localize. Past investigations of brain–behavior relationships have relied heavily on folk descriptions of function or personality. Think back to the discussion of phrenology in Chapter 1. Do you remember some of the functions that phrenologists were seeking to localize? Some examples of personality traits included "secretiveness," "destructiveness," and "mirthfulness." Some of the functions included "calculation," "comparison," and "language." With the benefit of hindsight, searching for the

Controversy

Ain't Misbehavin'—It's Genetic!

Although it has been accepted for a long time that characteristics such as height and hair color have a genetic basis, the idea that there is a genetic basis for psychological characteristics such as personality traits, intelligence, and sexual preference has met with considerable debate. However, there is accumulating evidence that there is a genetic component to personality traits, intelligence, and sexual orientation. There is even a suggestion that the tendency to undertake risk-taking behaviors or aggressive behaviors may have its roots in your genes.

Intelligence

A major study of the genetic basis of intelligence has been undertaken by Dr. T. Bouchard at the University of Minnesota. His studies (Bouchard & Loehlin, 2001; Bouchard & McGue, 2003) examine monozygotic twins (identical twins) who have been raised in different homes (typically as a result of adoption). His studies compare the twins who were reared apart (same genes, different environment) with their adoptive siblings (different genes, same environment). Among the many characteristics he has examined, Bouchard has found that the twins who are reared apart are more likely to perform the same as each other on intelligence tests as compared to their adoptive siblings or their adoptive parents. Bouchard has confirmed this result in over 100 pairs of twins and concluded that this is evidence that intelligence is largely a genetic characteristic.

Aggression

A number of prominent studies have looked for a genetic component for aggression and risk taking. For instance, the studies on twins who were reared apart have demonstrated that there is a genetic component to aggression (Coccaro, Bergeman, & McClearn, 1993). Other studies have looked at the genetic makeup of individuals who exhibit high levels of aggression (e.g., individuals who have been convicted of extremely violent crimes). Typically, these studies tend to find that aggression runs in families (Coccaro et al., 1993; Sierer, Torgersen, Gunderson, Livesley, & Kindler, 2002). However, because environment also runs in families, this is not a conclusive demonstration that aggression and risk taking are genetically based. However, a molecu-

lar biologist named Hans Brunner has found one clue to aggressive behavior in men; it is on the X chromosome (Brunner, Nelen, Breakefield, Ropers, & van Oost, 1993). Brunner studied a family that had high levels of incarceration and observed that men who had been convicted of violent crimes had a mutation on the X chromosome for the gene that was supposed to code for an enzyme that breaks down the neurotransmitter for serotonin. Subsequent studies have mutated the same gene in mice and found that these mice also behave in inappropriately aggressive ways (Brunner & Hen, 1997).

Sexual Orientation

Possibly the best-known and most controversial research in molecular biology has to do with sexual orientation. Sexual orientation is one of the fundamental ways in which men and women differ from each other. That is, a majority of men want their sex partners to be women, and most women want their sex partners to be men. However, homosexuality is a significant departure from this pattern. Research by Dean Hamer (1993) and colleagues (Hu et al., 1995; LeVay & Hamer, 1994; Pattatucci & Hamer, 1995) have demonstrated that for men, sexual orientation has a genetic basis and that, like the genetic basis of aggression, it is on the X chromosome. Hamer studied families in which homosexuality was confirmed (by the participant) and in which there was a pattern of male homosexuality that occurred only in the mother's family. He found a linkage at one part of the X chromosome, Xq28, that was present in most of the homosexual men and absent in most of the heterosexual men. Other studies (Mustanski, DuPree, Nievergelt, Bocklandt, Schork, & Hamer, 2005), however, have found candidate regions on chromosomes 7, 8, and 10. Mustanski and colleagues did that for some families, and there was some support for Xq28 linkage. However, they caution that sexuality is a very complex phenomena and thus, not likely resulting from the action of only one gene or set of genes. They also remind the reader that their samples were only taken from families in which two brothers self-identified as homosexual, which may make their sample different from families in which there is only one self-identified male or from families in which the person is female.

Taken together, there is a genetic basis to psychological characteristics. It is beyond the scope of this book to

Controversy

(Continued)

outline all of the psychological characteristics that appear to be mediated (in some part) by our genes, although it seems safe to say that just about any psychological trait that has been studied has some genetic component. However, research in this area has some serious ethical considerations that must be addressed. First, what are the legal ramifications of a genetic predisposition to a specific behavior? For instance, currently, homosexual people do not widely have the right to marry. If homosexuality is a biological or genetic trait (as are skin color and sex), then legally, homosexual individuals may not be discriminated against. Second, what are the responsi-

bilities of the individual who carries a currently undesirable trait? What are the responsibilities of society to that individual? For instance, if person X carries the aggression gene, is this person responsible for his or her actions? Given that we know that the environment can shape the expression of the genotype, should these individuals receive some type of therapy or behavioral treatment before they exhibit this characteristic? Finally, will it be acceptable to screen for these traits in fetuses, to either enhance or minimize these traits? The knowledge that is contained within the human genome will push these questions—and their answers—to the forefront of politics and will surely change our views of ourselves.

---

neuroanatomical correlates of many of these traits and functions appears to be fatally misguided. However, what information should we use as a guide to our investigation of the functional units within the brain?

If we focus our attention on investigating the neural circuits that are specialized to solve adaptive problems, we should be looking for circuits that (1) are complexly structured for a specific problem, (2) reliably develop in all normal humans, (3) develop without formal instruction, (4) are applied without conscious awareness, and (5) are distinct from more general processing abilities.

As you will discover later in this book, many functions that we describe satisfy all of these criteria, including visual object recognition, the ability to navigate through space, and the ability to learn oral/aural language. However, other functions that we describe clearly do not meet these criteria. For example, one should not expect to find a part of the brain that is dedicated to reading, driving a car, working for a large organization, programming a computer, playing the piano, or completing government forms (Tooby & Cosmides, 2000). Although many of these tasks challenge us and influence our ability to survive, reproduce, and acquire resources, we are not genetically endowed with the specific ability to complete them. This does not mean that we cannot learn the tasks. Clearly, we explicitly teach tasks such as reading, car driving, and piano playing. However, our ability to perform these tasks most likely relies on neural substrates that are not specialized for that particular function. Therefore, in our attempts to map the brain in terms of functionally specific areas, our attempt to define these functions should be guided by evolutionary theory:

There are an astronomical number of physical interactions and relationships in the brain, and blind empiricism rapidly drowns itself among the deluge of manic and enigmatic measurements . . . research techniques can abstract out of the welter of human cognitive performance a series of maps of the functional information-processing relationships that

1. What is the difference between the proximate cause and the ultimate cause of a behavior? Which type of cause is typically described in neuropsychology?

2. What is a behavioral adaptation? What are the properties of such an adaptation?

3. What is the Standard Social Science Model (SSSM) described by Tooby and Cosmides?

4. What are the properties of neural circuits that developed as adaptions to specific survival problems?

constitute our computational devices that evolved to solve this particular set of problems. (Tooby & Cosmides, 2000, p. 1176)

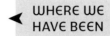 **WHERE WE HAVE BEEN**

We have described the modern synthesis, recognizing that genes are the means by which traits are inherited. The central mechanism of evolution is differential survival and reproduction due to physical or behavioral changes related to gene frequency. Behaviors that are subject to evolutionary selection pressures can be described in terms of their proximate or ultimate cause. Neuropsychology is largely, but not exclusively, the study of the proximate causes of behavior. However, evolutionary theory (and a focus on the ultimate cause of behavior) can serve as a useful guide for neuropsychological investigations of brain–behavior relationships.

Glossary

Adaptation—A "system of properties" or mechanism molded by natural selection because it helped solve to a specific adaptive problem posed by the physical, chemical, developmental, ecological, demographic, social, or informational environment.

Allele—An alternative form of a given gene.

Bipedal gait—The ability to walk on two legs.

Chromosome—Where an individual's genes are located.

Differential reproduction—Organisms that are the best suited for an environment will show enhanced survival and will reproduce at a greater rate than those that are less suited to the environment.

DNA (deoxyribonucleic acid)—Makes up chromosomes.

Dominant genes—Genes that are always expressed whenever they are present.

Endocast—A mold of the inside of the skull that looks much like the brain when it is covered with the meninges and that allows the skulls of mammals to be examined.

Evolutionary psychology—A psychological approach that attempts to apply the principles of evolution to human behavior.

Gene flow—The movement of genes through a population that results from mating; can be profound when there is extensive inbreeding.

Genes—Pieces of DNA that pass traits from generation to generation.

Genetic drift—The tendency for isolated populations to depart from the original genetic composition of the population which can produce evolutionary change.

Genotype—The genetic makeup of an individual.

Heterozygous—When both alleles for a trait are different.

Historical theory of evolution—The original theory of evolution.

Homozygous—When both alleles for a trait are the same.

Inbreeding—Mating between two related parents.

Inheritance—Passing differences in morphology from one generation to the next.

Intersexual selection—A type of sexual selection in which the members of one sex choose mates from the opposite sex on the basis of specific traits (e.g., men look for young and attractive women to mate with, and women place more importance on their mate's resources).

Intrasexual selection—A type of sexual selection in which the members of the same sex compete with each other for partners of the opposite sex (e.g., men might display their wealth more often to impress women, while women will enhance their youthfulness and attractiveness to impress men).

Modern synthetic theory of evolution—The current version of evolutionary theory.

Mutation—Spontaneous or random changes to a gene or genes.

Natural selection—Requires that all individuals are unique and that characteristics that give an animal a reproductive advantage will result in the magnification of these traits in the population.

Phenotypes—An expression of the genotype that you can see.

Polygenic trait—A trait that is controlled by multiple genes (often on different chromosomes).

Proximate cause—Describes the internal mechanisms that underlie a behavior; can also be characterized as the immediate cause of the behavior and can be addressed by asking "how" questions.

Random mutation—A mistake that occurs when genes are passed from generation to generation that is the original source of variation in genes.

Recessive genes—Genes that are expressed only when no dominant genes are present.

Replication—The process wherein DNA makes copies of itself.

Sexual selection—A form of selection in which the inheritance of a gene is based on the gene's ability to help an individual reproduce; there are two types of sexual selection: intersexual selection and intrasexual selection.

Tabula rasa—A blank slate; until recently, it was a commonly held belief that this is what the human brain resembled.

Ultimate cause—Describes the evolutionary basis behind a behavior, including a description of what makes a given behavior adaptive and can be addressed by asking "why" questions.

Variation—The differences in morphology that are characteristic of all individuals.

13

Neural Development and Developmental Disorders

It is easy to infer the existence of critical periods during which the wet cement of character can be set. It is less easy to conceive of how they work.
—MATT RIDLEY

When we think about development, we often focus on early childhood and the development of behaviors. As many of you know, behaviors such as walking often emerge at predictable ages. However, the brain has not completed its developmental journey at birth, and there is a long period of extended development that may be completed only sometime in adulthood. As we will learn in the first module, many of the striking behavioral changes that occur in childhood correspond with periods of brain growth or reorganization. The first module will describe the critical periods of development of the nervous system and how they relate to the variety of behavioral changes that are observed in infancy, childhood, and adolescence. Because much of what we have described to this point in the text relates to either acquired injuries of the CNS or disorders that occur primarily in adulthood or old age, the second module will discuss a number of CNS disorders that appear at birth or a little later in childhood.

WHERE WE ARE GOING ➤ The first module will describe prenatal and postnatal development of the central nervous system and how this relates to behavior. The second module will describe developmental disorders that appear at birth or in childhood.

MODULE **13.1**
Neural Development

Early Development

If you think about the fact that you started out as two haploid cells (a sperm and an egg), it is quite amazing that you are who you are now. Just how did the cells that make up your frontal lobe know to turn into frontal lobe neurons rather than skin cells of your left ring finger? How did your parietal lobe get connected correctly to your frontal and occipital lobes? This section will primarily examine prenatal development of the nervous system.

Early in embryonic life (approximately three weeks after conception), the **neural plate** forms from the **ectoderm** of the embryo. The neural plate is a patch of cells that are on the dorsal surface of the embryo, which eventually becomes the nervous system. The cells of the dorsal ectoderm in the neural plate are **stem cells** that are **pluripotent,** meaning that they have the potential to develop into different types of nervous system cells (because they are in the nervous system, they cannot turn into any other type of cell, such as skin cells).

As development progresses, the neural plate starts to form a groove, which by embryonic day 24 fuses to form the **neural tube.** The different sections of the neural tube become different parts of the nervous system, with the interior surface of the neural tube becoming the ventricles and central canal of the spinal cord. However, between the third and fifth months of gestation, rapid cell proliferation and neural migration are the dominant events. That is, the cells of the neural tube within the ventricular zone are rapidly dividing, a process called **proliferation,** and by embryonic day 40, there are three prominent bumps on the anterior portion of the neural tube. These bumps eventually form the forebrain, midbrain, and hindbrain of the central nervous system (CNS).

Cells also migrate from the interior ventricular zone to their final location by following certain types of glia. There are waves of proliferation and migration in the developing CNS. Beginning in the second month of gestation, the telencephalon undergoes tremendous growth, developing from the cortical plate. As migration occurs from the inside out, it is actually the deepest layer of neurons that develop first, and the subsequent layers of neurons must migrate through the already established neurons to reach their destination.

Once neurons migrate, they begin to grow axons and dendrites and to differentiate into their final form. Although development of axons and dendrites occurs both prenatally and postnatally, cell differentiation is essentially complete at birth. Furthermore, axons and dendrites must get to their appropriate targets and make functional synaptic connections. Although the exact mechanism underlying how axons grow toward their target is not known, the tips of growing axons and dendrites follow chemicals, arranging themselves in an orderly fashion in a position relative to their initial place on the cortical plate.

Problems with any phase of development can lead to significant abnormalities in the CNS (Table 13.1). Although the brain is particularly vulnerable during the last four to five months of gestation, failures at any point in CNS development can have significant impact on the final form of the brain. Adverse events can originate from problems within the neurons themselves, such as genetic or chromosomal abnormalities, or can be introduced by external factors. External events can include intrauterine

Table 13.1

Timing of Developmental Events and Malformations of the CNS Associated with Disruptions of Development

Embryonic Day	Developmental Event(s)	Malformation	Symptom
18	Neural groove appears	Craniorachischisis, anencephaly	Brain and spinal cord are not covered by skeleton or skin
22–23	Neural groove starts to form into a tube	Hydrocephalus	Enlargement of ventricles
24–26	Anterior neural tube starts to close	Anencephaly	Absence of cerebral hemispheres, diencephalons, and midbrain
26–28	Posterior neural tube starts to close	Spina bifida	Multiple and variable; generally a failure of parts of the CNS to be enclosed
32	Vascular circulation is forming	Microcephaly	Small cranium, with poor CNS development; low I.Q.
33–35	Telencephalon splits to make two hemispheres	Holoprosencephaly	Cortex develops as a single hemisphere
70–100	Corpus callosum begins formation	Agenesis of the corpus callosum	Absence or malformation of corpus callosum
70–100	Neuronal migration, synapse formation	Migration/proliferation problems	Abnormal gyral patterns, learning disabilities(?)

Source: Adapted from Nolte (1999).

trauma or exposure to toxins, such as lead or alcohol. The effects of these disruptions often depend on the nature, duration, and extent of the disruption. However, the type of CNS malformation can give us a clue as to when the disruption occurred.

For instance, one of the more common congenital malformations of the CNS occurs when the neural tube fails to close, occurring in about 1 in 1000 live births (Nolte, 1999). Complete failure of the closure of the neural tube is fatal, resulting in a condition known as **craniorachischisis.** Craniorachischisis is characterized by the CNS appearing as a groove in the top of the head and body. However, defective closure of the neural tube is rarely complete, and syndromes ranging from **spina bifida** to **anencephaly** result from partial closure of the neural tube. Anencephaly occurs when the rostral part of the neural plate does not fuse and is characterized by a general absence of the cerebral hemispheres. Although anencephaly is generally fatal (Fletcher, Dennis, & Northrup, 2000), not all neural tube defects are fatal. As an example, spina bifida is a disorder that is caused by a failure of the neural tube to close completely. There are a number of different subtypes of spina bifida, the symptoms of which depend on the part of the neural tube that did not close. However, for the most part, spina bifida results in neurological difficulties that are associated with locomotion rather than cognitive difficulties, which is consistent with the syndrome's having its primary effects on the spinal cord. Failure at later times during development can result in a host of other abnormalities, which vary in severity. Milder disruptions tend to occur later in development and can lead to more subtle behavioral effects, which may underlie a number of learning disabilities.

By the seventh month of prenatal development, most neurons have migrated and have differentiated into their final forms. However, this is just the beginning of a long period of brain growth and change. Neurons undergo a long period of **synaptogenesis** and **dendritic branching,** producing far more synapses and dendrites than are needed in the adult brain. However, both synaptogenesis and dendrite branching occur after birth—even, in some specific cases, into adulthood. Dendritic branching occurs slowly, with initial dendrites appearing as simple extensions exiting the cell body of the neuron. With time, the dendrites become more complex, adding branches and spines. It is on the dendritic spines that most dendritic synapses occur.

During early embryonic life, synaptogenesis, or synapse formation, is relatively sparse and occurs relatively independent of experience. However, between the period extending from shortly before birth to about 2 years of age, synapse formation enters a period of rapid growth. Shortly thereafter, a period of synapse reduction begins to occur. Synapse reduction reaches its maximal rate sometime during puberty. In fact, it appears that about 50% more neurons are produced in the developing brain than are required in the adult brain. Thus, death is actually a normal and critical feature of development, which occurs in predictable waves. Much of the neural death is apoptotic, or planned, programmed cell death. It is unclear what triggers

Self-Test

1. How is the following statement true? How is it false?: "Stem cells in the nervous system are pluripotent throughout the lifespan of the individual."

2. What are the diseases that result when the neural tube fails to close properly? Which ones are fatal? What is one common food additive that can help to prevent such diseases?

3. How does synaptic pruning and apoptosis ensure the functional development of the nervous system? Do these changes happen randomly?

apoptosis, although it is clear that apoptotic changes are controlled by genes. Synapses that do not make functional connections or that make incorrect connections are especially likely to die, leaving room for other synapses to sprout. Many of these apoptotic changes and synaptic pruning occurs after birth and may actually be very dependent on the environment and experiences of the individual.

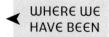

◄ **WHERE WE HAVE BEEN**   We have described the major points of embryonic, fetal, and prenatal development. Although there is much that is not understood about early development, many congenital neural disorders result from problems at particular phases of development.

WHERE WE ARE GOING ▶   As we have discussed briefly, CNS development does not end at birth. Between birth and adulthood, the cortical areas of the brain grow extensively. We will examine these patterns of development in an attempt to understand how CNS growth and development relate to the emergence of behavior.

Postnatal Development

One of the most striking features of any baby's early development is the emergence of behaviors such as sitting, walking, or speaking. These behaviors are correlated with the extensive growth in cortical areas of the brain, which increases its volume by four times between birth and adulthood (Johnson, 2003). In studying the relation between cortical growth and behavioral change, it is possible to approach the question from a number of different perspectives. One approach is to study the maturation of specific parts of the brain and observe whether or not certain behaviors become evident only when the brain reaches a certain level of maturation. Alternatively, you could reverse the question and observe whether or not the emergence of specific behaviors, such as walking, is associated with the development of specific aspects of the motor cortex (it is). As we will see in the following sections, understanding development of the brain and behavior requires examining the question from a number of perspectives.

However, we must acknowledge the important contribution that the environment plays in CNS development. As we learned previously, the prenatal environment can have significant effects on CNS. **Plastic change** is the ability of the CNS to alter itself in response to environmental stimuli. Further, there are **critical periods** of plastic change in which the environment can have a maximal effect on the CNS. The duration and timing of these critical periods vary by species, although it appears that longer-lived animals (such as humans) exhibit prolonged critical periods that often occur later in life, well beyond the prenatal period (Berardi, Pizzorusso, & Maffei, 2000).

The shaping of the CNS during these critical periods does not depend on random events in the environment. Rather, plasticity during critical periods occurs in response to specific experiences. These experiences can be classified as either experience-expectant or experience-dependent plasticity phenomena (Black, 1998). **Experience-expectant plastic changes** are those CNS changes that are dependent on experience(s) during the critical period for specific synapses to develop as they should. Much of the sensory cortex appears to have these experience-expectant critical periods, and numerous studies have demonstrated that if an organism does not experience sensory stimulation during the critical period, long-lasting impairments in the sensory modality occur (e.g., Berardi, Pizzorusso, Ratto, & Maffei, 2003). Further confirming the role of experience during the critical period, sensory impairments that occur after the critical period often have limited effects on the cortex (Berardi et al., 2000).

Experience-dependent plastic changes are those idiosyncratic experiences that occur during critical periods that also affect brain development (Black, 1998). For instance, it appears that musical training in childhood can have long-lasting changes on the size of the auditory cortex in adulthood (Pantev, Oostenvald, Engelien, Ross, Roberts, & Hoke, 1998). However, these changes were most profound in individuals who began practicing their instrument of choice before they were 9 years old. Similar effects have been observed with respect to the size of the motor cortex for individuals who play stringed instruments. That is, musicians had larger cortical representation of their left hand (the hand that is used to finger the notes on a stringed instrument) than did nonmusicians (Elbert, Panter, Wienbruch, Rockstroh, & Taub, 1995). Again, Elbert and colleagues report that this increase was proportionately related to the age at which the musicians began playing, suggesting that there are critical periods during which musical training can have maximal effects on the cortex. Furthermore, although these changes occur in tandem with individual experience, these changes are not random. That is, musical training affected parts of the brain associated with the playing of (and listening to) music. It appears that these changes were not observed throughout the CNS, although this was only indirectly tested in these studies. For instance, areas of the brain that were used equally by musicians and nonmusicians (e.g., the cortical representation of the right hand) did not differ between the two groups.

Volumes of cortical gray matter increase until about 4 years of age, with much of the postnatal growth and plastic change that occurs in the brain resulting from synaptogenesis, myelination of axons, and dendritic branching. Synaptogenesis and dendritic branching occur both prenatally and postnatally and are presumably maximal during critical periods (Doe & Sanes, 2000). Although the brain's ability to engage in plastic change is often reduced as we age, especially once the critical period has passed, there are significant exceptions to this statement. For instance, the types of plastic change that are required for learning extend well into adulthood. Even less plastic areas, such as areas of the sensory cortex, can change in response to significant environmental events (Berardi et al., 2003). Although the factors underlying plastic change are not completely understood, it appears that **neurotrophins** (chemicals, such as nerve growth factor, that are secreted by the brain that enhance the survival of neurons) and neurotransmitters, such as glutamate, play critical roles. Furthermore, both synaptogenesis and dendritic branching appear to be sensitive to experience-expectant and experience-dependent plasticity (Doe & Sanes, 2000).

Unlike cortical volume changes, white matter volumes increase steadily until about 20 years of age. Much of the cortex is not myelinated at birth; myelination begins shortly after birth and does not occur uniformly throughout the cortex. There are many examples of cortical areas that have completed myelination while other areas exhibit limited myelination. For instance, the primary motor and sensory areas have relatively complete myelination by 4 years of age, whereas the frontal cortex does not exhibit complete myelination until some time during the late teens.

Flechsig (1920, as cited in Finger, 1994) hypothesized that myelination corresponded to the emergence of behaviors. He hypothesized that simple motor and sensory behaviors emerge first, in part because these areas have completed myelination first. Similarly, more complex behaviors and the cortical areas associated with these behaviors are not myelinated until much later in life. Remember, however, that correlation does not infer causation. Thus, although there are numerous important correlations between CNS myelination and behavior, the sheer number of changes in the CNS (e.g., synaptogenesis) that occur simultaneously makes it difficult to determine which correlation is the meaningful one (Kolb & Fantie, 1997). That having been said, the relationship between myelination and the emergence of behavior is clearly interesting. As we will see, many of these questions are being studied in vivo with advanced neuroimaging techniques.

PARIETAL LOBE DEVELOPMENT. In comparison to the other lobes of the brain, relatively little is known about the development of the parietal lobes. The parietal lobe has inconsistent levels of development at birth; some parts of the parietal lobe are more mature than others. For instance, given the number of tactile reflexes present in newborns, somatosensory systems are likely functional at birth (Spreen, Risser, & Edgell, 1995; Teeter & Semrud-Clikeman, 1997), whereas other parietal lobe functions associated with visual perception and spatial ability may take much longer to develop. Further, myelination in spinal cord and thalamic centers begins prenatally and is relatively complete by 1 year of age, consistent with the observations that basic somatosensory function develops rapidly.

Babies who are 2 to 3 months of age exhibit large increases in glucose utilization in parietal lobes, increases that remain steady until about 2 to 3 years of age (Chugani, 1998; Teeter & Semrud-Clikeman, 1997). Presumably, these changes in glucose utilization correspond to improvements in visuospatial and visuosensorimotor skill (Chugani, 1998). Behaviorally, preschool children find tactile discrimination difficult. That is, children under the age of 6 are often unable to name or point to a finger that was just touched when they cannot see their hands, suggesting that although they can perceive touch, they have difficulties localizing the point on their hands. Other types of complex tactile perception (e.g., tactile discrimination of form) show significant increases in accuracy during childhood, with adultlike levels of performance occurring between 8 to 12 years of age (Benton, Hamsher, Varney, & Spreen, 1983). Thus, although basic tactile sensations mature early, complex tactile discriminations require more time to develop.

Furthermore, the degree to which sensory systems integrate with other functions, such as motor skill, depends on the maturation of other neural systems. The parietal lobe is also a component of the dorsal visual stream (the "where" and "how" pathway), the component that is involved with the processing of spatial information and directing behaviors toward certain points in space (Milner & Goodale, 1995). One important component of the dorsal visual stream is the processing of motion. Although babies as young as 7 weeks of age appear to prefer moving objects to stationary ones, infants first show sensitivity to directional motion sometime during the twelfth week of life, with adult levels of global motion processing occurring sometime after 4 years of age. Braddick and colleagues (2003) hypothesize that because global motion processing involves the coordination of motion and form processing, accurate global motion processing requires the participation of numerous cortical areas, including the slow to develop frontal lobes.

Individuals with Williams syndrome provide an important insight into the development of the parietal lobe and role that the connections between the parietal lobe and others have in mediating spatial behavior. Williams syndrome is a genetic condition in which some of chromosome 7 has been deleted. Individuals with Williams syndrome have mild to moderate cognitive impairments that are interesting because of the relative sparing of verbal ability and the significant difficulties that these individuals have with tasks of visuospatial ability (see Chapter 8). Although individuals with Williams syndrome have smaller brain volumes than controls do, the reduction in brain size is not uniform throughout the CNS. Individuals with Williams syndrome have relative sparing of the frontal and temporal lobes and disproportionate reductions in parietal and occipital lobes. It appears that there may also be significant reductions in white matter (Reiss et al., 2000). It has been hypothesized that the relative involvement of dorsal systems and impoverished connectivity among lobes that is apparent in Williams syndrome underlie the specific impairments in visuospatial ability (Galaburda & Bellugi, 2000). Because Williams syndrome results in congenital defects of the CNS, it may be that the missing genes on chromosome 7 may underlie typical development of parietal, occipital, and/or white matter in the CNS.

OCCIPITAL LOBE DEVELOPMENT. As was the case with the parietal lobe, development of the occipital lobe is incomplete at birth. Unlike what you may have heard, newborns do not have underdeveloped visual systems. Newborns have quite sophisticated visual systems, and they are capable of distinguishing between two-dimensional and three-dimensional stimuli. Newborns also have rudimentary form perception. Furthermore, infants become very competent with more complex stimuli, such as faces, very quickly (Slater & Kirby, 1998). In large part, competence with visual stimuli may depend on the myelination of the optic tract and requires the optic radiations to become functionally connected with the sensory organs and with other areas of the brain. At birth, myelination of the optic tract is moderate, whereas the optic radiations exhibit minimal amounts of myelination. However, by 3 months of age, both the optic tract and optic radiations exhibit heavy myelination, consistent with adult patterns of myelination (Spreen et al., 1995). Behaviorally, many visual behaviors change rapidly following birth. At about 6 weeks of age, infants begin to experience binocular vision, which becomes stable by about 6 months of age (Spreen et al., 1995).

As we learned in Chapter 6, development of the visual cortex is critically dependent on the environmental experiences of the individual. For instance, uncorrected congenital cataracts that deprive an infant of patterned visual experience result in irreversible changes in the visual cortex (Berardi et al., 2000). If the cataract is removed after the critical period, the now "normal" eye has only poor visual acuity, often exhibiting permanent **amblyopia,** and limited or no binocular vision (Berardi et al., 2000). Similar effects are observed when the eyes are misaligned, as in **strabismus.** That is, individuals who experience corrective measures for strabismus after the critical period often have impaired depth perception, presumably because of the loss of binocular cells in the visual cortex (Berardi et al., 2000). For humans, the critical

Neuropsychological Celebrity

Genie

Genie was deprived of many things early in her life. Most of the academic discourse about her focuses on how she was deprived of the opportunity to develop language skills early in her life, but that was the least of her troubles at the time. She endured years of abuse, spending most of her first thirteen years of life (except the first twenty months) locked in a room, tied to her potty chair, and fed only baby food. When she was discovered in 1970, she was immediately admitted to a hospital. She was only 54 inches tall and weighted a scant 62 pounds. She was unable to stand, chew, or vocalize.

During the years that followed, Genie received much better care, and she developed many of the skills that a young teenager should enjoy. However, her very late language acquisition became the focus of intense study and worldwide attention. The no-

tion that human language development has a critical period was a matter of academic debate that had not really been put to the test before. Testing Genie's capacity to develop language was not easy. At first, she was understandably uncooperative. However, after almost a year, it was clear that Genie's language comprehension skills far exceeded her ability (or willingness) to speak. After years of training, she learned to understand the differences between singular and plural nouns, the meaning of some prepositions, and a few other subtleties of grammar. However, her language skills never approached those of a normal adolescent. Specifically, her use of grammar was so poor that it did not meet some academics' definition of language.

Scientists who believed in a language critical period cautiously interpreted these findings as support for their position. However, others argued that her language deficits were not specific to language and that they were more likely the result of extreme trauma, neglect, and isolation.

period for binocular vision begins some time within the first few months of life and peaks between 1 and 3 years of age (Banks, Aslin, & Letson, 1975). When strabismus develops after the age of 4, there are no long-lasting effects on binocular vision once the strabismus is corrected (Banks et al., 1975), suggesting that the critical period ends sometime between the third and fourth years of life.

More complex visual tasks, which presumably rely on the participation of a number of different cortical areas, take longer to develop. For instance, simple face and emotion recognition is performed at adult levels by children between the ages of 6 and 8 years, whereas the ability to match emotional faces with cues provided by a cartoon situation did not approach adult levels until children were about 14 years old (Kolb, Wilson, & Taylor, 1992). Thus, although basic visual functions may be present relatively early, more complex tasks requiring the participation of the frontal lobes may not develop until the teens.

TEMPORAL LOBE DEVELOPMENT. To understand temporal lobe development, it is important to divide function into two main types: linguistic ability and hippocampally dependent memory function. This is particularly the case because the development of the temporal lobe appears to depend on the specific structure and the function that is being studied.

As you learned in Chapter 8, linguistic ability is multifaceted. The development of speech production and comprehension is the result of the cooperation and development of the frontal and temporal lobes. Language development requires the ability to perceive sounds, the ability to comprehend the meaning of sounds, and presumably the ability to coordinate the mouth and tongue to produce language sounds. It is well known that infants exhibit stereotypical stages of linguistic development that involve both the comprehension and production of speech (Table 13.2). Therefore, the development of linguistic competence involves the development of both the frontal and temporal lobes as well as the myelination of the connections among the lobes.

Although it is assumed that the auditory cortex is functional at birth, the auditory cortex may not make functional connections with other important language areas. In fact, both Wernicke's and Broca's areas undergo significant dendritic branching and extensive synaptic remodeling during the second year of life. Furthermore, between the ages of 1 and 2 years, a number of important commissural systems are undergoing myelination, including the corpus callosum, the anterior commissure, and the fornix (Hershkowitz, 2000). All of these areas are involved in connecting the right and left frontal and temporal lobes with each other and with increasing functional connectivity both ipsilaterally and bilaterally. Presumably, these CNS changes are related to the explosion in linguistic activity that occurs during this period. In fact, it appears that failure to experience linguistic stimulation at this time will result in permanent deficits in attaining adultlike linguistic skill, suggesting that this is the beginning of a critical period for language.

Finally, from 2 to 12 years of age, marked changes in dendritic arborization occur in speech areas in the brain (Kolb & Fantie, 1997). In other areas of the brain, dendritic arborization is sensitive to environmental factors, suggesting a means for the environment to affect language development. Certainly, there is evidence to suggest that there is tremendous variability in the development of speech and that the speech that children hear at home and at school affects the vocabulary and speech patterns that children actually use (e.g., Huttenloch, Levine, & Vevea, 1998). Therefore, Kolb and Fantie suggest that the correlation between neural maturation and linguistic ability may reflect idiosyncratic patterns of maturation of the speech areas that may have a large environmental component.

The hippocampus attains adult volumes around 7 to 10 months of age, and the hippocampus shows high levels of glucose utilization from birth, unlike the rest of the temporal lobe structures, which show relatively low levels of glucose utilization until about 4 years of age (Chugani, 1998). However, in the monkey, extensive synaptic remodeling and myelination of the hippocampus occur during the first 24 months of a monkey's life (Alvarado & Bachevalier, 2000). Furthermore, other structures in the limbic system exhibit a major growth spurt between 1 and 2 years of age (Herschkowitz, 2000). Therefore, although the hippocampus may appear to have adult volumes and glucose utilization at birth, many hippocampally dependent memory processes are not mature at birth. Finally, the hippocampus is one of the sites in adulthood that exhibits neurogenesis. Therefore, it may be that the memory functions of the hippocampus result from its ability to extend its developmental period throughout the life span.

Like many other areas of the brain, memory functions of the hippocampus rely on functional connections with the parietal and frontal lobes, and many hippocampally dependent memory functions develop over the course of the first five to seven

Table 13.2

Postnatal Development of Linguistic Functions

Age	Milestone
Birth to 2 months	Responds to human voice
	Tendency to move during pauses in speech
1 month	Differentiation of cries—can make noncrying sounds, often while eating
6 weeks	Cooing; cries to signal
3 months	Orients head to speech sounds
	Begins to babble or produce spontaneous production of speech sounds
	Begins to babble in response to speech
4 months	Begins to imitate tone
6 months	Echolalia (imitation of speech) begins
	Prosody begins to be present
9–12 months	Can express self and gain attention using gestures
	Can understand words in context (e.g., peek-a-boo)
12–18 months	Use of first recognizable word (often "No!")
	Rapidly gains a vocabulary of five to ten words
	Can understand words without addition of context
18–24 months	Vocabulary of 200–300 words, including
	• "My" and "mine"
	• Common everyday objects
	• Words for objects that are not present
	Speech consists of single- and two-word telegraphic sentences (e.g., "Me want")
	• Asks for names of objects
	Can respond to commands (e.g., "Where is your nose?")
	Responds to speech with speech
3 years	Vocabulary of 900–1000 words, including
	• Plurals
	• Past tenses
	• Body parts
	• Prepositions (e.g., "in," "on," "under")
	Speech consists of three- to four-word sentences (~90% intelligible)
4 years	Vocabulary > 1500 words, including
	• Animal names
	• Colors
	• Common objects
	Asks questions, forms complex sentences
5 years	Vocabulary 1500–2200 words, including
	• Opposites
	• Counting
	• Time references (e.g., yesterday, next week)
	Speech is grammatically correct
	May begin to read and write
6 years	Expressive vocabulary of 2600 words
	Receptive vocabulary of 20,000–24,000 words
Adult	Vocabulary > 50,000 words (usually attained by age 12)

Source: Adapted from Berk (2003) and Spreen et al. (1995).

years in humans (Alvarado & Bachevalier, 2000). As an example, although visual memory is functional at birth in primates, it does not reach adult levels of performance until about 5 years of age in humans (Alvarado & Bachevalier, 2000). Similarly, although episodic recollection can be demonstrated in children as young as 6 to 9 months of age, recall of autobiographical or episodic information does not usually appear until the child is about 4 years of age. Before this age, recollections tend to be incomplete and cue-dependent (Levine, 2004). In fact, most people experience childhood amnesia for events that occurred before the age of 3 or 4, suggesting that CNS systems for encoding, storing, and retrieving these memories are not yet functional.

Research with adults suggests that these autobiographical memories are subserved by a diverse number of areas, including cingulate, parietal, temporal, and prefrontal areas. As we will learn in the next section, the frontal lobes are among the last to mature. Areas of the prefrontal cortex associated with autobiographical memory increase in cortical thickness until the child is about 4 years old, which is consistent with the time frame for the emergence of stable autobiographical memory. Thus, many developmental features of memory are associated with development of the temporal lobe and with increases in connectivity among cortical areas.

FRONTAL LOBE DEVELOPMENT. As was the case for the other lobes of the brain, the functions of the frontal lobe are diverse. The role of the development of the frontal lobe in changes in language and memory was described in the preceding section. The following section will focus primarily on the development of functions of the frontal lobe that we have not described elsewhere: motor and executive function.

Similar to the functional diversity of the other lobes, areas of the frontal cortex differ in their development at birth. At birth, the prefrontal cortex is the least developed, reaching adult levels of myelination, glucose utilization, and cell differentiation sometime in the middle to late teen years (Kolb & Fantie, 1997; Segalowitz & Davies, 2004). Conversely, motor areas of the frontal lobes mature quickly, with primary and supplementary motor cortex exhibiting rapid development, often with significant maturation by 3 months of age. As a basic generalization, it appears that parts of the frontal lobes that are associated with later developing traits take longer to develop, whereas areas of the frontal cortex that are involved with more basic functions develop more quickly.

As was the case with language, motor development is associated with predictable milestones (Table 13.3). However, motor development follows **cephalocaudal** and **proximodistal** patterns of development. That is, the head is controlled before the arms and trunk are, but the arms and trunk are controlled before the legs are (cephalocaudal). The term *proximodistal* refers to the observation that motor skills develop in the head, trunk, and arms before they develop in the hands and fingers. As such, many gross motor skills develop before fine-motor skills. **Gross motor skills** are those involving the large muscles that are typically involved with walking, balance, or holding up the head, whereas **fine-motor skills** involve the small muscles and are typically used in the coordination of the hands and fingers.

At birth, the motor roots are highly myelinated, and by 6 months of age, many of the subcortical motor areas have at least moderate myelination. By 3 months of age, many of the secondary and tertiary motor areas of the frontal lobes exhibit

Table 13.3	Postnatal Development of Motor Skills
Age	**Milestone**
Birth	Reflexive movements: sucking, rooting, grasping (ulnar grasp, in which fingers press against palm)
6 weeks	When held upright, can keep head steady
2 months	When lying on stomach, can lift self by arms
3 months	Neonatal grasp reflex begins to disappear
	Can keep head up for long periods of time
	Begins to reach for objects
6 months	*Gross motor:* Can turn over, can sit briefly
	Fine motor: Grasps objects with both hands, can often reach with one arm, instead of both
9 months	*Gross motor:* Sits well, crawls
	Fine motor: Has a precision grip (thumb and forefinger grasp), plays pat-a-cake
12 months	*Gross motor:* Can stand unaided, walk with support, roll a ball
	Fine motor: Transfers objects between hands, drops and picks up toys
24 months	*Gross motor:* Can walk alone, can walk backwards, can walk up and down stairs (two feet on each step), can dance to music, can bend over and pick up objects
	Fine motor: can build a three-block tower, can turn pages in book, scribbles (whole arm movements), can throw a small ball, can partially dress
3 years	*Gross motor:* Runs, jumps, can walk up stairs (one foot per step), can stand on tiptoe, kicks a ball, can ride a tricycle
	Fine motor: Can dress self (may have problems with buttons, shoelaces), can string beads, can use scissors, uses a crayon with thumb and fingers, uses one hand consistently
4 years	*Gross motor:* Can walk on a line, can use the slide, can jump over objects, catches a bounced ball
	Fine motor: Can build a nine-block tower, can copy a circle, can make snakes, balls, and cookies out of clay or dough
5 years	*Gross motor:* Can skip, can do somersaults
	Fine motor: Can cut lines well, can print some capital letters
6 years	*Gross motor:* Can jump rope and skate
	Fine motor: Can cut shapes well, has adult grasp of pencil, can color in the lines, can write numbers

Source: Adapted from Berk (2003).

differentiated neurons and adult-type inhibition (Herschkowitz, 2000). Thus, although myelination of these tracts begins early, the differentiation and maturation of these areas extend well into early childhood. It is therefore tempting to suggest that the myriad of motor behaviors that appear during childhood are related to frontal lobe development. For instance, myelination of the pyramidal tracts occurs by the end of the first year and is often associated with walking (Spreen et al., 1995).

However, myelination is not the only change occurring in motor areas. One insight into how factors other than myelination affect motor development can be obtained by studying individuals with Rett syndrome. Rett syndrome occurs in one in every 10,000 to 15,000 live female births. Individuals with Rett syndrome appear to develop normally until sometime around their third to fourth month after birth, at which time a gene mutation, MECP2, begins to arrest brain development. Arrested brain development is most pronounced by the end of the first year and is most obvious within frontal and motor cortices. Symptoms of Rett syndrome are progressive, appear between 6 and 18 months of age, and include hypotonia (loss of muscle tone), loss of the use of hands, and apraxia. However, when pathologists examine the brains of girls with Rett syndrome, they do not find loss of myelin; rather, it appears that dendritic arborization in motor cortices is seriously reduced. This gene mutation also appears to affect neurotransmission, as there are numerous alterations in neurotransmitters in affected areas (Armstrong, 2001). Typical motor development relies on postnatal differentiation of neurons, synaptogenesis, dendritic arborization, neurotransmission, and myelination.

When solving a problem, individuals must choose appropriate strategies, to attend or ignore certain aspects of the problem, to spend more or less time on certain aspects of the problem, and to order the sequence of events so that the correct solution can be achieved. The frontal cortex contains these areas of the brain that are involved with controlling these cognitive processes and ordering them so that a solution is arrived at. These diverse activities are often referred to as executive function, an analogy to the organization of a company in which the executives (prefrontal cortex) organize and arrange solutions that other employees (e.g., motor cortex) then carry out. When examining the development of executive function, we can look at the types of problems that adults with prefrontal lesions have difficulty solving and observe whether or not similar difficulties are observed in children. Although this approach is not without problems (e.g., children may rely on strategies to solve problems that involve areas outside of the frontal lobes; Segalowitz & Davies, 2004), the research suggests that there are some very remarkable similarities in how individuals with immature frontal lobes and adults with frontal lesions behave.

Given that the prefrontal areas are among the last areas of the brain to develop, it is perhaps not surprising that children with immature frontal lobes have difficulties with tasks that rely on frontal lobe functions. As you know from Chapters 9 and 11, adults with frontal damage do not typically have significant changes in I.Q. scores, although they make very poor decisions. These deficits appear to be related to their inability to engage in different strategies for solving tasks and to switch among possible solutions; these individuals also appear to be impaired in their ability to produce multiple solutions for a problem. Further, they can exhibit striking differences in their ability to interact with others in social settings compared to normal adults.

Some of the most obvious neuropsychological deficits are observed when individuals with frontal deficits attempt to perform the Wisconsin Card Sorting Task. In this task, individuals can sort the cards according to a number of different rules, only some of which are correct at certain times during the test. Although many people with frontal lobe damage can frequently learn one rule for sorting, they often exhibit extreme difficulty in switching to a different rule when the first one is no longer correct (e.g., you first sort by color, and after a certain number of trials, you must switch to sorting by number). This deficit appears to be due to two factors: They have problems in shifting strategies, and they have difficulty in inhibiting incorrect responses (perseveration). Interestingly, children appear to have difficulties with the Wisconsin Card Sorting Task that change as they age (Kolb & Fantie, 1989; White, Nortz, Mandernach, Huntington, & Steiner, 2001). Children improve on the task as they age, with adultlike performance occurring sometime between 10 and 12 years of age (Teeter & Semrud-Clikeman, 1997). Younger children have more difficulty inhibiting previously correct responses (perseveration) and in switching strategies (e.g., Arffa, Lovell, Podell, & Goldberg, 1998; Bull & Scerif, 2001). Interestingly, children with I.Q.s in the gifted range tend to outperform their lower I.Q. peers, suggesting that some elements of executive function may mature earlier in bright children (Arffa et al., 1998).

Individuals with frontal lobe damage also tend to exhibit a loss of behavioral spontaneity, which is often tested by having the person generate lists of words or designs. In these tasks, the person is asked to generate as many words as they can that belong to a specific category (e.g., farm animals or words that begin with the letter *c*) in a specific length of time. In the design task, individuals are asked to generate as many different designs, similar to doodles in your notebook, as they can in a specific length of time. Individuals with frontal lobe damage often have extreme difficulty in generating these lists, suggesting that the problem is related to ability to engage in spontaneous acts rather than a problem with speech or doodling (Kolb & Whishaw, 2004). This is consistent with the difficulties that individuals with frontal lobe lesions have in their daily lives, as they often have difficulties beginning activities and are easily distracted. Children also exhibit difficulties in producing lists of words or making different doodles. However, in contrast to performance on the Wisconsin Card Sorting Task, significant difficulties with word fluency are observed well into the teen years (Kolb & Fantie, 1989). Although not quite the same as doodling, the drawing of clock faces appears to improve over childhood, with good drawings of clock faces occurring sometime in the twelfth year of age (Cohen, Ricci, Kibby, & Edmonds, 2000).

Recent results suggest that differences in performance on fluency tasks between adults and 12-year-old children are not due to differences in the areas that are activated (e.g., Gaillard, Balsamo, Ibrahim, Sachs, & Xu, 2003), although children may exhibit more general activation than adults (e.g., Gaillard, Hertz-Pannier, Mott, Barnett, LeBihan, & Theodore, 2000). Differences in ability in spontaneous acts may result from changes in connectivity between the frontal lobes and other cortical areas. However, this result is somewhat speculative, and this conclusion needs empirical support, presumably from additional studies of how the frontal lobe changes with age.

Among the most obvious deficits exhibited by individuals with frontal damage are the significant and numerous impairments in social situations. Because it is difficult to quantify these deficits, researchers have tended to focus on how individuals with frontal damage judge emotional expressions and how they self-regulate their behavior in social settings. As you might anticipate, adults with frontal lobe damage tend to have problems in producing emotional expressions and in judging the emotions that others portray. Similarly, individuals who have experienced early frontal

the **Real** world

Brain Development during Childhood

Human development is unique. No other species undergoes a process comparable to the protracted childhood and adolescence that humans (both children and their parents) must survive before a child enters adulthood. Are the physical changes in our brains during childhood and adolescent years uniquely human? Until a few years ago, the changes to our brain appeared to be unique in quantity but not necessarily in quality. However, a recent neuroimaging study by Giedd and colleagues (1999) changed all of that.

Before the study, it was well known that the relative amount of gray matter decreases between the ages of 4 and 20, whereas the relative amount of white matter increases. As we discussed earlier in the chapter, this myelination of the brain during development is especially pronounced in the frontal lobes, and it appears to correlate well with behavioral changes during those periods. However, the data supporting this "fact" was entirely cross-sectional (testing different people of different ages). Giedd and colleagues' study was the first longitudinal study of its kind, and it involved giving multiple MRIs (usually about two years apart) to the same people at different developmental periods. The participants received as many as five MRIs. The results were quite surprising. In addition to confirming that gray matter volume generally decreases and white matter volume generally increases during development, this finding was complicated by the observation that there is actually a small increase in gray matter volume *before* the decrease. Furthermore, this increase was regionally specific. Gray matter volume peaked in the frontal and parietal lobes at age 12 and in the temporal lobe at age 16; the occipital lobe continued to gain gray matter volume through age 20.

What is causing the increase in gray matter? There are a number of possibilities. It could be increases in dendritic arborization, increases in neuron size, or even changes in the glia. However, MRI does not have the spatial resolution to be able to test for these possibilities. This increase could be a second wave of overproduced synapses that are then pruned on the basis of the environment that is present at this later developmental stage. Regardless of the underlying cause, these changes appear to be uniquely human. Nonhuman primates tend to exhibit highly synchronous cortical development, during which all cortical regions develop at a similar pace over the same time. The changes that were observed in humans were very regionally specific. There is also no evidence of a second wave of brain development in nonhuman primates, which might help to account for the lengthy developmental course taken by humans.

---

injuries have life-long impairments in social functioning (Kolb & Fantie, 1997). Kolb, Wilson, and Taylor (1992) studied the ability of children to judge the emotion of a cartoon character from ambiguous drawings. They found that although 5- to 6-year-old children were able to recognize faces, they were unable to judge the emotion expressed on the face in an ambiguous situation. It was only the 14-year-old children who were able to perform this task at adult levels. Thus, judgments that are critical in social settings appear to rely on the development of frontal lobes, and this development appear to reach adult levels in the teen years.

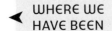

WHERE WE HAVE BEEN

The research presented in this section suggests that basic or early developing functions are associated with early development and myelination of underlying cortical and subcortical regions. For instance, the development of motor functions appears early, and the emergence of motor behaviors

1. What is the difference between experience-dependent and experience-expectant plasticity?
2. What are some of the factors that underlie plastic change? How do these factors relate to our lifelong ability to change behavior in response to the environment and our experiences?
3. Complete the following table

Lobe	Event	Timeline	Associated Behavior(s)
Parietal	myelination	_____	_____
	visuospatial skill	_____	_____
	dorsal stream maturation	_____	_____
Temporal	myelination	_____	_____
	auditory cortex maturation	_____	_____
	_____	_____	adultlike memory
Occipital	myelination	_____	_____
	binocular vision	_____	_____
	_____	_____	facial recognition
Frontal	myelination	_____	_____
	_____	_____	ability to switch strategies
	_____	_____	ability to accurately read emotions

4. How do cephalocaudal and proximodistal patterns of myelination in the frontal cortex appear in behavior?

such as walking is associated with myelination of cortical and subcortical motor areas. Conversely, more complex behaviors such as inhibition of previously rewarded strategies develop later in adolescence and rely on later-developing structures in the frontal lobes. Although it is tempting to view these correlations as potentially being causal, it is important to recognize that numerous changes are occurring throughout the brain in development. It is likely that ongoing neuroimaging studies will continue to provide important insights into how brain development is mirrored in behavior.

MODULE 13.2
Disorders of Development

When one considers how many things can go wrong during early development, it is a wonder that anyone turns out to be "normal" at all. The developing brain has many needs and even more enemies. Even though the brain accounts for only 2% of the body's weight, it receives 15% of the output from the heart, requires 20% of the body's available oxygen, and consumes 25% of the body's available glucose. Compromising these metabolic needs is disastrous at the best of times, but the demands during development can be even greater. As if these demands were not already enough, the developing brain is also vulnerable to what the expectant mother eats and breathes, the diseases to which she might be exposed during pregnancy, and the genes that both parents contributed. Amazingly, things usually go just fine, and the brain (along with the rest of the child) develops normally. This normal development was the primary focus of the previous twelve chapters. However, this module documents what happens when things go wrong during brain development.

WHERE WE
ARE GOING ➤ The brain is a fragile thing, and we are going to learn about the long list of threats to the normally developing brain. These include toxins, the lack of oxygen, infection, malnutrition, environmental insults, and genetic disorders.

Potential Causes of Developmental Abnormalities

STRUCTURAL ABNORMALITIES. Discussing structural abnormalities as a potential cause of developmental abnormalities is a bit like saying that the cause of darkness is a lack of light. Abnormal variation in the brain's structure certainly can lead to atypical behavioral development, but that does not really tell us what caused the structural defect in the first place. There are many potential causes, including damage from toxins, lack of oxygen, infections, malnutrition, or even genetic disorders. These are discussed in more detail later, but sometimes the cause of the structural abnormality is unknown. Depending on the severity and timing of the disruption, the result can vary from death to virtually undetectable symptoms.

At worst, abnormal nervous system development results in anencephaly, which is the complete lack of brain development. A drastic reduction in brain development

Current Controversy

Do Ultrasound Scans Cause Brain Damage?

Starting in the late 1990s, reports of the dangers of ultrasound scans started circulating around the Internet and popular media outlets, such as CNN. Most of the reports were quite conservative, but some were more alarmist, with titles such as "Ultrasound Scans May Harm Unborn Babies" and "Ultrasound Scans May Disrupt Fetal Brain Development." Where were these claims coming from? As it turns out, the studies on which these reports were based were not examinations of brain damage at all, but rather studies of laterality. For example, Helle Kieler of the Karolinska Institute in Stockholm, Sweden, has published a series of studies looking at the potential impact of ultrasound scans on the subsequent laterality (handedness in particular) of the developing child. In one of these studies, a group of almost 180,000 Swedish men born between 1973 and 1978 were followed. A relatively small number (almost 7000) had received diagnostic ultrasonic scans while in the womb,

whereas most of the men (over 172,000) did not. Kieler's research team found that the relatively young men (those born between 1976 and 1978) who had received ultrasound scans were much more likely (32%) to be left-handed than is normally observed in Swedish population (9%). Why only in the younger men? Perhaps because in 1976, it became much more common for women to have two ultrasound scans: one at 17 weeks of pregnancy and another at 37 weeks.

Does this mean that ultrasound scans cause brain damage? Certainly not, unless you equate left-handedness with being brain damaged (which some people do, including some members of the media). There is considerable evidence of higher rates of left-handedness among brain-damaged groups of individuals (reviewed in Chapter 4), but this does not mean that left-handedness is normally caused by brain damage. The underlying cause of the association between left-handedness and ultrasound is currently unknown, but the Swedish research group is recommending that expectant parents continue to get medically useful scans but avoid unnecessary ones.

is called **microcephaly,** a condition that can also be fatal. A third type of structural abnormality is **agenesis,** in which a specific structure of the brain fails to develop completely or sometimes at all. Depending on the structure that is involved, this can result in relatively mild symptoms (remember the discussion of **callosal agenesis** in Chapter 4). Finally, in the case of **dysgenesis,** a specific structure in the brain develops abnormally.

DAMAGE FROM TOXINS OR A LACK OF OXYGEN. A **teratogen** is an agent that can cause malformations of the developing brain. In most instances, the term is used to refer to a chemical. However, it can also refer to a virus or to ionizing radiation. Teratogens tend to exert very specific effects on the developing child, and the presence of one teratogen can greatly intensify the effect of another. In most cases, the effects of the teratogen are much weaker on the mother than on the fetus.

Chemical teratogens, such as mercury, lead, or PCBs, can be found "naturally" in the developing child's (or expectant mother's) environment. However, chemical teratogens can also be introduced into the child's body more deliberately, such as maternal alcohol or barbiturate use. In some cases, medications taken by expectant mothers have disastrous effects in the developing child. The most famous example of this is probably the anti–pregnancy sickness drug thalidomide, which in the early 1960s led to a wide range of defects. Babies who had been exposed to thalidomide as fetuses often suffered from blindness, deafness, and limb malformations.

Many common contagious maternal and even childhood diseases, such as influenza, mumps, chicken pox, or measles, can also serve as teratogens. Chronic diseases such as diabetes, asthma, and hypertension can also have teratogenic effects. Lately, there has been a lot of experimental work with infants who are infected with the human immunodeficiency virus (HIV). It appears that infants with HIV who have not yet developed acquired immune deficiency syndrome (AIDS) already exhibit cognitive impairments compared to controls (Chase et al., 2000). Finally, ionizing radiation can also be a teratogen, and just as is the case with other teratogens, the more the developing child is exposed, the greater is the effect of the agent.

The effects of teratogen exposure vary tremendously, and they depend on the type, duration, and dose of the exposure as well as the genetic makeup of the mother, the genetic makeup of the child, and the period of brain growth that is affected. The brain is most vulnerable to the effects of teratogens during the third through eighth weeks of prenatal development (when the brain cells are dividing and migrating most rapidly).

The brain is not only vulnerable to the presence of toxic substances, but it is even more vulnerable to the lack of a substance that it needs to grow and survive. Pound for pound, the brain uses more oxygen than any other part of the body. When you combine this trait with the fact that the brain cannot readily regenerate damaged cells (but there is limited capacity for this regeneration, as we will discuss further in Chapter 16), and the result is an organ that is particularly sensitive to damage from a lack of oxygen. A period of oxygen deprivation is called **anoxia** (lack of oxygen) or **hypoxia** (reduction of oxygen). There are many potential causes of anoxia or hypoxia during development, including abnormal compression, low blood pressure, carbon monoxide poisoning, or cardiac arrest (maternal or fetal). According to results from tests with animal models of prenatal hypoxia, relatively brief periods of hypoxia can cause neuronal loss and cerebral white matter damage. Chronic but mild placental problems in oxygen delivery can result in long-term deficits in neuronal connectivity that affect function postnatally, demonstrated in both the auditory and visual systems (Ress & Harding, 2004).

MALNUTRITION. There are many different types of malnutrition that can influence the developing brain; almost all of them share one symptom at birth; low birth weight, including a marked reduction in brain size at birth. This reduction in brain size appears to persist across an individual's lifetime. Using magnetic resonance imaging, a group of Chilean researchers found that malnourished children had smaller head circumferences and smaller brains than those of children who were not malnourished (Ivanovic et al., 2004). Diets that are lacking in calories result in a syndrome called **marasmus.** According to the World Health Organization, almost half of the deaths of children under 5 years of age in developing countries are associated with marasmus. For the most part, brain mass and morphology appear to be preserved during marasmus; however, there is some evidence of delays in psychomotor development.

Diets that are lacking in protein content (often high in carbohydrates) result in the syndrome known as **kwashiorkor.** This condition leads to cerebral atrophy, but in moderate cases, this atrophy may be reversible (Gunston, Burkimsher, Malan, & Sire, 1992). Severe kwashiorkor can result in permanent physical and mental disabilities.

HYDROCEPHALUS. Known colloquially as "water on the brain," **hydrocephalus** is caused by a large increase in the volume of cerebrospinal fluid (CSF). Therefore, the term *water on the brain* is a bit of misnomer (CSF is clear, but it is not water). Most of the buildup of CSF happens within the brain's ventricles, and this puts pressure on the brain. If the condition happens early in life, before the skull plates have fused, this increase in pressure leads to expansion of the head in all directions. The neurons surrounding the ventricles are the most vulnerable to damage, but when the condition is serious, even the neurons far away from the ventricles are at risk.

As you learned in Chapter 2, CSF is produced in the choriod plexus of the ventricles (mostly the lateral ventricles) and is later absorbed into the veins of the subarachnoid space. Initially, it was believed that hydrocephalus was simply a problem of oversupply of CSF. More recently, clinicians have suspected that the condition results from a blockage of the circulation of CSF. This blockage can occur at a number of different locations. If the obstruction is at the roof of the fourth ventricle, the entire ventricular system becomes enlarged. If it happens at the level of the cerebral aqueduct (the most common location of the blockage), this produces enlargement of the lateral and third ventricles. Finally, if the blockage occurs at the interventricular foramina between the lateral ventricles and third ventricle, one or both of the lateral ventricles become enlarged. Note that regardless of the location of blockage, the lateral ventricles are always enlarged. Therefore, the treatment of hydrocephalus can be the same, regardless of the cause.

Normally, when something is blocked, the solution is to try to unblock it. However, this is usually not practical in cases of hydrocephalus. In many cases, the exact location of the blockage is unknown. Even when the location is known, the act of trying to unblock it can produce further damage. After all, imagine if the blockage was at the cerebral aqueduct. How would a surgeon access the blockage? Only by cutting through the many neurons that are in the way! The most successful treatment of hydrocephalus has been the addition of a shunt (a tube and a valve) that drains excess fluid from the lateral ventricles through veins in the neck to the abdominal cavity. From here, the CSF can be removed from the brain and absorbed by the surrounding tissue in the abdomen. Modern shunts are relatively reliable, but it is not uncommon for them to require (surgical) adjustment or even replacement later in life.

Estimates of the prevalence of hydrocephalus vary tremendously, between .0025% and 0.5% in North American samples. When hydrocephalus does occur, it is more common in boys (almost two thirds of the cases). Left untreated, the condition can result in death. If treated early and successfully (i.e., the pressure is relieved), long-term symptoms such as mental retardation can sometimes be completely avoided. Unfortunately, the condition usually compromises a child's performance on visual-spatial and tactile perception tasks, including tasks that require rapid or precise sequenced movement and executive control (Wills, 1993). However, evaluating prognosis after hydrocephalus is complicated because the disorder is associated with many other problems, including tumors, bleeding, infection, brain trauma, and vascular malformations. Fortunately, diagnosing hydrocephalus is relatively easy. Because it is characterized by an expansion of the entire head, it can even be detected in utero by using an ultrasound scan.

GENETIC DISORDERS. The term *genetic disorder* can be a bit misleading, because genes do not code for disorders. Instead, mutations (additions, deletions, or dislocations) in your genes interfere with the normal manufacture of proteins, which can cause cells to malfunction. A famous example of a disorder caused by extra genetic material is **Down syndrome,** which is characterized by the trisomy (three copies instead of the normal two copies) of the twenty-first chromosome. This is the most common chromosomal disorder, and although some cases are inherited, the vast majority result from a developmental accident of the ovum, sperm, or zygote (Smith & Wilson, 1973).

Down syndrome is associated with cognitive impairments, but the extent of the impairment varies widely, from relatively mild to severe deficits in general intelligence. There are also highly characteristic physical anomalies that accompany the disorder, including a relatively small head, a protruding tongue, a flat nose, folds at the corners of the eyes, and possible defects of the heart, eye, or ear. There also appears to be a link with Alzheimer's disease; older individuals with Down syndrome often exhibit neuropathology very similar to that found in Alzheimer's.

Turner's syndrome affects young girls and is the result of a missing or abnormal second X chromosome. This abnormality happens at conception, and the vast majority of affected fetuses are spontaneously aborted or miscarried. However, the small minority of survivors exhibit characteristic physical and mental traits. As originally described by Turner in 1938, the syndrome is characterized by short stature and the failure to develop secondary sexual characteristics at puberty. It almost always results in ovarian failure, puffy hands and feet, unusually shaped ears, and a low posterior hairline. The condition is usually diagnosed quite early because of these characteristic physical traits. Estimates of prevalence in North America vary between 0.04% and 0.08%.

The neuropsychological profiles of girls with Turner's syndrome tend to be characterized by right hemispheric dysfunction but relatively preserved left hemisphere activity. Overall, this results in general I.Q. scores in the low-average range, although the preserved left hemispheric function can sometimes result in an I.Q. that appears to be normal. However, a more specific examination of the test scores generally reveals dysfunction of visual discrimination, visual-motor integration, route finding, mental rotation, design copying, visual attention, visual memory, and part–whole perception. These deficits tend not to involve verbal skills, so verbal I.Q.'s tend to look quite normal. Socially, girls with Turner's syndrome tend to show difficulty in adjusting to school life and participating in social interactions. Interpreting these problems is difficult because they could be related to cognitive deficits, or they could be related to a sense of abnormality, particularly in the area of sexual development.

Surprisingly, although the symptoms of Turner's syndrome appear to be related to right hemisphere function, neuroimaging tends to report bilateral abnormalities. According to MRI studies, girls with the syndrome tend to have smaller overall cerebral volumes, and proportionately smaller parieto-occipital regions, as well as lower volumes of some deeper structures, including the hippocampus. Curiously, one study also reported larger amygdala volumes in Turner's syndrome (Kesler, Garrett, Bender, Yankowitz, Zeng, & Reiss, 2004). Mostly similar results have been found with functional neuroimaging. In a PET study, girls with Turner's syndrome exhibited hypometabolism in both parietal lobes compared with controls (Elliott, Watkins, Messa, Liipe, & Chugani, 1996). Similar hypometabolism was also observed in occipital regions.

In terms of treatment, girls with Turner's syndrome almost always receive estrogen therapy, as their underdeveloped (or completely undeveloped) gonads will not produce sufficient estrogen. To combat the short stature that is often associated with the condition, most girls will also receive growth hormones. It is unclear whether these treatments mitigate the neuropsychological symptoms of the syndrome, although some specialized educational techniques can be helpful.

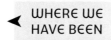 We have reviewed the many threats to normal brain development, such as toxins, the lack of oxygen, malnutrition, environmental insults, and genetic disorders.

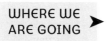 In the next module, we will review the neuropsychology of three major developmental disorders: developmental dyslexia, attention deficit disorder, and autism.

Developmental Dyslexia

As you learned in Chapter 8, dyslexia can be acquired as a result of brain damage. However, reading problems can also be developmental. The term **developmental dyslexia** traditionally refers to a significant discrepancy between reading ability and intelligence in children who have been receiving adequate reading instruction. By definition, the disorder is developmental in nature and therefore is not strictly associated with any particular traumatic event. There are two aspects of the definition that you should notice before you read further. First, the disorder is a relative one. If a child reads at a level well below the average for his or her age, this alone does not mean that the child is dyslexic; instead, the reading deficit must be selective. The second aspect that you should notice is how general the description of the deficit is. Popular culture tends to portray developmental dyslexia (usually simply referred to as *dyslexia*) as a disorder of reversing the order of numbers (such as substituting 93 for 39) or confusing reversible letters (such as *b*'s and *d*'s or *p*'s and *q*'s). Reversals of this type have certainly been documented in cases of developmental dyslexia, but as you will learn in the following paragraphs, this characterization of the disorder is mostly an inaccurate oversimplification.

However, the definition of the disorder that we provided in the preceding paragraph is a very broad one, and it probably describes an entire class of related disorders. So much of the research about this disorder is controversial, but there are a few points of general agreement. First of all, it has been well established that dyslexia is a behavioral disorder with a neurological basis and that dyslexia persists across an individual's lifetime (although some treatments can be helpful). Dyslexia appears to have a genetic origin in at least some cases; it runs in families, and there is a higher concordance of dyslexia in monozygotic twins than in dizygotic twins (Vellutino, 1987). The MZ concordance is far from 100%, however, suggesting that other factors must be at play. Sex differences are also present in both the incidence rates and the resultant severities of the disorder. Developmental dyslexia is much more common in males, and the females who suffer from the disorder tend to exhibit weaker symptoms (Gilger et al., 1992; Steenhuis, Bryden, & Schroeder, 1993).

Beyond these few points of general agreement, debates rage over the potential causes and types of developmental dyslexia and how the disorder should be treated. Currently, three major theories of dyslexia are under investigation (Ramus et al., 2003). The phonological theory posits that the primary impairment is in the representation, storage, and/or retrieval of speech sounds. Because learning to read requires the learning of arbitrary grapheme–phoneme correspondence rules, any deficit in the ability to encode or retrieve these associations would erode the very foundation of reading. There is considerable evidence in support of this theory. For example, when developmental dyslexics are given tests of phonological awareness in which they are required to segment or manipulate speech sounds, they perform particularly poorly. Similar impairments in verbal short-term memory have also been observed. However, developmental dyslexics also appear to be impaired in much more basic, nonlinguistic sensory tasks, such as tone discrimination, temporal order judgment, and gap detection (see Tallal et al., 1993). Therefore, the impairment might influence sensory processing even before phonological processing.

The **visual theory** of developmental dyslexia (Livingstone, Rosen, Drislane, & Galaburda, 1991; Lovegrove, Broling, Badcock, & Blackwood, 1980) characterizes the disorder as a primarily visual impairment, wherein the individual has difficulties processing the letters and words when reading text. In terms of the biological origins of the disorder, this theory postulates that the magnocellular visual pathway is selectively disrupted in developmental dyslexia. There is considerable evidence in favor of this theory, because dyslexic individuals exhibit abnormalities of the magnocellular layers of the lateral geniculate nucleus (Livingstone, Rosen, Drislane, & Galaburda,

1991). Consequently, these individuals have less sensitivity with magnocellular vision, including interpreting scenes of low spatial frequency and high temporal frequency (Cornelissen, Richardson, Mason, Fowler, & Stein, 1995). This theory does not preclude the possibility that there is a phonological deficit but rather postulates a lower-order mechanism that can give rise to the deficit.

A third possibility is the cerebellar theory of dyslexia (Nicolson, Fawcett, & Dean, 2001), sometimes called *automaticity theory*. Like the visual theory, the cerebellar theory identifies a potential biological origin of the disorder (a dysfunctional cerebellum). Because the cerebellum plays an important role in motor control (and, by extension, the articulation of speech), it is claimed that cerebellar dysfunction could lead to deficiencies in phonological representation. Furthermore, because the cerebellum plays an important role in the learning of highly automated motor tasks, this would also influence the normally overlearned task of grapheme–phoneme correspondences. Like the other two theories, the cerebellar theory draws support from a number of lines of evidence. Developmental dyslexics perform poorly on a wide variety of motor tasks, dual tasks, and other tasks that rely on cerebellar processing, such as time estimation (see Nicolson et al., 1995). Structural and functional imaging studies have also detected abnormal anatomy and metabolism in the cerebellar region of dyslexics (Brown et al., 2001; Rae et al., 1998). Attempts have been made to unify these three theories, and, of course, it remains possible that all three are correct in different cases. In other words, there might be three subtypes of developmental dyslexia. However, currently, none of the three theories accurately account for all the experimental evidence.

Attention Deficit Disorder (ADD)

Of all the conditions described in this module, **attention deficit disorder** (ADD) is probably the most talked about and the most controversial. Almost completely unheard of until recently, ADD has become a regular focus of media attention and has been at the center of many debates about social policy involving caregivers, health care providers, and educators. This exposure is well deserved. In North America, ADD is the most common behavioral disorder of childhood, estimated to affect 4% of all school-aged children. Between 30% and 50% of referrals for psychological services in the United States involve the diagnosis or treatment of ADD (Richters et al., 1995). Although the disorder appears to have an onset at preschool age, it is not strictly a disease of childhood. Instead, many adults also suffer from the condition, which some have even termed *adult attention deficit disorder*. Between 30% and 50% of children with ADD will exhibit symptoms well into adulthood.

The diagnostic features of ADD include a deficit of attention (inattention, distractibility), impulsivity, memory, and in some cases hyperactivity. Children with ADD often score badly on a wide variety of neuropsychological tests, but this does not necessarily mean that they have some sort of general impairment. Instead, when a central function such as attention is compromised, deficits on virtually every task with a significant attentional component can be observed. An analogy is that when there is serious language impairment, it is difficult to assess function because many neuropsychological tests require the use of language. In fact, the claim that children with

ADD have memory problems is itself controversial because the apparent memory deficits could simply be due to inattention during the memory tasks.

Experimental investigations of ADD have employed factor analytic techniques to identify at least two subtypes of ADD. One type is mostly characterized by attentional problems; the other is characterized mostly by motor hyperactivity. The first type is usually referred to as ADD or attention deficit disorder without hyperactivity (**ADD/noH**); the second type is called attention deficit hyperactivity disorder (ADHD). ADD/noH appears to be characterized by a sensitivity to interference and a difficulty in filtering out superfluous stimulation. In contrast, ADHD is characterized by a deficit in motor system inhibition. These two subtypes of the disorder often produce similar symptoms, but the mechanisms appear to be different.

As with many neuropsychological disorders, the best treatment for ADD appears to be a combination of pharmaceutical, educational, and environmental interventions. Treatment with psychostimulants has been the most popular method, and this leads to behavioral improvement in 70–90% of children with ADD. There are some interesting differences between the ADD/noH and ADHD groups, though. Both respond well to medication, but the dosage differs. There are also more children who do not respond at all to the medication among the ADHD group (Barkley, DuPaul, & McMurray, 1991). In addition to pharmaceutical treatments, children with either form of ADD also benefit from cognitive-behavioral interventions that target one's attention span and self-control.

Autism

Autism is a developmental disorder of early childhood characterized by abnormal social and communicative skills. The disorder was described independently by Kanner in 1943 and Asperger in 1944, and it is likely that several other earlier investigations described the same disorder using different names (such as dementia infantilis). However, a variant of Kanner's term *early infantile autism*, which described the abnormal social behavior, is the term that is currently used to describe this complicated disorder. The symptoms that are usually associated with the disorder are the restricted or delayed development of communicative skills, abnormal eating and sleeping behavior, small repertoires of repetitive activities, and sometimes even self-abusive behaviors. Unlike most infants, autistic babies tend not to desire to be held by their caregivers and might even resist being touched or held, shown by arching their backs.

Some autistic children grow to become very high-functioning adults, but others learn only minimal social skills and develop few (verbal and nonverbal) communicative skills. Most (about 75%) children with autism have I.Q.s that are significantly lower than normal. As is the case with so many developmental disorders, the condition is more common in males than in females. Curiously, the I.Q.s of the affected males are higher on average. Some autistic individuals have relatively preserved intelligence, and the higher the intelligence of the affected individual, the lower is the severity of the autistic symptoms.

An abnormally high (ten times the rate observed in the normal population) proportion of autistic individuals exhibit savant skills, that is, skills that are extraordinarily well developed, especially in light of limited capacity in other areas. These savant skills vary tremendously, but the most common ones involve feats of memory, calculation, artistic ability, musical ability, or calendar memory/calculation. For example, an autistic individual with a savant skill of calendar memory could correctly answer the question "What day of the week was November 1, 1972?" within seconds (it was a Wednesday). Although the movie *Rain Man* taught much of the public that some autistic individuals have savant skills, it also created the mistaken impression that all autistics have such skills. This is not the case. Only 10% of autistic individuals demonstrate these skills, compared with 1% in the general population (Munoz-Yunta, Ortiz-Alonso, Amo, Fernandez-Lucas, Maestu, Palau-Baduell, 2003).

Many recent investigations of autism have focused on the possibility that the disorder is a failure to develop a **theory of mind** (Baron-Cohen, 1995). This refers to the idea that people normally understand that other people have their own plans, thoughts, and consciousness. However, in autism, people might have difficulty understanding other people's beliefs, attitudes, and emotions. Support for this theory has come from investigations in which individuals are asked to guess about the beliefs of others, especially if false beliefs are involved (Brent, Rios, Happe, & Charman, 2004). For example, using two dolls (Anne and Sally), Baron-Cohen and colleagues (Baron-Cohen, Leslie, & Frith, 1985) taught a group of children (some of whom were autistic) to correctly identify each doll. Then, to test the children's understanding of others' beliefs, the two dolls were used to act out a scenario. The "Sally" doll placed a marble in her basket and then exited from the scene, leaving the basket behind. The "Anne" doll then took Sally's marble and put it in her own basket. On Sally's return, the experimenter would ask the child, "Where will Sally look for her marble?" Of course, the correct answer was that Sally would look in her own basket. If the child indicated that Sally would look in Anne's basket, this was taken as an indication that the child could not take Sally's false belief into account, failing the theory of mind test. Neurologically normal children performed very well on this test (twenty-three of twenty-seven children answered correctly), but only four of twenty of the children with autism correctly attributed a false belief to the Sally doll. Many variants of this type of test have produced similar results (Brent et al., 2004), suggesting that the social deficits that are observed in autistics are at least partially attributable to an inability to understand or predict what others are thinking.

What causes autism? There is fairly convincing evidence that at least one form of autism can be inherited. In the general population, 0.1% of children are autistic. The siblings of autistic children have a 3% chance of sharing the disorder (300 times more likely than the general population). Similarly, autism concordance is 300 times higher in monozygotic twins than in dizygotic twins, but the penetrance of the disorder is not 100% in monozygotic twins. There is very wide disagreement about the rates among monozygotic twins, with estimates ranging between 36% (Folstein and Rutter, 1977) and 96% (Bailey et al., 1995). Therefore, genetics cannot be the only factor in the development of autism (or every form of autism). The role of heredity may be in determining the vulnerability to the condition, which is triggered through other means. Some researchers suspect that autism is caused by prenatal exposure to toxins or even that the disorder is caused by a virus. These suspicions are not completely unwarranted. For instance, if a pregnant woman suffers from rubella during the first trimester of pregnancy, this significantly increases the odds that the child will

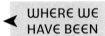

Self Test

1. What are some of the common causes of developmental abnormalities?

2. What are some of the common features of individuals with Down Syndrome? Turner's Syndrome? Why are only girls affected with Turner's syndrome?

3. What are the defining features of dyslexia? Compare and contrast the three major theories of dyslexia? Which one do you think explains dyslexia best? Why?

4. What are the defining features of ADD? What are the subtypes of ADD? How is it treated?

5. What are the defining features and potential causes of autism? What is the evidence that children with autism have difficulties in developing a theory of mind?

exhibit autism. There is even debate about whether the mumps, measles, and rubella vaccine that is routinely given to North American children puts them at greater risk of developing autism (Madsen and Vestergaard, 2004). However, the evidence for this link is not yet clear.

◄ **WHERE WE HAVE BEEN** We have reviewed the neuropsychology of three major developmental disorders: developmental dyslexia, attention deficit disorder, and autism. Developmental dyslexia is characterized by a discrepancy between reading ability and intelligence. Attention deficit disorder is characterized by problems with attention (inattention, distractibility), impulsivity, memory, and, in some cases, hyperactivity. Autism is a developmental disorder of early childhood characterized by abnormal social and communicative skills.

Glossary

Agenesis—A condition in which a specific structure fails to develop.

Amblyopia—A decrease in vision in one eye, also known as "lazy eye."

Anencephaly—A generally fatal failure of the rostral part of the neural plate to fuse; characterized by a general absence of the cerebral hemispheres.

Anoxia—A period of oxygen deprivation.

Apoptosis—Programmed cell death that is a regular part of development in the CNS.

Attention deficit disorder—A disorder characterized by deficits in attention and often accompanied by impulsivity and hyperactivity.

Autism—A developmental disorder characterized by abnormal social and communicative skills.

Cephalocaudal—Development of motor functions in which the head and trunk are controlled before the legs are.

Craniorachischisis—A fatal defect of the neural tube that results when there is a complete failure of the closure of the neural tube. The CNS appears as a groove in the top of the head and body.

Critical periods—Defined periods of time during development in which plastic change occurs easily.

Dendritic branching—The branching of dendrites that can result in increased numbers of synapses.

Down syndrome—A genetic disorder that is characterized by the trisomy of the twenty-first chromosome.

Dysgenesis—A condition in which a specific structure fails to develop completely or normally.

Ectoderm—The outermost of the three layers of cells that are in the early embryo; will form the nervous system and the epidermis of the skin.

Experience-dependent plastic change—Plastic changes that depend on idiosyncratic experiences that occur during critical periods that also affect brain development, such as the effects that musical training in childhood has on the cortex.

Experience-expectant plastic change—Plastic changes that depend on experience during the critical period for specific synapses to develop as they should. Much of the sensory cortex appears to have these experience expectant critical periods.

Fine-motor skills—Motor skills that involve the small muscles and are typically used in the coordination of the hands and fingers.

Gross motor skills—Motor skills that involve the large muscles that are typically involved with walking, balance, or holding the head up.

Hydrocephalus—A neurological disorder caused by a large increase in the volume of cerebrospinal fluid.

Hypoxia—A period of reduced oxygen supply.

Kwashiorkor—A syndrome that results from a diet that is lacking sufficient protein.

Marasmus—A syndrome that results from a diet lacking sufficient calories.

Microcephaly—A drastic reduction in brain development.

Neural plate—A patch of cells on the dorsal surface of the embryo that eventually become the nervous system.

Neural tube—The tube that is formed out of the ectoderm at embryonic day 24; will eventually become the spinal cord and brain.

Neurotrophins—Chemicals, such as nerve growth factor, that are secreted by the brain that enhance the survival of neurons.

Plastic change—Change in the nervous system that is a result of experience or the environment.

Pluripotent—Cells that can develop into different types of cells.

Proliferation—The process of cell division that results in new neurons.

Proximodistal—Development of motor skills that occur in head, trunk, and arms before occurring in the hands and fingers.

Spina bifida—A neural tube defect that is characterized by spinal cord defects; not necessarily fatal, though it can vary in its severity.

Stem cells—Embryonic cells that can develop into any type of cell in the body.

Strabismus—Misalignment of the eyes in which one or both eyes deviate toward the nose.

Synaptogenesis—The production of new synapses.

Teratogen—An agent that can cause malformations of the developing brain.

Theory of mind—The idea that people normally understand that other people have their own thoughts, plans, and consciousness.

Turner's syndrome—A disorder resulting from a missing or abnormal second X chromosome in young girls.

14

Human Brain Damage

Humpty Dumpty sat on a wall. Humpty Dumpty had a great fall.
All the king's horses and all the king's men
Couldn't put Humpty together again.

—MOTHER GOOSE

Muriel Lezak used the rhyme about Humpty Dumpty to introduce her chapter on neuropathology for neuropsychologists in her book *Neuropsychological Assessment.* Although she does not make direct reference to the quote in her chapter, the implication is quite clear. When a brain suffers significant damage, no amount of effort can restore the brain back to its original healthy state. This does not deny the importance of rehabilitation in recovery from brain damage (we will discuss that further in Chapter 16), but even successful rehabilitation is typically not a restoration to the previous state. Instead, rehabilitation usually requires the learning of new ways to do previously learned tasks. Recovery from brain damage often has more to do with compensation than with recovering or restoring lost function.

WHERE WE ARE GOING ➤ The nervous system is extremely fragile, and there are many ways in which one can damage it. A CNS lesion (meaning "to hurt") is an area of damaged neural tissue, including the loss of cells or discontinuity of previously present connections. The following sections detail some of the many ways in which the CNS can be lesioned. This topic can appear to be quite mechanical and depressing. However, the reader should be encouraged to learn that the prevention, treatment, and rehabilitation of brain damage have improved dramatically in recent years, and even more spectacular improvements appear to be on the horizon.

MODULE **14.1**
Causes of Brain Damage

Tumors

A **tumor** is mass of new and abnormal tissue that is not physiologically beneficial to its surrounding structures. Tumors are also called *neoplasms,* a term that literally means "new tissue." Some neurological texts describe tumors as **space-occupying lesions,** meaning that they are foreign objects that cause damage to the central nervous system (CNS) by putting pressure on it and occupying space that is normally occupied by the CNS. This term accurately reflects the damage that some types of tumors cause.

However, other types of tumors damage the surrounding tissues in ways other than exerting pressure. The brain is one of the most common sites for tumor growth, second only to the uterus. Tumors differ from one another in terms of what type of cell gives rise to the tumor, how rapidly they grow, whether they **infiltrate** and destroy the surrounding neural tissue or remain relatively **encapsulated,** and how likely they are to recur if they are removed. **Benign** tumors are not likely to recur; **malignant** ones are more likely to recur. The following sections detail some of the most common types of tumors that form within the CNS. There are four major types of brain tumors: those that originate from glial cells, the meninges, nervous tissue, or other parts of the body already infected with a tumor.

TUMORS ARISING FROM GLIAL CELLS. The most common type of tumors that form in the brain are **gliomas,** tumors that arise from glial cells. There are two main types of

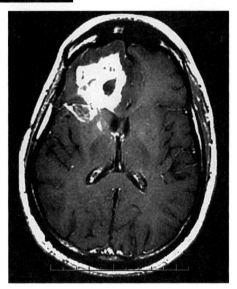

| Figure 14.1 | An MRI Scan of a Glioblastoma |

Source: Used by permission of John H. Sampson, Duke University Medical Center.

gliomas. **Astrocytomas** are tumors that arise from the growth of astrocytes. These tumors tend not to grow very quickly, and they are rarely malignant. Some astrocytomas are relatively well encapsulated, so the damage that they cause tends to come from compression of the surrounding tissues. Other astrocytomas infiltrate the surrounding neural tissue. The prognosis for individuals who have an astrocytoma removed surgically is generally quite good, provided that the tumor started to grow in a relatively surgically accessible location. Unfortunately, even slow-growing benign tumors can be extremely dangerous if they start to grow in relatively inaccessible locations. When surgical treatment is not practical, chemotherapy is typically used.

A second type of glioma is a **glioblastoma.** In many ways, these tumors are the opposite of astrocytomas. They grow quickly, and they are highly malignant. Instead of remaining relatively encapsulated, glioblastomas tend to infiltrate the surrounding tissues, making them very difficult to excise surgically without the removal of the relatively healthy surrounding neural tissue (see Figure 14.1). For this reason, chemotherapy is often used to treat gliobastomas.

A much less common type of glioma (2–6% of all gliomas) is the **medulloblastoma** (also called a primitive neuroectodermal tumor), another highly malignant infiltrating tumor. However, medulloblastomas tend to form around the cerebellum and brainstem early in life. Because of their malignant and infiltrating nature proximate to brainstem structures that are critical for supporting vegetative functions such as breathing, the prognosis for individuals who develop medulloblastomas tends to be relatively poor. Because of the location and nature of these tumors, chemotherapy is the most attractive treatment option.

TUMORS ARISING FROM THE MENINGES. **Meningiomas** are tumors that grow out of (and remain attached to) the meninges. More specifically, most meningiomas grow out of the dura mater, forming an ovoid shape (see Figure 14.2). Because they grow out of tissues found outside of the CNS, meningiomas tend to be reasonably well encapsulated. Therefore, the harmful effects of these tumors tend to result from pressure applied at the site of the tumor as well as sites distal from the tumor. Most types of meningiomas are relatively benign, but there are also some malignant varieties of the tumor. Regardless of type, surgery is typically the best treatment for meningiomas, particularly because of their encapsulated nature and partly because of their location on the surface of the brain. However, when the tumor is located in a relatively inaccessi-

| **Figure 14.2** | **An MRI Scan of a Meningioma** |

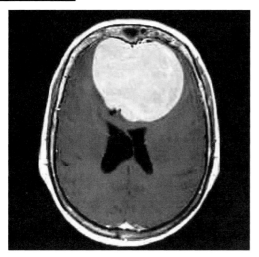

Source: Image courtesy of Leonard J. Tyminski.

ble part of the brain for surgery (such as between the hemispheres), chemotherapy or radiotherapy is used as a treatment.

METASTATIC TUMORS. Metastatic tumors (or *metastases*) are secondary tumors that form from migrated tumor tissue. The primary tumor site can be located in parts of the body such as the lungs, breasts, uterus, or kidneys. Although it is possible that the primary site of the tumor can be within the CNS, it is far more common for the original tumor to be located outside of the CNS. **Simple metastatic tumors** occur when only one tumor forms at one site. However, in most cases, there are **multiple metastatic tumors,** usually spreading from the lungs to the CNS. For simple metastatic tumors, surgical or radiological treatment can be quite effective. However, for multiple metastatic tumors, whole-brain radiotherapy or chemotherapy is most common, but the prognosis is generally quite poor.

NEUROPSYCHOLOGICAL EFFECTS OF TUMORS. The behavioral symptoms that arise from the formation of a tumor vary widely, just as the size, location, cell type, and growth rate of the tumors varies. For example, a small, slow-growing infiltrating astrocytoma located near the primary visual cortex might gradually start to cause blindness in part of a person's visual field. Tumors of the pituitary gland can have behavioral symptoms similar to those of a visual cortex tumor, despite having a very different location. Because of the proximity of the pituitary gland to the optic chiasm, pressure placed on the optic chiasm from pituitary tumors can also result in visual field defects.

A more rapidly growing meningioma that remains relatively well encapsulated between the two hemispheres could apply pressure to the primary motor and sensory cortices in this region, causing numbness and paresis to the feet and legs. Metastatic tumors that form in the left temporal lobe can cause speech disturbances, including receptive language problems, whereas tumors in the left parietal lobe can lead to apraxia. In addition to the brain damage caused by infiltration and compression, tumors can also cause epileptic seizures and release substances that are toxic to the brain. If the tumor releases toxins and is located in one of the ventricles (tumors often form in ventricles), the toxins can then be transported easily from the site of origin, producing lesions and behavioral deficits that are not confined to the region where the tumor is growing.

Cerebrovascular Disorders

A **cerebrovascular disorder** occurs when the blood supply to the brain is interrupted. The interruption itself can be sudden or gradual, complete or relative, permanent or transient. There are a number of different cerebrovascular disorders that differ along these dimensions, and they are reviewed below. The collective impact of these disorders should not be underestimated. They are the leading cause of disabling neurological damage and the third most common cause of death in the developed world. (Cancer is the leading cause, followed by heart attack; both of these conditions can also lead to neurological damage.) As a result of the impact of the lesions produced by these disorders, they are one of the primary sources of lesion evidence for clinical and experimental neuropsychologists who are seeking to make inferences about the function of areas of the brain.

The most commonly used term to describe cerebrovascular disorders is *stroke.* This term is not very specific; broadly defined, it is synonymous with the term *cerebrovascular disorder* described above. The more common and precise medical term for stroke is the term **cerebrovascular accident (CVA),** which refers to a class of cerebrovascular disorders, all of which result in interruptions to the brain's blood supply. This interruption can be quite sudden, or it can get gradually worse over a period of years before being detected. A CVA results in **cerebral ischemia,** which is a lack of blood supply to the brain. If the cerebral ischemia is severe or long-lasting enough to kill neurons, the damaged area is called an **infarct.** Infarcts can be very small if the CVA is restricted to small, minor arteries. However, if the interruption is in a major vessel (or perhaps the entire circulatory system, as in a heart attack), the resultant infarct can be very large. Interruptions in the blood supply can be caused by a variety of events, such as blocked cerebral arteries, broken cerebral arteries, or interruptions of blood supply outside of the CNS.

If a blood clot forms within a cerebral blood vessel, this clot is called a **thrombosis** (*thrombus* means "clot"). Thromboses can also form outside of the brain. If a thrombosis forms in the heart, it can cause a heart attack. The formation of a thrombosis can have several causes, but the most common one is **atherosclerosis,** in which fatty deposits build up inside the walls of blood vessels, constricting the vessel more and more and possibly even completely blocking it. Because the buildup of the fatty deposits tends to be gradual (although there are exceptions—I will never forget eating my first Monte Cristo sandwich, served with French fries!), the symptoms of cerebral thrombosis appear gradually. Furthermore, because atherosclerosis often forms where two relatively large arteries branch off from one single artery (called a **bifurcation**), the constriction of blood flow tends to influence relatively large areas of the brain, and the neuropsychological symptoms that result from the disorder are usually diffuse and gradual in nature.

An **embolism** is similar in form to a thrombosis. Both involve the blocking of an artery by the buildup of a substance. However, a thrombosis remains at the point of origin. An embolism is normally a clot (but can be another substance, such as a bubble of air or piece of fat) that travels in the bloodstream from one part of the body to another. Typically, the substance travels from a spot where the arteries are relatively large to a place where the arteries are smaller than the point of original formation, so a clot that previously did not completely block the flow of blood might suddenly do so at another location. The term *embolism* is derived from a word meaning "plug" or "wedge." Because the obstruction of blood flow is often quite sudden and complete (to the area irrigated by the blocked artery), embolisms can be extremely dangerous if the blockage is not relieved immediately. Depending on where they form, some embolisms can be treated surgically. There are also other treatments for embolisms, including the administration of anticoagulant drugs.

In some cases, the interruption in blood supply to the brain can be caused by the breakage of a blood vessel, called a **hemorrhage** (combining the root words for "blood" and "to burst forth"). The bursting of a blood vessel can happen for a variety of reasons. The presence of a thrombosis or embolism can cause blood pressure to build to a point that the walls of the artery cannot sustain, or the artery itself can be malformed, having a weak spot called an **aneurysm.** Other common causes of hemorrhages include abnormally high blood pressure, or **hypertension,** and the piercing of a blood vessel by a foreign or displaced object, such as a bullet. The damaging effects of cerebral hemorrhage are not limited to the interruption in blood supply. Not only is the supply of oxygen and glucose disrupted, but the blood itself is somewhat toxic to the neural tissue. (Recall our discussion on the blood–brain barrier in Chapter 2— CNS tissue does not normally come into direct contact with blood. Instead, there are two layers of cells that form the blood–brain barrier.)

To make matters even worse, the force of the bleeding can compromise the structural integrity of the brain regions surrounding the bleed, and if the bleed persists, the resulting pressure can cause compression injuries away from the site of the bleed. The resultant pressure can result in the displacement of neural centers that are critical for basic vegetative functions, such as the medulla oblongata's role in regulating heartbeat and breathing.

When the hemorrhage occurs within the brain, it is called an **intracerebral hemorrhage.** These bleeds are often caused by hypertension, and the damage that the bleeding produces is a result of the interruption of blood flow, toxicity of the uncontained blood, and pressure buildup at and away from the site of the bleed. This type of hemorrhage is unlikely to recur, but the prognosis for an individual who suffers from a single intracerebral hemorrhage is usually quite poor.

Another type of hemorrhage that can suddenly threaten the CNS is a **subarachnoid hemorrhage,** which is bleeding into the subarachnoid space (between the pia mater and arachnoid layer of the meninges). This type of bleed is also often the result of hypertension, but the primary threat posed to the brain is usually the pressure exerted by the bleed. Because the onset of a subarachnoid hemorrhage is usually sudden, so too are its symptoms. These include severe and sudden headache, nausea or even vomiting, and perhaps loss of consciousness. The pressure exerted on the brain by a subarachnoid hemorrhage tends to influence many different structures, so highly specific functional symptoms (such as aphasia or visual agnosia) tend not to accompany the bleed. Like intracerebral hemorrhages, subarachnoid hemorrhages tend not to recur, but the prognosis for an individual who suffers a single CVA of this type tends to be poor.

Some CVAs are caused by physical defects in the cerebral vasculature. These defects might be present at birth (called **congenital** defects); others can be caused by physical trauma. One type of congenital defect that places an individual at higher risk of a CVA is an **arteriovenus malformation (AVM).** AVMs are malformed arteries and vessels that have extra or missing connections, resulting in abnormal blood flow. These structures tend to form along the middle cerebral artery, and they tend to be somewhat weak. Some AVMs bleed at some point (or many points) in an individual's life, but many exist without incident throughout an otherwise healthy life. When AVMs do bleed, they do so in a rather different manner than the bleeds that we described in previous sections. Instead of suddenly releasing large amounts of blood in a very short time, AVMs tend to bleed very small amounts over long periods of time, and they tend to bleed more than once. Because they bleed less, the brain damage that is produced as a result of an AVM tends not to result from pressure at or away from the site. Instead, the damage tends to result from a lack of irrigation of a particular area coupled with the toxicity of the blood itself.

Another common defect in vasculature is called an aneurysm. This is an area of the artery that dilates because of local weakness, resulting in a balloonlike expansion. Some aneurysms are present very early in life, but others appear later, possibly as the result of trauma. Some bleed or even burst; others appear never to produce a noticeable problem. If an aneurysm starts to bleed slowly and this bleed is detected, the prognosis can be quite good. This is especially true if the aneurysm is easily accessible for surgery. However, if an aneurysm suddenly bursts (resulting in an intracranial hemorrhage), the rupture is often fatal. Fortunately, this is a relatively rare event. A number of different treatments are available for all of these vascular disorders. Various factors influence which treatment is used, including the size of the affected vessel, the location of the vessel (whether it is surgically accessible and whether other nearby vessels irrigate the same area), and other aspects of the person's medical history. For example, if a surgically inaccessible AVM is bleeding very slowly, the person's physician might elect to attempt to treat it by using drugs to alter blood pressure. However, if the person's blood pressure were already abnormally low, this course of treatment would not be chosen.

A more direct approach to treating cerebrovascular disorders is to treat them surgically, although the treatment of aneurysms is a contentious issue. Some argue that all aneurysms should be treated surgically, whether or not there is any evidence of bleeding. Others claim that the surgical treatment of aneurysms does more harm than good, on average, because most aneurysms do not burst and relatively few bleed (Bannister, 1992). Regardless, hemorrhaging areas such as a burst aneurysm can be treated by clipping them with small metal clips. The clips that are currently used for this procedure are typically not magnetic, which allows the person to have MRI examinations following the surgical procedure. Unfortunately, a number of individuals have died from hemorrhaging after an aneurysm clip was dislodged during an MRI exam because older types of aneurysm clips are vulnerable to magnetic fields.

There are other surgical interventions in addition to those that stop bleeding. A variety of draining procedures can be used to relieve intracranial pressure. Surgery can also be used to remove or break up thromboses or embolisms. The use of anticoagulant drugs can also be effective in treating blockages from thromboses or embolisms, but such treatment is concurrent with risk for starting a bleed that cannot be controlled.

Self-Test

1. What is the difference between a thrombosis and an embolism?

2. What is the difference between an infiltrating tumor and an encapsulated tumor? Which type is easier to treat and how?

3. When a vascular disorder is present, how does this damage the brain?

Head Injuries

TRAUMATIC BRAIN INJURY. Traumatic brain injury (TBI) is the leading cause of closed head injury, accounting for as many as 90% of the medically diagnosed head injuries each year (Satz et al., 1999). TBI is an acquired brain injury and does not include damage that was acquired due to congenital disorders (e.g., trisomy 21), degenerative disorders (e.g., Huntington's chorea), or birth trauma (e.g., perinatal asphyxia). In TBI, not all brain damage occurs as a result of the initial accident. In fact, ischemia (loss of oxygen due to loss of blood oxygenation, blood flow disruption, or blood pressure) accounts for about 88% of further brain damage after the initial insult (Young & Willatts, 1998).

It is estimated that between 1.5 million and 2 million people incur a TBI each year in the United States (Reynolds, Page, & Johnston, 2001) with one million people receiving medical treatment. Of those who require admission to the hospital (often for the most serious of injuries), 230,000 survive the injury. A further 70,000 to 90,000 people experience moderate head injuries (Moscato, Trevisan, & Willer, 1994). Young people (between 15 and 24 years of age) are at the highest risk for TBI, although middle-aged and older people often exhibit more serious symptoms (Moscato et al., 1994). Men are 1.8 times as likely to experience a TBI than women. These statistics likely underrepresent the true numbers of individuals sustaining TBI, as many individuals either do not seek treatment or are treated at other settings.

Individuals who survive beyond the acute phase of the injury do not have a greater risk of mortality. Using 1986 census data, Moscato and colleagues (1994) report that 65% of individuals with TBI had lived with TBI for five or more years, and 43% had lived with TBI for ten or more years (mean of 11.8 years). TBIs occur more often in the young, and the disabilities that are associated with TBI tend to reduce an individual's ability to work and remain independent (Lannoo et al., 2000). Therefore, this group represents a major challenge for neuropsychologists, health care providers, and occupational and physical therapists.

In fact, in 1985, it was estimated that the total lifetime cost of TBI was about $37.8 billion, and it rose in just three years to $44 billion (Max, MacKenzie, & Rice, 1991). Only 12% (or $4.5 billion) of the estimated $44 billion is associated with direct expenditures for hospital costs and costs associated with care, such as physiotherapy (Max et al., 1991). The National Institutes of Health (NIH) paint a different picture, suggesting that the average lifetime cost for a person with severe TBI ranges from $600,000 to $1,875,000. NIH also suggests that these numbers are underestimates and do not include lost earnings (which may be as high as $33 billion per year; Max et al., 1991), costs to social services, and/or the value of the time of caregivers. Regardless, for nonfatal injuries, these are very expensive injuries, especially for families, who often incur the highest proportion of these costs.

Many of these individuals are never examined for impairments to cognitive function. This is because the majority of patients with mild TBI recover within weeks to months following injury. It is estimated that approximately 15% of mild TBI patients are still disabled a year after injury (Satz et al., 1999). When TBI results in disability, the primary symptom is cognitive impairment (Moscato et al., 1994). Furthermore, individuals who exhibit cognitive deficits for more than one month tend to be those with severe TBI. Therefore, it is likely that our knowledge of the effects of TBI on cognitive function primarily reflect those with the most severe injuries (Malec, Buffington, Moessner, & Thompson, 1995).

In adults, the cognitive impairments that are associated with TBI are variable and depend on the severity of the injury. Common impairments associated with TBI include difficulties with executive skills (money and time management, organizational skills, and inhibition); short-term memory; and concentration. TBI-affected adults often have difficulties with the generalization of skills. That is, they may have difficulty in completing well-known tasks when there are small deviations from their normal routine (e.g., they can count out the correct change for the bus, but they cannot do so when they purchase a soda). Even when adults with TBI have normal intelligence, they may be incapable of independent living owing to their cognitive deficits. For instance, their inability to transfer learning from one environment to another may result in an inability to deal with novel situations that often occur in noninstitutional settings.

CLOSED VERSUS OPEN HEAD INJURY.   Most TBIs are **closed head injuries,** in which an individual receives a blow to the head but the blow does not penetrate the skull and meninges. However, when an object such as a bullet or a knife breaches the skull and meninges, this results in an **open head (or penetrating) injury.** One might imagine that open head injuries are typically much worse than closed head injuries, but this is not necessarily the case. In open head injuries, the resulting lesion tends to be at the point of impact, and the size of the lesion is proportional to the size of the object and the force that it exerts. Obviously, a gunshot wound to the head is often fatal, despite the fact that the bullet causing the wound is relatively small. However, people regularly survive open head injuries from knife wounds to the head—it is called neurosurgery! Even if a knife causes the penetrating wound, the damage that is caused by the event is usually somewhat localized to the point of entry, provided that no major vasculature is damaged.

This is not the case for closed head injuries. If someone suffers a major blow to the head, the blow typically causes some damage at the point of impact (called the **coup**). However, because the brain is essentially floating in cerebrospinal fluid, the sudden blow will also cause the brain to bounce against the opposite side of the skull from the impact, producing an injury called a **contre-coup** injury. Diffuse injuries throughout the rest of the brain can also be caused by this displacement, including the shearing of the brain as it rubs against some of the bony protrusions from the skull, called **fossae.** Buildup of blood and other fluids following closed head injury can also lead to high intracranial pressure, which can cause further brain damage. Thus, the type of damage following closed head injury is quite different from that following open head injury.

Interestingly, because widespread areas of the brain are immediately affected following a closed head injury, closed head injuries often result in a sudden loss of consciousness. Open head injuries often do not result in a loss of consciousness. Recall the story of Phineas Gage from Chapter 3: Despite the fact that a four-foot metal bar passed through his frontal lobes producing a massive open head injury, Phineas did not lose consciousness!

Infections

Just as other parts of the body are vulnerable to infection, so too is the CNS. Although the blood–brain barrier helps to protect the brain from pathogens, the brain cannot be completely isolated from these dangers while its metabolic needs are being met. Bacteria, viri (plural of *virus*), parasites, or even fungi can cause infections of the CNS. However, it is rather rare for the original source of infection to be within the CNS. Instead, most infections spread from other sites—often nearby sites such as the nose or ears. When the original infection originates within the CNS, the pathogen must first gain access to the CNS. This requires access through the meninges, which can happen as a result of an open head injury or even surgery if the environment is not completely sterile.

Infections can damage the brain in a variety of ways. The infection can disturb the cell membranes of the surrounding neurons, disrupt the metabolism of the surrounding neurons, or compromise the blood and oxygen supply to the neurons. Furthermore, the normal immune responses to infection (such as swelling and the formation of pus) can cause a buildup of pressure in the CNS, thereby further damaging the CNS.

Bacterial infections of the CNS are caused by the invasion of a microorganism that reproduces asexually. These organisms are often introduced through the bloodstream, and they affect the CNS in several negative ways. In addition to taking up resources such as oxygen, glucose, and space, some bacteria actually release toxins that kill surrounding nervous system tissue. Furthermore, the immune response to these infections can also have some harmful side effects.

Perhaps the best-known example of a bacterial infection of the CNS is **bacterial meningitis.** This potentially lethal condition involves an infection of the meninges. (For more on the meninges, look back to Chapter 2.) The symptoms of bacterial meningitis include the sudden onset of headache, high fever, and a stiff neck. Bacterial meningitis is typically treated with antibiotic medications.

The symptoms of bacterial meningitis are also observed in a variety of other, less severe disorders. One of these disorders is a less severe form of meningitis, called **viral meningitis.** A virus is an acellular, encapsulated entity composed of nucleic acids. This definition might not provide much help in picturing what a virus looks like or does, but perhaps describing some of the things that viri *don't do* would be helpful. Viri are not "alive" in the typical sense. They do not breathe, move, or grow. The most lifelike thing viri do is replicate, which they do with frightening efficiency. Using the synthetic machinery of the surrounding cells, viri make copy after copy of themselves.

Some viri appear to have a particularly high affinity for the cells of the nervous system. These viri are called **neurotropic.** When a virus invades the CNS, it is typically very difficult to treat. One cannot use medications such as antibiotics, because they are not effective against viri. In most instances, the infection must run its course, which can result in widespread lesions throughout the CNS. For example, the HIV/AIDS virus has very wide-ranging physiological and behavioral effects. Although some of these effects are due to the virus itself influencing the CNS, others are due to the disease's ability to compromise the immune system, thereby leaving the CNS vulnerable to infections that would normally be suppressed (Zillmer & Spiers, 2001).

Neurotoxins

Broadly defined, neurotoxins are substances that have the ability to destroy nervous system tissue. Chemically, neurotoxins can take many different forms, including organic solvents, pesticides, fuels, heavy metals, or other types of compounds. In most cases, the toxicity of a substance is dose-dependent. In sufficiently low doses, exposure to a substance (such as ethanol, the kind of alcohol that people most commonly drink) might not cause any permanent CNS damage. However, in larger doses, many substances become quite dangerous and possibly even fatal. The circumstances in which people expose their nervous system to neurotoxins are varied. Some people are injured at work, and some are injured during recreation. Some people are exposed during adventurous dining, and some people intentionally expose themselves.

Some of the most damaging neurotoxins are heavy metals, which include mercury (commonly found in items such as thermometers that people place in their mouths), lead (found in places you might not think of as metallic, such as older paints), and aluminum (commonly found in cookware). Perhaps the most famous (and fictional) account of mercury poisoning is provided in Lewis Carroll's *Alice's Adventures in Wonderland*. In the 1700s and 1800s, English hat makers used mercury to make hats. This practice was generally believed to poison the hatters, a generalization that was exemplified by the character of the Mad Hatter.

Lead poisoning also appears to have influenced many important historical events. For example, it now appears that some early explorers died in North America because their supplies were canned in vessels containing lead. One notable example is that of the Franklin expedition, which disappeared in 1845 with 129 men and two naval ships while searching for a northwest passage in the Canadian Arctic. Researchers have subsequently discovered many of the remains, and autopsies confirmed very high and likely toxic lead levels (Beattie & Geiger, 1987). In much of the developed world, current health standards have reduced much of our exposure to heavy metals. For example, lead is no longer used in paint, and unleaded gasoline has replaced the leaded variety, at least in Canada and the United States.

Other neurotoxins are ingested as part of a meal. One of the most famous examples of this happened in Prince Edward Island, Canada, in the summer of 1987 (Kolb & Whishaw, 1996). It was a particularly dry year, which resulted in a somewhat unusual diet for the mussels surrounding the island: They ate seaweed that grew inland, in relatively fresh water. Later that fall, many of these mussels were harvested and consumed. Many people became very ill after eating the mussels, and four people actually died. Postmortem examinations found temporal lobe damage. Other individuals who had become quite sick demonstrated symptoms that are typical of temporal lobe damage, such as memory impairments. On the basis of investigations of this group (and the mussels they ate), it is now believed that they ingested relatively high (in some cases lethal) doses of the neurotoxin **domoic acid.** This toxin, which is produced by seaweed, was ingested by the mussels and then passed along to the humans. (There are certainly risks associated with being high on the food chain!) Today, the seafood industry is much more mindful of this potential problem, and the domoic acid levels of shellfish are monitored much more closely.

the **Real** world

Signs of Stroke (or How to Tell a Subarachnoid Hemorrhage from a Migraine)

When I was a student in a neuropsychology class, another student asked the professor, "How can I tell if I am having a subarachnoid hemorrhage or just a migraine headache?" The professor replied, "If you wake up the next morning, it was just a migraine." The question was a good one, and there is no easy answer. If a person who is suffering from a subarachnoid hemorrhage (SAH) is seen by a physician while he or she is still conscious (which is often not the case—in many instances, people do not receive medical help for SAH until they have lost consciousness), the person will often complain of having the "worst headache of my life." However, any of us who have experienced headaches have also experienced "the worst headache of our lives," but few of us have suffered an SAH, making this diagnostic marker rather unhelpful. Another marker of SAH is nausea, including vomiting, which is also a common symptom of migraine. Unfortunately, this symptom has the tendency to send individuals to the washroom, a place where they can better cope with their nausea, but it is also a place where they are most often unattended. In fact, many of the individuals who die of SAH do so in the washroom, perhaps because they do not receive timely medical help. Other symptoms of SAH include disturbances in balance and consciousness. These symptoms make the brain vulnerable to other types of damage, such as a closed head injury from a fall. It is extremely difficult to diagnose some of these dangerous conditions on the basis of the behavioral symptoms alone. Neuroimaging is the most reliable diagnostic tool.

There are also numerous suspected neurotoxins that we encounter in our environment. These include exposure to low levels of pesticides. It should come as no surprise to you that pesticides can be harmful to one's nervous system. After all, what is the function of a pesticide? They are designed or chosen because of their capacity to kill certain organisms. There is mounting evidence that human exposure to pesticides, particularly repeated exposure, has impacts on the structural and functional integrity of the nervous system. Individuals with high or regular exposure to pesticides display difficulties with concentration, memory, language, and motor functions (Banich, 1997; Bosma, vax-Boxtel, Ponds, Houx, & Jolles, 2000; Overstreet, 2000, Stephens et al., 1995). It is still unknown what lower exposure levels do to CNS function.

In response to public concerns, many urban centers in North America are starting to restrict the use of pesticides. Some municipalities have even completely banned their use for noncommercial applications. However, this is not without problems. For instance, the West Nile virus, which is transmitted by mosquitoes, has spread rapidly throughout much of North America. Communities are therefore faced with a difficult decision: Spray pesticides to kill mosquitoes but risk exposing vulnerable people (often the same people who are vulnerable to West Nile, such as the elderly and the very young) to pesticides.

MODULE **14.2**
Neurological and Psychiatric Diseases

Until now, the chapters in this book have dealt with very typical neuropsychological topics. However, a large number of neurological and psychiatric diseases result from alterations in brain and/or brain chemistry. Neurological and psychiatric diseases can severely disrupt behavior, typically reflecting disruption of the nervous system. Furthermore, these diseases affect large numbers of people. For instance, neurological diseases such as epilepsy affect approximately 1.4 million Americans (Center for Disease Control, 1996), and psychiatric diseases such as schizophrenia are even more common. Both types of illness have significant impact on the costs of medical care. In the United States, schizophrenia alone affects approximately 2.2 million adults (Regier, Narrow, Rae, Manderschied, Locke, & Goodwin, 1993), and accounts for about 30% of all inpatient admissions, the equivalent of approximately 400,000 hospitalized individuals (Andreasen, 2000). It is therefore becoming increasingly important to understand the neural bases of these diseases and to examine the impact that these diseases have on cognitive function.

The focus of this module is to examine a number of diseases that have not been discussed in detail in other chapters. These diseases include the epilepsies, multiple sclerosis, amyotrophic lateral sclerosis, and schizophrenia. Primarily, this module will discuss what is known about how the brain is involved in these disorders and will describe the relevant behavioral features of these disorders. Also included in this module will be a discussion of what is currently unknown about the nature of the disorders and a brief synopsis of the types of problems that can occur in assessing individuals with these disorders.

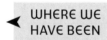

The preceding module described some of the many ways in which the CNS can suffer damage, including the formation of tumors, vascular disorders, introduction of toxins, and blows to the head.

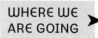

This module will discuss a number of neurological and psychiatric diseases and the types of neuropsychological effects that they have. The diseases that will be discussed include epilepsy, multiple sclerosis, amyotrophic lateral sclerosis, and schizophrenia. The discussions will feature a summary of the effects that these diseases have on the nervous system and the effects that these diseases have on neuropsychological function. Finally, this module will discuss a number of the issues surrounding these diseases.

The Epilepsies

Epilepsy is a disorder that is characterized by spontaneous, unpredictable, recurrent seizures. The hallmark diagnosis is two or more unprovoked seizures that are confirmed by electroencephalography (EEG). Epilepsy is often described in terms of two interrelated concepts: convulsions and seizures. Seizures describe the characteristic electrical activity of the brain that is associated with epilepsy (measured by EEG), whereas convulsions describe the behavioral manifestations of seizures (e.g., jerking of limbs). It is possible to have a seizure without a convulsion, but all convulsions have accompanying seizure activity. There are many types of epileptic seizures, and the frequency and form of seizures are quite variable. It is therefore thought to be more correct to refer to this disorder as the **epilepsies.** The epilepsies are among the oldest known neurological diseases and affect up to 5% of the population of the world. (Approximately 50,000,000 people per year are treated for epilepsy throughout the world.)

Epilepsy is thought to occur as a result of the brain's producing excessive excitatory neural activity, resulting in seizures and/or convulsions. The behavioral consequences of seizures can be quite limited (no noticeable change in behavior), minimal (small alterations in attention, similar to daydreaming), or severe (loss of consciousness). Seizures are usually described as either partial or generalized. **Partial seizures** are seizures in which the abnormal EEG activity is limited to one area of the brain. Partial seizures may or may not be accompanied by convulsions. **Partial-complex seizures,** sometimes referred to as *temporal lobe epilepsy,* are associated with involuntary complicated motor acts and impairments of consciousness during convulsions. **Generalized seizures** are known as *grand mal convulsions* and involve the whole brain in seizure activity. Typically, the generalized convulsion is two-phased: the **tonic phase,** which involves the loss of consciousness and falling with body rigidity, and the **clonic phase,** during which the body extremities jerk and twitch. When generalized seizures are prolonged and the individual does not regain consciousness, then the seizure is referred to as **status epilepticus.** Status epilepticus can result in brain damage and/or death if not treated.

Often, people with epilepsy will notice that their seizures can be triggered by certain events or stimuli. Although these stimuli vary from person to person, common triggers are flashing lights, sleep deprivation, stress, and certain types of drugs or foods. **Catamenial epilepsy** is a type of epilepsy that occurs only in women; the trigger is the changing hormone levels that occur across the menstrual cycle. Once individuals know their triggers, they tend to avoid these situations or stimuli.

Many people who have epilepsy may have experienced some type of traumatic incident (e.g., fever, head injury) before the development of epilepsy (Annegers & Coan, 2000). The severity of the traumatic event appears to be related to the probability of developing epilepsy, with a greater number of people with severe trauma to the brain developing epilepsy than those with milder brain injuries (Annegers & Coan, 2000; Asikainen, Kaste, & Sarna, 1999). Moreover, repeated episodes of seizure activity can result in brain damage. For instance, hippocampal degeneration and abnormal hippocampal organization are often observed in people who have partial-complex epilepsy. Although epilepsy can result from these kinds of brain injuries, much of the time the cause is **idiopathic,** or unknown.

Treatments for epilepsy aim to prevent or suppress seizures though the use of antiepileptic drugs. Most of the commonly used antiepileptic drugs enhance GABAergic neurotransmission (recall from Chapter 2 that GABA is an inhibitory neurotransmitter), suggesting that there may be some alteration in the brain's ability to inhibit neural activity. Conversely, drugs that enhance glutamatergic activity (an excitatory neurotransmitter) result in seizures. Thus, epilepsy may result from an imbalance between excitatory and inhibitory neural systems in the brain, which is somehow altered in individuals with epilepsy.

Unfortunately, drug treatment is not always successful (recall the case of H.M.), and sometimes surgery must be performed. Surgery is recommended only when the origin of the seizures is clear. That is, if the **focus** of the seizures is well localized, then a neurosurgeon may opt to remove that source of the seizure activity, especially if this area appears to be involved in spreading seizure activity to other areas of the brain. It is common for either the temporal or frontal lobes to be the source of focal epileptic activity. Thus, neurosurgeons who are going to remove the focus must carefully assess the potential for memory, linguistic, and motor impairments that may result from the surgery designed to treat the epilepsy.

Epilepsy can result in cognitive impairments, resulting from either the seizure activity itself (e.g., brain damage resulting from status epilepticus), the reason(s) underlying the seizures (e.g., tumors), or the associated changes in the brain as a result of epilepsy. Typically, the type of cognitive impairment is related to where the seizure activity originated. For instance, individuals with partial-complex epilepsy often display deficits in language, learning, and memory, presumably reflecting changes in the temporal lobes (Seidman, Stone, Jones, Harrison, & Mirsky, 1998). It is thought that the degree of cognitive impairment is related to the location of the seizures, the age of onset, and handedness. Specifically, left-handedness, frontal foci, and early onset epilepsy are associated with significantly greater cognitive impairments (Strauss et al., 1995). These cognitive impairments can be observed when the person is not experiencing seizure activity, suggesting that there may be significant changes in the brain beyond the ability to produce seizures.

Multiple Sclerosis and Amyotrophic Lateral Sclerosis

MULTIPLE SCLEROSIS. Multiple sclerosis (MS) is characterized by multiple areas of demyelination in the nervous system. This absence of myelin results in neurons that are no longer able to communicate effectively. (Recall from Chapter 2 that myelin insulates axons, allowing quick and accurate propagation of action potentials.) Demyelination can occur anywhere in the nervous system, and the symptoms of MS typically depend on the location of demyelination. For instance, demyelination in the descending motor systems may result in difficulty in motor movements, whereas demyelination in the optic nerve may result in blindness. Symptoms of MS tend to first appear in people between the ages of 20 and 40, and MS affects approximately 60 in 100,000 individuals. Although MS tends to be a progressive disease, it can go into remission for years. Because of its unpredictability and symptoms, MS is an extremely stressful condition.

The cause of MS is unknown, although there are a few clues that provide some insights into MS. First, MS appears to be a disease associated with cold climates; there is twice the incidence of MS in areas above the thirty-seventh parallel as below it. Furthermore, MS seems to occur in certain locations more often than others, suggesting some type of environmental trigger. It may be that the environmental trigger is a pathogen or virus. There also seems to be a genetic component in some people. Some researchers suggest that the genetic component is an inherited vulnerability to an environmental agent, rather than simply the disease itself being inherited. However, in all cases, it appears that the disease process involves an autoimmune response to the central nervous system. In individuals with MS, the immune cells of the body become sensitized to myelin and begin to attack it (in much the way that they attack infected tissue).

MS has been thought of as a disease that typically produces no cognitive deficits. However, recent research has begun to question that assumption. Although some individuals with MS exhibit no cognitive deficits, many individuals with MS (45–65%) do exhibit cognitive decline similar to dementia, though much less severe (DeSousa, Albert, & Kalman, 2002). The features of the cognitive impairments vary among individuals and tend to be more severe when the disease is active than when it is in remission (DeSousa et al., 2002). DeSousa and colleagues (2002) report that there are deficits in attention, memory, and language, as well as the expected deficits in motor speed and dexterity. Interestingly, the memory deficits appear to be related to the retrieval of information rather than recognition (which is intact), suggesting that the memory problem has to do with locating the information rather than with storing it initially. Imaging studies have shown that the degree of cognitive impairment is related to the degree to which MS has attacked the brain. Additionally, individuals with MS often show frontal lobe atrophy, and it is suggested that this atrophy underlies cognitive impairments in memory and executive function (Benedict, Bakshi, Simon, Priore, Miller, & Munschauer, 2002). Because MS attacks myelin, it may be that there is some degree of disconnection between the frontal lobes and subcortical structures such as the thalamus, which may also contribute to the cognitive deficits that are observed.

AMYOTROPHIC LATERAL SCLEROSIS. Amyotrophic lateral sclerosis (ALS) is also known as *Lou Gehrig's disease* because the great baseball player Lou Gehrig died from this disease in 1941. However, Charcot first described ALS in 1874. ALS is characterized by degeneration of the upper and lower motor neurons, which control movement of the muscles. ALS is a progressive and terminal disease, typically resulting in death 1.5 to 3 years from the time of first diagnosis (Murphy & Ringel, 1990). Symptoms of ALS tends to appear first as weakness in the limbs, followed by involvement of the muscles of the trunk and face (including muscles for swallowing and speaking). Eventually, the muscles that are responsible for breathing are affected, and the individual must resort to mechanical ventilation or will die. The incidence of ALS is between two and eleven individuals per 100,000, and it tends to affect men more often than women.

The cause of ALS is unknown, although there are a number of proposed causes. Some cases of ALS appears to be familial, but familial ALS accounts for only about 2% of the cases of ALS, suggesting that there must be other contributing factors. There are hypotheses that ALS results from excessive release of the neurotransmitter glutamate, neuronal stress, abnormal accumulation of the protein in the cell, abnormal genes, apoptosis (programmed cell death), and/or exposure to environmental toxins. Rather than focusing on just one cause, some researchers are now suggesting that ALS may result from a combination of these factors. That is, as with MS, it may be that a genetic predisposition combined with the unknown environmental factors result in a series of events that lead to the progressive degeneration of motor neurons. There is no cure for ALS, and treatments tend to focus on relieving symptoms of the disease.

Neuropsychological Celebrity

Stephen Hawking

Stephen Hawking is the current Lucasian Professor at Cambridge University in the United Kingdom, a professorship that has been held by many prominent mathematicians and physicists, including Sir Isaac Newton. Professor Hawking studies cosmology; that is, he studies the scientific laws that govern the universe. His research suggests that the universe and time had a beginning (the Big Bang) and that they will have an end (black holes). His research on black holes has also enabled their existence to be demonstrated. So why is Professor Hawking featured here?

When he was 21, Professor Hawking was diagnosed with ALS (he is now 60). Professor Hawking has been unable to feed himself since 1975 and has been unable to speak without assistance since 1985. Despite this, he is married and has three children and a grandchild. In addition, although he is unable to write or speak without assistance, he continues to make major contributions to science. As he writes, "I have had motor neuron disease for practically all my adult life. Yet it has not prevented me from having a very attractive family, and being successful in my work" (Hawking, 2001). Professor Hawking certainly demonstrates that not all individuals with neurological disorders exhibit cognitive impairments—often despite severe physical limitations.

The pattern of degeneration and the rate with which ALS progresses differ among individuals. However, damage to the upper motor neurons, located in the motor cortex of the brain, typically results in muscle **spasticity** and stiffness, whereas damage to the lower motor neurons, in the brainstem and spinal cord, results in muscle weakness, uncontrollable twitching of the muscles, and atrophy. Because it appeared that ALS affected only motor neurons, ALS has been thought of as a disease that was not associated with cognitive deficits. However, as with MS, recent research has begun to question that assumption. For instance, there are reports that some individuals with ALS experience declines in executive function and memory (Abe, 2000; Abe, Fujimura, Toyooka, Sakoda, Yorifugi, & Yanagihara, 1997; Abrahams et al., 1996). In these studies, the degree of cognitive decline was associated with the degree of frontal lobe atrophy. Furthermore, because ALS affects the muscles of the mouth, it was thought that any impairments in linguistic ability were primarily motor. However, recent studies have demonstrated that there are also nonmotoric linguistic impairments that may relate to atrophy of the temporal lobes (Strong, Grace, Orange, & Leeper, 1996; Wilson, Grace, Munoz, He, & Strong, 2001).

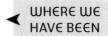 **WHERE WE HAVE BEEN** We have discussed the symptoms and neuropsychological effects of epilepsy, MS, and ALS. Research in this area suggests that the severity and type of cognitive impairment that occur with these diseases are often related to the extent and location of brain damage. Unfortunately, in the majority of individuals, the causes of these diseases and their cures are unknown.

WHERE WE ARE GOING The rest of this module will discuss schizophrenia and its effect on cognition. Although schizophrenia is commonly referred to as a psychiatric disease, as we will see, schizophrenia has significant effects on the brain and thus is not fundamentally different from the neurological diseases featured earlier in this module.

Schizophrenia

Schizophrenia is a diagnostic term that refers to a heterogeneous disorder that is not easily defined. As you no doubt know, schizophrenia does not involve having multiple personalities. Rather, the symptoms that occur in schizophrenia are classified as either positive or negative. **Positive symptoms** are behaviors that are present in the individual but should not be (e.g., hallucinations). Positive symptoms in schizophrenia include hallucinations (e.g., hearing voices or seeing things that are not present); delusions or patently unrealistic beliefs (e.g., that someone is controlling one's thoughts); disorganized speech (e.g., rapid switching of topics in speech, rambling or incoherent speech, also known as *word salad*); and grossly disorganized or bizarre behaviors (e.g., rapid and repetitive motor movements that appear to have no purpose). **Negative symptoms** are behaviors that are *not* present that should be (e.g., engaging in social interactions with others). Negative symptoms in schizophrenia include flattening of affect, social withdrawal, reduced speech, and reduced motivation. Many individuals exhibit both positive and negative symptoms, and their symptomatology may change over the course of their disease.

It is important to keep in mind that schizophrenia has no hallmark symptom; rather, diagnosis of schizophrenia is made by assessing the prevalence and duration of symptoms. In fact the DSM-IV (a diagnostic manual for categorizing type and presence of psychiatric or psychological disease) suggests that it is entirely possible that one individual who has been diagnosed with schizophrenia may present a completely different set of symptoms than another individual who has been diagnosed with schizophrenia (American Psychological Association, 1994). Because there is no single symptom that distinguishes schizophrenia from related disorders, some researchers suggest that schizophrenia must represent a group of disorders rather than a single disease.

The cause of schizophrenia is currently unknown, although there are many interesting hypotheses, including genetic factors, abnormal dopamine neurotransmission, maternal stress, and seasonal effects (for a review, see Andreasen, 1999). There are, however, a series of brain and behavioral abnormalities that are associated with schizophrenia. Again, as with everything to do with schizophrenia, we must keep in mind that these abnormalities do not occur in everyone with schizophrenia.

COGNITIVE FUNCTION IN PEOPLE WITH SCHIZOPHRENIA. In a review of over thirty-seven studies, Green and colleagues (Green, Kern, Braff, & Mintz, 2000) observed that there are consistent cognitive deficits that accompany schizophrenia. These deficits are observed in long-term memory (memory lasting more than a few minutes), working memory, vigilance (ability to maintain attention), and executive functioning (ability to plan actions and to monitor their success). In addition, some researchers have observed that people with schizophrenia have difficulty sequencing complex motor acts (similar to that of apraxics) and that they have difficulty integrating sensory information (Arango, Kirkpatrick, & Buchanan, 2000).

There are some who question these results. For example, although most people with schizophrenia exhibit these cognitive deficits, nearly 25% of people with schizophrenia appear to be within normal limits. However, others suggest that these "non-impaired" people with schizophrenia are actually impaired if you consider their level of functioning before the onset of their disease (Kremen, Seidman, Faraone, Toomey, & Tsuang, 2000; Kremen, Seidman, Faraone, & Tsuang, 2001).

Another common criticism of the research in this area is the testing of long-term chronically medicated people with schizophrenia, who may experience altered cognitive function, not as a consequence of their disease but because of their medication (e.g., Bilder et al., 2000). However, a large study of first-episode people with schizophrenia also observed significant cognitive impairments in both working memory and longer-term memory, executive function, motor skills, and ability to sustain attention during the testing session. Bilder and colleagues (2000) also found that the degree of cognitive impairment was related to the severity of the schizophrenic episode, suggesting that some of the failures to observe cognitive deficits in people with schizophrenia may be related to the relatively benign form of schizophrenia that these individuals exhibited.

GROSS STRUCTURAL ABNORMALITIES. It appears that a large subset of people with schizophrenia have enlarged lateral ventricles and/or cortical atrophy (Andreasen, 2000). Enlarged lateral ventricles and cortical atrophy are hallmarks of neural degeneration, which may result in some of the observed behavioral changes. Nonetheless, it is not clear whether these gross structural abnormalities are the cause of the disease or are caused by the disease! Some researchers have concluded that it is unlikely that a single gross change in brain structure could result in the wide array of symptoms that are associated with schizophrenia. Rather, these researchers point out that there are subtle changes in size of a variety of structures, including the hippocampus, thalamus, basal ganglia, cortex, and brainstem (Bogerts, 1993). The variability and extent of these changes may be more consistent with the variable pattern of symptoms associated with schizophrenia.

MICROSTRUCTURAL ABNORMALITIES. Rather than focusing on the gross structure of the brain, some researchers have chosen to focus on the microscopic investigation of the brains of people with schizophrenia (donated after they have died). These investigations often reveal abnormal organization of the neurons within the medial temporal lobe, including the neurons that make up the hippocampus (Altshuler, Conrad, Kovelman, & Scheibel, 1987; Jones, 2001) and the neurons within the frontal lobe (Jones, 2001). Others have found that there are developmental migrational problems with the organization of the cortex (Akil & Lewis, 1997; Beall & Lewis, 1992), with failure of cells to properly segregate within their appropriate layers of the cortex. Both the organizational and migrational observations suggest that schizophrenia may be a developmental problem as well as a degenerative one (as suggested by the cortical atrophy and ventricular enlargement observations).

FUNCTIONAL IMAGING. As we discussed in Chapter 3, functional imaging allows researchers to observe activity within the brain while an individual is engaged in a task.

Controversy

The Pros and Cons of Animal Research

Nonhuman animals are frequently the research subjects in a variety of areas, particularly the life sciences. Often, debate in this area concerns whether or not nonhuman animals can and should be used to understand human systems.

Nonhuman animals are often used for research in situations that cannot be ethically examined in humans (e.g., inducing brain lesions to examine the behavioral consequences). In fact, many of the advances in the life sciences in the last fifty years have resulted from research studying nonhuman animals. In psychology, treatment procedures such as aversion therapy, flooding, token economies, extinction therapies, desensitization, and time-out procedures were developed from the research performed by Hull, Pavlov, Skinner, and Thorndike, who studied nonhuman animals. In neuropsychology, much of what is known about the teratological and behavioral effects of drugs such as alcohol was first learned from studies on nonhuman animals. Much of what we know about the diseases that are featured in this module (and how to treat them) is based primarily on initial research with nonhuman animals.

Critiques of nonhuman animal research are varied, ranging from moral objections to claims about scientific limitations. One limitation that must be recognized is that although there are many similarities among mammalian species, there are also important differences. One obvious difference between humans and most other mammals is the complexity of the central nervous system. There are other, more subtle differences among species of mammals. For instance, humans who ingest the neurotoxin MPTP develop a permanent syndrome resembling Parkinson's disease. However, when rats ingest MPTP, the results are quite strikingly different: The rats eventually recover from the frozen state. These results suggest that there are important differences between rats and humans, especially in the basal ganglia, as revealed by the recovery of rats from MPTP neurotoxicity. Thus, although comparisons between human and nonhuman animals can be informative, care needs to be taken to ensure that differences are not minimized.

In this module, we have discussed four debilitating diseases for which we know very little about the cause or the cure. This is the case for most of the research discussed in this book; many of the people who are featured in this book are present because we cannot cure their deficits. Although this text is about what we do know about the brain, it should be apparent that there is much that we don't know. For instance, subtle questions such as how pharmacological treatments of depression work or what the mechanisms are that underlie how the print that you are reading right now is transformed into language within the brain are also currently unanswered. Given the large number of questions that still abound within the field of psychology and neuroscience, it seems reasonable to suggest that the nonhuman animal will continue to play a large part in understanding the nervous system.

Self-Test

1. What is the difference between partial-complex seizures and generalized seizures?

2. What are the causes of multiple sclerosis (MS) and amyotrophic lateral sclerosis (ALS)?

3. What types of symptoms are present in schizophrenia? Give two examples of each type of symptom.

4. What is the evidence that suggests that the epilepsies, schizophrenia, MS, and ALS result in cognitive change?

A number of functional imaging studies have observed abnormally low levels of activity in the frontal lobes, especially the prefrontal areas. Given the association between prefrontal areas and working memory, perhaps the known difficulties in working memory in people with schizophrenia are associated with disturbances in prefrontal processing (Beall & Lewis, 1992; Goldman-Rakic, 1999). A number of studies have also indicated that there may be an overproduction of dopamine receptors in the basal ganglia of people with schizophrenia and that there may be abnormal dopaminergic neurotransmission in the brains of people with schizophrenia (Laruelle & Abi-Dargham, 1999).

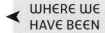

WHERE WE HAVE BEEN   There are many different potential causes of brain damage, and depending on demographic and genetic variables, one's risk for acquiring brain damage varies across the life span. Young children are much more likely to suffer TBI as the result of a fall, whereas older adolescents and young adults are more likely to suffer TBI as the result of a motor vehicle accident or violent episode. Later in life, neurological disorders such as the formation of tumors and cerebrovascular disorders affect more and more people. Throughout the life span, one's CNS is vulnerable to the effects of neurotoxins. Similarly, the likelihood of being affected by some neurological diseases varies throughout the life span and depending on one's genetics. Younger people (particularly males) have higher incidences of conditions such as epilepsy and schizophrenia, whereas older people have a higher risk of developing other neurodegenerative disorders. In all of these cases, clinical neuropsychologists can play a central role in evaluating the cognitive changes following these events, and they can also help to develop management and rehabilitation plans following brain injuries. These roles are the subject of Chapter 15.

Glossary

Amyotrophic lateral sclerosis (Lou Gehrig's disease)—A progressive neurodegenerative disease that is characterized by degeneration of the upper and lower motor neurons.

Aneurysm—Areas of veins or arteries that dilate because of local weaknesses, resulting in a balloonlike expansion.

Arteriovenus malformation (AVM)—Malformed arteries and vessels that have extra or missing connections, resulting in abnormal blood flow, which tend to form along the middle cerebral artery.

Astrocytomas—Slow-growing benign tumors that arise from the growth of astrocytes.

Atherosclerosis—A condition that occurs when fatty deposits build up inside the walls of blood vessels, which can constrict or completely block the blood vessel.

Bacterial meningitis—A potentially fatal bacterial infection of the central nervous system; symptoms include sudden onset of headache, high fever, and a stiff neck.

Benign—A type of tumor that is not likely to recur and has a good prognosis associated with it.

Bifurcation—The process of splitting in two.

Catamenial epilepsy—A form of epilepsy that occurs only in women and the trigger is the changing hormone levels that occur across the menstrual cycle.

Cerebral ischemia—A lack of blood supply to the brain.

Cerebrovascular accident (CVA)—A class of cerebrovascular disorders, all of which result in interruptions to the brain's blood supply.

Cerebrovascular disorder (stroke)—An interruption to the blood supply to the brain; often referred to as a *stroke*.

Clonic phase—The component of a generalized seizure that involves jerking of the body's extremities due to the contraction and relaxation of muscles.

Closed head injury—Occurs when an individual receives a blow to the head but the blow does not penetrate the skull and meninges.

Congenital—Present at birth.

Contre-coup—An injury to the brain that is opposite to the point of impact to the head.

Coup—An injury to the brain at the point of impact to the head.

Domoic acid—A neurotoxin that is found in marine algae and can be consumed by eating mussels (or other shellfish) that have eaten the algae.

Embolism—A clot, bubble, or piece of fat that moves along the length of a vein or artery, blocking the flow of blood.

Encapsulated—A term for a tumor that has clear borders.

Epilepsies—A neurological condition that is characterized by seizures and convulsions.

Focus—An isolated point of origin for a seizure.

Fossae—Bony protrusions from the skull.

Generalized seizures (grand mal convulsions)—Seizures that involve the whole brain in seizure activity.

Glioblastoma—A quick-growing malignant tumor.

Gliomas—Tumors that come from glial cells.

Hemorrhage—To bleed profusely.

Hypertension—Abnormally high blood pressure.

Idiopathic—Of unknown origin.

Infarct—An area of damage resulting from a CVA.

Infiltrate—A term for a tumor that moves into neural tissue with no clear boundaries.

Intracerebral hemorrhage—A hemorrhage that occurs within the brain.

Malignant—A type of tumor that is likely to recur and/or has a poor prognosis.

Medulloblastoma (primitive neuroectodermal tumor)—A rare but malignant infiltrating tumor that tends to occur in the cerebellum and brainstem early in life.

Meningiomas—An encapsulated tumor that grows out of (and remains attached to) the meninges.

Metastatic tumors (metastases)—Secondary tumors that form from migrated tumor tissue, typically originating in the lungs, breasts, uterus, or kidneys.

Multiple metastatic tumors—Metastatic tumors that spread and involve multiple sites and multiple tumors.

Multiple sclerosis—A neurodegenerative disease that is characterized by multiple areas of demyelination in the nervous system.

Negative symptoms—Symptoms of schizophrenia that are not present but should be (e.g., flattening of affect, social withdrawal).

Neurotropic—Having a particularly high affinity for the cells of the nervous system.

Open head (or penetrating) injury—Occurs when an object such as a bullet or a knife breaches the skull and meninges.

Partial-complex seizures (temporal lobe epilepsy)—Seizures that are associated with involuntary complicated motor acts and impairments of consciousness during convulsions.

Partial seizures—Seizures in which the abnormal EEG activity is limited to one area of the brain and which are not always accompanied by convulsions.

Positive symptoms—Symptoms of schizophrenia that are present in the individual but should not be (e.g., hallucinations).

Schizophrenia—A heterogeneous disorder that is characterized by bizarre behavior, distorted or disorganized thinking, and alterations of mood and thought processes.

Simple metastatic tumors—Rare cases in which metastasis involves only one tumor at a site.

Space-occupying lesions—Tissue that occupies space in the central nervous system, causing damage by putting pressure on the central nervous system.

Spasticity—Abnormal tightness or stiffness of a muscle.

Status epilepticus—A prolonged generalized seizure in which the individual is unconscious; can result in brain damage and/or death if not treated.

Subarachnoid hemorrhage—A hemorrhage into the subarachnoid space (between the pia mater and arachnoid layer of the meninges).

Thrombosis—A blood clot that remains at the point at which it was formed.

Tonic phase—The component of a generalized seizure that involves the loss of consciousness and falling with body rigidity.

Traumatic brain injury—An assault on the brain that causes injury ranging from mild to severe. The two main types of injury are "open head," caused by penetration of the brain, and "closed head."

Tumor (neoplasm)—A mass of new and abnormal tissue.

Viral meningitis—A viral infection of the central nervous system.

15 Neuropsychological Assessment

The only man who behaved sensibly was my tailor; he took my measurement anew every time he saw me, while all the rest went on with their old measurements and expected them to fit me.

—GEORGE BERNARD SHAW

MODULE **15.1**
Participants in a Neuropsychological Assessment

The goals of neuropsychological assessment have changed dramatically over the past fifty years. Before the advent of the neuroimaging techniques, neuropsychological assessment was concerned primarily with determining whether brain damage was present (sometimes called *organicity*). If there was evidence of damage, the neuropsychologist spent many hours of behavioral testing in an attempt to localize it. Now CT or MRI scanners have replaced those hours of behavioral testing, quickly locating the extent of damage, even in unconscious individuals.

Does this mean that clinical neuropsychologists are now obsolete? Certainly not! In response to technological advances, the nature and goals of neuropsychological assessments have changed dramatically. Clinical neuropsychologists now seek to diagnose conditions that are not readily detectable by using neuroimaging (e.g., early detection of Alzheimer's disease), to assess quality of life and to evaluate the client's capacity to succeed in his or her present environment (e.g., assessing whether the person will be able to return to work, whether the person should move from his or her own home to a managed care facility). Most recently, clinical neuropsychologists have become more involved in rehabilitation following brain injury.

WHERE WE ARE GOING ➤ The sections that follow detail the participants in neuropsychological assessment (the client, the neurologist, the radiologist, and the neuropsychologist) and the assessment tools that the neuropsychologist uses. This chapter is not meant to provide students with the tools necessary to perform neuropsychological assessments. Instead, this chapter details the goals and guiding principles of the assessment.

The Client

If you do a literature search for articles describing the results of a psychological assessment, you will notice that a variety of terms are used to describe the person being assessed. The person can be referred to as a *patient, subject, participant,* or *client.* If a physician writes the article or it is written from a medical perspective, the person is generally referred to as a *patient* (regardless of whether he or she is hospitalized at the time of assessment). Most research articles refer to the assessed individual as a *subject* (mostly in articles written before 1994) or as a *participant* (mostly in articles written after 1994). However, clinical neuropsychologists normally refer to the people they assess as their **clients.** Just as patients are regarded as consumers of medical services, clients are consumers of psychological services (such as assessment and treatment).

There is no "typical" neuropsychological client. As you learned in the previous chapters, nervous system damage (and the corresponding behavioral change) can have a wide variety of causes. Furthermore, people of all ages are vulnerable to nervous system damage. In younger people, nervous system damage often results from brain injuries acquired from events such as motor vehicle accidents or falls (Kraus et al., 1984). Some elderly people also suffer traumatic head injury, frequently as the result of a fall. This is particularly true in adults aged 65 to 70 years old (Goldstein, Levin,

Boake, & Lohrey, 1990). However, the nervous system damage suffered by older people is often the result of disease (e.g., dementia, the growth of a tumor, or a cerebrovascular accident). In the age group in between the very young and the very old, accidents involving motor vehicles account for most traumatic head injuries (Lezak, 1995).

Thus, the events that bring the client into contact with a clinical neuropsychologist can vary tremendously. Similarly, the settings in which clients are assessed and the goals of the assessments are variable. Medical personnel or family members might refer clients, the assessment might be prescribed by a court or insurance agency, or the client might voluntarily present himself or herself for assessment. Within a hospital setting, the referral to a neuropsychologist often comes from a neurologist.

The Neurologist

Neurology is the medical specialty that diagnoses, studies, and treats disorders of the CNS. Therefore, a **neurologist** is a special type of physician who diagnoses and treats disorders of the nervous system. This includes disorders of the CNS (brain and spinal cord) and PNS (nerves extending throughout the rest of the body). These disorders can be of unknown etiology or caused by trauma, infection, tumors, toxins, or metabolic disorders. Neurologists' education typically consists of two to four years of premedical university training, four years of medical school resulting in an M.D. (doctor of medicine) or D.O. (doctor of osteopathy) degree, and three years (or more) of specialty training in a neurology residency program.

Neurologists are trained to perform a detailed examination of the neurological structures throughout the body. Most of these examinations involve the testing of relatively basic sensory and motor functions, but in some cases, the neurologist also completes some testing of cognitive abilities. (We will discuss this type of testing in the next module.) Neurologists can also administer a lumbar puncture (spinal tap) to obtain cerebrospinal fluid for further testing. Acting in a consulting role, neurologists might help to diagnose and treat a neurological disorder while advising the primary care physician on the person's treatment. Although neurologists might recommend surgical treatment, they do not typically perform surgeries. Instead, when surgery is necessary, it is typically performed by a **neurosurgeon,** and the neurologist helps to monitor the surgically treated individuals.

The Radiologist

As you learned in Chapter 3, radiology was made possible because of a serendipitous discovery made by a physicist, Wilhelm Conrad Röntgen (1845–1923). While studying cathode rays, he noticed a glowing fluorescent screen on a nearby table. He quickly deduced that rays coming from his partially evacuated glass Hittorf-Crookes tube were causing the fluorescence, but these rays had a most unusual property: They penetrated the thick black paper that was wrapped around the tube. Subsequent experiments demonstrated that these **X-rays,** as he called them, could also penetrate other solid materials, including wood, metal, and human tissue. Röntgen was rewarded for his discovery with the first Nobel Prize in Physics in 1901.

Modern **radiologists** are a relatively rare group of physicians; according to the American Medical Association, only 1.2% of U.S. physicians specialize in radiology. Radiologists have specialized training in obtaining and interpreting images of the human body and/or treating conditions using radiological science. As is the case with neurologists, radiologists complete premedical training, medical training, and a residency in their speciality. Although in the early days of radiology, most radiology was accomplished by using X-rays, there are now a variety of ways of imaging the human body. Radiologists do not rely only on X-rays. For instance, individuals with head injuries often undergo a radiological examination (such as a CT scan or MRI), which is performed by a specially trained technologist. The scans are then reviewed and interpreted by the radiologist, who writes a report detailing the findings for the primary care physician or neurologist.

The Clinical Neuropsychologist

Clinical neuropsychology is "the branch of neuropsychology concerned with psychological assessment, management, and rehabilitation of neurological disease and injury" (Beaumont, 1996, p. 525). This includes explaining how patterns of behavioral impairments can be explained in terms of disruptions to the damaged neural components. This is qualitatively different from **experimental neuropsychology,** which focuses on how human behavior arises from brain activity. In contrast, **cognitive neuropsychology** is typically regarded as being less focused on the neural basis of the behavior and more focused on explaining behavior (and disruptions in behavior) in terms of functional brain units, regardless of their anatomical representation.

Therefore, the **clinical neuropsychologist** is a scientist-practitioner who seeks to assess, manage, and rehabilitate individuals who are suffering from neurological disorders, regardless of the cause. Unlike neurologists or radiologists, clinical neuropsychologists usually do not have medical training. Instead, they typically complete an undergraduate degree (B.A. or B.Sc.) in psychology (taking three to four years), a master's degree (M.A., M.Sc., or M.A.Sc.) in clinical psychology (taking one to three years), and by a doctorate degree (Ph.D. or Psy.D.) in clinical psychology (taking another two to six years). In addition to this training, clinical neuropsychologists typically complete internship programs in which they practice clinical skills under the supervision of one or more certified clinicians. There is considerable variability in the amount of time it takes to train to be a neuropsychologist, depending on where the training takes place. For example, some programs do not require the completion of a master's degree before completing doctoral training.

Self-Test

1. What type of training do neurologists typically have? Under what conditions does a person typically see a neurologist?

2. What type of training do radiologists typically have? Under what conditions does a person typically see a radiologist?

3. What is the difference between experimental neuropsychology and cognitive neuropsychology?

4. What is a clinical neuropsychologist?

5. When a neuropsychological assessment is requested, who typically makes the request?

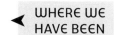 ◄ **WHERE WE HAVE BEEN**

The preceding module focused on the individuals that participate in a neuropsychological assessment. The role and functions of the physician, neurologist, and neuropsychologist were discussed.

We will now focus on the assessment itself. We will begin with a description of types of events that occur during a neuropsychological assessment and the goals of a neuropsychological assessment. Also provided are brief descriptions of some typical tests that are given during a neuropsychological assessment. Finally, we will discuss some of the important issues related to assessment.

Just as it is difficult to provide an account of a typical client in a neuropsychological assessment, it is difficult to describe the typical series of events that lead to the assessment because of the tremendous variability in the process. The health care professional who first assesses an individual with a neurological disorder is sometimes not a neurologist or even a physician. For example, after suffering a minor stroke to the left posterior parietal lobe, a person might start to have difficulties in reading and writing. It is not uncommon for the person to first book an appointment with an optometrist, claiming that his or her vision has started to deteriorate. Furthermore, even when people seek medical help for a condition that is caused by focal brain damage, the symptoms they describe can be secondary to the primary deficits. For example, an individual with a small right parietal lesion may start exhibiting hemispatial neglect of the left half of space (discussed in detail in Chapter 10) but may be unaware of their deficit (called a **lack of insight**). Because of the hemispatial neglect, the individual may collide with objects located in his or her left hemifield (such as a coffee table or other piece of furniture), bruising muscles or even breaking bones on the left side. After acquiring such an injury, the person may seek help from a physician, claiming that there is something wrong with his or her arm or leg. The secondary deficit is quite real and the complaint is legitimate, but the physician must be careful when performing examinations to seek the underlying cause.

Ideally, after suffering a brain injury, an individual promptly receives medical treatment by a general physician or emergency room attendant; this treatment is followed up by a neurological examination (including some sort of brain imaging). The brain imaging results are interpreted by a radiologist, who consults with a neurologist, after which the individual undergoes more thorough behavioral testing from a clinical neuropsychologist. The following sections detail many of the characteristics of the "ideal" series of events leading to a neuropsychological assessment. It is important to remember that in a perfect world, no one would ever need such an assessment. Furthermore, when such an assessment is necessary, the events that lead to it are frequently much more circuitous than those described next.

MODULE **15.2**
The Assessment

Many people have their first neurological exam in the emergency room. The initial exam may take the form of a series of questions and tests performed by a neurologist or emergency room physician. In its most basic form, the neurological exam is concerned with the reflexes, cranial nerve functioning, and the person's medical history. The physician also examines the person's muscle tone, ability to make gross movements, and to perceive stimuli. Depending on the severity of the symptoms, imaging (CT, MRI) of the nervous system may be ordered. Often, a neurological exam includes a test known as the Mini Mental State Exam (Folstein et al., 1975) or the Modified Mini Mental State Exam (Teng & Chui, 1987). Both tests look at how well people can answer a series of questions that are designed to briefly examine cognitive functions such as language (listening to the person speak as the person is telling you his or her medical history), orientation to location ("Do you know where you are?"), attention ("Can you count from 100 backwards by threes?"), mental status ("Do you know what day it is?"), and so on.

Although this brief exam is not as detailed as a full neuropsychological exam, it provides important insights into the person's functioning. Perhaps more important, physicians can perform these tests quickly, gaining a gross appreciation of the degree to which nervous system functions are impaired. Although this is a generalization, a preliminary neurology exam is intended primarily for determining the degree to which any nervous system injury (or disease) affects basic neurological functions. This is not to suggest that basic neurological functions are somehow less important than higher neurological functions. After all, the ability to use language (a higher cognitive function) could certainly be impaired by a more basic neurological function (such as the ability to maintain consciousness). As we mentioned above, depending on the severity of the injury, the person may then be referred to a neuropsychologist for further tests.

Alternatively, people with dementing illnesses or nontraumatic neurological impairment may first seek help from the family physician. The primary care physician may then perform basic tests of neurological function. Depending on the outcome of these tests and the severity of the symptoms, a referral to a neurologist may occur. Again, depending on the neurologist and the diagnosis, the person may then be referred to a neuropsychologist. For instance, some type of epilepsy may be responsible for the cognitive deficits, and the neurologist might determine that when this primary condition is treated with medication, there is no need for further assessment. Alternatively, the neurologist may suspect some type of progressive syndrome and may want to have the current level of cognitive functioning documented for future comparison.

Neuropsychological Assessment

Neuropsychological testing today is the detailed examination of cognitive functions. Briefly, a neuropsychological consultation consists of personal interview and the performance of a series of tests. The personal interview confirms the person's medical history and involves acquiring the person's description of any problems or highlighting any concerns the person might have about his or her cognitive functioning or the upcoming tests.

Neuropsychologists typically use a series of standardized cognitive tests. These tests are standardized in two ways: They are always administered to participants in the same way, and they are always scored in the same manner. Theoretically, if a person were to be given the same test by two different neuropsychologists, the person should receive the same score and should not notice any deviation in how the test was delivered. However, despite the intention to standardize testing procedures, there may be small deviations in how the test is delivered, and there may be day-to-day differences in the participant and his or her abilities.

Two general approaches have been taken in performing neuropsychological testing: one that advocates the use of a fixed battery (e.g., the Halstead-Reitan Battery) and one that advocates the use of a flexible selection of tests that depend on the reason for the assessment (e.g., memory deficits). Many neuropsychologists prefer to mix these approaches and include aspects of both in assessments. Typically, testing begins with some tests of general cognitive function (e.g., the Wechsler Adult Intelligence Test) and then, depending on the results of these tests, tests of more specific cognitive function will be given.

Together with the medical history and the neurologist's report, the results of the neuropsychological testing can be used to help with diagnosis, intervention, and rehabilitation. Regardless of the orientation of the neuropsychologist (fixed or flexible test batteries), Levin and Benton (1986) suggest that the are some common goals of neuropsychological assessment:

1. Neuropsychological assessments provide evidence of cognitive dysfunction (often mild). Although this evidence complements the data from other sources, neuropsychological testing frequently reveals subtle deficits that were not readily apparent from other sources. Neuropsychological testing might also provide a means for understanding ambiguous results from other assessments (e.g., radiology).

2. Neuropsychological assessments provide a profile of cognitive function for an individual at a specific time. This profile of cognitive function highlights both impaired and preserved cognitive function and can be used to document disease progression (or remission) and to plan rehabilitation. Furthermore, when someone is facing brain surgery, the cognitive profile of the individual can help to determine possible outcomes from surgery and to evaluate the extent to which cognitive function has changed following surgery.

3. As we discovered in the previous chapters, many types of diseases can result in changes in cognitive function. For instance, it was thought that Parkinson's disease resulted primarily in motor deficits and not changes in cognitive function. However, this is not necessarily the case, and the data that were obtained from the neuropsychological assessments of individuals with Parkinson's disease provided evidence that there is a pattern of cognitive decline that is associated with the progression of the disease. Neuropsychological assessments can also provide insights into the functions of different areas of the brain (e.g., the role of the basal ganglia in other cognitive functions).

4. Finally, the cognitive profile of the individual that a neuropsychological assessment provides can help to determine the reason for the cognitive impairment. Certain cognitive profiles are associated with specific conditions or diseases. Often, it is difficult to diagnose or differentiate among these diseases during their early stages. By examining an individual's cognitive profile, a neuropsychologist can

Controversy

Now That We Can Image the Brain, What Good Is a Neuropsychologist?

There are some who question the need for neuropsychologists now that we have excellent techniques for documenting the degree and location of central nervous system injury (e.g., structural neuroimaging). Before such imaging methods were readily available (i.e., pre-1960), neuropsychologists assessed individuals with brain damage using long and complicated test batteries that helped to identify behavioral deficits. On the basis of the pattern of these deficits, the neuropsychologist would then attempt to localize the lesion. In most cases, this is no longer necessary, as structural neuroimaging can usually inform clinicians

about the precise location of abnormalities. Neuroimaging has not made the clinical neuropsychologist obsolete; assessments that are meant to identify cognitive and sensorimotor deficits are still performed. For instance, a number of diseases result in subtle changes in the brain that are difficult to observe. The neuropsychologist works with the neurologist to confirm the presence of behavioral features associated with subtle brain injury. In addition, neuropsychologists provide important information about cognitive function for individuals who face brain surgery. A majority of assessments are done with the goal of a rehabilitation or management plan based on the pattern of observed deficits. Finally, the research conducted by neuropsychologists provides important insights into the brain and behavior.

---

determine the likely causes of the cognitive impairment and often can discount certain other diseases as a cause.

Fixed Test Batteries

There are a large number of tests that can be given during neuropsychological testing. Lezak (1995) provides a comprehensive list of neuropsychological tests (in just over 800 pages!). However, there are at least five tests or batteries of tests that are widely used in neuropsychological assessment: the Halstead-Reitan Battery, the Luria-Nebraska Neuropsychological Battery, the Wechsler Adult Intelligence Scale, the National Adult Reading Test, and the Wechsler Memory Scale. This section highlights the components of these five tests, along with their strengths and limitations.

The **Halstead-Reitan Battery (HRB)** is a set of tests that was first developed in the 1930s as a method to examine cognitive change following brain injury. In the 1950s, Reitan used the tests to examine the cognitive abilities of individuals with psychiatric disorders. Since its original development, the number of tests in the HRB has been reduced from seven to five core tests, with the potential to add an additional five tests depending on the preferences of the neuropsychologist (Reitan & Wolfson, 1993). The five core tests include a Category Test, in which participants are asked to solve problems that require abstract reasoning or hypotheses testing; a Tactual Performance Test, in which participants are asked to arrange variously shaped blocks into holes without using sight; a Rhythm Test, in which participants are asked to detect similarities and differences between rhythms; a Speech Sounds Perception Test, in which participants are asked to match spoken nonsense syllables with written forms; and a Finger Tapping Test, in which participants are asked to tap their index finger as quickly as possible for 10 seconds (Lezak, 1995). Often a trail-making test (a test in which the participant has to make a trail between stimuli in a specific order without having lines cross), an aphasia screening test (to test for language problems), and a grip strength test (to test for differences between the strength in either hand) are given. It is interesting to note that the HRB contains no direct tests of memory, although there are some who argue that memory is tested indirectly (e.g., Paniak & Finlayson, 1989).

The HRB does what it initially set out to do. It distinguishes those with brain damage from those who do not have brain damage. There is some conflicting evidence as to whether or not the HRB can localize lesions to areas of the brain (Lezak, 1995). However, with the advent of neuroimaging, the role of the neuropsychologist has changed from identifying the location and extent of brain injury to identifying the nature of the cognitive deficit produced by injury or disease. Therefore, the ability of the HRB to localize lesions is not critical. Unfortunately, the HRB does have problems discriminating those with psychiatric illness from those with brain damage (Lezak, 1995).

Although it is still widely used, the HRB as a whole tends not to be used as often as it once was, primarily because it takes a long time to administer (six to eight hours). Also, because of its large number of tasks requiring writing, pointing, or the manipulation of objects, it is not useful for individuals who have motor problems (which are common in many diseases or following brain injury). The core tests that make up the HRB are often used, especially by neuropsychologists who prefer to use flexible batteries of tests. The greatest strength of the HRB is the recognition that accurate cognitive profiles rely on the assessment of many types of behaviors.

The **Luria-Nebraska Neuropsychological Battery (LNNB)** was developed as an ideal test battery by Golden, Purisch, and Hammeke in 1985. The tests were selected from Christensen's (1979) compilation of the tests and examination techniques that were used by Luria (a famous Russian neuropsychologist). The LNNB includes tasks that measure receptive and expressive speech, motor, rhythm, tactile, visuospatial, writing, reading, arithmetic, and intellectual performance.

The LNNB is effective at discriminating individuals with brain damage from those who are neurologically normal. Although, like the HRB, it has difficulties discriminating individuals with psychiatric disorders from those with brain damage (e.g., Adams, 1980). In addition, there are some neuropsychologists who raise the concern that the LNNB is not sensitive enough to discriminate among those with subtle neurological impairments and those who are neurologically normal (e.g., Moses, Cardellino, & Thompson, 1983). Finally, some suggest that the most serious limitation of the LNNB is its failure to reliably identify the laterality of the lesion (Sears, Hirt, & Hall, 1984). Therefore, neuropsychologists who use the LNNB often use components only as a gross screening tool to determine whether there is neurological impairment.

The **Wechsler Adult Intelligence Test (WAIS-III)**, one of the most widely used tests in a neuropsychological battery, was not designed as a neuropsychological test (Lezak, 1995). Rather, David Wechsler developed the WAIS to test the intelligence of adults. The WAIS-III consists of two subtests: the verbal subtest and a performance subtest. Each subtest provides a separate I.Q. score, known as **Verbal I.Q. (VIQ)** and **Performance I.Q. (PIQ)** respectively. When the two tests are combined, a **Full-Scale Intelligence Quotient (FSIQ)** is obtained. The categorization of intelligence into two separate subscales indicates the recognition that intelligence is a multifaceted construct that is best assessed by a battery of tests.

Assessment of VIQ includes tests of information (e.g., "Who is the mayor of your city?"), comprehension (practical reasoning/interpretation of proverbs), similarities (abstraction and verbalization of properties common to objects), arithmetic reasoning, digit span (repetition and reversal of numbers presented serially), and vocabulary (definitions). Assessment of PIQ includes tests of digit symbols (pairing a digit to a symbol and transposing them in a matrix), picture completion (identification of missing features from line drawings), picture arrangement (ordering a series of cartoon drawings in a meaningful way), block designs (block construction of a given design), and object assembly (timed construction of puzzles). As you can see, PIQ relies much less on previously acquired information than does VIQ. However, it also appears that PIQ is more sensitive to age-related changes in cognition than are VIQ scores.

Performance on the subscales of the WAIS-III provides important insights into the basic cognitive functions and is usually sensitive enough to provide information about significant changes in cognitive function (Lezak, 1995). As was mentioned previously, although the WAIS-III was not designed to test neuropsychological function, significant discrepancies between VIQ and PIQ scores are often suggestive of some type of neurological impairment. (Most neurologically normal individuals have very similar VIQ and PIQ scores.) The tasks that make up the subscales test a variety of cognitive skills, and a detailed examination of the individual tests provides useful and important insights into a variety of cognitive functions.

The WAIS-III is a well-standardized test with versions that have been adapted and standardized for different cultures (e.g., in the U.S. form, people are asked to name the President, whereas in the British form, people are asked to name the Prime Minister). Furthermore, the WAIS-III is relatively reliable. However, many people suggest that the real problems with the WAIS-III have to do with its validity (Lezak, 1995). That is, some suggest that the idea of intelligence is a flawed and circular concept, resulting in questionable validity for any test of intelligence. Others have suggested that the WAIS-III is culturally and gender biased (both African Americans and women tend to perform more poorly than do Caucasian males). However, regardless of the limitations, performance on the WAIS-III is an excellent predictor of academic achievement (Lezak, 1995).

The **National Adult Reading Test** (**NART**) (Nelson, 1982) is a single-word reading test. People who take this test are asked to read aloud a series of English words, which are for the most part short and irregular (i.e., they do not obey the typical phoneme–grapheme correspondence rules) in their spelling (e.g., *aisle, yacht*). The test begins with items that are easier to pronounce (e.g., *debt*) and ends with harder words (e.g., *demesne*). The theory behind the NART is that vocabulary is correlated with intelligence and the ability to correctly pronounce irregular words suggests a familiarity with the word (Nelson & O'Connell, 1978). Irregular words are used because they do not follow the rules of phonics, and a person must therefore know how to pronounce the words rather than sounding them out.

In controls, the NART is good at predicting scores on the WAIS, although, perhaps predictably, the NART predicts VIQ better than PIQ (Crawford, Stewart, Cochrane, Foulds, Besson, & Parker, 1989). The NART is useful as a tool for neuropsychologists because it appears to be a good predictor of premorbid I.Q. (i.e., I.Q. before the brain injury). As we will see in the following section, it is rare that a neuropsychologist has any objective information regarding a person's cognitive profile before the person was injured or became ill. The NART is reliable and appears to be somewhat resistant to changes in I.Q. as a result of brain damage (with the obvious exception of people with reading or language difficulties).

The **Wechsler Memory Scale (WMS-III)** (The Psychological Corporation, 1997) is a widely used test that provides insight into memory function. In this test battery, memory is not conceptualized as a unitary function, as this battery includes subtests tapping logical memory, visual memory, and verbal memory. There are nine tests: Personal and Current Information ("Who is the President?"), Orientation ("What season is it?"), Mental Control (reciting the alphabet), Logical Memory (recall of stories read aloud), Digit Span (recall of series of digits), Visual Reproduction (drawing from memory), Verbal Paired Associate Learning (learning pairs of related or unrelated words), Figural Memory (recall of visually presented items), and Visual Paired Associates Learning (learning pairs of unrelated drawings). A number of these tasks test both immediate memory (memory for events that just occurred) and longer-term memory (memory for longer than twenty minutes).

The WMS-III is able to determine the presence of memory difficulties and does reliably distinguish those with brain damage resulting in memory impairment and those who are neurologically normal. Nevertheless, there are critics who point out that the WMS-III does not do a good job of distinguishing right hemisphere lesions from left hemisphere lesions. For instance, examinations of the verbal memory score (which you might predict would be more dependent on left hemisphere function) have failed to find reliable differences between those with left temporal lobectomies and those with right temporal lobectomies (Loring, Lee, Martin, & Meador, 1989). However, there are some who suggest that the WMS-III is a valuable tool that the WMS can distinguish among a variety of diseases (e.g., early-stage Alzheimer's disease) (Troster, Jacobs, Butters, Cullum, & Salmon, 1989).

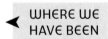 **WHERE WE HAVE BEEN**   The previous sections described the goals of assessment and the types of tests that are used during assessment. Some tests include the Halstead-Reitan Battery (overall cognitive function), the WAIS-III (intelligence), and the WMS-III (memory). Although many neuropsychologists use fixed batteries of tests, it is common to add additional tests to probe specific cognitive domains.

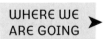 **WHERE WE ARE GOING**   The following sections will describe how a neuropsychologist chooses the tests that are used in assessment (including the benefits and limitations of fixed batteries of tests). Some common issues in neuropsychological testing will also be discussed, including how a neuropsychologist determines the level of functioning before brain injury and how to determine whether the client is motivated to do well during the assessment.

Which Test to Use?

In a very real sense, the choice of assessment tools is up to the neuropsychologist. The decision to use a test is often based on the reason for the referral to the neuropsychologist. If an individual is complaining of memory problems and seeks an assessment, the neuropsychologist might suspect that the person has some type of dementia and might choose to focus more on assessing memory skills than on testing language processing. However, it must be noted that many tests rely on skills that are not the primary focus of the test. For instance, in the trail-making task (described in the section on the HSB), participants have to manipulate a pencil to complete the task. It is easy to see that performance on this task might be impaired if an individual was paralyzed in the preferred hand and instead had to use the nonpreferred hand. (Try tracing a circle with your nonpreferred hand.) Neuropsychologists must be sensitive to these potential confounding factors, because the failure to notice even subtle behaviors can result in inaccurate conclusions about the nature of the cognitive deficit.

As we mentioned in the previous section, many neuropsychologists opt to perform a customized neuropsychological assessment that combines aspects of both fixed batteries of tests and other appropriate tests. Typically, such assessments begin with one or more of the fixed batteries of tests; then more specific tests are used to try and fully illustrate the nature of the cognitive deficit.

One advantage to using a fixed battery is that fixed batteries of tests are groups of related tests that are administered in a standardized fashion. That is, each individual is given the same series of tests with the same instructions, degree of assistance, and time constraints. Associated with standardization, fixed batteries provide the neuropsychologist with norms (a measure of how well neurologically normal individuals perform on the battery), which allows the neuropsychologist to compare the performance of their client with a group of similar people. Often, the more specialized tests tend not to have well-defined norms, requiring the neuropsychologist to rely on his or her experience with similar clients. Finally, standardized tests should allow comparison among tests. For instance, most people have very similar scores on both the NART and the VIQ subscale of the WAIS-III. Thus, if someone has completed the NART before his or her initial assessment, a neuropsychologist could compare current performance on the WAIS-III to determine whether there had been any cognitive decline since the time of taking the NART.

Some disadvantages of fixed batteries also relate to norms. Comparisons of current performance to a norm assumes that before brain damage the individual had "normal" cognitive function. This may or may not be true. Often, people who require neuropsychological assessment have had a long history of brain injury. As a final caution, a disadvantage of both fixed and flexible test batteries is that they do not take into account the individual's unique social, cultural, and medical history, which might alter test performance (Lezak, 1995).

Issues in Neuropsychological Assessment

There are a number of practical issues that must be addressed in performing or interpreting neuropsychological assessment. Interpretation of test scores might become pointless when the procedure for administering the test was not followed (e.g., not adhering to prescribed time limits) or when there are technical difficulties that occur during the testing session (e.g., a power outage). However, these concerns are related primarily to the skills of the individual neuropsychologist and do not tend to affect the discipline as a whole.

Some more general concerns about neuropsychology have to do with: the reliability and validity of the tests, the determination of preinjury cognitive functioning, the potential for psychiatric disorders to co-occur with brain damage, the effects that psychiatric disorders have on performance during the assessment, and the mental state of the participant during the testing session. Although the participant's mental state is, in part, what the assessment is trying to uncover, most neuropsychological tests are valid only when the participant is trying to do the best that he or she can on these tests. As we will see in the following paragraphs, there are a number of reasons why the outcome of an assessment might not provide a true picture of cognitive function.

RELIABILITY AND VALIDITY. Frequent criticisms of neuropsychological tests relate to their reliability and validity. However, it is interesting that both psychological and medical tests have varying degrees of validity and similar levels of reliability, yet rarely is the validity or reliability of medical tests questioned. There is quite a bit of evidence to suggest that neuropsychological testing provides valuable information that can inform rehabilitation practices and even subsequent medical treatment (Meyer et al., 2001). Significantly, neuropsychological tests are good predictors of everyday functional behaviors such as self-help skills, independent living, vocational ability, and employment following brain damage (Kubiszyn et al., 2000).

PREMORBID FUNCTIONING. Most of the tests described at the beginning of this module give information only about the current level of cognitive functioning and do not provide much insight into **premorbid functioning,** or how a person functioned before brain damage. That is, most people undergo neuropsychological assessment only after brain damage, and there is no means by which to objectively determine the individual's level of cognitive functioning. Although the NART is one test that purports to measure premorbid intelligence, deficits in cognitive functioning can often be restricted to areas other than intelligence as assessed by vocabulary. As a result, neuropsychologists also perform clinical interviews with their clients to learn about their clients' success in high school and/or college, their employment history, the type of employment they had, and their hobbies and interests. Although this information is useful background information, the neuropsychologist also uses it to infer the level of premorbid functioning. For instance, if a person held down a spatially demanding job (e.g., pilot or architect) or had a spatially challenging hobby (e.g., playing chess), it is reasonable to suspect that the person also had excellent levels of spatial ability before brain injury. Therefore, even a reduction in the spatial components of the WAIS-III to average would most likely reflect an impairment in spatial ability. However, any estimate of premorbid functioning might be in error and relies on assumptions regarding the typical person. It is difficult to estimate the absolute degree to which someone deviates from the typical performance. For example, among architects, some architects are average, some are below average, and some are geniuses. But how "smart" is the average architect?

PSYCHIATRIC DISORDERS. As you have seen in earlier chapters, a number of psychiatric disorders can affect performance on neuropsychological tests. For instance, depression is one of the most common comorbid conditions associated with brain-injured patients (e.g., Bay, 2000; Starkstein & Robinson, 1992). It is well documented that depression reduces motivation and subsequent performance on tasks (but see Satz et al., 1998, for a different viewpoint). The failure to assess the severity of the psychiatric condition, such as depression, can result in an invalid assessment of cognitive function.

In addition, the types of medications that individuals might be taking to treat psychiatric (and neurological) conditions are known to affect performance on cognitive tasks. That is, drugs that work to treat a large number of neurological and psychiatric illnesses do so by modifying the chemistry of the brain and thus its ability to function. An assessment that does not take into account the drugs (prescribed or not) that an individual is taking might also come to false conclusions about the cognitive profile of the client.

COMPLIANCE AND MALINGERING. Apart from brain damage or injury, there are a number of reasons why someone might not perform well on tests that are administered during an assessment. These reasons might relate to the psychiatric conditions discussed above as well as problems with getting the client to cooperate (**compliance**), problems with motivating the client to try to perform the tasks as well as he or she can, and/or deliberate exaggeration of a symptom.

When a client does not want to do well on a test or is deliberately answering the tasks incorrectly (also known as **malingering**), the neuropsychologist must often rely on information from the client's history and the overall pattern of cognitive performance. For instance, when a client performs much worse on all the tasks than is expected by the extent of brain damage, the possibility that the client is malingering must be considered. Most laypeople do not have the knowledge to successfully mimic the complex patterns of cognitive dysfunction that accompany brain damage. Instead, malingerers tend to exaggerate their performance and do poorly on every test that they are given, even ones on which they should be able to do well.

For instance, in Chapter 7, you learned that despite the profound anterograde amnesia exhibited by H.M., he has normal short-term memory. Someone who was faking amnesia would most likely be unaware of the differences between short-term and long-term memory and most likely would do poorly on all tests of memory. Unfortunately, unless the person admits that he or she is malingering, there is no way to know for certain that the individual is not experiencing these cognitive deficits (e.g., consider the possibility that the client exhibits a previously unreported syndrome).

In conclusion, neuropsychological testing provides important information that can give physicians, families, and clients a snapshot of how well (or poorly) a person is functioning.

Self-Test

1. Name three commonly used test batteries. What are the strengths and limitations of each of these batteries?

2. What are the advantages of using well-standardized tests?

3. List three goals of neuropsychological assessment.

4. Name three methods that a neuropsychologist might use to determine premorbid functioning. Can you think of some instances in which these methods might not provide true insight into premorbid functioning?

5. Consider the case of Patient X. You suspect that Patient X is malingering to obtain a large disability settlement. What are the features of a client who is malingering? What are the difficulties associated with detecting clients who malinger?

These snapshots can be used to inform subsequent treatment by occupational therapists as well as to make important decisions about living arrangements. Finally, as we will learn in Chapter 16, brain damage is rarely a static phenomenon. Neuropsychological assessments can provide a basis for the ongoing monitoring of a condition, helping to determine the degree to which there is improvement or change.

◄ **WHERE WE HAVE BEEN** This chapter detailed the participants in neuropsychological assessment, described the types of tests employed during the assessment, and discussed some of the strengths and weaknesses of these tests and the manner in which they are typically employed. The changing role of the neuropsychologist in light of relatively recent diagnostic procedures (such as neuroimaging) was also discussed. Instead of administering tests in hopes of localizing lesions, clinical neuropsychologists now assess clients with the goals of management and rehabilitation.

Glossary

Client (patient, subject, or participant)—The person who is the subject of an assessment.

Clinical neuropsychologist—A scientist-practitioner with a Ph.D. who seeks to assess, manage, and rehabilitate individuals who suffer from neurological disorders, regardless of their cause.

Clinical neuropsychology—A branch of neuropsychology that is involved with the assessment, management and rehabilitation of individuals who have neurological diseases or injury.

Cognitive neuropsychology—A branch of neuropsychology that is focused on explaining behavior (and disruptions in behavior) in terms of functional brain units, regardless of their anatomical representation.

Compliance—The degree to which a client performs the neuropsychological tests to the best of their ability.

Experimental neuropsychology—A branch of neuropsychology that examines how human behavior, both normal and that resulting from neurological damage, is produced by brain activity.

Full-Scale Intelligence Quotient (FSIQ)—The unitary measure of I.Q. that is obtained when VIQ is combined with PIQ. Large discrepancies between VIQ, PIQ, and FSIQ are often indicative of neural dysfunction.

Halstead-Reitan Battery (HRB)—A fixed battery of five core tests and five additional tests that differentiates brain-damaged individuals from neurologically normal individuals.

Lack of insight—A lack of acknowledgment of a deficit that often accompanies a nervous system injury.

Luria-Nebraska Neuropsychological Battery (LNNB)—A fixed battery of tests that measure receptive and expressive speech, motor, rhythm, tactile, visuospatial, writing, reading, arithmetic, and intellectual performance that are used to differentiate brain-damaged individuals from neurologically normal individuals.

Malingering—When clients deliberately exaggerate or feign symptoms to try to appear as though they have a neurological condition.

National Adult Reading Test (NART)—A single-word reading test that is useful for predicting VIQ.

Neurologist—A physician who has specialized training for diagnosing and treating disorders of the nervous system.

Neurosurgeon—A physician who performs surgery on the nervous system.

Performance I.Q. (PIQ)—A largely nonverbal subscale of the WAIS that includes tests of picture arrangement, block designs, object assembly, digit symbols, and so on.

Premorbid functioning—Often an estimate of the level of cognitive functioning before brain damage. Most often, this is estimated on the basis of education, profession, and hobbies as well as any available neuropsychological test data.

Radiologists—Physicians with specialized training in obtaining and interpreting images of the human body and/or treating conditions using radiological science.

Verbal I.Q. (VIQ)—A verbal subscale of the WAIS that includes tests of information, comprehension, similarities, arithmetic reasoning, and so on.

Wechsler Adult Intelligence Test (WAIS-III)—A battery of tests, both verbal and nonverbal problem solving, that were initially designed to measure intelligence.

Wechsler Memory Scale (WMS-III)—A widely used test of memory that consists of nine different tests of memory.

X-rays—A form of high-energy radiation that in low concentrations can be used to image structures (particularly bones) in the human body.

16

Recovery of Function

It is a good morning exercise for a research scientist to discard a pet hypothesis every day before breakfast.

—KONRAD LORENZ

You have probably taken courses in which you were told that you were born with all the neurons that you will ever have and any neurons that you lose are permanently gone. I have also frequently heard these claims outside of the classroom. When I was in high school, my mother often reminded me that neurons do not grow back. When I was in graduate school, it was dogma that, unlike neurons in the peripheral nervous system, neurons of the central nervous system do not regrow following damage. However, some of the most exciting research in neuroscience and neuropsychology has demonstrated that this truism is false. We now know that the normal adult brain produces new neurons and that neural death is a normal part of brain development.

Although much of the focus of the book (especially Chapter 14) has been on the behavioral effects of brain damage, recovery is a very important topic in neuropsychology. Understanding why and how recovery occurs (and why and when it does not) gives us the best hope to cure brain damage. Furthermore, understanding neural degeneration, regeneration, and organization in the intact central nervous system (CNS) will provide us with possible treatments and therapy that will improve quality of life following brain damage.

WHERE WE ARE GOING ➤	This module will focus on understanding how degeneration occurs in the central nervous system and possible remediation of damage by regeneration and reorganization. The second module will exam-

ine possible treatments for brain damage, including rehabilitation, strategies for inducing regeneration of neurons, and treatments that limit the initial brain damage.

MODULE **16.1**
Neural Degeneration, Regeneration, and Reorganization

When someone dies, there is often an autopsy. The purpose of the autopsy is not to somehow bring the person back to life, but rather to gain understanding by providing information about why the individual died. In fact, *autopsy* literally means "to see for oneself." A sign that says "Hic locus est ubi mors gaudet succurrere vitae" (translation: "This is the place where death rejoices to teach those who live") is frequently seen in autopsy rooms, which gives an insight into the information that an autopsy can provide. At one level, an autopsy provides specific information about the life and health of the individual as well as why the individual died. However, autopsies also give physicians and researchers valuable information about how various diseases and conditions affect the body, which can be translated into possible treatments for disease. Thus, as the sign suggests, death can provide the living with important insights.

These principles are also instructive for us, because many of the neurological diseases that have been covered in this book are caused by the death of neurons or glia. Understanding how and why neurons die and how various disease processes result in cell death will help us to develop treatments for these diseases. In addition, quite a few people suffer brain damage as a result of an accident. Realizing how the CNS responds to these insults (both acutely and long-term) may provide us with treatments for these people, either by preventing further damage following an accident or by encouraging the CNS to regenerate the damaged neurons.

Degeneration

In Chapter 14, we discussed the frequent causes of brain damage including stroke, tumors, and infection. However, we did not discuss how these diseases actually kill neurons and produce a lesion in the brain. All cells, including neurons, die in one of two ways: necrosis or apoptosis. **Necrosis** occurs when there is an overwhelming failure to maintain homeostasis within the neuron. **Apoptosis** is programmed neural death, in which the neuron uses its own machinery to ensure its own death. In a sense, necrosis can be thought of as neural manslaughter or homicide and apoptosis as neural suicide. See Figure 16.1 for the morphological differences between necrosis and apoptosis.

NECROSIS. When neurons completely lose their ability to regulate their internal environment (**homeostasis**), swelling and membrane bursting occur. The destruction of the membranes is not restricted to the membranes that encase the neuron itself; the membranes that encase the organelles (e.g., mitochondria and nucleus) and vesicles

---

Figure 16.1 **Ocular Dominance Columns with One Eye Patched**

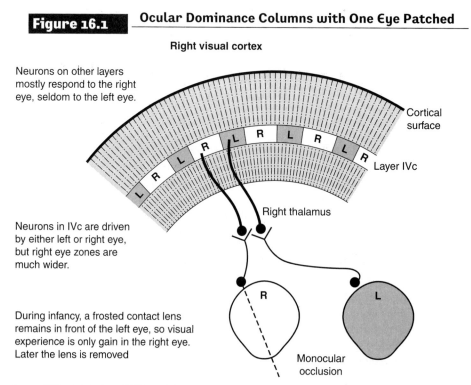

Source: William Calvin, http://williamcalvin.com/bk7/bk7ch11.htm, Figure 55. Reprinted with permission.

also burst. This bursting or **lysis** spills the contents of the neuron into the extracellular space, which obviously results in the death of the neuron. Necrosis, unlike apoptosis, is always an abnormal event. Necrosis is often associated with damage that occurs rapidly, such as mechanical damage to the neurons (such as occurs from tumors or from blows to the head), events that cause disruption to ion channels (e.g., anoxia or ischemia), or the results of infection (e.g., rabies, meningitis). However, necrosis can also follow damage that accumulates more slowly, such as secondary damage to nearby areas of the brain following stroke or a number of neurodegenerative diseases (e.g., Huntington's chorea). Thus, any type of disruption to homeostasis that cannot be compensated for by the neuron results in necrotic cell death.

One common cause of necrotic cell death is **ischemia,** or a disruption in blood flow that often results from a stroke or cerebrovascular accident. Ischemia is associated with disruptions in the energy pathways of the neuron, which in turn can affect ion channels that are important for homeostasis in the neuron. For instance, ischemia can reduce or terminate ATP production in the neuron. Because the sodium–potassium pump relies on ATP to power its opening and closing, failure to have available ATP will result in a stoppage of the sodium–potassium pump and thus the inability of the neuron to regulate levels of sodium and potassium following an action potential. There are other membrane pumps that regulate levels of water and calcium. Failure to maintain homeostatic levels of sodium and potassium will also disrupt the neuron's ability to regulate calcium and water, both of which can have disastrous effects for the neuron. Failure to regulate water can result in an accumulation of intracellular water, which results in the neuron's swelling and potentially breaking its membrane cover (although there are other pathways that are responsible for the observed inflammation in the neuron). Recall from Chapter 2 that cellular influx of calcium results in the release of neurotransmitters. Failure to regulate intracellular calcium concentrations can have severe consequences for the release of neurotransmitters. As we will see, the accumulation of intracellular calcium is thought to be responsible for much of the damage that occurs after the initial ischemic event.

Another common cause of brain damage is an acquired injury, such as occurs following traumatic brain injury (TBI). Both TBI and stroke, as well as neurodegenerative diseases such as Huntington's chorea, have elements of necrotic cell death, typically resulting from alterations in the release of glutamate (Fawcett, Rosser, & Dunnett, 2001). Recall from Chapter 2 that glutamate is an excitatory amino acid neurotransmitter that is involved in almost every fast excitatory event in the nervous system. However, glutamate itself is quite toxic to neurons and glia, an effect that is known as excitotoxicity (Olney, 1971). **Excitotoxicity** is the ability of specific compounds, such as glutamate, to both excite neurons and kill them. **Primary neural death,** or the death of neurons that occurs immediately after trauma, appears to occur when glutamate is released in excess. This activates a cascade of events that leads to even more release of glutamate and even more excitation of the cell. Primary cell death can result from the neuron's exhausting its resources and overwhelming homeostatic mechanisms.

Although it is certainly true that high concentrations of excitotoxins can result in neurons literally exciting themselves to death (e.g., Olney, 1990), some researchers have suggested that intracellular calcium also plays a major role in excitotoxic cell death (e.g., Choi, 1992). Research by Dennis Choi and colleagues suggest that **secondary neuronal death** (death of neurons following the primary event) results from a large-scale influx of calcium into the neuron. Glutamate can regulate a calcium channel; therefore, excess release of glutamate can result in a sustained and excessive influx of calcium. Beyond releasing even more glutamate, increases in intracellular calcium concentrations can trigger a wide range of intracellular events, including changes in second messengers and the production of free radicals. These changes are associated with the death of neural mitochondria, which results in the loss of energy production for the neuron. Furthermore, changes induced by calcium influx are associated with inflammation and membrane breakdown, a characteristic of necrosis. Thus, the cascade of events that lead to necrosis may rely on changes in intracellular concentrations of ions (such as calcium), changes in the ability of the neuron to produce energy (e.g., ATP), and damage to the organelles of the neuron (e.g., mitochondria).

APOPTOSIS. Apoptosis, or programmed cell death, was first named by A.H. Wylie, who delineated the differences between apoptosis and necrosis in a seminal paper in 1972. Before this, the importance of these differences was not widely understood (Dikranian et al., 2001). Although apoptosis and necrosis can be thought of as occurring at opposite ends of a continuum, the main difference between apoptosis and necrosis is that apoptosis is an active process that uses cellular energy to effect death. Unlike necrosis, apoptosis is typically characterized by dead cells in which the nucleus is condensed into a tangle of DNA fragments, as well as intact cell membranes. Also unlike necrosis, apoptosis is a feature of normal development of the neuron, and some theorists suggest that all neurons are on the verge of apoptotic cell death. Apoptosis can be initiated in a variety of ways, including damage to the DNA of the neuron, damage caused by free radicals, or withdrawal of tropic factors required for normal development. Even the presence of necrotic neurons can induce nearby neurons to undergo apoptosis. Although there are many pathways to apoptotic death, the process of apoptosis is typically regulated by genes, which trigger proteins known as caspases that are responsible for the destruction of the neuron (Chang, Putcha, Deshmukh, & Johnson, 2002; Sadowski-Debbing, Coy, Mier, Hug, & Los, 2002). Apoptosis has been implicated in the neural degeneration that is characteristic of a number of diseases, including Parkinson's disease, Huntington's chorea, Alzheimer's disease, and other types of dementia, multiple sclerosis, and amyotrophic lateralizing sclerosis (Honig & Rosenberg, 2000). However, apoptotic cell death has also been observed following acute events, such as stroke and TBI (Raghupathi, Graham, & McIntosh, 2000).

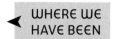

There are two mechanisms by which neurons die: apoptosis and necrosis. Necrosis is always pathological, whereas apoptosis occurs during the course of normal CNS development. Both types of cell death are observed in neurological disease.

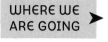

The next section will examine the factors that are associated with regeneration of neurons in the PNS and the CNS. Subsequent sections will explain principles of CNS reorganization, as well as possible treatments for brain damage and neurological disease that are related to the principles of degeneration, regeneration, and reorganization.

Regeneration

There are a number of possible events that could follow neural death, such as permanent loss of the neuron or regeneration of the neuron (neurogenesis). Frequently in the CNS, neurogenesis does not occur, resulting in a permanent loss of the neuron. As a compensatory mechanism, regeneration in the nervous system tends to involve a process known as **collateral sprouting,** in which undamaged neurons sprout new axon collaterals (side branches of axons) to innervate targets. However, if the entire neuron has not been damaged, there is also the possibility that the damaged portion (e.g., an axon) could regrow, which is known as **regenerative sprouting.**

COLLATERAL SPROUTING.   One of the first examples that regeneration could occur in the CNS was demonstrated by Raisman and colleagues (Raisman & Field, 1973). In this study, they examined synaptic responses to cutting one of two main inputs to the septum of the rat. Raisman observed that when one input to the septum was cut, there were immediate reductions in the number of synapses in the septum. However, over a two-week period, the number of synapses in the septum returned to prelesion levels, owing to collateral sprouting of the axons of the undamaged input. Thus, collateral sprouting of the undamaged axons demonstrated that the adult CNS was capable of producing new axons.

The ability of the CNS to demonstrate **plasticity** (the ability of the nervous system to change in response to events) through collateral sprouting is thought to underlie a number of normal processes, including development and somatosensory function. For instance, development of the primary visual cortex depends on the visual experiences of the individual during critical periods that occur rather early in life (e.g., Hubel, Wiesel, & Levay, 1977; LeVay, Wiesel, & Hubel, 1980). For instance, in the primary visual cortex (V1), inputs from the two eyes are separated in alternating columns of cortical tissue, known as ocular dominance columns. For most individuals with binocular vision, the width of the ocular dominance columns are equal (Figure 16.2). However, individuals who do not receive equal inputs from both eyes during development (e.g., individuals with amblyopia, or "lazy eye") do not exhibit this pattern. For instance, if the brain does not receive input from the left eye, then the ocular dominance columns for the right eye become larger. This effect does not occur in adults, suggesting that there is a critical period in which this plasticity can be exhibited. This type of plasticity is exhibited in many parts of the brain, including the sensory cortex, motor cortex, auditory cortex, and hippocampus. In fact, it may be that collateral sprouting is the basis for neural reorganization following injury (Fawcett et al., 2001).

REGENERATIVE SPROUTING.   In most animal species, regeneration of the axon is the norm. However, in mammalian species, regeneration usually occurs only within the peripheral nervous system (PNS). In fact, axotomy (cutting of an axon) in the PNS results in axon regrowth, with the regrown axons often traveling long distances to

Structural Changes of Cells Undergoing Necrosis or Apoptosis

Figure 16.2

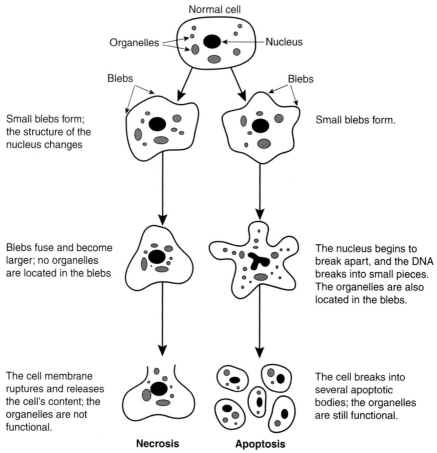

Source: Charles R. Goodlett and Kristin H. Horn, "Mechanisms of Alcohol-Induced Damage to the Developing Nervous System," www.niaaa.nih.gov/publications/arh25-3/175-184.htm, Figure 1.

make functional connections with their targets (e.g., muscles). Although the PNS often fully recovers from axotomy, the CNS typically does not. Events that lead to CNS axotomy (e.g., spinal cord injuries) result in the permanent loss of the axons and thus a permanent loss of function. Such was the case with Christopher Reeve (Figure 16.3), who suffered a severe spinal cord injury as the result of a fall during an equestrian competition in 1995, resulting in almost complete paralysis of his body below the neck. After his accident, Reeve was a prominent activist for spinal cord injuries and raised millions of dollars for spinal cord injury research before his death in 2004.

Given that PNS axons regenerate, what is different between the PNS and the CNS? One hypothesis posits that CNS axons are not capable of regeneration. A common way to study this hypothesis is to damage the dorsal roots of spinal nerves, because

Christopher Reeve, Who Suffered a Spinal Cord Injury

Figure 16.3

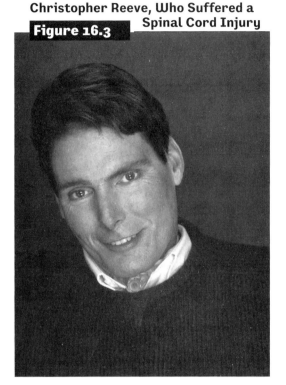

Source: Photo courtesy of the Christopher Reeve Paralysis Foundation.

they begin in the CNS and end in the PNS. When the dorsal root is damaged in the PNS, it successfully regenerates, which indicates that this neuron is capable of regeneration. However, when the dorsal root is damaged in the spinal cord, it will not regenerate, suggesting that although the axon has the potential to regenerate, the environment of the CNS does not permit regeneration.

One major difference between axons in the PNS and axons in the CNS is the type of glia that surround them. For instance, axons in the PNS are myelinated by Schwann cells, whereas axons in the CNS are myelinated by oligodendrocytes. If either Schwann cells or a piece of PNS nerve tissue (often the sciatic nerve) is transplanted into the CNS at the site of axotomy, the axons will grow through the transplant, stopping once they contact the CNS tissue on the other side of the transplant (e.g., Richardson, McGuinness, & Aguayo, 1982). These results provide further support for the idea that axons of the CNS can regenerate and that there is something about the environment of the CNS or its glia that prevents regeneration.

In fact, it appears that glia play an important role in the failure of CNS axons to regenerate. That is, both astrocytes and oligodendrocytes appear to actively inhibit axonal growth (Fawcett et al., 2001). However, it should be noted that there appears to be some type of position effect in the CNS. Even when axonal regeneration can be induced, it is strongest close to the PNS and in axons that typically interface with the PNS (Fawcett et al., 2001).

NEUROGENESIS. Although **neurogenesis** in adult amphibians has been recognized for some time, it was commonly believed that neurogenesis in the adult mammalian CNS did not occur. In mammals, much of the neurogenesis that occurs in an organism does so before birth, often during the second half of the embryo's life. Even when neurogenesis occurs following birth in mammals, it tends to be restricted to the perinatal period (the period immediately after birth). However, there are two areas of the mammalian CNS that demonstrate neurogenesis in adulthood: the neurons of the olfactory bulb and the neurons in the dentate gyrus of the hippocampus (Fawcett et al., 2001). New neurons in both the olfactory bulb and the dentate gyrus have been observed in primates and humans (e.g., Eriksson et al., 1998), suggesting that the CNS has a limited ability to produce new neurons. However, the rate of neurogenesis appears to be inhibited by age and by stress. That is, older individuals have lower rates of neurogenesis, as do stressed individuals. It has been suggested that the decrease in neurogenesis is related to the steroid hormone corticosterone, which is commonly associated with stress responses. Interestingly, steroid hormones are important factors in inflammatory responses (McEwen, 2001).

Where do new neurons come from? The first thing that you must know about neurons is that they are postmitotic. That is, unlike other cells in the body (e.g., the skin), neurons cannot use mitosis to divide and produce new copies of themselves. Instead, new neurons appear to come from populations of stem or precursor cells in the brain. Stem cells are cells that can become any type of cell in the body, whereas progenitor cells are "committed" stem cells. That is, progenitor cells come from stem cells and are committed to becoming a specific type of cell, such as a neuron or type of glia. Stem or progenitor cells have been found within the subgranular layer of the hippocampus and the floor and walls of the lateral ventricles (the subependymal zone) (e.g., Cayre, Malaterre, Scotto-Lomassese, Strambi, & Strambi, 2002). Cells in the subgranular layer divide, and some migrate a short distance to the dentate gyrus, where they emerge as new neurons. Cells in the subependymal zone divide, and some migrate a long distance to the olfactory bulbs, where they emerge as new neurons. It is important to remember that any division that stem or progenitor cells undertake occurs both in their home location and en route to their targets. There is then no further division once they reach their targets. It appears that the ability of the CNS to replace neurons from stem or progenitor cells decreases with age, which has interesting implications for neurodegenerative diseases that appear in the elderly.

Cells within the hippocampus or subependymal region appear to have characteristics of both stem cells and progenitor cells. That is, like stem cells, cells within the hippocampus and subependymal zone appear to be genuinely multipotential and can be transformed into neurons or glia. However, as is the case with progenitor cells, the type of cells that these cells become depends on their location within the CNS. That is, if a progenitor cell from the hippocampus is transplanted to the subependymal zone, it does not become a dentate granule neuron; instead, it becomes an olfactory bulb neuron (e.g., Gage, 2002). Finally, although there is evidence that there is stem or progenitor cell migration to the site of injuries, it is unclear what function these stem cells have. For instance, it appears that rather than becoming neurons at the site of injury, stem or progenitor cells transform into glia, which may further hinder the ability of the damaged neurons to recover. We will consider the implications of the ability of stem cells to produce new neurons in the next section.

◄ **WHERE WE HAVE BEEN** When neurons die, the brain can adopt a number of compensatory strategies. For instance, it can regenerate neurons (neurogenesis), or it can sprout new axon collaterals from surviving axons nearby (collateral sprouting). In addition, if only the axon of a neuron has been injured, there are some situations in which the axons can regrow, especially in the PNS. However, there appears to be some specific environmental component of the CNS, possibly CNS glia, that makes collateral sprouting and neurogenesis rather rare events.

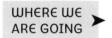 **WHERE WE ARE GOING** ► The next section will explain the principles of CNS reorganization. The subsequent module will investigate possible treatments for brain damage and neurological disease that are related to the principles of degeneration, regeneration, and reorganization.

Reorganization

As you saw in the previous module, many of the ways in which the brain can repair damage are very limited and/or occur only under experimental conditions. However, this belies the fact that individuals with brain damage frequently recover many of their lost abilities. This recovery is thought to be mediated by reorganization of cortical areas. Although the organization of the brain is fairly constant, there are instances in which the normal organization of the brain can be altered. When this type of plasticity occurs in adulthood, it is often referred to as *reorganization*. Reorganization can occur in adulthood in a variety of brain areas in response to such diverse events as injury, changes in the environment, enriched experiences, and exposure to chemicals (both endogenous and exogenous).

Furthermore, there is extensive documentation that the cortical representation areas, such as the primary motor cortex and primary somatosensory cortex, can be altered by sensory input and experience. Alterations have been observed following either **enrichment,** which is the addition of something to the environment (e.g., educational experiences), or **deprivation,** which is the removal of something from the environment (e.g., loss of a limb). For instance, when animals are placed into an enriched environment, increased cortical thickness (Sirevaag, Black, Shafron, & Greenough, 1988) and increased numbers of new neurons in the hippocampus (Kempermann, Kuhn, & Gage, 1998) are observed. It has also been observed that lesions of the nerves that innervate facial whiskers in rats (deprivation of feedback) resulted in a decrease in the representation of these whiskers in the primary motor cortex. In addition, within hours of the lesion, the primary motor cortex had been reorganized, and areas that had previously represented whiskers now represented areas of the adjacent forelimb and eyes (Sanes & Donoghue, 2000).

In humans, it is well documented that reorganization of the motor and somatosensory cortices can accompany either peripheral damage or enriched experiences. For instance, a study by Ramachandran and colleagues (Ramachandran, 1993; Ramachandran & Rogers-Ramachandran, 2000) examined the tactile discrimination abilities of amputees. In these studies, individuals who had experienced the amputation of one hand were asked to indicate the location of light touches on their bodies. For instance, if the individual was touched on the right ear with a cotton swab, he or she was expected to report that the right ear had been touched. For the most part, the amputees exhibited very accurate tactile discrimination. However, sometimes following touches to the face, the amputees would indicate that their missing limb had been touched (which is obviously impossible). Ramachandran interpreted the phantom limb (also see Chapter 6 for a discussion of phantom limb) as the result of an expansion of the area of the somatosensory homunculus to occupy the part of the cortex that had previously represented the missing limb.

Other studies have demonstrated that this degree of plasticity can be observed following spinal cord injury, temporary changes in sensory feedback, and repetitive movements (Sanes & Donoghue, 2000). It is interesting to note that this type of plasticity may occur in everyday life. For instance, individuals who practice complex motor movements tend to have larger representations of the muscles involved to produce these movements. For instance, individuals who play stringed instruments tend to use their left hand to finger the notes and the right hand to pluck, strum, or bow the instrument, so playing a stringed instrument involves different motoric requirements for the hands. Interestingly, imaging studies of skilled string players tend to observe that the cortical representation of the left hand is larger than that of controls (Elbert, Pantev, Wienbruch, Rockstroh, & Taub, 1995). This change is the smallest for the left thumb, which tends to perform the fewest skilled movements, suggesting that these changes are experience dependent. These changes have also been observed during learning, giving support to the position that experience is responsible for these changes (Pascual-Leone, 2001; Pascual-Leone, Grafman, & Hallett, 1994).

It is also important to note that it may be difficult to determine whether an effect of experience is due to enrichment or deprivation, because these conditions are not mutually exclusive. For instance, an individual who is blind may experience the loss of visual information (deprivation) but may learn to cope with this loss using techniques that many of us do not experience, which is enrichment (e.g., Braille). Braille readers experience a great deal of cortical reorganization, including a greater representation of the reading finger that depends on proficiency with Braille (Pascual-Leone, Cammarota, Wasserman, Brasil-Neto, Cohen, & Hallett, 1993; Pascual-Leone, Wassermann, Sadato, & Hallett, 1995). However, what is surprising is that there are some imaging studies that suggest that Braille readers often experience activation in the visual cortex even though they are blind (Cohen et al., 1997). Furthermore, transcranial magnetic stimulation of visual areas of blind people resulted in the disruption of their Braille reading (Cohen et al., 1997). These researchers suggest that one consequence of early blindness is that areas that are ordinarily used for vision are reorganized to process different somatosensory information. Taken as a whole, these results suggest that reorganization of the cortex may occur both within and between cortical areas.

How does this reorganization occur? There is evidence to suggest that reorganization is a function of plasticity mechanisms that involve neurotransmitter systems, collateral sprouting, and dendritic arborization. For instance, somatosensory cortical reorganization can be affected by altering levels of neurotransmitters, including glutamate, GABA, and nitric oxide (for review, see Johansson, 2000). As you learned in the previous section, changes in visual experience affect the organization of ocular dominance columns by affecting the degree to which collateral sprouting occurs. In addition, as you learned in Chapter 8, dendritic arborization is constantly changing in response to experience. It is interesting to note that the degree of dendritic arborization has been related to education, linguistic ability, and occupation (e.g., Jacobs, Schall, & Scheibel, 1993; Scheibel, Conrad, Perdue, Tomiyasu, & Wechsler, 1990). For instance, individuals with more education had greater dendritic branching in cortical language areas than did those with less education. In addition, individuals with greater linguistic skill also had greater dendritic branching in cortical language areas. Finally, individuals who performed tasks requiring high levels of finger dexterity (e.g., typists) also showed greater dendritic branching. However, Schiebel cautions that their studies were based on a small sample and that further research is necessary to replicate their results.

Taken together, these studies suggest that enriched experience can increase dendritic arborization. You must remember, though, that these studies are only

the **Real** world

Do You Recover from Brain Damage Better When You Are Young?

In the previous section, you learned that the ability of the brain to either produce new neurons or engage in collateral sprouting was enhanced in younger brains. In Chapter 8, you learned that fewer new synapses and dendritic branches were formed in elderly brains. Given that collateral sprouting, dendritic arborization (or the branching of dendrites), and neurogenesis are all means by which the brain can compensate for damage, does it follow that younger brains recover from damage better than older brains do? Like many answers in this text, the answer to this question is "It depends." The first extensive investigation of this question was performed by Margaret Kennard, who observed the effects of motor cortex lesions in monkeys. She observed that recovery of motor function was better when the lesions were performed in infancy rather than adulthood (Kennard, 1940). Now called the **Kennard effect,** the ability of the young to recover from brain damage more thoroughly than adults has been observed in several species. Although Kennard described the effect and hypothesized that recovery must be dependent on some type of change in the cortex, she did not study what these changes might be.

The properties of the Kennard effect have been extensively studied by Bryan Kolb and colleagues, who have found that rats with lesions of the frontal cortex recovered better when the lesions occurred at 7–10 days of age as compared to those in adulthood (Kolb & Whishaw, 1981). In addition, Kolb has demonstrated that functional recovery in adults was related to the degree of dendritic branching (Kolb & Whishaw, 1998) and that functional recovery was associated with widespread changes in dendritic branching (Kolb, Gibb, & van der Kooy, 1994). Kolb and Whishaw (1998) conclude that functional recovery following brain damage in infancy is associated with greater changes in cortical organization than in adulthood. These changes in cortical organization may be the basis for the Kennard effect.

However, there appear to be limits on the Kennard effect. For instance, children with brain injury to the frontal lobes during the perinatal period experience greater behavioral deficits than do those who experience later damage—either in later infancy or in adulthood (Kolb & Gibb, 1999). Similar effects can be observed in rats (e.g., Kolb & Gibb, 1993). That is, rats that received frontal lesions before 10 days of age failed to exhibit the degree of functional recovery that was observed when the frontal lesion occurred at 10 days of age. In addition, the rats who experienced the very early lesions exhibited dendritic atrophy and a reduction in synapse count; in contrast, rats that received their lesions at 10 days of age exhibited profound dendritic arborization and extensive cortical remodeling (Kolb & Gibb, 1999). Kolb and Whishaw (1998) suggest that before 10 days of age, the brain is still undergoing significant and basic developmental organization (e.g., neural differentiation in the cortex). Lesions that occur prior to the completion of basic developmental organization of the cortex cannot be compensated for. At about 10 days of life, neurons are more mature and are beginning to send profuse numbers of dendrites throughout other areas of the cortex. Lesions at this time can be compensated for because neurons are predisposed to increase the numbers of dendrites, which can compensate for lost neurons. Kolb and Gibb (1999) suggest that good functional recovery occurs when brain damage is associated with compensatory dendritic arborization (e.g., at 10 days of age) where this age is a critical period for optimal dendritic arborization. In humans, the period associated with greatest functional recovery is between the ages of 1–5 years of age. However, as was observed with rats, brain damage that occurs before 1 year of age tends to be associated with widespread significant behavioral deficits. Thus, although age is associated with the degree of functional recovery, younger is not always better.

Self-Test

1. Compare and contrast the two mechanisms of cell death.

2. What is the evidence for neurogenesis in the CNS? Where does neurogenesis occur in the CNS?

3. What is the evidence that suggests that the CNS is capable of repairing itself following injury?

4. What factors contribute to the failure of the CNS to repair itself following injury?

correlational, so it is possible that this effect can be interpreted differently. That is, rather than dendritic arborization reflecting changes resulting from experience, it is possible that individuals with greater dendritic arborization seek out these experiences. Regardless, it appears that there is a wide diversity in the means by which plasticity reorganizes the cortex.

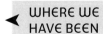

◄ WHERE WE HAVE BEEN

Currently, brain damage results in a permanent loss of neurons. However, despite this loss, individuals often experience limited recovery of function. Neurogenesis and collateral sprouting appear to be relatively rare events in the CNS, so one possible mechanism for this recovery is reorganization of the remaining cortical areas. It appears that the brain is capable of plastic reorganization of cortical areas and that reorganization of cortical areas occurs routinely in the neurologically normal brain. Furthermore, it is likely that changes in neurotransmitter systems, dendritic arborization, and collateral sprouting all play a role in the reorganization of the cortex.

WHERE WE ARE GOING ►

The next module will investigate possible treatments for brain damage and neurological disease that are related to the principles of degeneration, regeneration, and reorganization.

MODULE **16.2**
Therapeutic Interventions

As we learned in the previous module, brain damage is often associated with some recovery. This recovery can take place within hours of the insult, or it may occur more slowly over a period of months or years. Initial recovery within hours of the event is thought to be related to edema (swelling), which often accompanies any injury to the body. However, once this initial period has passed, functional recovery can still occur and is often associated with extensive physiotherapy, occupational and speech therapy, and/or cognitive rehabilitation.

This module will focus on examining the treatments that are currently available and on techniques that hold promise for maximizing functional recovery following brain damage. However, as we learned in the previous module, it should be possible (at least in theory) to replace damaged neurons, which should be accompanied by functional recovery. Therefore, this module will also explain some experimental treatments that show much promise for the repair and/or replacement of dead neurons.

Rehabilitation

Following brain damage, rehabilitation is one of the most readily available treatments, typically occurring once the acute phase of the injury is past. Rehabilitation efforts are aimed at developing behavioral and cognitive strategies for dealing with deficits and are often individually tailored to the specific client. The goal of rehabilitation is to enhance effective functioning in daily activities. This can be as simple as retraining individuals to ensure competence in self-care (e.g., bathing and grooming) or as involved as retraining individuals for work experience. Common methods of rehabilitation include training individuals to do the following:

1. Avoid situations in which they may experience difficulty.
2. Find different behaviors to replace lost ones.
3. Rely on remaining skills to accomplish tasks.
4. Use errorless learning techniques to improve learning situations.

Furthermore, it is important to ensure that their families have adequate support, training, and counseling to effectively deal with the behavioral changes that may result from brain injury (Fawcett et al., 2001).

Regardless of the goals of rehabilitation, what evidence is there that rehabilitation techniques are effective in helping individuals cope with, and overcome, the functional consequences of their injury? What are the likely mechanisms underlying recovery of function that is achieved through rehabilitation?

Before we can consider whether or not rehabilitation is effective, we need to consider the process of behavioral or functional recovery. For instance, although many of the functional gains that are achieved with rehabilitation can be attributed to compensation (new behaviors replacing impaired ones), some degree of functional recovery can be attributed to remaining neural plasticity. Recall from the previous module that the degree of recovery exhibited by rats that were lesioned in adulthood was associated with the degree to which dendritic arborization occurred (reorganization). Thus, simple substitution of intact behaviors for ones that were lost (compensation) is not likely to account for the complete spectrum of recovery that is observed. Thus, the experiences that are provided in rehabilitation exhibit superficial similarity with enriched environments, suggesting that rehabilitation itself may alter the course of recovery.

As was hypothesized, many brain-damaged individuals learn to perform tasks differently using compensatory mechanisms, as well as frequently exhibiting partial recovery of the impaired function (Fawcett et al., 2001). In fact, Kolb and Gibb (1999) suggest that compensatory mechanisms are dissociable from true recovery of function. Furthermore, Kolb and Gibb (1999) hypothesize that small lesions result in recovery of function through participation of proximal neural circuits. By contrast, larger lesions result in the loss of circuits that could participate in recovery, and the brain must rely on different mechanisms to achieve functional recovery.

Kolb and Gibb (1999) suggest that larger lesions result in only partial recovery that is mainly the result of behavioral and neural compensation. Presumably, recovery from larger lesions is mediated by the processes that underlie cortical reorganization. Studies in a variety of species, including humans, support this hypothesis. For instance, two groups of monkeys were given unilateral motor cortex lesions for the areas representing their wrist, forearm, and digits. Monkeys that were forced to use their affected arm and hand exhibited some recovery of function as well as some sparing of the motor cortex for these areas. Monkeys that were not forced to use their affected arm exhibited no such behavioral or cortical sparing (Nudo & Milliken, 1996). Similar effects have been observed in humans who exhibit hemiparesis following brain injury (Taub et al., 1993). That is, individuals who continued physical therapy for their affected arm for two years following injury exhibited greater improvement than did those who terminated physiotherapy. Together, these results suggest that there are elements of cortical reorganization and compensation that underlie improvements in motor function. In addition, these types of improvements have been observed for functions including language, perception, memory, and other cognitive skills (e.g., McGlynn, 1990; Ottenbacher & Jannell, 1993).

Assessment of the effectiveness of rehabilitation techniques must take into account the different categories of behavioral change that can occur following brain injury—those involving the loss of an ability (e.g., aphasia) and those involving the addition of new, often unwanted behaviors (e.g., loss of social inhibitions). These types of behaviors may be differentially susceptible to recovery. Thus, any evaluation of rehabilitation programs may be affected by the types of behaviors that are monitored. There is also evidence to suggest that the age of the person and the type and degree of impairment can affect the degree to which rehabilitation is effective. Thus, although there was variation (e.g., one study reported improved function for only 65% of the studied individuals) in the degree to which rehabilitation improved function, it does appear that rehabilitation programs can positively affect the effects of brain damage. The mechanisms of this recovery are only now beginning to be understood. However, preliminary results suggest that both compensation and reorganization of remaining brain areas are responsible for recovery following rehabilitation (e.g., Chollet, DiPiero, Wise, Brooks, Dolan, & Frakowiak, 1991). Finally, it should be emphasized that rehabilitative efforts are relatively new, and controlled studies of their effectiveness are only now beginning.

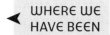 Techniques in rehabilitation are frequently associated with some degree of functional recovery. However, the degree of functional recovery appears to be associated with the size and location of the lesion. Small lesions may promote functional recovery through enhanced dendritic sprouting and cortical reorganization of adjacent areas. Large lesions typically involve some type of behavioral and neural compensation, rather than simple cortical reorganization.

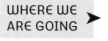 The next section will investigate the pros and cons of neural transplantation. Following that, treatments involving the use of stem cells, genetic therapy, and therapeutic drugs will be discussed.

Transplantation

When an organ is damaged beyond its ability to repair itself, transplantation of the affected organ is often the viable medical option. Although we have learned that the brain has a limited capability for repair, there are still a number of situations in which this is not likely to be effective. For instance, brain damage that results in the complete loss of a complete population of neurons is a situation in which the remaining areas are unlikely to be able to reorganize or compensate for the lost neurons. Similarly, diseases that are marked by progressive neural loss (e.g., Alzheimer's disease), also result in widespread brain damage that cannot be compensated for. It may be preferable in these situations to examine the feasibility of transplanting neural tissue into the CNS to replace the tissue that has been lost.

Unlike the rest of the body, the brain is an immune-protected site, which means that the brain is separate from the immune system that is active in the rest of the body. As such, the brain cannot undertake the same sorts of immune responses that characterize transplantation of other organs, which may lead to rejection of the tissue. Thus, one major hurdle of standard organ transplants—prevention of organ rejection—is avoided in the brain. However, other significant challenges remain; including providing an adequate supply of blood to the transplanted tissue, ensuring the survival of transplanted tissue, and ensuring that the transplanted tissue forms functional connections with the CNS. These challenges are made more difficult by the negative environment of the adult CNS, which typically does not permit regeneration. As we will see, successful transplantation relies on the age and type of transplanted tissue and on the location of the tissue graft within the CNS (the location must provide metabolic support for the graft). Successfully transplanted tissue tends to be fetal tissue that is suspended in solution and injected into the striatum. Fetal neural tissue is predisposed to seek out targets to enervate, and it is this property of embryonic tissue that is exploited in transplantation.

To date, much of the work involving transplanted neural tissue has been to graft dopaminergic neural tissue into the CNS of individuals with Parkinson's disease. Recall from Chapter 6 that Parkinson's disease is characterized by the loss of dopaminergic neurons that originate in the substantia nigra and project to the striatum. On the basis of techniques developed in rats by Bjorklund and colleagues (e.g., Bjorklund, Schmidt, & Stenevi, 1980), several hundred humans who are affected by Parkinson's disease have received transplanted neural tissue. Although other types of transplants are available, most individuals receive stereotaxic injections of embryonic brain tissue into their caudate nucleus or putamen. In the very best of cases, individuals are able to resume independent life and go off the medication that was used to treat Parkinson's disease (e.g., Lindvall, 2000). Imaging studies of these individuals demonstrate that there are progressive changes in their dopaminergic function and that there is often substantial reinnervation of the brain by the grafted tissue (Lindvall, 2000). At the very least, over two thirds of treated individuals experience clinically significant improvements in their response to medication and motor function (Lindvall, 2000).

Currently, this treatment is only experimental, and research is focused on improving transplantation techniques as well as understanding why improvements are not observed for all treated individuals (Lindvall, 2000). However, there is the possibility that with improvements, this technique will change from a treatment to a cure for Parkinson's disease. In addition, the techniques that are used in transplanting neural tissue may be applicable to other neurodegenerative diseases, raising the possibility that transplantation may be an effective treatment for these diseases as well.

Stem Cells

As you learned at the beginning of this module, the adult brain is capable of limited neurogenesis in specific locations of the brain. This neurogenesis is accomplished through existing progenitor or stem cells that are located within the lateral ventricles and hippocampus. The role of these stem or progenitor cells is unknown, although research by Gage has related the number of new neurons in the hippocampus to experience, suggesting a role in learning (Gage, 2002). However, stem or progenitor cells do not appear to play a significant role in the genesis of new neurons at the site of damage. Despite the lack of self-repair within the adult CNS, a tremendous amount of research is being conducted into the application of exogenously derived stem cells to repair damage. Stem cells are **multipotential**—that is, they have the ability to differentiate into different types of neurons and glia—and have the ability to replicate themselves. Unlike neurons in the adult nervous system, stem cells can continue to make new copies of themselves. These properties of stem cells are very attractive and may hold the key to repairing damage within the CNS.

Much of the research into stem cells is only at a preliminary stage. The goals of the research tend to revolve around whether or not stem cells can be divided indefinitely and how to control their differentiation into different types of neurons and glia. It seems likely that once these basic questions are understood, stems cells will have therapeutic value in the treatment of brain damage, most likely through transplantation into the CNS. For instance, hippocampal progenitor cells were transplanted into rats that had experienced ischemic damage to the hippocampus (Sinden, Stroemer, Grigoryan, Patel, French, & Hodges, 2000). The treated rats (the ones that received stem cell transplants) exhibited improvements in performance of the Morris water maze (a task that relies on hippocampal function). In addition, histology confirmed that these stem cells repopulated the areas of the hippocampus that were damaged by ischemia. Further studies have demonstrated that this type of recovery can be observed in other areas of the brain, including the motor cortex (Sinden et al., 2000) and basal ganglia (Svendsen, Clarke, Rosser, & Dunnett, 1996). However, it does appear that there are limits to the multipotentiality of stem or progenitor cells, as hippocampal progenitor cells were unable to reinnervate areas of the basal ganglia (Sinden et al., 2000). Thus, stem cells are an exciting area of research that shows much therapeutic promise for the treatment of brain damage.

Genetic Engineering

Many neurodegenerative diseases are based either entirely on genetic factors (e.g., Huntington's chorea) or have some genetic component (e.g., schizophrenia). In addition, cell death through apoptosis appears to have a genetic aspect, which may underlie changes that occur in the nervous system due to normal aging. **Genetic engineering** is the development of techniques that alter the genotype of cells (or complete organisms) that affect the expressed phenotype of the cell. When genetic engineering is applied to the treatment of a genetic disease of the nervous system, it has two main goals: the treatment of the affected individual and the prevention of the transmission of the disease to offspring. Specifically, the treatment of the affected individual may be accomplished either by blocking the expression of a faulty gene or by inserting a functional allele in place of the defective one. **Gene therapy** is related to genetic engineering, although gene therapy tends to focus on inserting genes that enhance the production of selected molecules (e.g., insulin) rather than the insertion or deletion

Current Controversy

Using Stem Cells and Fetal Tissue to Repair Damage

Before the transplantation of stem cells or embryonic brain tissue can proceed, the tissue must be obtained. Often, tissue for these techniques is obtained from human embryos, although stem cells can be retrieved from adult human brains after death. Typically, embryos are obtained from elective or spontaneous abortions and from embryos that were part of infertility treatments (e.g., in vitro fertilization) that are no longer needed. Because abortion is a contentious issue, many of the objections to stem cell research and the transplantation of embryonic tissue revolve around the question of when a human life begins. Although there are legal definitions of when human life begins, these definitions are not universally accepted. There is also concern that making use of aborted fetuses will provide an impetus for abortion. For instance, there have been cases in which babies were deliberately conceived so that they could be potential bone marrow donors for older siblings who were in need of a transplant. There is also the fear that scientists will create and harvest human embryos just for research.

There are also concerns over intellectual property rights. That is, if someone donates an embryo and this embryo is used to develop a cure for a disease, who should profit from the discovery? Currently, there are numerous patents on the human genome that have relied on the goodwill of unacknowledged donors. Furthermore, treatments involving stem cells or embryonic tissue are bound to be expensive and beyond the means of many of the donors. Therefore, within a health care system that does not provide universal accessibility, individuals who made these treatments possible may not themselves have access to them.

To address these concerns and others, guidelines for the use of stem cells and embryonic tissue are being developed in the United States. In Canada, guidelines for stem cell research have already been adopted. They emphasize the need for the donor to provide informed consent at two times: when the embryo is collected and again when the embryo is to be used for research. Included in the contract is the guarantee that the donors may change their mind as to the status of the use of the embryo in research. Furthermore, when embryos are obtained from abortion, the decision to have an abortion must be separated from the decision to donate tissue. When embryos are obtained from infertility treatments, there must not be pressure on the woman or the parents to have embryos created just for research. To avoid inadvertent coercion, neither the fertility specialist nor the physician who provides the abortion may take part in stem cell research. Individuals who donate embryos cannot be compensated in any form, either directly or indirectly. Genetic material from any other species cannot be placed in human embryos (as is the case with transgenic mice). Finally, the creation of embryos solely for research is prohibited, as is the creation of embryos by using cloning techniques. Although these guidelines do not solve the question of when human life begins, they do go a long way toward ensuring that some of the potential problems with stem cell research are avoided.

On August 9, 2001, President George W. Bush gave a speech announcing the position of the U.S. government on stem cell research. This quote statement nicely sums up the problems of stem cell research: "As I thought through this issue I kept returning to two fundamental questions. First, are these frozen embryos human life and therefore something precious to be protected? And second, if they're going to be destroyed anyway, shouldn't they be used for a greater good, for research that has the potential to save and improve other lives?"

---

of genes themselves. Gene therapy is thus able to bypass the problems that are associated with attempting to get certain types of molecules across the blood–brain barrier.

The major challenge to any form of gene therapy is to ensure that the genes are incorporated into the genome of the target cells in a stable fashion. Genes are typically inserted into the CNS or specific neurons using viruses, which are inherently good at using the machinery of the cell to reproduce themselves. Researchers remove the parts of the virus that make it produce disease and insert the copies of the genes (**transfection**) that they would like to infect a neuron with. Typically, neurons are infected with the mutated virus in vitro (outside of the nervous system), and neurons that express the changed genome can then be placed into suspension and placed back into the nervous system. Transfection of neurons can also be performed by injecting the virus directly into the CNS. Research in this area is only preliminary, although there has been success in using viruses to deliver genes to enhance the synthesis of dopamine in monkeys with damage to the basal ganglia (e.g., During et al., 1998) and to enhance the production of trophic factors (factors that enhance neuron growth) in nonhuman animals following damage to the CNS (e.g., Geschwind, Hartnick, Liu, Amat, Van De Water, & Federoff, 1996). Given this success, some researchers are planning to begin clinical trials with humans to test gene therapy as a treatment for Parkinson's disease (During, Kaplitt, Stern, & Eidelberg, 2001).

However, there are problems with gene therapy as it exists today. For instance, the expression of the infected genes often decreases back to baseline after a period of months in vivo (Fawcett et al., 2001). Other problems associated with transfection include low efficiency and toxicity. For instance, often only a small percentage of neurons exhibit the altered gene activity, suggesting that only a few neurons were successfully infected with the mutated virus. In addition, injections of the mutated virus are often quite toxic, which is thought to reflect an immune response produced in reaction to the virus. However, for currently incurable diseases that have a genetic component, gene therapy and genetic engineering offer new methods by which these diseases may be treated.

Self-Test

1. How is recovery of function following neuropsychological rehabilitation thought to occur? Is this recovery a unitary phenomenon?

2. Name two problems that are associated with each of the following techniques: (a) rehabilitation, (b) gene therapy, and (c) transplantation.

3. What are the properties of stem cells that make them attractive in transplantation?

4. What are the ethical concerns associated with the use of fetal tissue and stem cells?

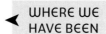

◄ **WHERE WE HAVE BEEN**   Techniques in rehabilitation are frequently associated with some degree of functional recovery. Techniques are also being developed that aim to treat brain damage by taking advantage of the properties of stem cells, fetal tissue, and viruses. Although most of these techniques are only experimental at the moment, they offer real hope for a cure.

Glossary

Apoptosis—Programmed neural death, whereby the neuron uses its own machinery, and thus cellular energy, to ensure its own death. Apoptosis is a feature of normal development of the neuron, typically regulated by genes, which trigger proteins known as caspases. Apoptosis can be initiated by damage to the DNA of the neuron, damage caused by free radicals, withdrawal of tropic factors required for normal development, or even the presence of nectrotic neurons nearby.

Collateral sprouting—A process by which undamaged neurons sprout new axon collaterals (side branches of axons) as a means to compensate for the permanent loss of a neuron.

Deprivation—The removal of something from the environment (e.g., loss of a limb).

Enrichment—The addition of something to the environment (e.g., educational experiences).

Excitotoxicity—The ability of specific compounds, such as glutamate, to both excite neurons and kill them.

Gene therapy—Related to genetic engineering, gene therapy tends to focus on inserting genes that enhance the production of selected molecules (e.g., insulin) rather than the insertion or deletion of genes themselves.

Genetic engineering—The development of techniques that alter the genotype of cells (or complete organisms) that affect the expressed phenotype of the cell.

Homeostasis—Regulation of a cell's internal environment.

Ischemia—A disruption in blood flow that often results from a stroke or cerebrovascular accident. It is associated with disruptions in the energy pathways of the neuron, which in turn can affect ion channels that are important for homeostasis in the neuron. Ischemia is a common cause of necrotic cell death.

Kennard effect—The ability of the young to recover from brain damage more thoroughly than adults, which has been observed in several species.

Lysis—A process of necrosis in which the cell membrane of the neuron breaks open, spilling the contents of the neuron into the extracellular space.

Multipotential—The ability of stem cells to differentiate into different types of neurons and glia.

Necrosis—A means by which neurons die, occurring when there is an overwhelming failure to maintain homeostasis within the neuron. It is always an abnormal event, often being associated with damage that occurs rapidly (e.g., tumors, meningitis) as well as with damage that accumulates more slowly (e.g., stroke/neurodegenerative diseases).

Neurogenesis—The formation of new neuronal cells. The neurons of the olfactory bulb and the neurons of the dentate gyrus of the hippocampus have recently been found to produce a limited number of new neurons, even in adulthood. However, stress and age have been found to be two limiting factors of neurogenesis.

Plasticity—The ability of the nervous system to change in response to events; collateral sprouting is an example of plasticity.

Primary neural death—The death of neurons that occurs immediately following trauma, appearing to occur when glutamate is released in excess, activating a cascade of events that leads to even more release of glutamate and even more excitation of the cell. Primary cell death can result from the neuron exhausting its resources and overwhelming homeostatic mechanisms.

Regenerative sprouting—An activity that only occurs in the PNS but not the CNS of mammals. This results in a permanent loss of structure and thus a permanent loss of function (paralysis below the site of injury) in the CNS.

Secondary neuronal death—The death of neurons following the primary event, resulting from a large-scale influx of calcium into the neuron.

Transfection—The process of removing the parts of the virus that make it produce disease while inserting copies of the genes with which the researcher would like to infect a neuron.

References

Abe, K. (2000). Cognitive function in amyotrophic lateral sclerosis. *Amyotrophic Lateral Sclerosis and Other Motor Neuron Disorders, 1*(5), 343–347.

Abe, K., Fujimura, H., Toyooka, K., Sakoda, S., Yorifuji, S., & Yanagihara, T. (1997). Cognitive function in amyotrophic lateral sclerosis. *Journal of the Neurological Sciences, 148*(1), 95–100.

Abrahams, S., Goldstein, L. H., Kew, J. J., Brooks, D. J., Lloyd, C. M., Frith, C. D., et al. (1996). Frontal lobe dysfunction in amyotrophic lateral sclerosis: A PET study. *Brain, 119*(Pt. 6), 2105–2120.

Acredolo. L. P. (1976). Frames of reference used by children for orientating in unfamiliar spaces. In G. Moore & R. Golledge (Eds.), *Environmental knowing* (pp. 165–172). Stroudsburg, PA: Dowden, Hutchinson, & Ross.

Adams, K. M. (1980). In search of Luria's battery: A false start. *Journal of Consulting and Clinical Psychology, 48*, 522–524.

Adolphs, R., Tranel, D., & Damasio, A. R. (1998). The human amygdala in social judgment. *Nature, 393*(6684), 470–474.

Adolphs, R., Tranel, D., Damasio, H., & Damasio, A. R. (1995). Fear and the human amygdala. *Journal of Neuroscience, 15*(9), 5879–5891.

Adolphs, R., Tranel, D., Hamann, S., Young, A. W., Calder, A. J., Phelps, E. A., et al. (1999). Recognition of facial emotion in nine individuals with bilateral amygdala damage. *Neuropsychologia, 37*(10), 1111–1117.

Aggleton, J. P., Bland, J. M., Kentridge, R. W., & Neave, N. J. (1994). Handedness and longevity: Archival study of cricketers. *British Medical Journal, 309*(6970), 1681–1684.

Aggleton, J. P., Kentridge, R. W., & Neave, N. J. (1993). Evidence for longevity differences between left handed and right handed men: An archival study of cricketers. *Journal of Epidemiology and Community Health, 47*(3), 206–209.

Aguirre, G. K., & D'Esposito, M. (1999). Topographical disorientation: A synthesis and taxonomy. *Brain, 122*(9), 1613–1628.

Akil, M., & Lewis, D. A. (1997). Cytoarchitecture of the entorhinal cortex in schizophrenia. *American Journal of Psychiatry, 154*(7), 1010–1012.

Albert, M. L. (1973). A simple test of visual neglect. *Neurology, 23*(6), 658–664.

Alcock, J. (2001). *Animal behavior: An evolutionary approach* (7th ed.). Sunderland, MA: Sinauer Associates.

Alison, A. (2001). Into the mind of a killer. *Nature, 410*(6826), 296–298.

Allain, P., Etcharry-Bouyx, F., & Le Gall, D. (2001). A case study of selective impairment of the central executive component of working memory after a focal frontal lobe damage. *Brain and Cognition, 45*(1), 21–43.

Altshuler, L. L., Conrad, A., Kovelman, J. A., & Scheibel, A. (1987). Hippocampal pyramidal cell orientation in schizophrenia: A controlled neurohistologic study of the Yakovlev collection. *Archives of General Psychiatry, 44*(12), 1094–1098.

Alvarado, M. C., & Bachevalier, J. (2000). Revisiting the maturation of medial temporal lobe memory functions in primates. *Learning and Memory, 7*(5), 244–256.

American Psychological Association. (1994). *Diagnostic and Statistical Manual of Mental Disorders* (4th ed., pp. 285–286). Washington, D.C.: Author.

Anderson, J. M., Gilmore, R., Roper, S., Crosson, B., Bauer, R. M., Nadeau, S., et al. (1999). Conduction aphasia and the arcuate fasciculus: A re-examination of the Wernicke-Geschwind model. *Brain and Language, 80*(1), 1–12.

Andreasen, N. C. (1999). Understanding the causes of schizophrenia. *New England Journal of Medicine, 340*(8), 645–647.

Andreasen, N. C. (2000). Schizophrenia: The fundamental questions. *Brain Research Review, 31*(2–3), 106–112.

Andres, P., & Van der Linden, M. (2001). Supervisory attentional system in patients with focal frontal lesions. *Journal of Clinical and Experimental Neuropsychology, 23*(2), 225–239.

Andrew, J. (1978). Laterality on the tapping test among legal offenders. *Journal of Clinical Child Psychology, 7*, 149–150.

Annegers, J. F., & Coan, S. P. (2000). The risks of epilepsy after traumatic brain injury. *Seizure, 9*(7), 453–457.

Annett, M. (1972). The distribution of manual asymmetry. *British Journal of Psychology, 63*(3), 343–358.

Annett, M. (1978). Genetic and nongenetic influences on handedness. *Behavior Genetics, 8*(3), 227–249.

Annett, M., & Kilshaw, D. (1984). Lateral preference and skill in dyslexics: Implications of the right shift theory. *Journal of Child Psychology and Psychiatry and Allied Disciplines, 25*(3), 357–377.

Annett, M., & Manning, M. (1990). Arithmetic and laterality. *Neuropsychologia, 28*(1), 61–69.

Appell, J., Kertesz, A., & Fisman, M. (1982). A study of language functioning in Alzheimer patients. *Brain and Language, 17*(1), 73–91.

Arffa, S., Lovell, M., Podell, K., & Goldberg, E. (1998). Wisconsin Card Sorting Test performance in above average and superior school children: Relationship to intelligence and age. *Archives of Clinical Neuropsychology, 13*(8), 713–720.

Armstrong, D. D. (2001). Rett syndrome neuropathology review, 2000. *Brain Development, 23*(S.1), S72–S76.

Arnold, M. B. (1960). *Emotion and personality. Volume I: Psychological aspects* (pp. xiv, 296). New York: Columbia University Press.

Asbjornsen, A. E., & Bryden, M. P. (1996). Biased attention and the fused dichotic words test. *Neuropsychologia, 34*(5), 407–411.

Asikainen, I., Kaste, M., & Sarna, S. (1999). Early and late posttraumatic seizures in traumatic brain injury rehabilitation patients: Brain injury factors causing late seizures and influence of seizures on long-term outcome. *Epilepsia, 40*(5), 584–589.

Asperger, H. (1944). Die autistischen Psychopathen im Kindersalter. Archiv fuer Psychiatrie und Nervenkrankheiten. *Journal of Autism, 15*(389), 117–176.

Asthana, H. S., & Mandal, M. K. (2001). Visual-field bias in the judgment of facial expression of emotion. *Journal of General Psychology, 128*(1), 21–29.

Astur, R. S., Ortiz, M. L., & Sutherland, R. J. (1998). A characterization of performance by men and women in a virtual Morris water task: A large and reliable sex difference. *Behavioural Brain Research, 93*(1–2), 185–190.

Augustine, J. R. (1996). Circuitry and functional aspects of the insular lobe in primates including humans. *Brain Research Reviews, 22*(3), 229–244.

Ay, H., Buonanno, F. S., Price, B. H., Le, D. A., & Koroschetz, W. J. (1998). Sensory alien hand syndrome: Case report and review of the literature. *Journal of Neurology, Neurosurgery and Psychiatry, 65*(3), 366–369.

Baddeley, A. D. (1998). *Human memory: Theory and practice* (2nd ed.). Boston: Allyn & Bacon.

Baddeley, A. D., Grant, S., Wight, E., & Thomson, N. (Eds.). (1975). *Imagery and visual working memory*. London, England: Academic Press.

Baddeley, A. D., & Hitch, G. (Eds.). (1974). *Working memory* (Vol. 8). Hillsdale, NJ: Lawrence Erlbaum.

Bailey, A., Le Couteur, A., Gottesman, I., Bolton, P., Simonoff, E., Yuzda, F. Y., et al. (1995). Autism as a strongly genetic disorder: Evidence from a British twin study. *Psychological Medicine, 25*, 63–77.

Bakan, P. (1991). Handedness and maternal smoking during pregnancy. *International Journal of Neuroscience, 56*(1–4), 161–168.

Bakan, P., Dibb, G., & Reed, P. (1973). Handedness and birth stress. *Neuropsychologia, 11*(3), 363–366.

Baker, E., Blumstein, S. E., & Goodglass, H. (1981). Interaction between phonological and semantic factors in auditory comprehension. *Neuropsychologia, 19*(1), 1–15.

Bakker, D. J., & Van der Kleij, P. C. M. (1978). Development of lateral asymmetry in the perception of sequentially touched fingers. *Acta Psychologica, 42*, 357–365.

Banich, M. (1997). *Neuropsychology: The mental bases of mental function*. New York: Houghton-Mifflin.

Banks, M. S., Aslin, R. N., & Letson, R. D. (1975). Sensitive period for the development of human binocular vision. *Science, 190*(4215), 675–677.

Bannister, R. (1992). Disorders of the cerebral circulation. In R. Bannister (Ed.), *Brain and Bannister's clinical neurology* (7th ed.). New York: Oxford University Press.

Barbur, J. L., Weiskrantz, L., & Harlow, J. A. (1999). The unseen color aftereffect of an unseen stimulus: Insight from blindsight into mechanisms of color afterimages. *Proceedings of the National Academy of Sciences of the United States of America, 96*(20), 11637–11641.

Barkley, R. A., DuPaul, G. J., McMurray, M. B. (1991). Attention deficit disorder with and without hyperactivity: Clinical response to three dose levels of methylphenidate. *Pediatrics, 87*(4), 519–531.

Baron-Cohen, S. (1995). *Mindblindness*. Cambridge, MA: MIT Press.

Baron-Cohen, S., Leslie, A. M., Frith, U. (1985). Does the autistic child have a "theory of mind"? *Cognition, 21*(1), 37–46.

Barrash, J. (1998). A historical review of topographical disorientation and its neuroanatomical correlates. *Journal of Clinical and Experimental Neuropsychology, 20*(6), 807–827.

Barrett, A. M., Schwartz, R. L., Crucian, G. P., Kim, M., & Heilman, K. M. (2000). Attentional grasp in far extrapersonal space after thalamic infarction. *Neuropsychologia, 38*(6), 778–784.

Bartels, A., & Zeki, S. (2000). The neural basis of romantic love. *Neuroreport, 11*(17), 3829–3834.

Barry, R. J., & James, A. L. (1978). Handedness in autistics, retardates, and normals of a wide age range. *Journal of Autism and Developmental Disorders, 8*(3), 315–323.

Bartl-Storck, C., & Mueller, G. (1999). Beeintraechtigung der Problemloesefaehigkeit bei Broca-Aphasie [Deficits in problem solving in patients with Broca's Aphasia]. *Sprache and Kognition, 18*(3–4), 98–112.

Bartol, C. (1999). *Criminal behavior: A psychosocial approach*. New Jersey: Prentice-Hall.

Baumann, B., & Bogerts, B. (2001). Neuroanatomical studies on bipolar disorder. *British Journal of Psychiatry, 41*(Suppl.), S142–S147.

Bavelier, D., Corina, D., Jezzard, P., Clark, V., Karni, A., Lalwani, A., et al. (1998). Hemispheric specialization for English and ASL: Left invariance-right variability. *Neuroreport, 9*(7), 1537–1542.

Bay, E. J. (2000). The biobehavioral correlates of posttraumatic brain injury depression. *Journal of Neuroscience Nursing, 32*(3), 169–176.

Beall, M. J., & Lewis, D. A. (1992). Heterogeneity of layer II neurons in human entorhinal cortex. *Journal of Comparative Neurology, 321*(2), 241–266.

Bear, M. F. (2001). *Neuroscience: Exploring the brain*. Baltimore: Lippincott Williams & Wilkins.

Bearden, C. E., Hoffman, K. M., & Cannon, T. D. (2001). The neuropsychology and neuroanatomy of bipolar affective disorder: A critical review. *Bipolar Disorders, 3*(3), 106–150, 151–153.

Beattie, O., & Geiger, J. (1987). *Frozen in time.* London, England: Bloomsbury.

Beaubrun, G., & Gray, G. E. (2000). A review of herbal medicines for psychiatric disorders. *Psychiatric Services, 51*(9), 1130–1134.

Beaumont, J. G. (1996). Neuropsychology. In J. G. Beaumont, P. M. Kenealy, & M. J. Rogers (Eds.), *The Blackwell dictionary of neuropsychology.* Oxford, UK: Blackwell Publishers.

Beauvois, M. F., & Saillant, B. (1985). Optic aphasia for colours and colour agnosia: A distinction between visual and visuo-verbal impairments in the processing of colours. *Cognitive Neuropsychology, 2*(1), 1–48.

Beisteiner, R., Windischberger, C., Lanzenberger, R., Edward, V., Cunnington, R., Erdler, M., et al. (2001). Finger somatotopy in human motor cortex. *Neuroimage, 13*(6, Pt. 1), 1016–1026.

Belliveau, J. W., Kennedy, D. N., Jr., McKinstry, R. C., Buchbinder, B. R., Weisskoff, R. M., Cohen, M. S., et al. (1991). Functional mapping of the human visual cortex by magnetic resonance imaging. *Science, 254*(5032), 716–719.

Bemporad, B., & Kinsbourne, M. (1983). Sinistrality and dyslexia: A possible relationship between subtypes. *Topics in Learning and Learning Disabilities, 3*(1), 48–65.

Benbow, C. P. (1986). Physiological correlates of extreme intellectual precocity. *Neuropsychologia, 24*(5), 719–725.

Benbow, C. P. (1988). Sex differences in mathematical reasoning ability in intellectually talented preadolescents: Their nature, effects, and possible causes. *Behavioral and Brain Sciences, 11*(2), 169–232.

Benbow, C. P., & Stanley, J. C. (1980). Sex differences in mathematical ability: Fact or artifact? *Science, 210*(4475), 1262–1264.

Benedict, R. H., Bakshi, R., Simon, J. H., Priore, R., Miller, C., & Munschauer, F. (2002). Frontal cortex atrophy predicts cognitive impairment in multiple sclerosis. *Journal of Neuropsychiatry and Clinical Neuroscience, 14*(1), 44–51.

Benson, D. F. (1984). Alexia and the neural basis of reading. *Annals of Dyslexia, 34,* 3–13.

Benson, D. F. (1996). Alexia. In J. G. Beaumont, P. M. Kenealy, & M. J. C. Rogers (Eds.), *The Blackwell dictionary of neuropsychology* (pp. 128–133). Cambridge, MA: Blackwell Publishers.

Benson, D. F., Gardner, H., & Meadows, J. C. (1976). Reduplicative paramnesia. *Neurology, 26*(2), 147–151.

Benson, D. F., & Greenberg, J. P. (1969). Visual form agnosia: A specific defect in visual discrimination. *Archives of Neurology, 20*(1), 82–89.

Benson, D. F., Sheremata, W. A., Bouchard, R., Segarra, J. M., Price, D., & Geschwind, N. (1973). Conduction aphasia. A clinicopathological study. *Archives of Neurology, 28*(5), 339–346.

Benton, A. L., Hamsher, K. D., Varney, N. R., & Spreen, O. (1983). *Contributions to neuropsychological assessment: A clinical manual.* New York: Oxford University Press.

Benton, A. L., & Meyers, R. (1956). An early description of the Gerstmann syndrome. *Neurology, 6,* 838–842.

Berardi, N., Pizzorusso, T., & Maffei, L. (2000). Critical periods during sensory development. *Current Opinion in Neurobiology, 10*(1), 138–145.

Berardi, N., Pizzorusso, T., Ratto, G. M., & Maffei, L. (2003). Molecular basis of plasticity in the visual cortex. *Trends in Neuroscience, 26*(7), 369–378.

Berk, L. (2003). *Development through the lifespan: International edition* (3rd ed.). Boston: Allyn and Bacon.

Berthier, M. L. (1995). Transcortical sensory aphasia: Dissociation between naming and comprehension. *Aphasiology, 9*(5), 431–451.

Berthier, M. L. (1999). *Transcortical aphasias.* Hove, England: Psychology Press/Taylor and Francis.

Berthier, M. L., Starkstein, S. E., Leiguarda, R., Ruiz, A., Mayberg, H. S., Wagner, H., et al. (1991). Transcortical aphasia. Importance of the nonspeech dominant hemisphere in language repetition. *Brain, 114*(Pt. 3), 1409–1427.

Bilder, R. M., Goldman, R. S., Robinson, D., Reiter, G., Bell, L., Bates, J. A., et al. (2000). Neuropsychology of first-episode schizophrenia: Initial characterization and clinical correlates. *American Journal of Psychiatry, 157,* 549–559.

Binkofski, F., Kunesch, E., Classen, J., Seitz, R. J., & Freund, H. J. (2001). Tactile apraxia. Unimodal apractic disorder of tactile object exploration associated with parietal lobe lesions. *Brain, 124*(1), 132–144.

Biro, V., & Novotny, I. (1991). On laterality in alcoholics: A probe study (P. Tkac, Trans.). *Studia Psychologica, 33*(3–4), 125–128.

Bisazza, A., Rogers, L. J., & Vallortigara, G. (1998). The origins of cerebral asymmetry: A review of evidence of behavioural and brain lateralization in fishes, reptiles and amphibians. *Neuroscience and Biobehavioral Reviews, 22*(3), 411–426.

Bishop, D. V. (1986). Is there a link between handedness and hypersensitivity? *Cortex, 22*(2), 289–296.

Bishop, K. M., & Wahlsten, D. (1997). Sex differences in the human corpus callosum: Myth or reality? *Neuroscience and Biobehavioral Reviews, 21*(5), 581–601.

Bisiach, E. (1988). The (haunted) brain and consciousness. In A. Marcel & E. Bisiach (Eds.), *Consciousness in contemporary science.* New York: Oxford University Press.

Bisiach, E. (1999). Unilateral neglect and related disorders. In G. Denes & L. Pizzamiglio (Eds.), *Handbook of clinical and experimental neuropsychology.* Hove, England: Psychology Press/Lawrence Erlbaum.

Bisiach, E., & Luzzatti, C. (1978). Unilateral neglect of representational space. *Cortex, 14*(1), 129–133.

Bjorklund, A., Schmidt, R. H., & Stenevi, U. (1980). Functional reinnervation of the neostriatum in the adult rat by use of intraparenchymal grafting of dissociated cell suspensions from the substantia nigra. *Cell Tissue Research, 212*(1), 39–45.

Black, D., Young, C. C., Pei, W. C., & de Chardin, T. (1933). Fossil man in China. *Memoirs of the Geological Survey, Series A, No. 11.*

Black, J. E. (1998). How a child builds its brain: Some lessons from animal studies of neural plasticity. *Preventive Medicine, 27*(2), 168–171.

Blair, R. J. R., Morris, J. S., Frith, C. C., Perrett, D. I., & Dolan, R. J. (1999). Dissociable neural responses to facial expressions of sadness and anger. *Brain, 122*(5), 883–893.

Blau, A. (1946). The master hand: A study of right and left sidedness and its relation to laterality and language. *American Orthopsychiatric Association Research Monographs (No. 5).*

Blest, A. D. (1957). The function of eye-spot patterns in the Lepidoptera. *Behavior, 11,* 257–309.

Blumberg, H. P., Stern, E., Martinez, D., Ricketts, S., de Asis, J., White, T., et al. (2000). Increased anterior cingulate and caudate activity in bipolar mania. *Biological Psychiatry, 48*(11), 1045–1052.

Blumenfeld, Z., Dirnfeld, M., Abramovici, H., Amit, A., Bronshtein, M., & Brandes, J. M. (1992). Spontaneous fetal reduction in multiple gestations assessed by transvaginal ultrasound. *British Journal of Obstetrics and Gynaecology, 99*(4), 333–337.

Bogaert, A. F. (1997). Genital asymmetry in men. *Human Reproduction, 12*(1), 68–72.

Bogen, J. E. (2000). Split-brain basics: Relevance for the concept of one's other mind. *Journal of the American Academy of Psychoanalysis, 28*(2), 341–369.

Bogerts, B. (1993). Recent advances in the neuropathology of schizophrenia. *Schizophrenia Bulletin, 19*(2), 431–445.

Bornstein, B. (1963). Prosopagnosia. In L. Halpern (Ed.), *Problems of dynamic neurology* (pp. 283–318). Jerusalem, Israel: Hadasseh Medical Organization.

Borod, J. C. (1992). Interhemispheric and intrahemispheric control of emotion: Focus on unilateral brain damage. *Journal of Consulting and Clinical Psychology, 60*(3), 339–348.

Borod, J. C., & Caron, H. S. (1980). Facedness and emotion related to lateral dominance, sex and expression type. *Neuropsychologia, 18,* 237–241.

Borod, J. C., Caron, H. S., & Koff, E. (1981). Asymmetry of facial expression related to handedness, footedness, and eyedness: A quantitative study. *Cortex, 17*(3), 381–390.

Borod, J. C., Haywood, C. S., & Koff, E. (1997). Neuropsychological aspects of facial asymmetry during emotional expression: A review of the normal adult literature. *Neuropsychology Review, 7*(1), 41–60.

Borod, J. C., Koff, E., & White, B. (1983). Facial asymmetry in posed and spontaneous expressions of emotion. *Brain and Cognition, 2*(2), 165–175.

Borod, J. C., Koff, E., Yecker, S., Santschi, C., & Schmidt, J. M. (1998). Facial asymmetry during emotional expression: Gender, valence, and measurement technique. *Neuropsychologia, 36*(11), 1209–1215.

Borod, J. C., St. Clair, J., Koff, E., & Alpert, M. (1990). Perceiver and poser asymmetries in processing facial emotion. *Brain and Cognition, 13*(2), 167–177.

Borod, J. C., Vingiano, W., & Cytryn, F. (1989). Neuropsychological factors associated with perceptual biases for emotional chimeric faces. *International Journal of Neuroscience, 45*(1–2), 101–110.

Bottini, G., Cappa, S., Geminiani, G., & Sterzi, R. (1990). Topographic disorientation: A case report. *Neuropsychologia, 28*(3), 309–312.

Botvinick, M., & Cohen, J. (1998). Rubber hands "feel" touch that eyes see. *Nature, 391*(6669), 756.

Bouchard, T. J., Jr., & Loehlin, J. C. (2001). Genes, evolution, and personality. *Behavior Genetics, 31*(3), 243–273.

Bouchard, T. J., Jr., & McGue, M. (2003). Genetic and environmental influences on human psychological differences. *Journal of Neurobiology, 54*(1), 4–45.

Boucher, J. (1977). Hand preference in autistic children and their parents. *Journal of Autism and Developmental Disorders, 7*(2), 177–187.

Boucher, J., Lewis, V., & Collis, G. (1990). Hand dominance of parents and other relatives of autistic children. *Developmental Medicine and Child Neurology, 32*(4), 304–313.

Bourin, M., Chue, P., & Guillon, Y. (2001). Paroxetine: A review. *CNS Drug Reviews, 7*(1), 25–47.

Bowers, D., & Heilman, K. M. (1980). Pseudoneglect: Effects of hemispace on a tactile line bisection task. *Neuropsychologia, 18*(4-sup-5), 491–498.

Brackenridge, C. J. (1981). Secular variation in handedness over ninety years. *Neuropsychologia, 19*(3), 459–462.

Bradbury, M. W. B. (1979). *The concept of a blood-brain barrier.* New York: John Wiley and Sons.

Bradshaw, J. L. (1996). Gail D. Poizner, Klima, and Bellugi's (1987) deaf agrammatic signer: Form and function in the specialisation of the left cerebral hemisphere for speech and language. In C. Code, C. W. Wallesh, Y. Joanette, et al. (Eds.), *Classic cases in neuropsychology.* East Sussex, England: Psychology Press.

Bradshaw, J. L., & Mattingley, J. B. (1995). *Clinical neuropsychology: Behavioral and brain science.* San Diego, CA: Academic Press.

Bradshaw, J. L., & Nettleton, N. C. (1983). *Human Cerebral Asymmetry.* Engelwood Cliffs, NJ: Prentice-Hall.

Brauen, W. (1891). Zeitschrift für Anatomie und Entwicklungsgeschichte. *Arch. f. Anatomie, 253.*

Braun, A. R., Balkin, T. J., Wesensten, N. J., Gwadry, F., Carson, R. E., Varga, M., et al. (1998). Dissociated pattern of activity in visual cortices and their projections during human rapid eye movement sleep. *Science, 279*(5347), 91–95.

Brent, E., Rios, P., Happe, F., & Charman, T. (2004). Performance of children with autism spectrum disorder on advanced theory of mind tasks. *Autism, 8*(3), 283–299.

Brinton, D. (1896). Left-handedness in North American aboriginal art. *American Anthropologist, 9*, 175–181.

Brinton, R. D. (2001). Cellular and molecular mechanisms of estrogen regulation of memory function and neuroprotection against Alzheimer's disease: Recent insights and remaining challenges. *Learning Memory, 8*(3), 121–133.

Brito-Marques, P. R., Mello, R. V., & Montenegro, L. (2001). Classic Pick's disease type with ubiquitin-positive and tau-negative inclusions: Case report. *Arq Neuropsiquiatr, 59*(1), 128–133.

Broca, P. (1865). Sur le siège de la faculté du language articulé. *Bulletins et Mémoires de la Société d'Anthropologie, 6*, 337–393.

Broca, P. (1875). Sur les trous parietaux et sur la perforation congenitale, double et symmetrique des parietaux. *Bull. Soc. Anthrop. Paris, Sér, 2*(10), 326.

Broca, P. (1876). Sur les trépanations préhistoriques. *Bull. Soc. Anthrop. Paris, Sér, 2*(11), 236, 431.

Broca, P. (1965). On the speech center. In R. J. Herrnstein & E. G. Boring (Eds.), *A source book in the history of psychology* (M. D. Boring, Trans.) (pp. 223–229). Cambridge, MA: Harvard University Press. (Original work published in 1861)

Brooks, L. R. (1967). The suppression of visualization by reading. *Quarterly Journal of Experimental Psychology, 19*(4), 289–299.

Brown, J. (1958). Some tests of the decay theory of immediate memory. *Quarterly Journal of Experimental Psychology, 10*, 12–21.

Brown, J. W. (1975). The problem of repetition: A study of "conduction" aphasia and the "isolation" syndrome. *Cortex, 11*(1), 37–52.

Brown, J. W. (1988). *Agnosia and apraxia: Selected papers of Liepmann, Lange, & Potzl.* Hillsdale, NJ: Lawrence Erlbaum.

Brown, P., Will, R. G., Bradley, R., Asher, D. M., & Detwiler, L. (2001). Bovine spongiform encephalopathy and variant Creutzfeldt-Jakob disease: Background, evolution, and current concerns. *Emerging Infectious Diseases, 7*(1), 6–16.

Brown, S., & Nicholls, M. E. (1997). Hemispheric asymmetries for the temporal resolution of brief auditory stimuli. *Perception and Psychophysics, 59*(3), 442–447.

Bruder, G. E., Quitkin, F. M., Stewart, J. W., Martin, C., Voglmaier, M. M., & Harrison, W. M. (1989). Cerebral laterality and depression: Differences in perceptual asymmetry among diagnostic subtypes. *Journal of Abnormal Psychology, 98*, 177–186.

Brunner, D., & Hen, R. (1997). Insights into the neurobiology of impulsive behavior from serotonin receptor knockout mice. *Annals of the New York Academy of Science, 836*, 81–105.

Brunner, H. G., Nelen, M., Breakefield, X. O., Ropers, H. H., & van Oost, B. A. (1993). Abnormal behavior associated with a point mutation in the structural gene for monoamine oxidase A. *Science, 262*(5133), 578–580.

Bryden, M. P., & MacRae, L. (1988). Dichotic laterality effects obtained with emotional words. *Neuropsychiatry, Neuropsychology, and Behavioral Neurology, 1*(3), 171–176.

Bryden, M. P., McManus, I. C., & Bulman-Fleming, M. B. (1994). Evaluating the empirical support for the Geschwind-Behan-Galaburda model of cerebral lateralization. *Brain and Cognition, 26*(2), 103–167.

Buchanan, T. W., Lutz, K., Mirzazade, S., Specht, K., Shah, N. J., Zilles, K., et al. (2000). Recognition of emotional prosody and verbal components of spoken language: An fMRI study. *Cognitive Brain Research, 9*(3), 227–238.

Budiansky, S. (1998). *If a lion could talk: Animal intelligence and the evolution of consciousness.* New York: The Free Press.

Bull, R., & Scerif, G. (2001). Executive functioning as a predictor of children's mathematics ability: Inhibition, switching, and working memory. *Developmental Neuropsychology, 19*(3), 273–93.

Bulman-Fleming, M. B., & Bryden, M. P. (1994). Simultaneous verbal and affective laterality effects. *Neuropsychologia, 32*(7), 787–797.

Burgess, P. W., & Shallice, T. (1996a). Bizarre responses, rule detection and frontal lobe lesions. *Cortex, 32*(2), 241–259.

Burgess, P. W., & Shallice, T. (1996b). Response suppression, initiation and strategy use following frontal lobe lesions. *Neuropsychologia, 34*(4), 263–272.

Burton, L. A., Wagner, N., Lim, C., & Levy, J. (1992). Visual field differences for clockwise and counterclockwise mental rotation. *Brain and Cognition, 18*, 192–207.

Buss, D. M. (1999). *Evolutionary psychology: The new science of the mind.* Boston: Allyn & Bacon.

Calvin, W. H. (1983). A stone's throw and its launch window: Timing precision and its implications for language and hominid brains. *Journal of Theoretical Biology, 104*(1), 121–135.

Calvin, W. H. (2002). *A brain for all seasons: Human evolution and abrupt climate change.* Chicago: University of Chicago Press.

Cammalleri, R., Gangitano, M., D'Amelio, M., Raieli, V., Raimondo, D., & Camarda, R. (1996). Transient topographical amnesia and cingulate cortex damage: A case report. *Neuropsychologia, 34*(4), 321–326.

Campain, R., & Minckler, J. (1976). A note on the gross configurations of the human auditory cortex. *Brain and Language, 3*(2), 318–323.

Cannon, W. B. (1927). The James-Lange theory of emotions. *American Journal of Psychology, 39,* 115–124.

Cappa, S. F., & Vignolo, L. A. (1999). The neurological foundations of language. In G. Denes & L. Pizzamiglio (Eds.), *Handbook of clinical and experimental neuropsychology.* Hove, England: Psychology Press/Taylor and Francis.

Capruso, D. X., & Levin, H. S. (1992). Cognitive impairment following closed head injury. *Neurologic Clinics, 10*(4), 879–893.

Carlson, N. R. (2001). *Physiology of behavior.* Toronto, Canada: Allyn & Bacon.

Carlson, S., Martinkauppi, S., Rama, P., Salli, E., Korvenoja, A., & Aronen, H. J. (1998). Distribution of cortical activation during visuospatial n-back tasks as revealed by functional magnetic resonance imaging. *Cerebral Cortex, 8*(8), 743–752.

Carmon, A., & Bechtoldt, H. P. (1969). Dominance of the right cerebral hemisphere for stereopsis. *Neuropsychologia, 7*(1), 29–39.

Carr, D. B., Goate, A., & Morris, J. C. (1997). Current concepts in the pathogenesis of Alzheimer's disease. *American Journal of Medicine, 103*(3A), 3S–10S.

Carter-Saltzman, L. (1980). Biological and sociocultural effects on handedness: Comparison between biological and adoptive families. *Science, 209*(4462), 1263–1265.

Cayre, M., Malaterre, J., Scotto-Lomassese, S., Strambi, C., & Strambi, A. (2002). The common properties of neurogenesis in the adult brain: From invertebrates to vertebrates. *Comparative Biochemistry and Physiology B, Biochemistry Molecular Biology, 132*(1), 1–15.

Center for Disease Control. (1996). *Vital and Health Statistics Series, 10*(200), 82.

Chamberlain, H. D. (1928). Inheritance of left-handedness. *Journal of Heredity, 19,* 557–559.

Chan, J. L., & Liu, A. B. (1999). Anatomical correlates of alien hand syndromes. *Neuropsychiatry, Neuropsychology, and Behavioral Neurology, 12*(3), 149–155.

Chang, L. (1995). In vivo magnetic resonance spectroscopy in HIV and HIV-related brain diseases. *Reviews in the Neurosciences, 6*(4), 365–378.

Chang, L. K., Putcha, G. V., Deshmukh, M., & Johnson, E. M. (2002). Mitochondrial involvement in the point of no return in neuronal apoptosis. *Biochimie, 84*(2–3), 223–231.

Chase, C., Ware, J., Hittelman, J., Blasini, I., Smith, R., Llorente, A., et al. (2000). Early cognitive and motor development among infants born to women infected with human immunodeficiency virus. *Pediatrics, 106*(2), E25.

Chenery, H. J., Murdoch, B. E., & Ingram, J. C. L. (1996). An investigation of confrontation naming performance in Alzheimer's dementia as a function of disease severity. *Aphasiology, 10*(5), 423–441.

Cherry, E. C. (1953). Some experiments on the recognition of speech, with one and two ears. *Journal of the Acoustical Society of America, 25,* 975–979.

Choi, D. W. (1992). Excitotoxic cell death. *Journal of Neurobiology, 23*(9), 1261–1276.

Chollet, F., DiPiero, V., Wise, R. J., Brooks, D. J., Dolan, R. J., & Frackowiak, R. S. (1991). The functional anatomy of motor recovery after stroke in humans: A study with positron emission tomography. *Annals of Neurology, 29*(1), 63–71.

Chong, S. A., Mahendran, R., Machin, D., Chua, H. C., Parker, G., & Kane, J. (2002). Tardive dyskinesia among Chinese and Malay patients with schizophrenia. *Journal of Clinical Psychopharmacology, 22*(1), 26–30.

Christensen, J. M., & Sacco, P. R. (1989). Association of hair and eye color with handedness and stuttering. *Journal of Fluency Disorders, 14,* 37–45.

Christensens, A. L. (1979). *Luria's neuropsychological investigation* (2nd ed.). Copenhagen, Denmark: Munksgard.

Chugani, H. T. (1998). A critical period of brain development: Studies of cerebral glucose utilization with PET. *Preventive Medicine, 27*(2), 184–188.

Clarke, A. R., Jackson, G. S., & Collinge, J. (2001). The molecular biology of prion propagation. *Philosophical Transactions of the Royal Society of London Series B: Biological Sciences, 356*(1406), 185–195.

Clementz, B. A., Iacono, W. G., & Beiser, M. (1994). Handedness in first-episode psychotic patients and their first-degree biological relatives. *Journal of Abnormal Psychology, 103*(2), 400–403.

Coccaro, E. F., Bergeman, C. S., & McClearn, G. E. (1993). Heritability of irritable impulsiveness: A study of twins reared together and apart. *Psychiatry Research, 48*(3), 229–242.

Cockayne, E. A. (1938). The genetics of transposition of vicera. *Quarterly Journal of Medicine, 31,* 479–493.

Cohen, L. G., Celnik, P., Pascual-Leone, A., Corwell, B., Falz, L., Dambrosia, J., et al. (1997). Functional relevance of cross-modal plasticity in blind humans. *Nature, 389*(6647), 180–183.

Cohen, M. J., Ricci, C. A., Kibby, M. Y., & Edmonds, J. E. (2000). Developmental progression of clock face drawing in children. *Neuropsychology Development and Cognition Section C, Child Neuropsychology, 6*(1), 64–76.

Cohen, M. S., Kosslyn, S. M., Breiter, H. C., DiGirolamo, G. J., Thompson, W. L., Anderson, A. K., et al. (1996). Changes in cortical activity during mental rotation. A mapping study using functional MRI. *Brain, 119*(Pt. 1), 89–100.

Colby, C. L., Duhamel, J. R., & Goldberg, M. E. (1995). Oculocentric spatial representation in parietal cortex. *Cerebral Cortex, 5*(5), 470–481.

Collette, F., Van der Linden, M., Delfiore, G., Degueldre, C., Luxen, A., & Salmon, E. (2001). The functional anatomy of inhibition processes investigated with the hayling task. *Neuroimage, 14*(2), 258–267.

Corballis, M. C. (1991). *The lopsided ape.* New York: Oxford University Press.

Corballis, M. C. (2002). *From hand to mouth: The origins of language.* Princeton, NJ: Princeton University Press.

Coren, S. (1989). Left-handedness and accident-related injury risk. *American Journal of Public Health, 79*(8), 1040–1041.

Coren, S. (1994). Twinning is associated with an increased risk of left-handedness and inverted writing hand posture. *Early Human Development, 40*(1), 23–27.

Coren, S. (1995). Differences in divergent thinking as a function of handedness and sex. *American Journal of Psychology, 108*(3), 311–325.

Coren, S., & Halpern, D. F. (1991). Left-handedness: A marker for decreased survival fitness. *Psychological Bulletin, 109*(1), 90–106.

Coren, S., & Halpern, D. F. (1993). A replay of the baseball data. *Perceptual and Motor Skills, 76*(2), 403–406.

Coren, S., & Porac, C. (1977). Fifty centuries of right-handedness: The historical record. *Science, 198,* 631–632.

Coren, S., & Searleman, A. (1987). Left sidedness and sleep difficulty: The alinormal syndrome. *Brain and Cognition, 6*(2), 184–192.

Cornelissen, P., Richardson, A., Mason, A., Fowler, S., & Stein, J. (1995). Contrast sensitivity and coherent motion detection measured at photopic luminance levels in dyslexics and controls. *Vision Research, 35,* 1483–1494.

Cornette, L., Dupont, P., Rosier, A., Sunaert, S., Van Hecke, P., Michiels, J., et al. (1998). Human brain regions involved in direction discrimination. *Journal of Neurophysiology, 79*(5), 2749–2765.

Corteen, R. S., & Wood, B. (1972). Autonomic responses to shock-associated words in an unattended channel. *Journal of Experimental Psychology, 94*(3), 308–313.

Cosi, V., Citterio, A., & Pasquino, C. (1988). A study of hand preference in myasthenia gravis. *Cortex, 24*(4), 573–577.

Coslett, H. B. (1997). Consciousness and attention. *Seminars in Neurology, 17*(2), 137–144.

Coslett, H. B., Bowers, D., & Heilman, K. M. (1987). Reduction in cerebral activation after right hemisphere stroke. *Neurology, 37*(6), 957–962.

Cotzias, G. C., Papavasiliou, P. S., & Gellene, R. (1969). Modification of Parkinsonism: Chronic treatment with L-Dopa. *New England Journal of Medicine, 280*(7), 337–345.

Cowey, A., & Stoerig, P. (1991). The neurobiology of blindsight. *Trends in Neurosciences, 14*(4), 140–145.

Cowey, A., & Wilkinson, F. (1991). The role of the corpus callosum and extra striate visual areas in stereoacuity in macaque monkeys. *Neuropsychologia, 29*(6), 465–479.

Craddock, N., Dave, S., & Greening, J. (2001). Association studies of bipolar disorder. *Bipolar Disorders, 3*(6), 284–298.

Crawford, J. R., Stewart, L. E., Cochrane, R. H., Foulds, J. A., Besson, J. A., & Parker, D. M. (1989). Estimating premorbid IQ from demographic variables: Regression equations derived from a UK sample. *Br J Clin Psychol, 28*(Pt. 3), 275–278.

Crichton-Browne, J. (1880). A plea for the minute study of mania. *Brain, 81,* 347–362.

Crick, F., & Koch, C. (1990). Some reflections on visual awareness. *Cold Spring Harbor symposia on quantitative biology, 55,* 953–962.

Culver, C. M. (1969). Test of right-left discrimination. *Perceptual and Motor Skills, 29*(3), 863–867.

Cynader, M., & Regan, D. (1978). Neurones in cat parastriate cortex sensitive to the direction of motion in three-dimensional space. *Journal of Physiology, 274,* 549–569.

Damasio, A. (1999). *The feeling of what happens: Body and emotion in the making of consciousness.* San Diego, CA: Harcourt.

Damasio, A. R. (1989). Time-locked multiregional retroactivation: A systems-level proposal for the neural substrates of recall and recognition. *Cognition, 33*(1–2), 25–62.

Damasio, A. R. (1994). *Descartes' error. Emotion, reason and the human brain.* New York: G. P. Putnam's Sons.

Damasio, A. R., Bellugi, U., Damasio, H., Poizner, H., & Van Gelder, J. (1986). Sign language aphasia during left-hemisphere Amytal injection. *Nature, 322*(6077), 363–365.

Damasio, A. R., Damasio, H., & Van Hoesen, G. W. (1982). Prosopagnosia: Anatomic basis and behavioral mechanisms. *Neurology, 32*(4), 331–341.

Damasio, H. (1998). Neuroanatomical correlates of the aphasias. In M. T. Sarno (Ed.), *Acquired Aphasia.* San Diego, CA: Academic Press.

Damasio, H., & Damasio, A. R. (1980). The anatomical basis of conduction aphasia. *Brain, 103*(2), 337–350.

Damasio, H., Grabowski, T., Frank, R., Galaburda, A. M., & Damasio, A. R. (1994). The return of Phineas Gage: Clues about the brain from the skull of a famous patient. *Science, 264*(5162), 1102–1105.

Damasio, H., Grabowski, T. J., Tranel, D., Hichwa, R. D., & Damasio, A. R. (1996). A neural basis for lexical retrieval. *Nature, 380*(6574), 499–505.

Danta, G., Hiton, R. C., & O'Boyle, D. J. (1978). Hemispheric function and binocular depth perception. *Brain, 101,* 569–590.

Dart, R. A. (1949). The predatory implemental technique of Australopithicus. *American Journal of Physical Anthropology, 7,* 1–38.

Darwin, C. (1872). *The expression of the emotions in man and animals* (3rd ed). New York: Oxford University Press.

David, A., Malmberg, A., Lewis, G., Brandt, L., & Allebeck, P. (1995). Are there neurological and sensory risk factors for schizophrenia? *Schizophrenia Research, 14*(3), 247–251.

Davidoff, J. (1996). Lewandowsky's case of object-colour agnosia. In C. Code, C. W. Wallesh, Y. Joanette, et al. (Eds.), *Classic cases in neuropsychology* (pp. 349–361). East Sussex, UK: Psychology Press.

Davis, A., & Annett, M. (1994). Handedness as a function of twinning, age and sex. *Cortex, 30*(1), 105–111.

Dawson, T. M. (2000). Parkinson's disease: Clinical manifestations and treatment. *International Review of Psychiatry, 12*(4), 263–269.

Day, L. B., & MacNeilage, P. F. (1996). Postural asymmetries and language lateralization in humans (Homo sapiens). *Journal of Compararive Psychology, 110*(1), 88–96.

Deacon, T. (1997). *The symbolic species: The co-evolution of language and the human brain.* London, England: Penguin Press.

Decety, J., & Jeannerod, M. (1995). Mentally simulated movements in virtual reality: Does Fitts's law hold in motor imagery? *Behavioural Brain Research, 72*(1–2), 127–134.

Deiber, M. P., Passingham, R. E., Colebatch, J. G., Friston, K. J., Nixon, P. D., & Frackowiak, R. S. (1991). Cortical areas and the selection of movement: A study with positron emission tomography. *Experimental Brain Research, 84*(2), 393–402.

Déjerine, J. (1891). Sur un cas de cécité verbale agraphie, suive d'autopsie. *Mémoire de la Société Biologique, 3*, 197–201.

Déjerine, J. (1892). Contribution à l'étude anatomoclinique et clinique des différentes variéts de cécité verbale. *Mémoire de la Société Biologique, 4*, 61–90.

Delacour, J. (1995). An introduction to the biology of consciousness. *Neuropsychologia, 33*(9), 1061–1074.

Delaney, J. S., Lacroix, V. J., Leclerc, S., & Johnston, K. M. (2000). Concussions during the 1997 Canadian Football League season. *Clinical Journal of Sport Medicine, 10*(1), 9–14.

Delis, D. C., Robertson, L. C., & Efron, R. (1986). Hemispheric specialization of memory for visual hierarchical stimuli. *Neuropsychologia, 24*(2), 205–214.

Dellatolas, G., Annesi, I., Jallon, P., Chavance, M., & Lellouch, J. (1990). An epidemiological reconsideration of the Geschwind-Galaburda theory of cerebral lateralization. *Archives of Neurology, 47*(7), 778–782.

Dellatolas, G., Luciani, S., Castresana, A., Remy, C., Jallon, P., Laplane, D., et al. (1993). Pathological left-handedness: Left-handedness correlatives in adult epileptics. *Brain, 116*(Pt. 6), 1565–1574.

Denes, G. (1999). Disorders of body awareness and body knowledge. In G. Denes & L. Pizzamiglio (Eds.), *Handbook of clinical and experimental neuropsychology* (pp. 497–506). Hove, England: Psychology Press/Erlbaum.

Denes, G., Cappelletti, J. Y., Zilli, T., Porta, F. D., & Gallana, A. (2000). A category-specific deficit of spatial representation: The case of autotopagnosia. *Neuropsychologia, 38*(4), 345–350.

Dennis, W. (1958). Early graphic evidence of dextrality in man. *Pereceptual and Motor Skills, 8*, 147–149.

DeRenzi, E. (1985). Disorders of spatial orientation. In J. A. M. Frederiks (Ed.), *Handbook of clinical neurology* (Vol. 1)(45) (pp. 405–422). Amsterdam, the Netherlands: Elsevier Science Publishers.

DeRenzi, E. (1999). Agnosia. In G. Denes & L. Pizzamiglio (Eds.), *Handbook of clinical and experimental neuropsychology.* Hove, England: Psychology Press/Taylor and Francis.

DeRenzi, E., Faglioni, P., & Villa, P. (1977). Topographical amnesia. *Journal of Neurology, Neurosurgery and Psychiatry, 40*(5), 498–505.

DeRenzi, E., & Spinnler, H. (1967). Impaired performance on color tasks in patients with hemispheric damage. *Cortex, 3*(2), 194–217.

Desimone, R., Albright, T. D., Gross, C. G., & Bruce, C. (1984). Stimulus-selective properties of inferior temporal neurons in the macaque. *Journal of Neuroscience, 4*(8), 2051–2062.

Desimone, R., Schein, S. J., Moran, J., & Ungerleider, L. G. (1985). Contour, color and shape analysis beyond the striate cortex. *Vision Research, 25*(3), 441–452.

DeSousa, E. A., Albert, R. H., & Kalman, B. (2002). Cognitive impairments in multiple sclerosis: A review. *American Journal of Alzheimers Disease and Other Dementias, 17*(1), 23–29.

D'Esposito, M., Detre, J. A., Alsop, D. C., Shin, R. K., Atlas, S., & Grossman, M. (1995). The neural basis of the central executive system of working memory. *Nature, 378*(6554), 279–281.

Detwiler, L. A., & Rubenstein, R. (2000). Bovine spongiform encephalopathy: An overview. *Asaio Journal, 46*(6), S73–S79.

Deutsch, G., Bourbon, W. T., Papanicolaou, A. C., & Eisenberg, H. M. (1988). Visuospatial tasks compared via activation of regional cerebral blood flow. *Neuropsychologia, 26*, 445–452.

Deutsch, J. A., & Deutsch, D. (1963). Attention. Some theoretical considerations. *Psychological Review, 70*(1), 51–61.

DeYoe, E. A., Felleman, D. J., Van Essen, D. C., & McClendon, E. (1994). Multiple processing streams in occipitotemporal visual cortex. *Nature, 371*(6493), 151–154.

DeYoe, E. A., & Van Essen, D. C. (1988). Concurrent processing streams in monkey visual cortex. *Trends in Neurosciences, 11*(5), 219–226.

Diamond, A. S. (1959). *The history and origin of language.* London, England: Methuen.

diGiovanni, M., D'Alessandro, G., Baldini, S., Cantalupi, D., & Bottacchi, E. (1992). Clinical and neuroradiological findings in a case of pure word deafness. *Italian Journal of Neurological Sciences, 13*(6), 507–510.

Dikranian, K., Ishimaru, M. J., Tenkova, T., Labruyere, J., Qin, Y. Q., Ikonomidou, C., et al. (2001). Apoptosis in the in vivo mammalian forebrain. *Neurobiology of Disease, 8*(3), 359–379.

Dillon, K. M. (1989). Lateral preference and students' worries: A correlation. *Psychological Reports, 65*(2), 496–498.

Dixon, M. (1999). Tool and bird exemplar identification in a patient with category-specific visual agnosia. *Brain and Cognition, 40*(1), 97–100.

Dixon, M., Bub, D. N., & Arguin, M. (1997). The interaction of object form and object meaning in the identification performance of a patient with category-specific visual agnosia. *Cognitive Neuropsychology, 14*(8), 1085–1130.

Dixon, M. J., Bub, D. N., Chertkow, H., & Arguin, M. (1999). Object identification deficits in dementia of the Alzheimer type: Combined effects of semantic and visual proximity. *Journal of the International Neuropsychological Society, 5*(4), 330–345.

Dixon, M. J., Koehler, D., Schweizer, T. A., & Guylee, M. J. (2000). Superior single dimension relative to "exclusive" or categorization performance by a patient with category-specific visual agnosia: Empirical data and an alcove simulation. *Brain and Cognition, 43*(1–3), 152–158.

Dixon, M. J., Piskopos, M., & Schweizer, T. A. (2000). Musical instrument naming impairments: The crucial exception to the living/nonliving dichotomy in category-specific agnosia. *Brain and Cognition, 43*(1–3), 158–164.

Doe, C. Q., & Sanes, J. R. (2000). Development: Neural development at the millennium. *Current Opinion in Neurobiology, 10*(1), 31.

Dogil, G., Ackermann, H., Grodd, W., Haider, H., Kamp, H., Mayer, J., et al. (2002). The speaking brain: A tutorial introduction to fMRI experiments in the production of speech, prosody and syntax. *Journal of Neurolinguistics, 15*(1), 59–90.

Dolado, A. M., Castrillo, C., Urra, D. G., & De-Seijas, E. V. (1995). Alien hand sign or alien syndrome? *Journal of Neurology, Neurosurgery and Psychiatry, 59*(1), 100–101.

Dolan, R. J., Morris, J. S., & de Gelder, B. (2001). Crossmodal binding of fear in voice and face. *Proceedings of the National Academy of the Sciences of the United States of America, 98*(17), 10006–10010.

Drevets, W. C., Price, J. L., Bardgett, M. E., Reich, T., Todd, R. D., & Raichle, M. E. (2002). Glucose metabolism in the amygdala in depression: Relationship to diagnostic subtype and plasma cortisol levels. *Pharmacology, Biochemistry, and Behavior, 71*(3), 431–447.

Du, L., Faludi, G., Palkovits, M., Bakish, D., & Hrdina, P. D. (2001). Serotonergic genes and suicidality. *Crisis, 22*(2), 54–60.

During, M. J., Kaplitt, M. G., Stern, M. B., & Eidelberg, D. (2001). Subthalamic GAD gene transfer in Parkinson disease patients who are candidates for deep brain stimulation. *Human Gene Therapy, 12*(12), 1589–1591.

During, M. J., Samulski, R. J., Elsworth, J. D., Kaplitt, M. G., Leone, P., Xiao, X., et al. (1998). In vivo expression of therapeutic human genes for dopamine production in the caudates of MPTP-treated monkeys using an AAV vector. *Gene Therapy, 5*(6), 820–827.

Durnford, M., & Kimura, D. (1971). Right hemisphere specialization for depth perception reflected in visual field differences. *Nature, 231*(5302), 394–395.

Dursteller, M. R., & Wurtz, R. H. (1988). Pursuit and optokinetic deficits following lesions of cortical areas MT and MST. *Journal of Neurophysiology, 60,* 940–965.

Dutton, D. G., & Aron, A. P. (1974). Some evidence for heightened sexual attraction under conditions of high anxiety. *Journal of Personality and Social Psychology, 30*(4), 510–517.

Efron, R., Crandall, P. H., Koss, B., DiVenyi, P. L., & Yund, E. W. (1983). Central auditory processing: III. The "cocktail party" effect and anterior temporal lobectomy. *Brain and Language, 19*(2), 254–263.

Eglinton, E., & Annett, M. (1994). Handedness and dyslexia: A meta-analysis. *Perceptual and Motor Skills, 79*(3, Pt. 2), 1611–1616.

Ehringer, H., & Hornykiewicz, O. (1960). Distribution of noradrenaline and dopamine (3-hydroxytyramine) in the human brain and their behavior in the presence of disease affecting the extrapyramidal system. In J. Marks (Ed.), *The treatment of Parkinsonism with L-dopa.* Lancaster, England: MTP Medical and Technical Publishing.

Ehrlichman, H., Zoccolotti, P., & Owen, D. (1982). Perinatal factors in hand and eye preference: Data from the Collaborative Perinatal Project. *International Journal of Neuroscience, 17*(1), 17–22.

Eiberg, H., & Mohr, J. (1987). Major genes of eye color and hair color linked to LU and SE. *Clinical Genetics, 31*(3), 186–191.

Eidelberg, D., & Galaburda, A. M. (1982). Symmetry and asymmetry in the human posterior thalamus: I. Cytoarchitectonic analysis in normal persons. *Archives of Neurology, 39*(6), 325–332.

Ekman, P. (1998). *What the face reveals: Basic and applied studies of spontaneous expression using the Facial Action Coding System (FACS).* New York: Oxford University Press.

Ekman, P., & Friesen, W. V. (1971). Constants across cultures in the face and emotion. *Journal of Personality and Social Psychology, 17*(2), 124–129.

Ekman, P., Friesen, W. V., & Simons, R. C. (1985). Is the startle reaction an emotion? *Journal of Personality and Social Psychology, 49*(5), 1416–1426.

Elbert, T., Pantev, C., Wienbruch, C., Rockstroh, B., & Taub, E. (1995). Increased cortical representation of the fingers of the left hand in string players. *Science, 270*(5234), 305–307.

Elias, L. J., & Bryden, M. P. (1998). Footedness is a better predictor of language lateralization than handedness. *Laterality, 3*(1), 41–51.

Elias, L. J., Bryden, M. P., & Bulman-Fleming, M. B. (1998). Footedness is a better predictor than is handedness of emotional lateralization. *Neuropsychologia, 36*(1), 37–43.

Elias, L. J., Bulman-Fleming, M. B., & Guylee, M. J. (1999). Complementarity of cerebral function among individuals with atypical laterality profiles. *Brain and Cognition, 40*(1), 112–115.

Elias, L. J., Bulman-Fleming, M. B., & McManus, I. C. (1999). Visual temporal asymmetries are related to asymmetries in linguistic perception. *Neuropsychologia. 37*(11), 1243–1249.

Elias, L. J., Bulman-Fleming, M. B., & McManus, I. C. (2000). Linguistic lateralization and interhemispheric transfer time. *Brain and Cognition, 43*(1), 181–185.

Eliot, R. S., & Buell, J. C. (1981). Environmental and behavioral influences in the major cardiovascular disorders. In S. M. Weiss, J. A. Herd, & B. H. Fox (Eds.), *Perspectives on behavioral medicine* (pp. 22–39). New York: Academic Press.

Elliott, T. K., Watkins, J. M., Messa, C., Liipe, B., & Chugani, H. (1996). Positron emission tomography and neuropsychological correlations in children with Turner's syndrome. *Developmental Neuropsychology, 12,* 365–386.

Ellis, A. W., Young, A. W., & Critchley, E. M. (1989). Loss of memory for people following temporal lobe damage. *Brain, 112*(Pt. 6), 1469–1483.

Ellis, H. D., & Florence, M. (1990). Bodamer's (1947) paper on prosopagnosia. *Cognitive Neuropsychology, 7*(2), 81–105.

Ellis, L., & Ames, M. A. (1989). Delinquency, sidedness, and sex. *Journal of General Psychology, 116*(1), 57–62.

Elston, G. N., & Rosa, M. G. (1998). Complex dendritic fields of pyramidal cells in the frontal eye field of the macaque monkey: Comparison with parietal areas 7a and LIP. *Neuroreport, 9*(1), 127–131.

Emmerling, M. R., Morganti-Kossmann, M. C., Kossmann, T., Stahel, P. F., Watson, M. D., Evans, L. M., et al. (2000). Traumatic brain injury elevates the Alzheimer's amyloid peptide A beta 42 in human CSF: A possible role for nerve cell injury. *Annals of the New York Academy of Sciences, 903,* 118–122.

Ende, G., Braus, D. F., Walter, S., Weber-Fahr, W., & Henn, F. A. (2000). The hippocampus in patients treated with electroconvulsive therapy: A proton magnetic resonance spectroscopic imaging study. *Archives of General Psychiatry, 57*(10), 937–943.

Erhan, H., Borod, J. C., Tenke, C. E., & Bruder, G. E. (1998). Identification of emotion in a dichotic listening task: Event-related brain potential and behavioral findings. *Brain and Cognition, 37*(2), 286–307.

Eriksson, P. S., Perfilieva, E., Bjork-Eriksson, T., Alborn, A. M., Nordborg, C., Peterson, D. A., et al. (1998). Neurogenesis in the adult human hippocampus. *Nature Medicine, 4*(11), 1313–1317.

Esquirol, J. E. D. (1814). Mental maladies (E. K. Hunt, Trans., 1845). New York: Hafner.

Etkoff, N. K. L. (1984). Selective attention to facial identity and facial emotion. *Neuropsychologia, 22,* 281–295.

Ettlinger, G., Blakemore, C. B., Milner, A. D., & Wilson, J. (1972). Agenesis of the corpus callosum: A behavioral investigation. *Brain, 95*(2), 327–346.

Eustache, F., Desgranges, B., Aupee, A. M., Guillery, B., & Baron, J. C. (2000). Functional neuroanatomy of amnesia: Positron emission tomography studies. *Microscopy Research and Technique, 51*(1), 94–100.

Ewart, A. K., Morris, C. A., Atkinson, D., Jin, W., Sternes, K., Spallone, P., et al. (1993). Hemizygosity at the elastin locus in a developmental disorder, Williams syndrome. *Nature Genetics, 5*(1), 11–16.

Exner, S. (1881). *Untersuchungen über die Lokalisation der Funktionen in der Grosshirnrinde des Menschen.* Vienna, Austria: Wilhelm Braumuller.

Falek, A. (1959). Handedness: A family study. *American Journal of Human Genetics, 11,* 52–62.

Farah, M. (2001). Consciousness. In B. Rapp (Ed.), *The handbook of cognitive neuropsychology: What deficits reveal about the human mind.* Philadelphia: Psychology Press/Taylor and Francis.

Farah, M. J. (1990). *Visual agnosia: Disorders of object recognition and what they tell us about normal vision.* Cambridge, MA: MIT Press.

Farah, M. J. (2000). *The cognitive neuroscience of vision.* Malden, MA: Blackwell.

Farah, M. J., Hammond, K. M., Levine, D. N., & Calvanio, R. (1988). Visual and spatial mental imagery: Dissociable systems of representation. *Cognitive Psychology, 20*(4), 439–462.

Farah, M. J., & McClelland, J. L. (1991). A computational model of semantic memory impairment: Modality specificity and emergent category specificity. *Journal of Experimental Psychology: General, 120*(4), 339–357.

Farah, M. J., Monheit, M. A., & Wallace, M. A. (1991). Unconscious perception of "extinguished" visual stimuli: Reassessing the evidence. *Neuropsychologia, 29*(10), 949–958.

Fawcett, J. W., Rosser, A. E., & Dunnett, S. B. (2001). *Brain damage, brain repair.* New York: Oxford University Press.

Faymonville, M. E., Fissette, J., Mambourg, P. H., Roediger, L., Joris, J., & Lamy, M. (1995). Hypnosis as adjunct therapy in conscious sedation for plastic surgery. *Regional Anaesthesia, 20*(2), 145–151.

Feehan, M., Stanton, W. R., McGee, R., Silva, P. A., & Moffitt, T. E. (1990). Is there an association between lateral preference and delinquent behavior? *Journal of Abnormal Psychology, 99*(2), 198–201.

Feinberg, T. E., & Roane, D. M. (2000). Misidentification syndromes. In M. J. Farah (Ed.), *Patient-based approaches to cognitive neuroscience. Issues in clinical and cognitive neuropsychology.* Cambridge, MA: MIT Press.

Feldman, R. S., Meyer, J. S., Quenzer, L. F. (1997). *Principles of neuropsychopharmacology.* Sunderland, MA: Sinauer.

Fenton, W. S. (2000). Prevalence of spontaneous dyskinesia in schizophrenia. *Journal of Clinical Psychiatry, 61*(Suppl. 4), 10–14.

Ferber-Viart, C., Duclaux, R., Collet, L., & Guyonnard, F. (1995). Influence of auditory stimulation and visual attention on otoacoustic emissions. *Physiology and Behavior, 57*(6), 1075–1079.

Ferreira, C. T., Verin, M., Pillon, B., Levy, R., Dubois, B., & Agid, Y. (1998). Spatio-temporal working memory and frontal lesions in man. *Cortex, 34*(1), 83–98.

Finger, S. (1994). *Origins of neuroscience: A history of explorations into brain function.* London, England: Oxford University Press.

Finlay, D. C., Peto, T., Payling, J., Hunter, M., Fulham, W. R., & Wilkinson, I. (2000). A study of three cases of familial related agenesis of the corpus callosum. *Journal of Clinical and Experimental Neuropsychology, 22*(6), 731–742.

Fischer, M., Ryan, S. B., Dobyns, W. B. (1992). Mechanisms of interhemispheric transfer and patterns of cognitive function in acallosal patients of normal intelligence. *Archives of Neurology, 49,* 271–277.

Fitzsimons, M., Sheahan, N., & Staunton, H. (2001). Gender and the integration of acoustic dimensions of prosody: Implications for clinical studies. *Brain and Language, 78*(1), 94–108.

Fletcher, J. M., Dennis, M., & Northrup, H. (2000). Hydrocephalus. In K. O. Yeates, M. D. Ris, & H. J. Taylor (Eds.), *Pediatric neuropsychology. Research, theory, and practice.* New York: Guilford Press.

Fletcher, P. C., Shallice, T., Frith, C. D., Frackowiak, R. S., & Dolan, R. J. (1996). Brain activity during memory retrieval. The influence of imagery and semantic cueing. *Brain, 119*(Pt. 5), 1587–1596.

Folstein, M. F., Folstein, S. E., & McHugh, P. R. (1975). "Mini-mental state." A practical method for grading the cognitive state of patients for the clinician. *Journal of Psychiatric Research, 12*(3), 189–198.

Folstein, S., & Rutter, M. (1977). Genetic influences and infantile autism. *Nature, 265,* 726–728.

Folstein, S. E. (1991). The psychopathology of Huntington's disease. *Research Publications Association for Research in Nervous and Mental Disease, 69,* 181–191.

Fontenot, D. J. (1973). Visual field differences in the recognition of verbal and nonverbal stimuli in man. *Journal of Comparative and Psychological Psychology, 85,* 564–569.

Forster, R. (1890). Uber Rindenblindheit [On cortical blindness]. *Graefe's Archiv fur Opthalmologie, 36,* 94–108.

Foundas, A. L., Daniels, S. K., & Vasterling, J. J. (1998). Anomia: Case studies with lesion localization. *Neurocase, 4*(1), 35–43.

Freed, D. M., & Corkin, S. (1988). Rate of forgetting in H. M.: 6-month recognition. *Behavioral Neuroscience, 102*(6), 823–827.

Freedman, M., Alexander, M. P., & Naeser, M. A. (1984). Anatomic basis of transcortical motor aphasia. *Neurology, 34*(4), 409–417.

Freund, C. S. (1991). On optic aphasia and visual agnosia. *Cognitive Neuropsychology, 8*(1), 21–38.

Frith, C. D., & Friston, K. J. (1996). Studying brain function with neuroimaging. In M. D. Rugg (Ed.), *Cognitive neuroscience.* Cambridge, MA: MIT Press.

Funnell, E., & Sheridan, J. (1992). Categories of knowledge? Unfamiliar aspects of living and nonliving things. *Cognitive Neuropsychology, 9*(2), 135–153.

Gage, F. H. (2002). Neurogenesis in the adult brain. *Journal of Neuroscience, 22*(3), 612–613.

Gabrielli, W. F., Jr., & Mednick, S. A. (1980). Sinistrality and delinquency. *Journal of Abnormal Psychology, 89*(5), 654–661.

Gaillard, W. D., Balsamo, L. M., Ibrahim, Z., Sachs, B. C., & Xu, B. (2003). fMRI identifies regional specialization of neural networks for reading in young children. *Neurology, 60*(1), 94–100.

Gaillard, W. D., Hertz-Pannier, L., Mott, S. H., Barnett, A. S., LeBihan, D., & Theodore, W. H. (2000). Functional anatomy of cognitive development: fMRI of verbal fluency in children and adults. *Neurology, 54*(1), 180–185.

Galaburda, A. M. (1980). La region de Broca: Observations anatomiques faites un siècle après la mort de son decouvrer. *Revue de Neurologie (Paris), 136,* 609–616.

Galaburda, A. M. (1995). Anatomic basis of cerebral dominance. In R. J. Davidson & K. Hugdahl (Eds.), *Brain asymmetry.* Cambridge, MA: MIT Press.

Galaburda, A. M., & Bellugi, U. (2000). V. Multi-level analysis of cortical neuroanatomy in Williams syndrome. *Journal of Cognitive Neuroscience, 12*(Suppl. 1), 74–88.

Galaburda, A. M., LeMay, M., Kemper, T. L., & Geschwind, N. (1978). Right-left asymmetries in the brain: Structural differences between the hemispheres may underlie cerebral dominance. *Science, 199*(4331), 852–856.

Galea, L. A., & McEwen, B. S. (1999). Sex and seasonal differences in the rate of cell proliferation in the dentate gyrus of adult wild meadow voles. *Neuroscience, 89*(3), 955–964.

Gallagher, P., Allen, D., & MacLachlan, M. (2001). Phantom limb pain and residual limb pain following lower limb amputation: A descriptive analysis. *Disability and Rehabilitation: An International Multidisciplinary Journal, 23*(12), 522–530.

Galletti, C., Battaglini, P. P., & Fattori, P. (1990). 'Real-motion' cells in area V3A of macaque visual cortex. *Experimental Brain Research, 82*(1), 67–76.

Galliford, D., James, E. F., & Woods, G. E. (1964). Laterality in atheioid cerebral palsied children. *Developmental Medicine and Child Neurology, 6,* 261–263.

Gangestad, S. W., & Yeo, R. A. (1994). Parental handedness and relative hand skill: A test of the developmental instability hypothesis. *Neuropsychology, 8*(4), 572–578.

Garavan, H., Kelley, D., Rosen, A., Rao, S. M., & Stein, E. A. (2000). Practice-related functional activation changes in a working memory task. *Microscopy Research and Technique, 51*(1), 54–63.

Garde, M. M., & Cowey, A. (2000). "Deaf hearing": Unacknowledged detection of auditory stimuli in a patient with cerebral deafness. *Cortex, 36*(1), 71–80.

Gardner, H. (1974). *The Shattered Mind.* New York: Vintage Books.

Gaulin, S. J. C., & McBurney, D. H. (2001). *Psychology. An evolutionary approach.* Upper Saddle River, NJ: Prentice-Hall.

Gazzaniga, M. S. (2000). Cerebral specialization and interhemispheric communication: Does the corpus callosum enable the human condition? *Brain, 123*(Pt. 7), 1293–1326.

Gazzaniga, M. S., Bogen, J. E., & Sperry, R. W. (1965). Observations on visual perception after disconnection of the cerebral hemispheres in man. *Brain, 88*(2), 221–236.

Gazzaniga, M. S., Bogen, J. E., & Sperry, R. W. (1967). Dyspraxia following division of the cerebral commissures. *Archives of Neurology, 16*(6), 606–612.

Gazzaniga, M. S., Ivry, R. B., & Mangun, G. R. (1998). *Cognitive neuroscience: The biology of the mind.* New York: W. W. Norton.

Gazzaniga, M. S., Ivry, R., & Mangun, G. R. (2002). *Cognitive neuroscience.* New York: W. W. Norton.

Gazzaniga, M. S., & Sperry, R. W. (1967). Language after section of the cerebral commissures. *Brain, 90*(1), 131–148.

Gedda, L., Sciacca, A., Brenci, G., Villatico, S., Bonanni, G., Gueli, N., et al. (1984). Situs viscerum specularis in monozygotic twins. *Acta Geneticae et Medicae Gemellologiae, 33*(1), 81–85.

Gerendai, I., & Halasz, B. (1997). Neuroendocrine asymmetry. *Frontiers in Neuroendocrinology, 18*(3), 354–381.

Gerstmann, J. (1924). Fingeragnosie. Eine umschriebene Storung der Orientierung am eigene Korper. *Wien Klin Wschr, 37,* 1010–1012.

Gerstmann, J. (1930). Zur Symptomomatologie der Hirnlasionen im Ubergangs-region der unteren Parietal-und mittleren Okzipitalhirnwindung. *Dt Z Nervheilk, 116,* 46–49.

Geschwind, D. H., Iacoboni, M., Mega, M. S., Zaidel, D. W., et al. (1995). Alien hand syndrome: Interhemispheric motor disconnection due to a lesion in the midbody of the corpus callosum. *Neurology, 45*(4), 802–808.

Geschwind, M. D., Hartnick, C. J., Liu, W., Amat, J., Van De Water, T. R., & Federoff, H. J. (1996). Defective HSV-1 vector expressing BDNF in auditory ganglia elicits neurite outgrowth: Model for treatment of neuron loss following cochlear degeneration. *Human Gene Therapy, 7*(2), 173–182.

Geschwind, N. (1983). Biological associations of left-handedness. *Annals of Dyslexia, 33,* 29–40.

Geschwind, N., (1984). Cerebral dominance in biological perspective. *Neuropsychologia, 22*(6), 675–683.

Geschwind, N., & Behan, P. (1982). Left-handedness: Association with immune disease, migraine, and developmental learning disorder. *Proceedings of the National Academy of Sciences of the United States of America, 79*(16), 5097–5100.

Geschwind, N., & Behan, P. (1984). Laterality, hormones, and immunity. In N. Geschwind & A. M. Galaburda (Eds.), *Cerebral dominance: The biological foundations* (pp. 211–224). Cambridge, MA: Harvard University Press.

Geschwind, N., & Galaburda, A. M. (1985a). Cerebral lateralization. Biological mechanisms, associations, and pathology: I. A hypothesis and a program for research. *Archives of Neurology, 42*(5), 428–459.

Geschwind, N., & Galaburda, A. M. (1985b). Cerebral lateralization. Biological mechanisms, associations, and pathology: II. A hypothesis and a program for research. *Archives of Neurology, 42*(6), 521–552.

Geschwind, N., & Galaburda, A. M. (1985c). Cerebral lateralization. Biological mechanisms, associations, and pathology: III. A hypothesis and a program for research. *Archives of Neurology, 42*(7), 634–654.

Geschwind, N., & Galaburda, A. M. (1987). *Cerebral lateralization.* London, England: MIT Press.

Geschwind, N., & Levitsky, W. (1968). Human brain: Left-right asymmetries in temporal speech region. *Science, 161*(837), 186–187.

Ghika-Schmid, F., Ghika, J., Vuilleumier, P., Assal, G., Vuadens, P., Scherer, K., et al. (1997). Bihippocampal damage with emotional dysfunction: Impaired auditory recognition of fear. *European Neurology, 38*(4), 276–283.

Giedd, J. N., Blumenthal, J., Jeffries, N. O., Castellanos, F. X., Liu, H., Zijdenbos, A., et al. (1999). Brain development during childhood and adolescence: A longitudinal MRI study. *Nature Neuroscience, 2*(10), 861–863.

Giese, A., & Kretzschmar, H. A. (2001). Prion-induced neuronal damage: The mechanisms of neuronal destruction in the subacute spongiform encephalopathies. *Current Topics in Microbiology and Immunology, 253,* 203–217.

Gilbert, A. N., & Wysocki, C. J. (1992). Hand preference and age in the United States. *Neuropsychologia, 30*(7), 601–608.

Gilbert, P. (2001). Evolution and social anxiety. The role of attraction, social competition, and social hierarchies. *Psychiatric Clinics of North America, 24*(4), 723–751.

Gilger, J. W., Pennington, B. F., Green, P., Smith, S. M., & Smith, S. D. (1992). Reading disability, immune disorders and non-right-handedness: Twin and family studies of their relations. *Neuropsychologia, 30*(3), 209–227.

Gilles de la Tourette, G. E. (1885). Etude sur une affection nerveuse caractérisée par l'inccordination motrice accompagnée d'écholalie et coprolalie. *Archives of Neurology, 9*, 19–42.

Glazer, W. M. (2000). Review of incidence studies of tardive dyskinesia associated with typical antipsychotics. *Journal of Clinical Psychiatry, 61*(Suppl. 4), 15–20.

Glucksberg, S., & Cowen, G. N. (1970). Memory for non-attended auditory material. *Cognitive Psychology, 1*(2), 149–156.

Golbin, A., Golbin, Y., Keith, L., & Keith, D. (1993). Mirror imaging in twins: Biological polarization, an evolving hypothesis. *Acta Geneticae Medicae et Gemellologiae, 42*(3–4), 237–243.

Golden, C. J., Purisch, A. D., & Hammeke, T. A. (1985). *Luria-Nebraska Neuropsychological Battery: Forms I and II.* Los Angeles: Western Psychological Services.

Golden, G. S. (1990). Tourette syndrome: Recent advances. *Neurologic Clinics, 8*(3), 705–714.

Goldman, P. S., Lodge, A., Hammer, L. R., Semmes, J., & Mishkin, M. (1968). Critical flicker frequency after unilateral temporal lobectomy in man. *Neuropsychologia, 6*, 355–366.

Goldman-Rakic, P. S. (1987). Motor control function of the prefrontal cortex. *Ciba Foundation Symposium, 132*, 187–200.

Goldman-Rakic, P. S. (1999). The physiological approach: Functional architecture of working memory and disordered cognition in schizophrenia. *Biological Psychiatry, 46*(5), 650–661.

Goldman-Rakic, P. S., Bates, J. F., & Chafee, M. V. (1992). The prefrontal cortex and internally generated motor acts. *Current Opinion in Neurobiology, 2*(6), 830–835.

Goldstein, F. C., Levin, H. S., Boake, C., & Lohrey, J. H. (1990). Facilitation of memory performance through induced semantic processing in survivors of severe closed-head injury. *Journal of Clinical and Experimental Neuropsychology, 12*(2), 286–300.

Good, C. D., Johnsrude, I., Ashburner, J., Henson, R. N., Friston, K. J., & Frackowiak, R. S. (2001). Cerebral asymmetry and the effects of sex and handedness on brain structure: A voxel-based morphometric analysis of 465 normal adult human brains. *Neuroimage, 14*(3), 685–700.

Goodale, M. A., & Milner, A. D. (1992). Separate visual pathways for perception and action. *Trends in Neuroscience, 15*(1), 20–25.

Goodale, M. A., Milner, A. D., Jakobson, L. S., & Carey, D. P. (1991). A neurological dissociation between perceiving objects and grasping them [see comments]. *Nature, 349*(6305), 154–156.

Goodwin, R. S., & Michel, G. F. (1981). Head orientation position during birth and in infant neonatal period, and hand preference at nineteen weeks. *Child Development, 52*(3), 819–826.

Gordon, A. (1926). Remarks on astereognosis. *Journal of Nervous and Mental Disease, 64*, 359–361.

Gorelick, P. B., & Ross, E. D. (1987). The aprosodias: Further functional-anatomical evidence for the organisation of affective language in the right hemisphere. *Journal of Neurology, Neurosurgery and Psychiatry, 50*(5), 553–560.

Gorno-Tempini, M. L., Pradelli, S., Serafini, M., Pagnoni, G., Baraldi, P., Porro, C., et al. (2001). Explicit and incidental facial expression processing: An fMRI study. *Neuroimage, 14*(2), 465–473.

Gorski, R. A., Harlan, R. E., Jacobson, C. D., Shryne, J. E., & Southam, A. M. (1980). Evidence for the existence of a sexually dimorphic nucleus in the preoptic area of the rat. *Journal of Comparative Neurology, 193*(2), 529–539.

Gotestam, K. O. (1990). Lefthandedness among students of architecture and music. *Perceptual and Motor Skills, 70*(3 Pt. 2), 1323–1327; discussion 1345–1346.

Gould, J. A. (1981). Human homing: An elusive phenomenon. *Science, 212*, 1061–1064.

Gracco, V. L., & Abbs, J. H. (1986). Variant and invariant characteristics of speech movements. *Experimental Brain Research, 65*(1), 156–166.

Graham, C. J., & Cleveland, E. (1995). Left-handedness as an injury risk factor in adolescents. *Journal of Adolescent Health, 16*(1), 50–52.

Graham, C. J., Dick, R., Rickert, V. I., & Glenn, R. (1993). Left-handedness as a risk factor for unintentional injury in children. *Pediatrics, 92*(6), 823–826.

Graves, R., Landis, T., & Simpson, C. (1985). On the interpretation of mouth asymmetry. *Neuropsychologia, 23*(1), 121–122.

Green, M. F., Kern, R. S., Braff, D. L., & Mintz, J. (2000). Neurocognitive deficits and functional outcome in schizophrenia: Are we measuring the right stuff? *Schizophrenia Bulletin, 26*(1), 119–136.

Grimshaw, G. M., Bryden, M. P., & Finegan, J. K. (1995). Relations between prenatal testosterone and cerebral lateralization in children. *Neuropsychology, 9*(1), 68–79.

Grossi, D., Fragassi, N. A., Orsini, A., DeFalco, F. A., Sepe, O., et al. (1984). Residual reading capability in a patient with alexia without agraphia. *Brain and Language, 23*(2), 337–348.

Grossi, D., Trojano, L., Chiacchio, L., Soricelli, A., Mansi, A., Postiglione, A., et al. (1991). Mixed transcortical aphasia: Clinical features and neuroanatomical correlates: A possible role of the right hemisphere (with 1 color plate). *European Neurology, 31*(4), 204–211.

Grossman, E., Donnelly, M., Price, R., Pickens, D., Morgan, V., Neighbor, G., et al. (2000). Brain areas involved in perception of biological motion. *Journal of Cognitive Neuroscience, 12*(5), 711–720.

Guidetti, V., Moschetta, A., Ottaviano, S., Seri, S., & Fornara, R. (1987). Random dominance and childhood migraine: A new marker? A controlled study of laterality in children with migraine. *Functional Neurology, 2*(1), 59–68.

Guillain, G., & Bize, P. R. (1932). Astereognosie pure par lesion corticale parietale traumatique [Pure astereognosia by traumatic parietal cortical lesion]. *Revue Neurologique, 39,* 502–509.

Gunston, G. D., Burkimsher, D., Malan, H., Sive, A. A. (1992). Reversible cerebral shrinkage in kwashiorkor: An MRI study. *Archives of Disease in Childhood, 67*(8), 1030–1032.

Gur, R. C., Packer, I. K., Hungerbuhler, J. P., Reivich, M., Obvist, W. M. D., Amarnek, W. S., et al. (1980). Differences in the distribution of gray and white matter in human cerebral hemispheres. *Science, 207*(4436), 1226–1228.

Gusella, J. F., Wexler, N. S., Conneally, P. M., Naylor, S. L., Anderson, M. A., Tanzi, R. E., et al. (1983). A polymorphic DNA marker genetically linked to Huntington's disease. *Nature, 306*(5940), 234–238.

Guylee, M. J., Elias, L. J., Bulman-Fleming, M. B., & Dixon, M. J. (2000). Tactile gap detection and language lateralization. *Brain and Cognition, 43*(1–3), 234–238.

Haass, C., & Kahle, P. J. (2001). Parkin and its substrates. *Science, 293*(5528), 224–225.

Haggard, M. P., & Parkinson, A. M. (1971). Stimulus and task factors as determinants of ear advantages. *Quarterly Journal of Experimental Psychology, 23*(2), 158–177.

Hakim, H., Verma, N. P., & Greiffenstein, M. F. (1988). Pathogenesis of reduplicative paramnesia. *Journal of Neurology, Neurosurgery and Psychiatry, 51*(6), 839–841.

Halligan, P. W., Hunt, M., Marshall, J. C., & Wade, D. T. (1995). Sensory detection without localization. *Neurocase, 1*(3), 259–266.

Halpern, D. F., & Coren, S. (1988). Do right-handers live longer? *Nature, 333*(6170), 213.

Haltia, M. (2000). Human prion diseases. *Annals of Medicine, 32*(7), 493–500.

Hamann, S. B., & Squire, L. R. (1997). Intact perceptual memory in the absence of conscious memory. *Behavioral Neuroscience, 111*(4), 850–854.

Hamer, D. (1993). Sexual orientation. *Nature, 365*(6448), 702.

Hammond, G. R. (1981). Finer temporal acuity for stimuli applied to the preferred hand. *Neuropsychologia, 19*(2), 325–329.

Hansen, C. H., & Hansen, R. D. (1988). Finding the face in the crowd: An anger superiority effect. *Journal of Personality and Social Psychology, 54*(6), 917–924.

Harburg, E. (1981). Handedness and drinking-smoking types. *Perceptual and Motor Skills, 52*(1), 279–282.

Harburg, E., Feldstein, A., & Papsdorf, J. D. (1978). Handedness and smoking. *Perceptual and Motor Skills, 47*(3, Pt. 2), 1171–1174.

Hardyck, C., & Petrinovich, L. F. (1977). Left-handedness. *Psychological Bulletin, 84*(3), 385–404.

Hare, R. D. (1991). *Manual for the Hare Psychopathy Checklist-revised.* Toronto, Canada: Multi-Health Systems.

Hare, R. D., & Forth, A. E. (1985). Psychopathy and lateral preference. *Journal of Abnormal Psychology, 94*(4), 541–546.

Harlow, J. M., & Miller, E. (1993). Recovery from the passage of an iron bar through the head. *History of Psychiatry, 4,* 271–281.

Harris, G. J., Aylward, E. H., Peyser, C. E., Pearlson, G. D., Brandt, J., Roberts-Twillie, J. V., et al. (1996). Single photon emission computed tomographic blood flow and magnetic resonance volume imaging of basal ganglia in Huntington's disease. *Archives of Neurology, 53*(4), 316–324.

Harris, L. J. (1980). Left-handedness: Early theories, facts, and fancies. In J. Herron (Ed.), *Neuropsychology of left-handedness.* Toronto, Canada: Academic Press.

Harris, L. J. (1993). Do left-handers die sooner than right-handers? Commentary on Coren and Halpern's (1991) "Left-handedness: A marker for decreased survival fitness." *Psychological Bulletin, 114*(2), 203–234, 235–247.

Harris, L. J., & Gitterman, S. R. (1978). University professors' self-descriptions of left-right confusability: Sex and handedness differences. *Perceptual and Motor Skills, 47*(3, Pt. 1), 819–823.

Harvey, M., & Milner, A. D. (1995). Balint's patient. *Cognitive Neuropsychology, 12*(3), 261–264.

Haseltine, E. (2002). Phantom sensations. *Discover, 23*(3), 88.

Haskell, S. G., Richardson, E. D., & Horwitz, R. I. (1997). The effect of estrogen replacement therapy on cognitive function in women: A critical review of the literature. *Journal of Clinical Epidemiology, 50*(11), 1249–1264.

Hatta, T., & Kawakami, A. (1994). Handedness and incidence of disease in a new Japanese cohort. *Psychologia: An International Journal of Psychology in the Orient, 37*(3), 188–193.

Hauser, R. A., Freeman, T. B., Snow, B. J., Nauert, M., Gauger, L., Kordower, J. H., et al. (1999). Long-term evaluation of bilateral fetal nigral transplantation in Parkinson disease. *Archives of Neurology, 56*(2), 179–187.

Hawking, S. (2001). On living with a disability [Online]. Retrieved June 7, 2005, from www.flipsideshow.com/Documents/News050402.htm.

Haxby, J. V., Horwitz, B., Ungerleider, L. G., Maisog, J. M., Pietrini, P., & Grady, C. L. (1994). The functional organization of human extrastriate cortex: A PET-rCBF study of selective attention to faces and locations. *Journal of Neuroscience, 14*(11, Pt. 1), 6336–6353.

Hecaen, H., & Angelergues, R. (1962). Agnosia for faces (Prosopagnosia). *Archives of Neurology Chicago, 7*(2), 92–100.

Heilman, K. M., & Bowers, D. (1995). "Apperceptive visual agnosia: A case study": Reply. *Brain and Cognition, 28*(2), 178–179.

Heilman, K. M., Bowers, D., Coslett, H. B., Whelan, H., & Watson, R. T. (1985). Directional hypokinesia: Prolonged reaction times for leftward movements in patients with right hemisphere lesions and neglect. *Neurology, 35*(6), 855–859.

Heilman, K. M., & Rothi, L. J. G. (1993). Apraxia. In K. M. Heilman (Ed.), *Clinical neuropsychology* (pp. 141–146). New York: Oxford University Press.

Heilman, K. M., Watson, R. T., & Rothi, L. J. G. (2000). Disorders of skilled movements. In M. J. Farah & T. E. Feinberg (Eds.), *Patient-based approaches to cognitive neuroscience. Issues in clinical and cognitive neuropsychology* (pp. 335–343). Cambridge, MA: MIT Press.

Heilman, K. M., Watson, R. T., & Valenstein, E. (2000). Neglect I: Clinical and anatomic issues. In M. J. Farah (Ed.), *Patient-based approaches to cognitive neuroscience. Issues in clinical and cognitive neuropsychology* (pp. 115–123). Cambridge, MA: MIT Press.

Heller, W., & Levy, J. (1981). Perception and expression of emotion in right-handers and left-handers. *Neuropsychologia, 19*(2), 263–272.

Henderson, V. W. (1986). Anatomy of posterior pathways in reading: A reassessment. *Brain and Language, 29,* 119–133.

Herrero, J. V., & Hillix, W. A. (1990). Hemispheric performance in detecting prosody: A competitive dichotic listening task. *Perceptual and Motor Skills, 71*(2), 479–486.

Herschkowitz, N. (2000). Neurological bases of behavioral development in infancy. *Brain Development, 22*(7), 411–416.

Hicks, R. A., & Dusek, C. M. (1980). The handedness distributions of gifted and non-gifted children. *Cortex, 16*(3), 479–481.

Hicks, R. A., Johnson, C., Cuevas, T., Deharo, D., & Bautista, J. (1994). Do right-handers live longer? An updated assessment of baseball player data. *Perceptual and Motor Skills, 78*(3, Pt. 2), 1243–1247.

Hicks, R. A., Pass, K., Freeman, H., Bautista, J., & Johnson, C. (1993). Handedness and accidents with injury. *Perceptual and Motor Skills, 77*(3, Pt. 2), 1119–1122.

Hicks, R. A., & Kinsbourne, M. (1976). Human handedness: A partial cross-fostering study. *Science, 192*(4242), 908–910.

Hillis, A. E., & Caramazza, A. (1995). A framework for interpreting distinct patterns of hemispatial neglect. *Neurocase: Case Studies in Neuropsychology, Neuropsychiatry, and Behavioural Neurology, 1*(3), 189–207.

Hillyard, S. A., Hink, R. F., Schwent, V. L., & Picton, T. W. (1973). Electrical signs of selective attention in the human brain. *Science, 182*(4108), 177–179.

Hinkin, C. H., & Cummings, J. L. (1996). Agraphia. In J. G. Beaumont, P. M. Kenealy, & M. J. C. Rogers (Eds.), *The Blackwell dictionary of neuropsychology* (pp. 128–133). Cambridge, MA: Blackwell.

Hochberg, F. H., & le-May, M. (1975). Arteriographic correlates of handedness. *Neurology, 25*(3), 218–222.

Hoffman, M. A. & Swaab, D. F. (1994). The human hypothalamus: Comparative morphometry and photoperiodic influences. *Brain Research, 93,* 133–147.

Hoffstein, V., Chan, C. K., & Slutsky, A. S. (1993). Handedness and sleep apnea. *Chest, 103*(6), 1860–1862.

Holloway, R. L. (1980). Indonesian "solo" (Ngandong) endocranial reconstructions: Some preliminary observations and comparisons with Neanderthal and homo erectus groups. *American Journal of Physical Anthropology, 53,* 285–295.

Holloway, R. L. (1981). Volumetric and asymmetry determinations on recent hominid endocasts: Spy I and II, Djebel Ihroud I, and the Sale homo erectus specimens, with some notes on Neanderthal brain size. *American Journal of Physical Anthropology, 55*(3), 385–393.

Holloway, R. L. (1982). *Homo erectus* brain endocasts: Volumetric and morphological observations with some comments on cerebral asymmetries. In H. de Lumley (Ed.), *L'Homo erectus et la Place de l'Homme de Tautavel parmi les Hominidés Fosiles 1er Congrès International de Paléontologie Humaine, Nice, Prètirage:* Vol. 1. (pp. 355–369). Nice, France: Louis-Jean.

Holloway, R. L., & De La Coste-Lareymondie, M. C. (1982). Brain endocast asymmetry in pongids and hominids: Some preliminary findings on the paleontology of cerebral dominance. *American Journal of Physical Anthropology, 58*(1), 101–110.

Holmes, G. (1919). Disturbances of visual space perception. *British Medical Journal, 2,* 230–233.

Honig, L. S., & Rosenberg, R. N. (2000). Apoptosis and neurologic disease. *American Journal of Medicine, 108*(4), 317–330.

Hood, S. D., Argyropoulos, S. V., & Nutt, D. J. (2000). Agents in development for anxiety disorders: Current status and future potential. *CNS Drugs, 13*(6), 421–431.

Hoormann, J., Falkenstein, M., & Hohnsbein, J. (2000). Early attention effects in human auditory-evoked potentials. *Psychophysiology, 37*(1), 29–42.

Hu, S., Pattatucci, A. M., Patterson, C., Li, L., Fulker, D. W., Cherny, S. S., et al. (1995). Linkage between sexual orientation and chromosome Xq28 in males but not in females. *Nature Genetics, 11*(3), 248–256.

Hubble, J. P., Kurth, J. H., Glatt, S. L., Kurth, M. C., Schellenberg, G. D., Hassanein, R. E. S., et al. (1998). Gene-toxin interaction as a putative risk factor for Parkinson's disease with dementia. *Neuroepidemiology, 17*(2), 96–104.

Hubel, D. H., Wiesel, T. N., & LeVay, S. (1977). Plasticity of ocular dominance columns in monkey striate cortex. *Philosophical Transactions of the Royal Society of London Series B, Biological Sciences, 278*(961), 377–409.

Hubel, D. H., Wiesel, T. N., & Stryker, M. P. (1977). Orientation columns in macaque monkey visual cortex demonstrated by the 2-deoxyglucose autoradiographic technique. *Nature, 269*(5626), 328–330.

Hudson, P. T. W. (1975). The genetics of handedness: A reply to Levy and Nagylaki. *Neuropsychologia, 13,* 331–339.

Hugdahl, K., Satz, P., Mitrushina, M., & Miller, E. N. (1993). Left-handedness and old age: Do left-handers die earlier? *Neuropsychologia, 31*(4), 325–333.

Hughlings-Jackson, J. (1870). On voluntary and automatic movements. *British Medical Journal, 2,* 641–642.

Hughlings-Jackson, J. (1931). *Selected writings of John Hughlings Jackson: Vol. 1 and 2* (J. Taylor, Ed., pp. 8–36). London, England: Hodder and Stoughton.

Hull, A. M. (2002). Neuroimaging findings in post-traumatic stress disorder: Systematic review. *British Journal of Psychiatry, 181,* 102–110.

Humphreys, G. W., & Riddoch, M. J. (1993). Interactions between object and space systems revealed through neuropsychology. In D. E. Meyer (Ed.), *Attention and performance 14: Synergies in experimental psychology, artificial intelligence, and cognitive neuroscience* (pp. 143–162). Cambridge, MA: MIT Press.

Huntington, D. (1872). On Chorea. *Medical Surgical Reporter, 26,* 317–321.

Huttenlocher, J., Levine, S., & Vevea, J. (1998). Environmental input and cognitive growth: A study using time-period comparisons. *Child Development, 69*(4), 1012–1029.

Hyde, T. M., Stacey, M. E., Coppola, R., Handel, S. F., Rickler, K. C., & Weinberger, D. R. (1995). Cerebral morphometric abnormalities in Tourette's syndrome: A quantitative MRI study of monozygotic twins. *Neurology, 45*(6), 1176–1182.

Ironside, J. W. (2000). Pathology of variant Creutzfeldt-Jakob disease. *Archives of Virology* (Suppl. 16), 143–151.

Isojaervi, J. I., & Tokola, R. A. (1998). Benzodiazepines in the treatment of epilepsy in people with intellectual disability. *Journal of Intellectual Disability Research, 42*(Suppl. 1), 80–92.

Ivanovic, D. M., Leiva, B. P., Perez, H. T., Olivares, M. G., Diaz, N. S., Urrutia, M. S., et al. (2004). Head size and intelligence, learning, nutritional status and brain development. *Neuropsychologia, 42*(8), 1118–1131.

Ivry, R. B., & Lebby, P. C. (1993). Hemispheric differences in auditory perception are similar to those found in visual perception. *Psychological Science, 4*(1), 41–45.

Izard, C. E. (1992). Basic emotions, relations among emotions, and emotion-cognition relations. *Psychological Review, 99*(3), 561–565.

Jackson, H. (1905). *Ambidexterity.* London, England: Keagan Paul.

Jacobs, B., Schall, M., & Scheibel, A. B. (1993). A quantitative dendritic analysis of Wernicke's area in humans. II. Gender, hemispheric, and environmental factors. *Journal of Comparative Neurology, 327*(1), 97–111.

Jacobs, L. F., Gaulin, S. J., Sherry, D. F., & Hoffman, G. E. (1990). Evolution of spatial cognition: Sex-specific patterns of spatial behavior predict hippocampal size. *Proceedings of the National Academy of Sciences of the United States of America, 87*(16), 6349–6352.

Jakobson, L. S., Archibald, Y. M., Carey, D. P., & Goodale, M. A. (1991). A kinematic analysis of reaching and grasping movements in a patient recovering from optic ataxia. *Neuropsychologia, 29*(8), 803–809.

James, W. (1890). *The principles of psychology* (2 vols.). New York: Henry Holt.

Jankovic, J. (2001). Tourette's syndrome. *New England Journal of Medicine, 345*(16), 1184–1192.

Jankowiak, J., & Albert, M. L. (1994). Lesion localization in visual agnosia: Japanese: A case study. *Cognitive Neuropsychology, 13*(6), 823–848.

Jasnos, T. M., & Hakmiller, K. L. (1975). Some effects of lesion level, and emotional cues on affective expression in spinal cord patients. *Psychological Reports, 37*(3, Pt. 1), 859–870.

Jeannerod, M., & Decety, J. (1995). Mental motor imagery: A window into the representational stages of action. *Current Opinions in Neurobiology, 5*(6), 727–732.

Jeanty, P., Rodesch, F., Verhoogen, C., & Struyven, J. (1981). The vanishing twin. *Ultrasonics, 2,* 25–31.

Jerison, H. J. (1990). Fossil evidence of the evolution of the brain. In E. G. Jones & A. Peters (Eds.), *Cerebral cortex Vol 8A, Part 1: Comparative structure and evolution of cerebral cortex* (pp. 285–309). New York: Plenum Press.

Jewell, G., & McCourt, M. E. (2000). Pseudoneglect: A review and meta-analysis of performance factors in line bisection tasks. *Neuropsychologia, 38*(1), 93–110.

Johanson, D., & Edgar, B. (1996). *From Lucy to language.* New York: Simon and Schuster.

Johansson, B. B. (2000). Brain plasticity and stroke rehabilitation. The Willis lecture. *Stroke, 31*(1), 223–230.

Johnson, M. H. (2003). Development of human brain functions. *Biological Psychiatry, 54*(12), 1312–1316.

Jones, I., & Craddock, N. (2001). Candidate gene studies of bipolar disorder. *Annals of Medicine, 33*(4), 248–256.

Jones, L. B. (2001). Recent cytoarchitechtonic changes in the prefrontal cortex of schizophrenics. *Frontiers in Bioscience, 6,* E148–E153.

Jonides, J., Smith, E. E., Koeppe, R. A., Awh, E., Minoshima, S., & Mintun, M. A. (1993). Spatial working memory in humans as revealed by PET. *Nature, 363,* 623–624.

Jordan, H. E. (1911). The inheritance of left-handedness. *American Breeder's Magazine, 2*(1–2).

Jordan, H. E. (1922). The crime against left-handedness. *Good Health, 57,* 378–383.

Joseph, A. B., O'Leary, D. H., Kurland, R., & Ellis, H. D. (1999). Bilateral anterior cortical atrophy and subcortical atrophy in reduplicative paramnesia: A case-control study of computed tomography in 10 patients. *Canadian Journal of Psychiatry, 44*(7), 685–689.

Jovin, T. G., Vitti, R. A., & McCluskey, L. F. (2000). Evolution of temporal lobe hypoperfusion in transient global amnesia: a serial single photon emission computed tomography study. *Journal of Neuroimaging, 10*(4), 238–241.

Kandel, E. R., Schwartz, J. H., & Jessell, T. M. (2000). *Principles of neural science* (4th ed.). New York: McGraw-Hill.

Kattouf, V.-M. (1996). Alexia without agraphia: A disconnection syndrome. *Journal of Optometric Vision Development, 27*(4), 236–242.

Kay, D. W. (1994). The diagnosis and grading of dementia in population surveys: Measuring disability. *Dementia, 5*(5), 289–294.

Keats, S. (1965). *Cerebral palsy.* Springfield, IL: Thomas.

Kegl, J., & Poizner, H. (1997). Crosslinguistic/crossmodal syntactic consequences of left-hemisphere damage: Evidence from an aphasic signer and his identical twin. *Aphasiology, 11*(1), 1–37.

Keillor, J. M., Barrett, A. M., Crucian, G. P., Kortenkamp, S., & Heilman, K. M. (2002). Emotional experience and perception in the absence of facial feedback. *Journal of the International Neuropsychological Society, 8*(1), 130–135.

Kempermann, G., Kuhn, H. G., & Gage, F. H. (1998). Experience-induced neurogenesis in the senescent dentate gyrus. *Journal of Neuroscience, 18*(9), 3206–3212.

Kempler, D., Metter, E. J., Jackson, C. A., Hanson, W. R., Riege, W. H., Mazziotta, J. C., et al. (1988). Disconnection and cerebral metabolism: The case of conduction aphasia. *Archives of Neurology, 45*(3), 275–279.

Kennard, M. A. (1940). Relation of age to motor impairment in man and in subhuman primates. *Archives of Neurology and Psychiatry, 44,* 377–397.

Kesler, S. R., Garrett, A., Bender, B., Yankowitz, J., Zeng, S. M., Reiss, A. L. (2004). Amygdala and hippocampal volumes in Turner syndrome: A high-resolution MRI study of X-monosomy. *Neuropsychologia, 42*(14), 1971–1978.

Kessler, J., Markowitsch, H. J., Rudolf, J., & Heiss, W. D. (2001). Continuing cognitive impairment after isolated transient global amnesia. *International Journal of Neuroscience, 106*(3–4), 159–168.

Ketonen, L. M. (1998). Neuroimaging of the aging brain. *Neurologic Clinics, 16*(3), 581–598.

Kety, S. S., & Schmidt, C. F. (1945). The determination of cerebral blood flow in man by the use of nitrous oxide in low concentrations. *American Journal of Physiology, 143,* 53–66.

Kiehl, K. A., Smith, A. M., Hare, R. D., Mendrek, A., Forster, B. B., Brink, J., et al. (2001). Limbic abnormalities in affective processing by criminal psychopaths as revealed by functional magnetic resonance imaging. *Biological Psychiatry, 50*(9), 677–684.

Kim, H., & Levine, S. C. (1991). Inferring patterns of hemispheric specialization for individual subjects from laterality data: A two-task criterion. *Neuropsychologia, 29*(1), 93–105.

Kimura, D. (1967). Functional asymmetry of the brain in dichotic listening. *Cortex, 3,* 163–168.

Kimura, D. (1969). Spatial localization in left and right visual fields. *Canadian Journal of Psychology, 23*(6), 445–458.

Kimura, D. (1996). Sex, sexual orientation and sex hormones influence human cognitive function. *Current Opinions in Neurobiology, 6*(2), 259–263.

Kimura, D., & Archibald, Y. (1974). Motor functions of the left hemisphere. *Brain, 97*(2), 337–350.

King, F. L., & Kimura, D. (1972). Left-ear superiority in dichotic perception of vocal nonverbal sounds. *Canadian Journal of Psychology, Vol. 26*(2), 111–116.

Kinsbourne, M. (1988). Integrated field theory of consciousness. In A. J. Marcel & E. Bisiach (Eds.), *Consciousness in contemporary science.* Oxford, UK: Clarendon Press.

Kirveskari, P., & Alanen, P. (1989). Right-left asymmetry of maximum jaw opening. *Acta Odontologica Scandinavica, 47*(2), 101–103.

Kitterle, F. L., Christman, S., & Hellige, J. B. (1990). Hemispheric differences are found in the identification, but not the detection, of low versus high spatial frequencies. *Perception and Psychophysics, 48*(4), 297–306.

Kitterle, F. L., Hellige, J. B., & Christman, S. (1992). Visual hemispheric asymmetries depend on which spatial frequencies are task relevant [see comments]. *Brain and Cognition, 20*(2), 308–314.

Kjaer, T. W., Law, I., Wiltschiotz, G., Paulson, O. B., & Madsen, P. L. (2002). Regional cerebral blood flow during light sleep—a h(2)(15)o-pet study. *Journal of Sleep Research, 11*(3), 201–207.

Klar, A. J. (1996). A single locus, RGHT, specifies preference for hand utilization in humans. *Cold Spring Harbor Symposia on Quantitative Biology, 61,* 59–65.

Klein, R. M., & Dick, B. (2002). Temporal dynamics of reflexive attention shifts: A dual-stream rapid serial visual presentation exploration. *Psychological Science, 13*(2), 176–179.

Kleinert, R., Cervos-Navarro, J., Kleinert, G., Walter, G. F., & Steiner, H. (1987). Predominantly cerebral manifestation in Urbach-Wiethe's syndrome (lipoid proteinosis cutis et mucosae): A clinical and pathomorphological study. *Clinical Neuropathology, 6*(1), 43–45.

Kleinschmidt-DeMasters, B. K., & Gilden, D. H. (2001). Varicella-Zoster virus infections of the nervous system: Clinical and pathologic correlates. *Archives of Pathology Labrotory Medicine, 125*(6), 770–780.

Kleist, K. (1934). *Gehirnpathologie vornehmlich auf Grund der Kriegserfahrungen.* Leipzig, Germany: Barth.

Klüver, H. & Bucy, P. C. (1939). Preliminary analysis of functions of the temporal lobes in monkeys. *Arch Neurol Psychiatry, 42*, 979–1000.

Knowlton, B. J., Mangels, J. A., & Squire, L. R. (1996). A neostriatal habit learning system in humans. *Science, 273*(5280), 1399–1402.

Knowlton, B. J., Squire, L. R., & Gluck, M. A. (1994). Probabilistic classification learning in amnesia. *Learning Memory, 1*(2), 106–120.

Kohen-Raz, R. (1986). *Learning disabilities and postural control.* London, England: Freund.

Kolb, B., & Fantie, B. (1989). Development of the child's brain and behavior. In C. R. Reynolds & E. Fletcher-Janzen (Eds.), *Handbook of clinical child neuropsychology* (pp. 17–39). New York: Plenum.

Kolb, B., & Fantie, B. (1997). Development of the child's brain and behavior. In C. R. Reynolds, & E. Fletcher-Janzen (Eds.). *Handbook of clinical child neuropsychology.* (pp. 17–39). New York: Plenum.

Kolb, B., & Gibb, R. (1993). Possible anatomical basis of recovery of function after neonatal frontal lesions in rats. *Behavioral Neuroscience, 107*(5), 799–811.

Kolb, B., & Gibb, R. (Eds.). (1999). *Neuroplasticity and recovery of function after brain injury.* New York: Cambridge University Press.

Kolb, B., Gibb, R., & van der Kooy, D. (1994). Neonatal frontal cortical lesions in rats alter cortical structure and connectivity. *Brain Research, 645*(1–2), 85–97.

Kolb, B., & Whishaw, I. Q. (1981). Neonatal frontal lesions in the rat: Sparing of learned but not species-typical behavior in the presence of reduced brain weight and cortical thickness. *Journal of Comparative Physiology and Psychology, 95*(6), 863–879.

Kolb, B., & Whishaw, I. Q. (1990). *Fundamentals of human neuropsychology.* New York: W. H. Freeman.

Kolb, B., & Whishaw, I.Q. (1996). *Fundamentals of human neuropsychology* (4th ed.). New York: W. H. Freeman.

Kolb, B., & Whishaw, I. Q. (1998). Brain plasticity and behavior. *Annual Review of Psychology, 49*, 43–64.

Kolb, B., & Whishaw, I. Q. (2003). *Fundamentals of human neuropsychology.* (5th ed.). New York: Worth Publishers.

Kolb, B., Wilson, B., & Taylor, L. (1992). Developmental changes in the recognition and comprehension of facial expression: Implications for frontal lobe function. *Brain and Cognition, 20*(1), 74–84.

Koller, W. C. (1991). Environmental risk factors in Parkinson's disease. In G. Bernardi (Ed.), *The basal ganglia III. Advances in behavioral biology* (Vol. 39, pp. 717–722). New York: Plenum Press.

Kooistra, C. A., & Heilman, K. M. (1988). Motor dominance and lateral asymmetry of the globus pallidus. *Neurology, 38*(3), 388–390.

Korsakoff, S. S. (1887). Disturbance of psychic functions in alcoholic paralysis and its relation to the disturbance of the psychic sphere in multiple neuritis of non-alcoholic origin. *Vestnik Psichiatrii, 4,* Fasicle 2.

Kramer, E. L., & Sanger, J. J. (1990). Brain imaging in acquired immunodeficiency syndrome dementia complex. *Seminars in Nuclear Medicine, 20*(4), 353–363.

Kramer, M. A., Albrecht, S., & Miller, R. A. (1985). Handedness and the laterality of breast cancer in women. *Nursing Research, 34*(6), 333–337.

Krasyuk, A. E., & Rivchina, Z. A. (1968). On clinical variants of apraxia. *Zhurnal Nevropatologii i Psikhiatrii, 68*(12), 1793–1795.

Krause, T., Kurth, R., Ruben, J., Schwiemann, J., Villringer, K., Deuchert, M., et al. (2001). Representational overlap of adjacent fingers in multiple areas of human primary somatosensory cortex depends on electrical stimulus intensity: An MRI study. *Brain Research, 899* (1-2), 36–46.

Kremen, W. S., Seidman, L. J., Faraone, S. V., Toomey, R., & Tsuang, M. T. (2000). The paradox of normal neuropsychological function in schizophrenia. *Journal of Abnormal Psychology, 109*(4), 743–752.

Kremen, W. S., Seidman, L. J., Faraone, S. V., & Tsuang, M. T. (2001). Intelligence quotient and neuropsychological profiles in patients with schizophrenia and in normal volunteers. *Biological Psychiatry, 50*(6), 453–462.

Kroll, J. F., & Potter, M. C. (1984). Recognizing words, pictures, and concepts: A comparison of lexical, object, and reality decisions. *Journal of Verbal Learning and Verbal Behavior, 23*(1), 39–66.

Kubiszyn, T. W., Meyer, G. J., Finn, S. E., Eyde, L. D., Kay, G. G., Moreland, K. L., et al. (2000). Empirical support for psychological assessment in clinical health care settings. *Professional Psychology: Research and Practice, 31*(2), 119–130.

Kugu, N., & Bolayir, E. (2001). Ankiyete bozukluklarinda PET ve SPECT bulgulari. PET and SPECT findings in anxiety disorders. *Klinik Psikofarmakoloji Buelteni, 11*(2), 132–142.

Kujawa, S. G., & Liberman, M. C. (1999). Long-term sound conditioning enhances cochlear sensitivity. *Journal of Neurophysiology, 82*(2), 863–873.

Kunst-Wilson, W. R., & Zajonc, R. B. (1980). Affective discrimination of stimuli that cannot be recognized. *Science, 207*(4430), 557–558.

Kutas, M. (2000). Current thinking on language structures. In M. S. Gazzaniga (Ed.), *Cognitive neuroscience: A reader.* Oxford, UK: Blackwell.

LaBerge, D. L. (1990). Attention. *Psychological Science, 1*(3), 156–162.

Landis, T., Cummings, J. L., Benson, D. F., & Palmer, E. P. (1986). Loss of topographic familiarity: An environmental agnosia. *Archives of Neurology, 43*(2), 132–136.

Landy, H. J., Keith, L., & Keith, D. (1982). The vanishing twin. *Acta Geneticae Medicae et Gemellologiae, 31*(3–4), 179–194.

Landy, H. J., Weiner, S., Corson, S. L., Batzer, F. R., & Bolognese, R. J. (1986). The "vanishing twin": Ultrasonographic assessment of fetal disappearance in the first trimester. *American Journal of Obstetrics and Gynecology, 155*(1), 14–19.

Lane, R. D., Caruso, A. C., Brown, V. L., Axelrod, B., Schwartz, G. E., Sechrest, L., et al. (1994). Effects of non-right-handedness on risk for sudden death associated with coronary artery disease [see comments]. *American Journal of Cardiology, 74*(8), 743–747.

Lane, R. D., Reiman, E. M., Ahern, G. L., Schwartz, G. E., & Davidson, R. J. (1997). Neuroanatomical correlates of happiness, sadness, and disgust. *American Journal of Psychiatry, 154*(7), 926–933.

Langston, J. W. (1985). MPTP neurotoxicity: An overview and characterization of phases of toxicity. *Life Sciences, 36*(3), 201–206.

Lanius, R. A., Williamson, P. C., Boksman, K., Densmore, M., Gupta, M., Neufeld, R. W., et al. (2002). Brain activation during script-driven imagery induced dissociative responses in PTSD: A functional magnetic resonance imaging investigation. *Biological Psychiatry, 52*(4), 305–311.

Lanius, R. A., Williamson, P. C., Hopper, J., Densmore, M., Boksman, K., Gupta, M. A., et al. (2003). Recall of emotional states in posttraumatic stress disorder: An fMRI investigation. *Biological Psychiatry, 53*(3), 204–210.

Lannoo, E., Van Rietvelde, F., Colardyn, F., Lemmerling, M., Vandekerckhove, T., Jannes, C., et al. (2000). Early predictors of mortality and morbidity after severe closed head injury. *Journal of Neurotrauma, 17*(5), 403–414.

Laruelle, M., & Abi-Dargham, A. (1999). Dopamine as the wind of the psychotic fire: New evidence from brain imaging studies. *Journal of Psychopharmacology, 13*(4), 358–371.

Lashley, K. S. (1963). *Brain mechanisms and intelligence.* New York: Dover. (Original work published 1929.)

Lashley, K. S., & Franz, S. I. (1917). The effects of cerebral destruction upon habit-formation and retention in the albino rat. *Psychbiology, 1,* 71–139.

Lassen, N. A., & Ingvar, D. H. (1961). The blood flow of the cerebral cortex determined by radioactive krypton-85. *Experientia, 17,* 42–45.

Lassonde, M., Sauerwein, H. C., & Lepore, F. (1995). Extent and limits of callosal plasticity: Presence of disconnection symptoms in callosal agenesis. *Neuropsychologia, 33*(8), 989–1007.

Lawton, C. A. (1994). Gender differences in way-finding strategies: Relationship to spatial ability and spatial anxiety. *Sex Roles, 30*(11–12), 765–779.

Leboyer, M., Osherson, D. N., Nosten, M., & Roubertoux, P. (1988). Is autism associated with anomalous dominance? *Journal of Autism and Developmental Disorders, 18*(4), 539–551.

Lecours, A. R. (1999). Frank Benson's teachings on acquired disorders of written language (with addenda). *Aphasiology, 13*(1), 21–40.

Lecours, A. R., & Lhermitte, F. (1969). Phonemic paraphasias: Linguistic structures and tentative hypotheses. *Cortex, 5*(3), 193–228.

LeDoux, J. (1996). *The emotional brain.* New York: Simon and Schuster.

Lehmkuhl, G., Poeck, K., & Willmes, K. (1983). Ideomotor apraxia and aphasia: An examination of types and manifestations of apraxic symptoms. *Neuropsychologia, 21*(3), 199–212.

LeMay, M. (1976). Morphological cerebral asymmetries of modern man, fossil man, and nonhuman primate. *Annals of the New York Academy of Sciences, 280,* 349–366.

LeMay, M. (1977). Asymmetries of the skull and handedness. Phrenology revisited. *Journal of Neuroscience, 32*(2), 243–253.

LeMay, M., & Culebras, A. (1972). Human brain-morphologic differences in the hemispheres demonstrable by carotid arteriography. *New England Journal of Medicine, 287*(4), 168–170.

Leon-Carrion, J., Rodriguez-Duarte, R., Barroso-Martin, J. M., Machuca, F., Dominguez-Morales, M. R., Murillo, F., et al. (1996). The attentional system in brain injury survivors. *International Journal of Neuroscience, 85*(3–4), 231–236.

LeVay, S., & Hamer, D. H. (1994). Evidence for a biological influence in male homosexuality. *Scientific American, 270*(5), 44–49.

LeVay, S., Wiesel, T. N., & Hubel, D. H. (1980). The development of ocular dominance columns in normal and visually deprived monkeys. *Journal of Comparative Neurology, 191*(1), 1–51.

Levi, S. (1976). Ultrasonic assessment of the high rate of human multiple pregnancy in the first trimester. *Journal of Clinical Ultrasound, 4*(1), 3–5.

Levin, H. S., & Benton, A. L. (1986). Neuropsychological assessment. In A. B. Barker and R. J. Joynt (Eds.), *Clinical neurology: Vol. 1.* New York: Harper and Row.

Levine, B. (2004). Autobiographical memory and the self in time: Brain lesion effects, functional neuroanatomy, and lifespan development. *Brain and Cognition, 55*(1), 54–68.

Levine, D. N., Warach, J., & Farah, M. (1985). Two visual systems in mental imagery: Dissociation of "what" and "where" in imagery disorders due to bilateral posterior cerebral lesions. *Neurology, 35*(7), 1010–1018.

Levinson, R. W., Ekman, P., & Friesen, W. V. (1990). Voluntary facial action generates emotion-specific autonomic nervous system activity. *Psychophysiology, 27,* 363–384.

Levy, J. (1969). Possible basis for the evolution of lateral specialization of the human brain. *Nature, 224*(219), 614–615.

Levy, J., Trevarthen, C., & Sperry, R. W. (1972). Reception of bilateral chimeric figures following hemispheric deconnexion. *Brain, 95*(1), 61–78.

Lewin, J., Kohen, D., & Mathew, G. (1993). Handedness in mental handicap: Investigation into populations of Down's syndrome, epilepsy and autism. *British Journal of Psychiatry, 163,* 674–676.

Lewis, J. L. (1970). Semantic processing of unattended messages using dichotic listening. *Journal of Experimental Psychology, 85*(2), 225–228.

Lezak, M. D. (1995). *Neuropsychological assessment* (3rd ed.). New York: Oxford University Press.

Liepmann, H. (1977). The Liepmann syndrome of apraxia (motor asymboly) based on a case of unilateral apraxia (W. H. O. Bohne, K. Liepmann & D. A. Rottenberg, Trans.). In D. A. Rottenberg & F. H. Hochberg (Eds.), *Neurological classics in modern translation.* New York: Hafner Press. (Original work published 1900.)

Liepmann, H. (1980). The left hemisphere and action. In *Research bulletin* (p. 506). London, Ontario: Department of Psychology, University of Western Ontario. (Original work published 1905.)

Lindvall, O. (2000). Neural transplantation in Parkinson's disease. *Novartis Foundation Symposium, 231,* 110–123.

Linn, M. C., & Petersen, A. C. (1985). Emergence and characterization of sex differences in spatial ability: A meta-analysis. *Child Development, 56*(6), 1479–1498.

Lisanby, S. H., Maddox, J. H., Prudic, J., Devanand, D. P., & Sackeim, H. A. (2000). The effects of electroconvulsive therapy on memory of autobiographical and public events. *Archives of General Psychiatry, 57*(6), 581–590.

Livingstone M., Rosen G., Drislane F., & Galaburda A. (1991). Physiological and anatomical evidence for a magnocellular defect in developmental dyslexia. *Proceedings of the National Academy of Science, 88,* 7943–7947.

Loftus, E. F. (1997). Creating false memories. *Scientific American, 277*(3), 70–75.

Loftus, E. F. (1998). The private practice of misleading deflection. *American Psychologist, 53,* 484–485.

Logie, R. H., Zucco, G. M., & Baddeley, A. D. (1990). Interference with visual short-term memory. *Acta Psychologica, 75*(1), 55–74.

Lombroso, C. (1903). Left-handedness and left-sidedness. *North American Review, 177,* 440–444.

London, W. P. (1989). Left-handedness and life expectancy. *Perceptual and Motor Skills, 68*(3, Pt. 2), 1040–1042.

London, W. P., & Albrecht, S. A. (1991). Breast cancer and cerebral laterality. *Perceptual and Motor Skills, 72*(1), 112–114.

Longden, K., Ellis, C., & Iversen, S. D. (1976). Hemispheric differences in the discrimination of curvature. *Neurospychologia, 14,* 195–202.

Lonton, A. P. (1976). Hand preference in children with myelomeningocele and hydrocephalus. *Developmental Medicine and Child Neurology, 18*(6, Suppl. 37), 143–149.

Loring, D. W., Lee, G. P., Martin, R. C., & Meador, K. J. (1989). Verbal and visual memory index discrepancies from the Wechsler Memory Scale-Revised: Cautions in interpretation. *Psychological Assessment, 1,* 198–202.

Lovell, M. R., Iverson, G. L., Collins, M. W., McKeag, D., & Maroon, J. C. (1999). Does loss of consciousness predict neuropsychological decrements after concussion? *Clinical Journal of Sport Medicine, 9*(4), 193–198.

Lovegrove, W. J., Bwoling, A., Badcock, B., & Blackwood, M. (1980). Specific reading disability: Differences in contrast sensitivity as a function of spatial frequency. *Science, 210,* 439–440.

Lucas, J. A., Rosenstein, L. D., & Bigler, E. D. (1989). Handedness and language among the mentally retarded: Implications for the model of pathological left-handedness and gender differences in hemispheric specialization. *Neuropsychologia, 27*(5), 713–723.

Luria, A. R. (1966). *Higher cortical functions in man.* New York: Basic Books.

Luria, A. R. (1973). *The working brain.* London, England: Penguin.

Luzzatti, C., & Verga, R. (1996). Reduplicative paramnesia for places with preserved memory and perceptual skills: "Reduplication" or "adapation" disorder. In P. W. Halligan & J. C. Marshall (Eds.), *Method in madness: Case studies in cognitive neuropsychiatry.* Hove, England: Psychology Press.

Lysakowski, A., Standage, G. P., & Benevento, L. A. (1988) An investigation of collateral projections of the dorsal lateral geniculate nucleus and other subcortical structures to cortical areas V1 and V4 in the macaque monkey: A double label retrograde tracer study. *Experimental Brain Research, 69,* 651–661.

MacLeod, C. M., & MacDonald, P. A. (2000). Interdimensional interference in the Stroop effect: Uncovering the cognitive and neural anatomy of attention. *Trends in Cognitive Sciences, 4*(10), 383–391.

Macmillan, M. (2000). Restoring Phineas Gage: A 150th retrospective. *Journal of the History of the Neurosciences, 9*(1), 46–66.

MacNeilage, P. F. (1991). The "postural origins" theory of primate neurobiological asymmetries. In N. A. Krasnegor, R. L. Schiefelbusch, & M. G. Studdart-Kennedy (Eds.),

Biological and behavioral determinants of language development. Hillsdale, NJ: Lawrence Erlbaum.

MacNiven, E. (1994). Increased prevalence of left-handedness in victims of head trauma. *Brain Injury, 8*(5), 457–462.

Madsen, K. M., & Vestergaard, M. (2004). MMR vaccination and autism: What is the evidence for a causal association? *Drug Safety, 27*(12), 831–840.

Maeshima, S. I., Komai, N., Kinoshita, Y., Ueno, M., Nakai, E., Naka, Y., et al. (1992). Transcortical sensory aphasia following the unilateral left thalamic infarction: A case report. *Journal of Neurolinguistics, 7*(3), 251–257.

Magoun, H. W. (1966). Discussion of brain mechanisms in speech. In E. C. Carterette (Ed.), *Brain function: Speech, language, and communication.* Los Angeles: University of California Press.

Maguire, E. A., Frackowiak, R. S. J., & Frith, C. D. (1997). Recalling routes around London: Activation of the right hippocampus in taxi drivers. *Journal of Neuroscience, 17*(18), 7103–7110.

Maguire, E. A., Frith, C. D., Burgess, N., Donnett, J. G., & O'Keefe, J. (1998). Knowing where things are parahippocampal involvement in encoding object locations in virtual large-scale space. *Journal of Cognitive Neuroscience, 10*(1), 61–76.

Maguire, E. A., Gadian, D. G., Johnsrude, I. S., Good, C. D., Ashburner, J., Frackowiak, R. S., et al. (2000). Navigation-related structural change in the hippocampi of taxi drivers [see comments]. *Proceeding of the National Academy of Sciences of the United States of America, 97*(8), 4398–4403.

Maier, M. (1995). In vivo magnetic resonance spectroscopy. Applications in psychiatry. *British Journal of Psychiatry, 167*(3), 299–306.

Maison, S., Micheyl, C., & Collet, L. (2001). Influence of focused auditory attention on cochlear activity in humans. *Psychophysiology, 38*(1), 35–40.

Malec, J. F., Buffington, A. L., Moessner, A. M., & Thompson, J. M. (1995). Maximizing vocational outcome after brain injury: Integration of medical and vocational hospital-based services. *Mayo Clinic Proceedings, 70*(12), 1165–1171.

Mangun, G. R., & Hillyard, S. A. (1988). Spatial gradients of visual attention: Behavioral and electrophysiological evidence. *Electroencephalography and Clinical Neurophysiology, 70*(5), 417–428.

Mangun, G. R., Hillyard, S. A., & Luck, S. J. (1993). Electrocortical substrates of visual selective attention. In D. Meyer & S. Kornblum (Eds.), *Attention and performance XIV* (pp. 219–243). Cambridge, MA: MIT Press.

Manoach, D. S. (1994). Handedness is related to formal thought disorder and language dysfunction in schizophrenia. *Journal of Clinical and Experimental Neuropsychology, 16*(1), 2–14.

Manoach, D. S., Maher, B. A., & Manschreck, T. C. (1988). Left-handedness and thought disorder in the schizophrenias. *Journal of Abnormal Psychology, 97*(1), 97–99.

Mann, V. A., Sasanuma, S., Sakuma, N., & Masaki, S. (1990). Sex differences in cognitive abilities: A cross-cultural perspective. *Neuropsychologia, 28*(10), 1063–1077.

Maquet, P. (2005). Current status of brain imaging in sleep medicine. *Sleep Med Rev, 9*(3), 155–156.

Maquet, P., Peters, J., Aerts, J., Delfiore, G., Degueldre, C., Luxen, A., et al. (1996). Functional neuroanatomy of human rapid-eye-movement sleep and dreaming. *Nature, 383*(6596), 163–166.

Marcel, A. J. (1998). Blindsight and shape perception: Deficit of visual consciousness or of visual function? *Brain, 121*(8), 1565–1588.

Marie, P. (1906). Que faut-il penser des aphasies sous-corticales? *Sem Med, 42,* 493–500.

Markow, T. A. (1992). Human handedness and the concept of developmental stability. *Genetica, 87*(2), 87–94.

Markowitsch, H. J., Calabrese, P., Wurker, M., Durwen, H. F., Kessler, J., Babinsky, R., et al. (1994). The amygdala's contribution to memory: A study on two patients with Urbach-Wiethe disease. *Neuroreport, 5*(11), 1349–1352.

Marks, I. M. (1987). *Fears, phobias, and rituals: Panic, anxiety, and their disorders.* New York: Oxford University Press.

Marlowe, W. B., Mancall, E. L., & Thomas, J. J. (1975). Complete Kluver-Bucy syndrome in man. *Cortex, 11*(1), 53–59.

Marquez, S., Zubiaur, M., Serrano, I., & Delgado, J. (1989). Hemispheric asymmetry and visual perception: Absence of laterality effects in iconic storage. *Medical Science Research, 17*(24), 1019–1020.

Marshall, D., & Zimbardo, P. G. (1979). Affective consequences of inadequately explained physiological arousal. *Journal of Personality and Social Psychology, 37,* 970–988.

Martin, G. N. (1998). *Human neuropsychology.* Hemel Hempstead, England: Prentice-Hall.

Martin, J. H. (1996). *Neuroanatomy text and atlas.* Stamford, CN: Appleton and Lange.

Marx, J. (1996). Searching for drugs that combat Alzheimer's. *Science, 273*(5271), 50–53.

Marzi, C. A. (1999). Neuropsychology of attention. In G. Denes (Ed.), *Handbook of clinical and experimental neuropsychology* (pp. 509–524). Hove, England: Psychology Press/Taylor and Francis.

Masson, C. (2000). Transient global amnesia. *Presse Medicale, 29*(30), 1677–1682.

Matser, E. J., Kessels, A. G., Lezak, M. D., Jordan, B. D., & Troost, J. (1999). Neuropsychological impairment in amateur soccer players. *Journal of the American Medical Association, 282*(10), 971–973.

Mattingley, J. B., Bradshaw, J. L., Nettleton, N. C., & Bradshaw, J. A. (1994). Can task specific perceptual bias be distinguished from unilateral neglect? *Neuropsychologia, 32*(7), 805–817.

Max, W., MacKenzie, E. J., & Rice, D. P. (1991). Head injuries: Costs and consequences. *Journal of Head Trauma and Rehabilitation, 6*(2), 76–91.

Mazzoni, M., Del-Torto, E., Vista, M., & Moretti, P. (1993). Transient topographical amnesia: A case report. *Italian Journal of Neurological Sciences, 14*(9), 633–636.

McCarthy, A., & Brown, N. A. (1998). Specification of left-right asymmetry in mammals: Embryo culture studies of stage of determination and relationships with morphogenesis and growth. *Reproductive Toxicology, 12*(2), 177–184.

McCarthy, R. A., & Warrington, E. K. (1987). The double dissociation of short-term memory for lists and sentences: Evidence from aphasia. *Brain, 110*(Pt. 6), 1545–1563.

McCarthy, R. A., & Warrington, E. K. (1990). *Cognitive neuropsychology: A clinical introduction.* San Diego, CA: Academic Press.

McCrae, D., & Trolle, E. (1956). The defect of function in visual agnosia. *Brain, 79,* 94–110.

McCreadie, R. G., Thara, R., Padmavati, R., Srinivasan, T. N., & Jaipurkar, S. D. (2002). Structural brain differences between never-treated patients with schizophrenia, with and without dyskinesia, and normal control subjects: A magnetic resonance imaging study. *Archives of General Psychiatry, 59*(4), 332–336.

McDowell, I. (2001). Alzheimer's disease: Insights from epidemiology. *Aging (Milano), 13*(3), 143–162.

McEwen, B. S. (2001). Plasticity of the hippocampus: Adaptation to chronic stress and allostatic load. *Annals of the New York Academy of Sciences, 933,* 265–277.

McGlynn, S. M. (1990). Behavioral approaches to neuropsychological rehabilitation. *Psychological Bulletin, 108*(3), 420–441.

McKeever, W. F. (1986). Tachistoscopic methods in neuropsychology. In H. J. Hannay (Ed.), *Experimental techniques in neuropsychology* (pp. 167–211). New York: Oxford University Press.

McLean, J. M., & Cuirczak, F. M. (1982). Bimanual dexterity in major league baseball players: A statistical study. *New England Journal of Medicine, 307,* 1278–1279.

McManus, I. C. (1980). Handedness in twins: A critical review. *Neuropsychologia, 18*(3), 347–355.

McManus, I. C. (1985). Handedness, language dominance and aphasia: A genetic model. *Psychological Medicine, Monograph Supplement 8,* 1–40.

McManus, I. C., & Bryden, M. P. (1992). The genetics of handedness, cerebral dominance and lateralization. In I. Rapin & S. J. Segalowitz (Eds.), *Handbook of neuropsychology, Vol. 6: Developmental neuropsychology* (pp. 115–144). Amsterdam, The Netherlands: Elsevier Science.

McManus, I. C., & Humphrey, N. K. (1973). Turning the left cheek. *Nature, 243,* 271–272.

McMullen, P. A., Fisk, J. D., Phillips, S. J., & Maloney, W. J. (2000). Apperceptive agnosia and face recognition. *Neurocase, 6*(5), 403–414.

Mebert, C. J., & Michel, G. F. (1980). Handedness in artists. In J. Herron (Ed.), *The neuropsychology of left-handedness* (pp. 273–279). New York: Academic Press.

Mellet, E., Tzourio, N., Crivello, F., Joliot, M., Denis, M., & Mazoyer, B. (1996). Functional anatomy of spatial mental imagery generated from verbal instructions. *Journal of Neuroscience, 16*(20), 6504–6512.

Mendez, M. (2001). Visuospatial deficits with preserved reading ability in a patient with posterior cortical atrophy. *Cortex, 37*(4), 535–543.

Mendez, M. F. (1995). The neuropsychiatric aspects of boxing. *International Journal of Psychiatry in Medicine, 25*(3), 249–262.

Merckelbach, H., Muris, P., & Kop, W. J. (1994). Handedness, symptom reporting, and accident susceptibility. *Journal of Clinical Psychology, 50*(3), 389–392.

Merikle, P. (2000). Subliminal Perception. In A. E. Kazdin (Ed.), *Encyclopedia of psychology.* New York: Oxford University Press.

Mesulam, M. M. (1981). A cortical network for directed attention and unilateral neglect. *Annals of Neurology, 10*(4), 309–325.

Meyer, D. E., Schvaneveldt, R. W., & Ruddy, M. G. (1974). Functions of graphemic and phonemic codes in visual word-recognition. *Memory and Cognition, 2*(2), 309–321.

Meyer, G. J., Finn, S. E., Eyde, L. D., Kay, G. G., Moreland, K. L., Dies, R. R., et al. (2001). Psychological testing and psychological assessment: A review of evidence and issues. *American Psychologist, 56*(2), 128–165.

Meyers, S., & Janowitz, H. D. (1985). Left-handedness and inflammatory bowel disease. *Journal of Clinical Gastroenterology, 7*(1), 33–35.

Miller, E. (1971). Handedness and the pattern of human ability. *British Journal of Psychology, 62*(1), 111–112.

Miller, G. A. (1956). The magical number seven plus or minus two: Some limits on our capacity for processing information. *Psychological Review, 63,* 81–97.

Miller, R. (1996). *Axonal conduction delay and human cerebral laterality: A psychobiological theory.* London, England: Harwood Academic Publishers.

Mills, L., & Rollman, G. B. (1979). Left hemisphere selectivity for processing duration in normal subjects. *Brain and Language, 7*(3), 320–335.

Mills, L., & Rollman, G. B. (1980). Hemispheric asymmetry for auditory perception of temporal order. *Neuropsychologia, 18*(1), 41–48.

Milner, A. D., & Goodale, M. A. (1995). *The visual brain in action*. Oxford, UK: Oxford University Press.

Mishkin, M., Ungerleider, L. G., & Macko, K. A. (1983). Object vision and spatial vision: Two cortical pathways. *Trends in Neurosciences, 6*(10), 414–417.

Monk, D., & Brodaty, H. (2000). Use of estrogens for the prevention and treatment of Alzheimer's disease. *Dementia and Geriatric Cognitive Disorders, 11*(1), 1–10.

Monrad-Krohn, G. H. (1947). Dysprosody of altered "melody of language." *Brain, 70,* 405–415.

Montague, D. P., & Walker-Andrews, A. S. (2001). Peek-a-boo: A new look at infants' perception of emotion expressions. *Developmental Psychology, 37*(6), 826–838.

Moreno, C. R., Borod, J. C., Welkowitz, J., & Alpert, M. (1990). Lateralization for the expression and perception of facial emotion as a function of age. *Neuropsychologia, 28*(2), 199–209.

Morera, A., Gonzalez-Feria, L., Valenciano, R., & Sabat, M. C. (1989). Apraxia del vestir: Estandarizacion de una prueba en sujetos normales [Dressing apraxia: Standardization of a task in healthy subjects]. *Revista de Psiquiatria de la Facultad de Medicina de Barcelona, 16*(3), 121–126.

Morera-Fumero, A., & Rodriguez, F. (1990). Pure apraxia for dressing: A case report. *European Journal of Psychiatry, 4*(3), 133–137.

Morris, J. S., Friston, K. J., Buchel, C., Frith, C. D., Young, A. W., Calder, A. J., et al. (1998). A neuromodulatory role for the human amygdala in processing emotional facial expressions. *Brain, 121*(Pt. 1), 47–57.

Morris, J. S., Friston, K. J., & Dolan, R. J. (1997). Neural responses to salient visual stimuli. *Proceedings of the Royal Society of London: Series B, Biological Sciences, 264*(1382), 769–775.

Morris, J. S., Frith, C. D., Perrett, D. I., Rowland, D., Young, A. W., Calder, A. J., et al. (1996). A differential neural response in the human amygdala to fearful and happy facial expressions. *Nature, 383*(6603), 812–815.

Morris, R. D., & Romski, M. A. (1993). Handedness distribution in a nonspeaking population with mental retardation. *American Journal of Mental Retardation, 97*(4), 443–448.

Morris, R. G., Garrud, P., Rawlins, J. N., & O'Keefe, J. (1982). Place navigation impaired in rats with hippocampal lesions. *Nature, 297*(5868), 681–683.

Moscato, B. S., Trevisan, M., & Willer, B. S. (1994). The prevalence of traumatic brain injury and co-occurring disabilities in a national household survey of adults. *Journal of Neuropsychiatry and Clinical Neuroscience, 6*(2), 134–142.

Moscovitch, M. (1979). Information processing and the cerebral hemispheres. In M. S. Gazzaniga (Ed.), *Handbook of behavioral neurology: Vol. 2* (pp. 379–446). New York: Plenum Press.

Moscovitch, M. (1994). Memory and working with memory: Evaluation of a component process model and comparisons with other models. In D. L. Schacter & E. Tulving (Eds.), *Memory systems* (pp. 269–310). Cambridge, MA: MIT Press.

Moscovitch, M., & Olds, J. (1982). Asymmetries in spontaneous facial expressions and their possible relation to hemispheric specialization. *Neuropsychologia, 20*(1), 71–81.

Moscovitch, M., Strauss, E., & Olds, J. (1981). Handedness and dichotic listening performance in patients with unipolar endogenous depression who received ECT. *American Journal of Psychiatry, 138*(7), 988–990.

Moser, D. J., Cohen, R. A., Malloy, P. F., Stone, W. M., & Rogg, J. M. (1998). Reduplicative paramnesia: Longitudinal neurobehavioral and neuroimaging analysis. *Journal of Geriatric Psychiatry and Neurology, 11*(4), 174–180.

Moses, J. A., Cardellino, J. P., & Thompson, L. L. (1983). Discrimination of brain damage from chronic psychosis by the Luria-Nebraska Neuropsychological Battery: A closer look. *Journal of Consulting and Clinical Psychology, 51,* 441–449.

Motter, B. C., & Mountcastle, V. B. (1981). The functional properties of light-sensitive neurons of the posterior parietal cortex studied in waking monkeys: Foveal sparing and opponent vector organziation. *Journal of Neuroscience, 1,* 3–26.

Mountcastle., V. B., Lynch, J. C., Georgopoulus, A., Sakata, H., & Acuna, C. (1975). Posterior parietal association cortex of the monkey: Command functions for operations within extrapersonal space. *Journal of Neurophysiology, 38,* 871–908.

Mueller, J. H., Grove, T. R., & Thompson, W. B. (1993). Test anxiety and handedness. *Bulletin of the Psychonomic Society, 31*(5), 461–464.

Munoz-Yunta, J. A., Ortiz-Alonso, T., Amo, C., Fernandez-Lucas, A., Maestu, F., Palau-Baduell, M. (2003). Savant or idiot savant syndrome. *Review of Neurology, 36,* S157–S161.

Murai, T., Toichi, M., Sengoku, A., Miyoshi, K., & Morimune, S. (1997). Reduplicative paramnesia in patients with focal brain damage. *Neuropsychiatry, Neuropsychology, and Behavioral Neurology, 10*(3), 190–196.

Murdoch, B. D., & Reef, H. E. (1986). Lateral dominance and visual evoked potentials in albinos. *Perceptual and Motor Skills, 62*(3), 867–872.

Murdoch, B. E., Chenery, H. J., Wilks, V., & Boyle, R. S. (1987). Language disorders in dementia of the Alzheimer type. *Brain and Language, 31*(1), 122–137.

Murphy, J. R., & Ringel, S. P. (1990). Survival prediction in amyotrophic lateral sclerosis. *Muscle Nerve, 13*(7), 657–658.

Mustanski, B. S., Dupree, M. G., Nievergelt, C. M., Bocklandt, S., Schork, N. J., & Hamer, D. H. (2005). A genomewide scan of male sexual orientation. *Human Genetics, 116*(4), 272–278.

Nagaratnam, N., & Nagaratnam, K. (2000). Acute mixed transcortical aphasia with bihemispheric neurological deficits following diffuse cerebral dysfunction. *Aphasiology, 14*(9), 893–899.

Navon, D. (1977). Forest before trees: The precedence of global features in visual perception. *Cognitive Psychology, 9*(3), 353–383.

Nebes, R. D. (1971). Handedness and the perception of part-whole relationship. *Cortex, 7*(4), 350–356.

Neiser, U. (1967). *Cognitive psychology.* New York: Appleton-Century-Crofts.

Nelson, H. E. (1982). *The National Adult Reading Test (NART): Test manual.* Windsor, Berks, UK: NFER-Nelson.

Nelson, H. E., & O'Connell, A. (1978). Dementia: The estimation of premorbid intelligence levels using the National Adult Reading Test. *Cortex, 14*, 234–244.

Neville, H. J., & Mills, D. L. (1997). Epigenesis of language. *Mental Retardation and Developmental Disabilities Research Reviews, 3*(4), 282–292.

Newland, G. A. (1981). Differences between left- and right-handers on a measure of creativity. *Perceptual and Motor Skills, 53,* 787–792.

Newman, H. H. (1931). Differences between conjoined twins: In relation to a general theory of twinning. *Journal of Heredity, 22,* 201–207.

Newton, F. H., Rosenberg, R. N., Lampert, P. W., & O'Brien, J. S. (1971). Neurologic involvement in Urbach-Wiethe's disease (lipoid proteinosis). A clinical, ultrastructural, and chemical study. *Neurology, 21*(12), 1205–1213.

Nichelli, P. (1999). Visuospatial and imagery disorders. In G. Denes & L. Pizzamiglio (Eds.), *Handbook of clinical and experimental neuropsychology* (pp. 453–477). Hove, England: Psychology Press/Erlbaum.

Nicholls, M. E., & Atkinson, J. (1993). Hemispheric asymmetries for an inspection time task: A general left hemisphere temporal advantage? *Neuropsychologia, 31*(11), 1181–1190.

Nicholls, M. E., Clode, D., Wood, S. J., & Wood, A. G. (1999). Laterality of expression in portraiture: Putting your best cheek forward. *Proceedings of the Royal Society of London: Series B, Biological Sciences, 266*(1428), 1517–1522.

Nicholls, M. E., & Cooper, C. J. (1991). Hemispheric differences in the rates of information processing for simple nonverbal stimuli. *Neuropsychologia, 29*(7), 677–684.

Nicholls, M. E., Wolfgang, B. J., Clode, D., & Lindell, A. K. (2002). The effect of left and right poses on the expression of facial emotion. *Neuropsychologia, 40*(10), 1662–1665.

Nicholls, M. E. R. (1996). Temporal processing asymmetries between the cerebral hemispheres: Evidence and implications. *Laterality, 1,* 97–137.

Nicholls, M. E. R., Bradshaw, J. L., & Mattingley, J. B. (1999). Free-viewing perceptual asymmetries for the judgement of brightness, numerosity and size. *Neuropsychologia, 37*(3), 307–314.

Nicolson, R. I., Fawcett, A. J., & Dean, P. (2001). Dyslexia, development and the cerebellum. *Trends in Neuroscience, 24,* 515–516.

Niederlandova, Z. (1967). Left-handedness in strabismus. *Cesk Oftalmol, 23*(1), 9–13.

Niedermeyer, E. (1994). Consciousness: Function and definition. *Clinical Electroencephalography, 25*(3), 86–93.

Nielsen, J. M. (1946). *Agnosia, apraxia, aphasia: Their value in cerebral localization* (2nd ed.). New York: Hoeber.

Nilsson, M., Perfilieva, E., Johansson, U., Orwar, O., & Eriksson, P. S. (1999). Enriched environment increases neurogenesis in the adult rat dentate gyrus and improves spatial memory. *Journal of Neurobiology, 39*(4), 569–578.

Nofzinger, E. A., Buysse, D. J., Miewald, J. M., Meltzer, C. C., Price, J. C., Sembrat, R. C., et al. (2002). Human regional cerebral glucose metabolism during non-rapid eye movement sleep in relation to waking. *Brain, 125*(Pt. 5), 1105–1115.

Nolte, J. (1999). *The human brain. An introduction to its functional anatomy* (4th ed.). St. Louis, MO: Mosby.

Norman, D. A., & Shallice, T. (Eds.). (1986). *Attention to action: Willed and automatic control of behaviour: Vol. 4.* New York: Plenum Press.

Novak, V., Kangarlu, A., Abduljalil, A., Novak, P., Slivka, A., Chakeres, D., et al. (2001). Ultra high field MRI at 8 Tesla of subacute hemorrhagic stroke. *Journal of Computer Assisted Tomorgaphy, 25*(3), 431–435.

Nudo, R. J., & Milliken, G. W. (1996). Reorganization of movement representations in primary motor cortex following focal ischemic infarcts in adult squirrel monkeys. *Journal of Neurophysiology, 75*(5), 2144–2149.

Obeso, J. A., Guridi, J., & DeLong, M. (1997). Surgery for Parkinson's disease. *Journal of Neurology, Neurosurgery and Psychiatry, 62*(1), 2–8.

O'Callaghan, M. J., Burn, Y. R., Mohay, H. A., Rogers, Y., & Tudehope, D. I. (1993). The prevalence and origins of left hand preference in high risk infants, and its implications for intellectual, motor and behavioural performance at four and six years. *Cortex, 29*(4), 617–627.

O'Connell, S. M. (1995). Empathy in chimpanzees: Evidence for theory of mind? *Primates, 36,* 397–410.

Odani, S. (1935). A case of alexia. *Japanese Journal of Experimental Psychology, 2,* 333–348.

Ohman, A., Flykt, A., & Esteves, F. (2001). Emotion drives attention: Detecting the snake in the grass. *Journal of Experimental Psychology General, 130*(3), 466–478.

Ohman, A., & Mineka, S. (2001). Fears, phobias, and pre-paredness: Toward an evolved module of fear and fear learning. *Psychological Review, 108*(3), 483–522.

O'Keefe, J., & Dostrovsky, J. (1971). The hippocampus as a spatial map. Preliminary evidence from unit activity in the freely-moving rat. *Brain Research, 34,* 171–175.

Oldfield, R. C. (1971). The assessment and analysis of hand-edness: The Edinburgh inventory. *Neuropsychologia, 9*(1), 97–113.

Olney, J. W. (1971). Glutamate-induced neuronal necrosis in the infant mouse hypothalamus. An electron microscopic study. *Journal of Neuropathol and Experimental Neurology, 30*(1), 75–90.

Olney, J. W. (1990). Excitotoxicity: An overview. *Canada Diseases Weekly Report, 16* (Suppl. 1E), 47–57, 47–48.

Olsen, J. (1995). Is left-handedness a sensitive marker of pre-natal exposures or indicators of fetal growth? *Scandinavian Journal of Social Medicine, 23*(4), 233–235.

Olsson, B., & Rett, A. (1986). Shift to righthandedness in Rett syndrome around age 7. *American Journal of Medical Genetics* (Suppl. 1), 133–141.

Orbach, J. (1998). *The neuropsychological theories of Lashley and Hebb: Contemporary perspectives fifty years after Hebb's The Organization of Behavior: Vanuxem Lectures and selected theoretical papers of Lashley.* Lanham, MD: University Press of America.

Ostrosky-Solis, F., Quintanar, L., Madrazo, I., Drucker-Colin, R., Franco-Bourland, R., & Leon-Meza, V. (1991). Neuropsychological effects of brain autograft of adrenal medullary tissue for the treatment of Parkinson's disease. *Neurology, 1988*(38), 1442–1450.

Otsuki, M., Soma, Y., Sato, M., Homma, A., & Tsuji, S. (1998). Slowly progressive pure word deafness. *European Neurology, 39*(3), 135–140.

Ottenbacher, K. J., & Jannell, S. (1993). The results of clinical trials in stroke rehabilitation research. *Archives of Neurology, 50*(1), 37–44.

Overstreet, D. H. (2000). Organophosphate pesticides, cholinergic function and cognitive performance in advanced age. *Neurotoxicology, 21*(1–2), 75–81.

Owen, A. M. (2000). The role of the lateral frontal cortex in mnemonic processing: The contribution of functional neuroimaging. *Experimental Brain Research, 133*(1), 33–43.

Oyebode, F., & Davison, K. (1990). Handedness and epileptic schizophrenia. *British Journal of Psychiatry, 156,* 228–230.

Paganini-Hill, A., & Henderson, V. W. (1994). Estrogen deficiency and risk of Alzheimer's disease in women. *American Journal of Epidemiology, 140,* 256–261.

Pallis, C. A. (1955). Impaired identification of faces and places with agnosia for colours. Report of a case due to cerebral embolism. *Journal of Neurology, Neurosurgery and Psychiatry, 18,* 218–224.

Paniak, C. E., & Finlayson, A. J. (1989). Does the Halstead-Reitan Battery assess 'memory' functioning? *Journal of Clinical and Experimental Neuropsychology, 11,* 631–644.

Pantev, C., Oostenveld, R., Engelien, A., Ross, B., Roberts, L. E., & Hoke, M. (1998). Increased auditory cortical representation in musicians. *Nature, 392*(6678), 811–814.

Pascual-Leone, A. (2001). The brain that plays music and is changed by it. *Annals of the New York Academy of Sciences, 930,* 315–329.

Pascual-Leone, A., Cammarota, A., Wassermann, E. M., Brasil-Neto, J. P., Cohen, L. G., & Hallett, M. (1993). Modulation of motor cortical outputs to the reading hand of braille readers. *Annals of Neurology, 34*(1), 33–37.

Pascual-Leone, A., Grafman, J., & Hallett, M. (1994). Modulation of cortical motor output maps during development of implicit and explicit knowledge. *Science, 263*(5151), 1287–1289.

Pascual-Leone, A., Wassermann, E. M., Sadato, N., & Hallett, M. (1995). The role of reading activity on the modulation of motor cortical outputs to the reading hand in Braille readers. *Annals of Neurology, 38*(6), 910–915.

Paterson, A., & Zangwill, O. L. (1944). Disorders of visual space perception associated with lesions of the right cerebral hemisphere. *Brain, 67,* 331–358.

Peiterson, E. (1974). Measurement of vestibulo-spinal responses in man. In H. H. Kornhuber (Ed.), *Handbook of sensory physiology.* Berlin, Germany: Springer-Verlag.

Pelisson, D., Prablanc, C., Goodale, M. A., & Jeannerod, M. (1986). Visual control of reaching movements without vision of the limb. II. Evidence of fast unconscious processes correcting the trajectory of the hand to the final position of a double-step stimulus. *Experimental Brain Research, 62*(2), 303–311.

Penfield, W., & Boldrey, E. (1937). Somatic motor and sensory representations in cerebral cortex of man as studied by electrical stimulation. *Brain, 60,* 389–443.

Penfield, W., & Jasper, H. (1954). *Epilepsy and the functional anatomy of the human brain.* Boston: Little, Brown.

Penfield, W., & Rasmussen, T. (1950). *The cerebral cortex of man as studied by electrical stimulation.* New York: Macmillan.

Pennington, B. F., Smith, S. D., Kimberling, W. J., Green, P. A., & Haith, M. M. (1987). Left-handedness and immune disorders in familial dyslexics. *Archives of Neurology, 44*(6), 634–639.

Perani, D., & Cappa, S. (1995). Neuroimaging methods in dementia. *Alzheimer's Research, 1,* 177–182.

Perani, D., & Cappa, S. F. (1999). Neuroimaging methods in neuropsychology. In G. Denes & L. Pizzamiglio (Eds.), *Handbook of clinical and experimental neuropsychology.* Hove, England: Psychology Press/Taylor and Francis.

Perani, D., Di Piero, V., Lucignani, G., Gilardi, M. C., Pantano, P., Rossetti, C., et al. (1988). Remote effects of subcortical cerebrovascular lesions: A SPECT cerebral perfusion study. *Journal of Cerebral Blood Flow and Metabolism, 8*(4), 560–567.

Perani, D., Di Piero, V., Vallar, G., Cappa, S., Messa, C., Bottini, G., et al. (1988). Technetium-99m HM-PAO-SPECT study of regional cerebral perfusion in early Alzheimer's disease. *Journal of Nuclear Medicine, 29*(9), 1507–1514.

Perrett, D. I., Rolls, E. T., & Caan, W. (1982). Visual neurones responsive to faces in the monkey temporal cortex. *Experimental Brain Research, 47*(3), 329–342.

Perry, R. B. (1904). Conceptions and misconceptions of consciousness. *Psychological Review, 11*(4–5), 282–296.

Persson, P. G., & Ahlbom, A. (1988). Relative risk is a relevant measure of association of left-handedness with inflammatory bowel disease. *Neuropsychologia, 26*(5), 737–740.

Persson, P. G., & Allebeck, P. (1994). Do left-handers have increased mortality? *Epidemiology, 5*(3), 337–340.

Peters, A., Palay, S. L., & Webster, H. deF. (1991). *The fine structure of the nervous system* (3rd ed.). New York: Oxford University Press.

Peters, M. (1995). Handedness and its relation to other indices of cerebral lateralization. In R. J. Davidson & K. Hugdahl (Eds.), *Brain asymmetry* (pp. 183–214). Cambridge, MA: MIT Press.

Peters, M., & Perry, R. (1991). No link between left-handedness and maternal age and no elevated accident rate in left-handers. *Neuropsychologia, 29*(12), 1257–1259.

Peterson, J. M. (1979). Left-handedness: Differences between student artists and scientists. *Perceptual and Motor Skills, 48*(3, Pt. 1), 961–962.

Peterson, J. M., & Lansky, L. M. (1977). Left-handedness among architects: Partial replication and some new data. *Perceptual and Motor Skills, 45*(3, Pt. 2), 1216–1218.

Peterson, L. R., & Peterson, M. J. (1959). Short term retention of individual verbal items. *Journal of Experimental Psychology, 58,* 193–198.

Phillips, M. L., Young, A. W., Scott, S. K., Calder, A. J., Andrew, C., Giampietro, V., et al. (1998). Neural responses to facial and vocal expressions of fear and disgust. *Proceedings of the Royal Society of London: Series B, Biological Sciences, 265*(1408), 1809–1817.

Phillips, M. L., Young, A. W., Senior, C., Brammer, M., Andrew, C., Calder, A. J., et al. (1997). A specific neural substrate for perceiving facial expressions of disgust. *Nature, 389*(6650), 495–498.

Phillips, W. A., & Baddeley, A. D. (1971). Reaction time and short-term visual memory. *Psychonomic Science, 22*(2), 73–74.

Pick, A. (1892) Ueber die biziehungen der senilen hirntumoren. *Archive fur psychhologie und nervenkrankheiten, 47,* 558–569.

Pick, H. L., Jr., & Rieser, J. J. (1982). Children's cognitive mapping. In M. Poetgal (Ed.), *Spatial abilities: Development and physiological foundations.* New York: Academic Press.

Pieczuro, A. C., & Vignolo, L. A. (1967). Studio speimentale sulla aprassia ideomotoria. *Sistema Nervoso, 19,* 131–143.

Pietrini, P., Furey, M. L., Graff-Radford, N., Freo, U., Alexander, G. E., Grady, C. L., et al. (1996). Preferential metabolic involvement of visual cortical areas in a subtype of Alzheimer's disease: Clinical implications. *American Journal of Psychiatry, 153*(10), 1261–1268.

Pinel, J. P. J. (1997). *Biopsychology.* Boston: Allyn & Bacon.

Pinel, J. P. J. (2003). *Biopsychology* (5th ed.). Toronto, Canada: Allyn & Bacon.

Pinker, S. (1994). *The language instinct.* New York: William Morrow.

Pinker, S. (2002). *The blank slate: The modern denial of human nature.* New York: Penguin Putnam.

Pipe, M. E. (1988). Atypical laterality and retardation. *Psychological Bulletin, 104*(3), 343–347.

Piran, N., Bigler, E. D., & Cohen, D. (1982). Motoric laterality and eye dominance suggest unique pattern of cerebral organization in schizophrenia. *Archives of General Psychiatry, 39*(9), 1006–1010.

Plaut, D. C., McClelland, J. L., & Seidenberg, M. S. (1995). Reading exception words and pseudowords: Are two routes really necessary? In J. P. Levy, D. Bairaktaris, J. Bullinaria, & P. Cairns (Eds.), *Connectionist models of memory and language* (pp. 145–159). London, England: UCL Press.

Podoll, K., & Robinson, D. (2000). Macrosomatognosia and microsomatognosia in migraine art. *Acta Neurologica Scandinavica, 101*(6), 413–416.

Poizner, H., Klima, E. S., & Bellugi, U. (1987). *What the hands reveal about the brain.* Cambridge, MA: MIT Press.

Pollmann, S., & von Cramon, D. Y. (2000). Object working memory and visuospatial processing: Functional neuroanatomy analyzed by event-related fMRI. *Experimental Brain Research, 133*(1), 12–22.

Polymeropoulos, M. H. (2000). Genetics of Parkinson's disease. *Annals of the New York Academy of Sciences, 920,* 28–32.

Posner, M. I., Boies, S. J., Eichelman, W. H., & Taylor, R. L. (1969). Retention of visual and name codes of single letters. *Journal of Experimental Psychology, 79*(1, Pt. 2), 1–16.

Posner, M. I., & Petersen, S. E. (1990). The attention system of the human brain. *Annual Review of Neuroscience, 13,* 25–42.

Povinelli, D. J., Nelson, K. E., & Boysen, S. T. (1990). Inferences about guessing and knowing by chimpanzees. *Journal of Comparative Psychology, 104,* 203–210.

Povinelli, D. J., Parks, K. A., & Novak, M. A. (1991). Do rhesus monkeys (Macaca mulatta) attribute knowledge and ignorance to others? *Journal of Comparative Pyschology, 105*(4), 318–325.

Powls, A., Botting, N., Cooke, R. W., & Marlow, N. (1996). Handedness in very-low-birthweight (VLBW) children at 12 years of age: Relation to perinatal and outcome variables. *Developmental Medicine and Child Neurology, 38*(7), 594–602.

Previc, F. H. (1991). A general theory concerning the prenatal origins of cerebral lateralization in humans. *Psychological Review, 98*(3), 299–334.

Previc, F. H. (1996). Nonright-handedness, central nervous system and related pathology, and its lateralization: A reformulation and synthesis. *Developmental Neuropsychology, 12*(4), 443–515.

Profet, M. (1991). The function of allergy: Immunological defense against toxins. *Quarterly Review of Biology, 66,* 23–62.

Psychological Corporation, The. (1997). *WAIS-III and WMS-III technical manual.* San Antonio, TX: The Psychological Corporation.

Quigg, M., & Fountain, N. B. (1999). Conduction aphasia elicited by stimulation of the left posterior superior temporal gyrus. *Journal of Neurology, Neurosurgery and Psychiatry, 66*(3), 393–396.

Rafal, R., Smith, J., Krantz, J., Cohen, A., & Brennan, C. (1990). Extrageniculate vision in hemianopic humans: Saccade inhibition by signals in the blind field. *Science, 250*(4977), 118–121.

Raghupathi, R., Graham, D. I., & McIntosh, T. K. (2000). Apoptosis after traumatic brain injury. *Journal of Neurotrauma, 17*(10), 927–938.

Raine, A., Lencz, T., Bihrle, S., LaCasse, L., & Colletti, P. (2000). Reduced prefrontal gray matter volume and reduced autonomic activity in antisocial personality disorder. *Archives of General Psychiatry, 57*(2), 119–127.

Raisman, G., & Field, P. M. (1973). A quantitative investigation of the development of collateral reinnervation after partial deafferentation of the septal nuclei. *Brain Research, 50*(2), 241–264.

Raju, T. N. (1999). The Nobel chronicles. 1979: Allan MacLeod Cormack (b 1924); and Sir Godfrey Newbold Hounsfield (b 1919). *Lancet, 354*(9190), 1653.

Ramachandran, V. S. (1993). Behavioral and magnetoencephalographic correlates of plasticity in the adult human brain. *Proceedings of the National Academy of Sciences of the United States of America, 90*(22), 10413–10420.

Ramachandran, V. S. (1995). Anosognosia in parietal lobe syndrome. *Consciousness and Cognition, 4*(1), 22–51.

Ramachandran, V. S., & Rogers-Ramachandran, D. (2000). Phantom limbs and neural plasticity. *Archives of Neurology, 57*(3), 317–320.

Ramachandran, V. S., Stewart, M., & Rogers-Ramachandran, D. C. (1992). Perceptual correlates of massive cortical reorganization. *Neuroreport, 3*(7), 583–586.

Ramaley, F. (1913). Inheritance of left-handedness. *American Naturalist, 47,* 334–339.

Ramus, F., Rosen, S., Dakin, S. C., Day, B. L., Castellote, J. M., White, S., et al. (2003). Theories of developmental dyslexia: Insights from a multiple case study of dyslexic adults. *Brain, 126*(Pt. 4), 841–865.

Ranson, S. W. (1934). The hypothalamus: Its significance for visceral innervation and emotional expression. *Transactions of the College of Physicians, Philadelphia Service, 4*(2), 222–242.

Rapcsak, S. Z., Gonzalez-Rothi, J., & Heilman, K. M. (1987). Phonological alexia with optic and tactile anomia: A neuropsychological and anatomical study. *Brain and Language, 31*(1), 109–121.

Rapcsak, S. Z., Krupp, L. B., Rubens, A. B., & Reim, J. (1990). Mixed transcortical aphasia without anatomic isolation of the speech area. *Stroke, 21*(6), 953–956.

Rasmussen, T., & Milner, B. (1977). The role of early left-brain injury in determining lateralization of cerebral speech functions. *Annals of the New York Academy of Sciences, 299,* 355–369.

Ratcliff, G. (1979). Spatial thought, mental rotation and the right cerebral hemisphere. *Neuropsychologia, 17,* 49–54.

Rauch, S. L., Savage, C. R., Alpert, N. M., Miguel, E. C., Baer, L., Breiter, H. C., et al. (1995). A positron emission tomographic study of simple phobic symptom provocation. *Archives of General Psychiatry, 52*(1), 20–28.

Raymer, A. M., Foundas, A. L., Maher, L. M., Greenwald, M. L., Morris, M., Rothi, L. S., (1997). Cognitive neuropsychological analysis and neuroanatomic correlates in a case of acute anomia. *Brain and Language, 58*(1), 137–156.

Records, M. A., Heimbuch, R. C., & Kidd, K. K. (1977). Handedness and stuttering: A dead horse? *Journal of Fluency Disorders, 2,* 271–282.

Reed, C. L., & Caselli, R. J. (1994). The nature of tactile agnosia: A case study. *Neuropsychologia, 32*(5), 527–539.

Rees, S., & Harding, R. (2004). Brain development during fetal life: Influences of the intra-uterine environment. *Neuroscience Letters, 6;361(1–3),* 111–114.

Regier, D. A., Narrow, W. E., Rae, D. S., Manderscheid, R. W., Locke, B. Z., & Goodwin, F. K. (1993). The de facto US mental and addictive disorders service system: Epidemiologic catchment area prospective 1-year prevalence rates of disorders and services. *Archives of General Psychiatry, 50*(2), 85–94.

Reiss, A. L., Eliez, S., Schmitt, J. E., Straus, E., Lai, Z., Jones, W., et al. (2000). IV. Neuroanatomy of Williams syndrome: A high-resolution MRI study. *Journal of Cognitive Neuroscience, 12*(Suppl. 1) 65–73.

Reitan, R. M., & Wolfson, D. (1993) *The Halstead-Reitan Neuropsychological Test Battery: Theory and clinical interpretation.* Tucson, AZ: Neuropsychology Press.

Rempel-Clower, N. L., Zola, S. M., Squire, L. R., & Amaral, D. G. (1996). Three cases of enduring memory impairment after bilateral damage limited to the hippocampal formation. *Journal of Neuroscience, 16*(16), 5233–5255.

Reynolds, W. E., Page, S. J., & Johnston, M. V. (2001). Coordinated and adequately funded state streams for rehabilitation of newly injured persons with TBI. *Journal of Head Trauma and Rehabilitation, 16*(1), 34–46.

Rezaie, P., & Lantos, P. L. (2001). Microglia and the pathogenesis of spongiform encephalopathies. *Brain Research Reviews, 35*(1), 55–72.

Ricaurte, G. A., Langston, J. W., Delanney, L. E., Irwin, I., Peroutka, S. J., & Forno, L. S. (1986). Fate of nigrostriatal neurons in young mature mice given 1-methyl-4-phenyl-1,2,3,6-tetrahydropyridine: A neurochemical and morphological reassessment. *Brain Research, 376*(1), 117–124.

Richardson, P. M., McGuinness, U. M., & Aguayo, A. J. (1982). Peripheral nerve autografts to the rat spinal cord: Studies with axonal tracing methods. *Brain Research, 237*(1), 147–162.

Richters, J. E., Arnold, L. E., Jensen, P. S., Abikoff, H., Conners, C. K., Greenhill, L. L., et al. (1995). NIMH collaborative multisite multimodal treatment study of children with ADHD: I. Background and rationale. *Journal of the American Academy of Child and Adolescent Psychiatry, 34*(8), 987–1000.

Riddoch, M. J., & Humphreys, G. W. (1987). A case of integrative visual agnosia. *Brain, 110*(Pt. 6), 1431–1462.

Riecker, A., Ackermann, H., Wildgruber, D., Dogil, G., & Grodd, W. (2000). Opposite hemispheric lateralization effects during speaking and singing at motor cortex, insula and cerebellum. *Neuroreport, 11*(9), 1997–2000.

Rieger, C. (1909). *Ueber Apparate in dem Hirn. Arbeiten aus der Psychiatrischen Klinik zu Wuerzburg, Heft 5.* Jena, Germany: Gustav Fischer.

Rife, D. C. (1940). Handedness with a special reference to twins. *Genetics, 25,* 178–186.

Ringo, J. L., Doty, R. W., Demeter, S., & Simard, P. Y. (1994). Time is of the essence: A conjecture that hemispheric specialization arises from interhemispheric conduction delay. *Cerebral Cortex, 4*(4), 331–343.

Risse, G. L., Gates, J., Lund, G., Maxwell, R. & Rubens, A. (1989). Interhemispheric transfer in patients with incomplete section of the corpus callosum: Anatomic verification with magnetic resonance imaging. *Archives of Neurology, 46*(4), 437–443.

Rizzolatti, G., Luppino, G., & Matelli, M. (1998). The organization of the cortical motor system: New concepts. *Electroencephalography and Clinical Neurophysiology, 106*(4), 283–296.

Roberts, W. A. (1998). *Principles of animal cognition.* Boston: McGraw-Hill.

Robinson, R. G. (1985). Lateralized behavioral and neurochemical consequences of unilateral brain injury in rats. In S. G. Glick (Ed.), *Cerebral lateralization in nonhuman species.* Orlando, FL: Academic Press.

Rogers, M. J. C. (1996). Apraxia. In J. G. Beaumont, P. M. Kenealy, & M. J. C. Rogers (Eds.), *The Blackwell dictionary of neuropsychology* (pp. 100–106). Oxford: Blackwell Publishers.

Roland, P. E., & Zilles, K. (1996). Functions and structures of the motor cortices in humans. *Current Opinions in Neurobiology, 6*(6), 773–781.

Rondal, J. (1980). Language delay and language difference in moderately and severely retarded children. *Special Education in Canada, 54,* 27–32.

Ross, E. D. (1993). Nonverbal aspects of language. *Neurologic Clinics, 11*(1), 9–23.

Ross, E. D. (2000). Affective prosody and the aprosodias. In M.-M. Mesulam (Ed.), *Principles of behavioral and cognitive neurology* (pp. 316–331). New York: Oxford University Press.

Ross, G., Lipper, E., & Auld, P. A. (1992). Hand preference, prematurity and developmental outcome at school age. *Neuropsychologia, 30*(5), 483–494.

Ross, G., Lipper, E. G., & Auld, P. A. (1987). Hand preference of four-year-old children: Its relationship to premature birth and neurodevelopmental outcome. *Develpmental Medicine and Child Neurology, 29*(5), 615–622.

Rossor, M. N. (2001). Pick's disease: A clinical overview. *Neurology, 56*(11, Suppl. 4), S3–S5.

Roth, M., Decety, J., Raybaudi, M., Massarelli, R., Delon-Martin, C., Segebarth, C., et al. (1996). Possible involvement of primary motor cortex in mentally simulated movement: A functional magnetic resonance imaging study. *Neuroreport, 7*(7), 1280–1284.

Rothwell, J. (1994). *Control of human voluntary movement.* London, England: Chapman & Hall.

Rothwell, J. C., Traub, M. M., Day, B. L., Obeso, J. A., Thomas, P. K., & Marsden, C. D. (1982). Manual motor performance in a deafferented man. *Brain, 105*(Pt. 3), 515–542.

Rubens, A. B., & Benson, D. F. (1971). Associative visual agnosia. *Archives of Neurology, 24*(4), 305–316.

Ruff, R. L., & Volpe, B. T. (1981). Environmental reduplication associated with right frontal and parietal lobe injury. *Journal of Neurology, Neurosurgery and Psychiatry, 44*(5), 382–386.

Rugg, M. D., Milner, A. D., Lines, C. R., & Phalp, R. (1987). Modulation of visual event-related potentials by spatial and non-spatial visual selective attention. *Neuropsychologia, 25*(1-A), 85–96.

Russell, J. A. (1995). Facial expressions of emotion: What lies beyond minimal universality? *Psychological Bulletin, 118*(3), 379–391.

Sacchett, C., & Humphreys, G. W. (1992). Calling a squirrel a squirrel but a canoe a wigwam: A category-specific deficit for artefactual objects and body parts. *Cognitive Neuropsychology, 9*(1), 73–86.

Sackeim, H. A., & Gur, R. C. (1978). Lateral asymmetry in intensity of emotional expression. *Neuropsychologia, 16,* 473–481.

Sadowski-Debbing, K., Coy, J. F., Mier, W., Hug, H., & Los, M. (2002). Caspases—Their role in apoptosis and other physiological processes as revealed by knock-out studies. *Archivum Immunologiae Et Therapiae Experimentalis, 50,* 19–34.

Saffran, E. M., Schwartz, M. F., & Marin, O. S. (1980). The word order problem in agrammatism: II. Production. *Brain and Language, 10*(2), 263–280.

Saigal, S., Rosenbaum, P., Szatmari, P., & Hoult, L. (1992). Non-right handedness among ELBW and term children at eight years in relation to cognitive function and school performance. *Developmental Medicine and Child Neurology, 34*(5), 425–433.

Saint Cyr, J., Taylor, A., & Lang, A. (1988). Procedural learning and neostriatal dysfunction in man. *Brain, 111,* 941–959.

Sakurai, Y., Ichikawa, Y., & Mannen, T. (2001). Pure alexia from a posterior occipital lesion. *Neurology, 56*(6), 778–781.

Salk, L. (1966). Thoughts on the concept of imprinting and its place in early human development. *Canadian Psychiatric Association Journal, 11,* 295–305.

Salk, L. (1973). The role of the heartbeat in the relations between mother and infant. *Scientific American, 228*(5), 24–29.

Sandifer, P. H. (1946). Anosognosia and disorders of body scheme. *Brain, 69,* 122–137.

Sanes, J. N., & Donoghue, J. P. (2000). Plasticity and primary motor cortex. *Annual Review of Neuroscience, 23,* 393–415.

Sasanuma, S., Ito, H., Patterson, K., & Ito, T. (1996). Phonological alexia in Japanese: A case study. *Cognitive Neuropsychology, 13,* 823–848.

Satori, G., & Job, R. (1988). The oyster with four legs: A neuropsychological study on the interaction of visual and semantic information. *Cognitive Neuropsychology, 5,* 105–132.

Satz, P. (1972). Pathological left-handedness: An explanatory model. *Cortex, 8*(2), 121–135.

Satz, P., Forney, D. L., Zaucha, K., Asarnow, R. R., Light, R., McCleary, C., et al. (1998). Depression, cognition and functional correlates of recovery outcome after traumatic brain injury. *Brain Injury, 12*(7), 537–553.

Satz, P., Orsini, D. L., Saslow, E., & Henry, R. (1985). The pathological left-handedness syndrome. *Brain and Cognition, 4*(1), 27–46.

Satz, P. S., Alfano, M. S., Light, R. F., Morgenstern, H. F., Zaucha, K. F., Asarnow, R. F., et al. (1999). Persistent Post-Concussive Syndrome: A proposed methodology and literature review to determine the effects, if any, of mild head and other bodily injury. *Journal of Clinical and Experimental Neuropsychology, 21*(5), 620–628.

Schacter, D. L. (1996). Illusory memories: A cognitive neuroscience analysis. *Proceedings of the National Academy of Sciences of the United States of America, 93*(24), 13527–13533.

Schacter, D. L., McAndrews, M. P., & Moscovitch, M. (1988). Access to consciousness: Dissociations between implicit and explicit knowledge in neuropsychological syndromes. In L. Weiskrantz (Ed.), *Thought without language* (pp. 242–278) Oxford: Oxford University Press.

Schachter, S., & Singer, J. E. (1962). Cognitive, social and physiological determinants of emotional state. *Psychological Review, 69,* 379–399.

Schachter, S. C., & Ransil, B. J. (1996). Handedness distributions in nine professional groups. *Perceptual and Motor Skills, 82*(1), 51–63.

Scheibel, A., Conrad, T., Perdue, S., Tomiyasu, U., & Wechsler, A. (1990). A quantitative study of dendrite complexity in selected areas of the human cerebral cortex. *Brain and Cognition, 12*(1), 85–101.

Schieber, M., & Hibbard, L. (1993). How somatotopic is the motor cortex hand area? *Science, 261,* 489–492.

Schieber, M. H. (1990). How might the motor cortex individuate movements? *Trends in Neuroscience, 13*(11), 440–445.

Schiff, B. B., & Lamon, M. (1989). Inducing emotion by unilateral contraction of facial muscles: A new look at hemispheric specialization and the experience of emotion. *Neuropsychologia, 27*(7), 923–935.

Schiff, B. B., & Lamon, M. (1994). Inducing emotion by unilateral contraction of hand muscles. *Cortex, 30*(2), 247–254.

Schneck, J. M. (1977). Sleep paralysis and microsomatognosia with special reference to hypnotherapy. *International Journal of Clinical and Experimental Hypnosis, 25*(2), 72–77.

Schott, A. (1931). [Left-handedness and heredity]. *Zeitschrift für die Gesamte Neurologie und Psychiatrie, 135,* 1–322.

Schwartz, M. (1988). Handedness, prenatal stress and pregnancy complications. *Neuropsychologia, 26*(6), 925–929.

Scott, S. K., Young, A. W., Calder, A. J., Hellawell, D. J., Aggleton, J. P., & Johnson, M. (1997). Impaired auditory recognition of fear and anger following bilateral amygdala lesions. *Nature, 385*(6613), 254–257.

Scoville, W. B., & Milner, B. (2000). Loss of recent memory after bilateral hippocampal lesions. 1957 [classical article]. *Journal of Neuropsychiatry and Clinical Neurosciences, 12*(1), 103–113.

Searleman, A., & Fugagli, A. K. (1987). Suspected autoimmune disorders and left-handedness: Evidence from individuals with diabetes. Crohn's disease and ulcerative colitis. *Neuropsychologia, 25*(2), 367–374.

Searleman, A., Porac, C., & Coren, S. (1989). Relationship between birth order, birth stress, and lateral preferences: A critical review. *Psychological Bulletin, 105*(3), 397–408.

Sears, J. D., Hirt, M. L., & Hall, R. W. (1984). A cross-validation of the Luria-Nebraska Neuropsychological Battery. *Journal of Consulting and Clinical Psychology, 52,* 309–310.

Segal, N. L. (1989). Origins and implications of handedness and relative birth weight for IQ in monozygotic twin pairs. *Neuropsychologia, 27*(4), 549–561.

Segalowitz, S. J., & Davies, P. L. (2004). Charting the maturation of the frontal lobe: An electrophysiological strategy. *Brain and Cognition, 55*(1), 116–133.

Seidenberg, M. S., & McClelland, J. L. (1989). A distributed, developmental model of word recognition and naming. *Psychological Review, 96*(4), 523–568.

Seidman, L. J., Stone, W. S., Jones, R., Harrison, R. H., & Mirsky, A. F. (1998). Comparative effects of schizophrenia and temporal lobe epilepsy on memory. *Journal of the International Neuropsychological Society, 4*(4), 342–352.

Seitz, R. J., Stephan, K. M., & Binkofski, F. (2000). Control of action as mediated by the human frontal lobe. *Experimental Brain Research, 133*(1), 71–80.

Selnes, O. A. (2001). A historical overview of contributions from the study of deficits. In B. Rapp (Ed.), *The handbook of cognitive neuropsychology: What deficits reveal about the human mind.* (pp. 23–41). Philadephia: Psychology Press/Taylor and Francis.

Seltzer, B., Burres, M. J., & Sherwin, I. (1984). Left-handedness in early and late onset dementia. *Neurology, 34*(3), 367–369.

Semmes, J., Weinstein, S., Ghent, L., & Teuber, H. L. (1960). *Somatosensory changes after penetrating brain wounds in man* (pp. xiii, 91). Cambridge, MA: Harvard University Press.

Sergent, J. (1983). Role of the input in visual hemispheric asymmetries. *Psychological Bulletin, 93*(3), 481–512.

Servos, P., Engel, S. A., Gati, J., & Menon, R. (1999). fMRI evidence for an inverted face representation in human somatosensory cortex. *Neuroreport, 10*(7), 1393–1395.

Shaldubina, A., Agam, G., & Belmaker, R. H. (2001). The mechanism of lithium action: State of the art, ten years later. *Progress in Neuropsychopharmacology Biological Psychiatry, 25*(4), 855–866.

Shallice, T., & Burgess, P. (1996). The domain of supervisory processes and temporal organization of behaviour. *Philosophical Transactions of the Royal Society of London: Series B, Biological Sciences, 351*(1346), 1405–1411; discussion 1411–1412.

Sheline, Y. I., Sanghavi, M., Mintun, M. A., & Gado, M. H. (1999). Depression duration but not age predicts hippocampal volume loss in medically healthy women with recurrent major depression. *Journal of Neuroscience, 19*(12), 5034–5043.

Shelton, P. A., Bowers, D., Duara, R., & Heilman, K. M. (1994). Apperceptive visual agnosia: A case study. *Brain and Cognition, 25*(1), 1–23.

Shepard, R. N., & Metzler, J. (1971). Mental rotation of three-dimensional objects. *Science, 171*(3972), 701–703.

Sheppard, G. M. (1994). *Neurobiology* (3rd ed.). New York: Oxford University Press.

Sherry, D. F. (1997). Cross-species comparisons. *Ciba Foundation Symposia, 208,* 181–189.

Shiah, I. S., & Yatham, L. N. (2000). Serotonin in mania and in the mechanism of action of mood stabilizers: A review of clinical studies. *Bipolar Disorders, 2*(2), 77–92.

Shulman, G. L., Ollinger, J. M., Akbudak, E., Conturo, T. E., Snyder, A. Z., Petersen, S. E., et al. (1999). Areas involved in encoding and applying directional expectations to moving objects. *Journal of Neuroscience, 19*(21), 9480–9496.

Shumaker, S. A., Reboussin, B. A., Espeland, M. A., Rapp, S. R., McBee, W. L., Dailey, M., et al. (1998). The women's health initiative memory study (WHIMS): A trial of the effect of estrogen therapy in preventing and slowing the progression of dementia. *Controlled Clinical Trials, 19,* 604–621.

Siever, L. J., Torgersen, S., Gunderson, J. G., Livesley, W. J., & Kendler, K. S. (2002). The borderline diagnosis III: Identifying endophenotypes for genetic studies. *Biological Psychiatry, 51*(12), 964–968.

Signoret, J. L., Castaigne, P., Lhermitte, F., Abelanet, R., & Lavorel, P. (1984). Rediscovery of Leborgne's brain: Anatomical description with ct scan. *Brain and Language, 22*(2), 303–319.

Simos, P. G., Breier, J. I., Wheless, J. W., Maggio, W. W., Fletcher, J. M., Castillo, E. M., et al. (2000). Brain mechanisms for reading: The role of the superior temporal gyrus in word and pseudoword naming. *Neuroreport, 11*(11), 2443–2447.

Simpson, D. (1998). HIV rounds at Cornell: Selected neurologic complications of HIV disease. *AIDS Patient Care STDS, 12*(3), 209–215.

Sinden, J. D., Stroemer, P., Grigoryan, G., Patel, S., French, S. J., & Hodges, H. (2000). Functional repair with neural stem cells. *Novartis Foundation Symposia, 231,* 270–283.

Singer, H. S., Reiss, A. L., Brown, J. E., Aylward, E. H., Shih, B., Chee, E., et al. (1993). Volumetric MRI changes in basal ganglia of children with Tourette's syndrome. *Neurology, 43*(5), 950–956.

Singer, H. S., Wendlandt, J., Krieger, M., & Giuliano, J. (2001). Baclofen treatment in Tourette syndrome: A double-blind, placebo-controlled, crossover trial. *Neurology, 56*(5), 599–604.

Sirevaag, A. M., Black, J. E., Shafron, D., & Greenough, W. T. (1988). Direct evidence that complex experience increases capillary branching and surface area in visual cortex of young rats. *Brain Research, 471*(2), 299–304.

Sirigu, A., Duhamel, J. R., & Poncet, M. (1991). The role of sensorimotor experience in object recognition. A case of multimodal agnosia. *Brain, 114*(Pt. 6), 2555–2573.

Sittig, O. (1921). Störungen im Verhalten gegenüber Farben bei Aphasischen. *Monastschrift für psychiatrie und Neurologie, 49,* 159–187.

Slater, A., & Kirby, R. (1998). Innate and learned perceptual abilities in the newborn infant. *Experimental Brain Research, 123*(1–2), 90–94.

Smidt, G. L., Arora, J. S., & Johnston, R. C. (1971). Accelerographic analysis of several types of walking. *American Journal of Physical Medicine, 50*(6), 285–300.

Smith, D. W., & Wilson, A. A. (1973). *The child with Down's syndrome (Mongolism)*. Philadelphia: Saunders.

Smith, E. E., & Jonides, J. (1998). Neuroimaging analyses of human working memory. *Proceedings of the National Academy of Sciences of the United States of America, 95*(20), 12061–12068.

Smith, E. E., & Jonides, J. (1999). Storage and executive processes in the frontal lobes. *Science, 283*(5408), 1657–1661.

Smith, J. (1987). Left-handedness: Its association with allergic disease. *Neuropsychologia, 25*(4), 665–674.

Smulders, T. V., Sasson, A. D., & DeVoogd, T. J. (1995). Seasonal variation in hippocampal volume in a food-storing bird, the black-capped chickadee. *Journal of Neurobiology, 27*(1), 15–25.

Smulders, T. V., Shiflett, M. W., Sperling, A. J., & DeVoogd, T. J. (2000). Seasonal changes in neuron numbers in the hippocampal formation of a food-hoarding bird: The black-capped chickadee. *Journal of Neurobiology, 44*(4), 414–422.

Snyder, T. J. (1991). Self-rated right/left confusability and objectively measured right-left discrimination. *Developmental Neuropsychology, 7*(2), 219–230.

Soper, H. V., Satz, P., Orsini, D. L., Van Gorp, W. G., & Green, M. F. (1987). Handedness distribution in a residential population with severe or profound mental retardation. *American Journal of Mental Deficiency, 92*(1), 94–102.

Souques, A. (1928). Quelques cas d'anarthrie de Pierre Marie [Certain cases of the anarthria of Pierre Marie]. *Revista de Neurologia, 35,* 319–368.

Sperling, G. (1960). The information available in brief visual presentation. *Psychological Monographs, 74*(11, Whole No. 498), 29.

Sperling, G. (1963). A model for visual memory tasks. *Human Factors, 5,* 19–31.

Sperling, G. (1967). Successive approximations to a model for short term memory. *Acta Psychologica, 27,* 285–292.

Spinnler, H. (Ed.). (1991). *The role of attention disorders in the cognitive deficits of dementia*. Amsterdam, The Netherlands: Elsevier.

Spivak, B., Segal, M., Mester, R., & Weizman, A. (1998). Lateral preference in post-traumatic stress disorder. *Psychological Medicine, 28*(1), 229–232.

Spreen, O., Risser, A. H., & Edgell, D. (1995). *Developmental neuropsychology*. New York: Oxford University Press.

Springer, S. (1986). Dichotic listening. In H. J. Hannay (Ed.), *Experimental techniques in neuropsychology* (pp. 138–166). New York: Oxford University Press.

Squire, L. R. (1992). Memory and the hippocampus: A synthesis from findings with rats, monkeys, and humans. *Psychological Review, 99*(2), 195–231. [Published erratum appears in *Psychological Review, 99*(3), 582].

Stanton, W. R., Feehan, M., Silva, P. A., & Sears, M. R. (1991). Handedness and allergic disorders in a New Zealand cohort. *Cortex, 27*(1), 131–135.

Starkstein, S. E., Brandt, J., Folstein, S., Strauss, M., Berthier, M. L., Pearlson, G. D., et al. (1988). Neuropsychological and neuroradiological correlates in Huntington's disease. *Journal of Neurology, Neurosurgery and Psychiatry, 51*(10), 1259–1263.

Starkstein, S. E., & Robinson, R. G. (1992). Neuropsychiatric aspects of cerebral vascular disorders. In S. C. Yudofsky & R. E. Hales (Eds.), *Textbook of neuropsychiatry* (2nd ed.). Washington, D.C.: American Psychiatric Press.

State, M. W., Pauls, D. L., & Leckman, J. F. (2001). Tourette's syndrome and related disorders. *Child and Adolescent Psychiatric Clinics of North America, 10*(2), 317–331.

Steenhuis, R. E., Bryden, M. P., & Schroeder, D. H. (1993). Gender, laterality, learning difficulties and health problems. *Neuropsychologia, 31*(11), 1243–1254.

Stehling, M. K., Turner, R., & Mansfield, P. (1991). Echo-planar imaging: Magnetic resonance imaging in a fraction of a second. *Science, 254*(5028), 43–50.

Stengel, E. (1930). Morphologische und cytoarchiektonische Studien uber deb Bau der unteren Frontalwindung bei Normalen und Taubstummen Ihre indivuellen und Seitenunterschiede. *Zeitschrift fur die gesamte Neurologie und Psychiatrie, 130,* 631.

Stephens, R., Spurgeon, A., Calvert, I. A., Beach, J., Levy, L. S., Berry, H., et al. (1995). Neuropsychological effects of long-term exposure to organophosphates in sheep dip. *Lancet, 345*(8958), 1135–1139.

Stoerig, P., & Cowey, A. (1997). Invited review. Blindsight in man and monkey. *Brain, 120*(3), 535–559.

Stolboun, D. E. (1934). Stereognostic disorders. *Sovetskaya Nevropatologiya, Psikhiatriya, i Psikhohigiena, 3* (No. 6), 52–66.

Stoll, A. L., Renshaw, P. F., Yurgelun-Todd, D. A., & Cohen, B. M. (2000). Neuroimaging in bipolar disorder: What have we learned? *Biological Psychiatry, 48*(6), 505–517.

Stracciari, A. (1992). Transient topographical amnesia. *Italian Journal of Neurological Sciences, 13*(7), 593–596.

Stracciari, A., Lorusso, S., & Pazzaglia, P. (1994). Transient topographical amnesia. *Journal of Neurology, Neurosurgery and Psychiatry, 57*(11), 1423–1425.

Strakowski, S. M., DelBello, M. P., Adler, C., Cecil, D. M., & Sax, K. W. (2000). Neuroimaging in bipolar disorder. *Bipolar Disorders, 2*(3, Pt. 1), 148–164.

Strauss, E., Loring, D., Chelune, G., Hunter, M., Hermann, B., Perrine, K., et al. (1995). Predicting cognitive impairment in epilepsy: Findings from the Bozeman epilepsy consortium. *Journal of Clinical and Experimental Neuropsychology, 17*(6), 909–917.

Strauss, E., & Moscovitch, M. (1981). Perception of facial expressions. *Brain and Language, 13*(2), 308–332.

Strauss, E., Semenza, C., Hunter, M., Hermann, B., Barr, W., Chelune, G., et al. (2000). Left anterior lobectomy and category-specific naming. *Brain and Cognition, 43*(1–3), 403–406.

Strehlow, U., Haffner, J., Parzer, P., Pfuller, U., Resch, F., & Zerahn-Hartung, C. (1996). [Handedness and cognitive abilities: Findings in a representative sample of adolescents and young adults]. *Z Kinder Jugendpsychiatr Psychother, 24*(4), 253–264.

Stringer, A. Y., & Hodnett, C. (1991). Transcortical motor aprosodia: Functional and anatomical correlates. *Archives of Clinical Neuropsychology, 6*(1–2), 89–99.

Strong, M. J., Grace, G. M., Orange, J. B., & Leeper, H. A. (1996). Cognition, language, and speech in amyotrophic lateral sclerosis: A review. *Journal of Clinical and Experimental Neuropsychology, 18*(2), 291–303.

Stroop, J. R. (1935). Studies of interference in serial verbal reactions. *Journal of Experimental Psychology, 18*, 643–662.

Subbiah, I., & Caramazza, A. (2000). Stimulus-centered neglect in reading and object recognition. *Neurocase: Case Studies in Neuropsychology, Neuropsychiatry, and Behavioural Neurology, 6*(1), 13–31.

Svendsen, C. N., Clarke, D. J., Rosser, A. E., & Dunnett, S. B. (1996). Survival and differentiation of rat and human epidermal growth factor-responsive precursor cells following grafting into the lesioned adult central nervous system. *Experimental Neurology, 137*(2), 376–388.

Sweeney, J. A., Kmiec, J. A., & Kupfer, D. J. (2000). Neuropsychologic impairments in bipolar and unipolar mood disorders on the CANTAB neurocognitive battery. *Biological Psychiatry, 48*(7), 674–684.

Tabert, M. H., Borod, J. C., Tang, C. Y., Lange, G., Wei, T. C., Johnson, R., et al. (2001). Differential amygdala activation during emotional decision and recognition memory tasks using unpleasant words: An fMRI study. *Neuropsychologia, 39*(6), 556–573.

Takarae, Y., & Levin, D. T. (2001). Animals and artifacts may not be treated equally: Differentiating strong and weak forms of category-specific visual agnosia. *Brain and Cognition, 45*(2), 249–264.

Takayama, Y., Sugishita, M., Hirose, S., & Akiguchi, I. (1994). Anosodiaphoria for dressing apraxia: Contributory factor to dressing apraxia. *Clinical Neurology and Neurosurgery, 96*(3), 254–256.

Tallal, P., Miller, S., & Fitch, R. H. (1993). Neurobiological basis of speech: A case for the preeminence of temporal processing. *Annals of the New York Academy of Sciences, 682*, 27–47.

Taras, J. S., Behrman, M. J., & Degnan, G. G. (1995). Left-hand dominance and hand trauma. *Journal of Hand Surgery* [Am], *20*(6), 1043–1046. [Published erratum appears in *Journal of Hand Surgery* [Am], *21*(2), 336.]

Tassi, P., & Muzet, A. (2001). Defining the states of consciousness. *Neuroscience and Biobehavioral Reviews, 25*(2), 175–191.

Tatemichi, T. K., Desmond, D. W., Paik, M., Figueroa, M., Gropen, T. I., Stern, Y., et al. (1993). Clinical determinants of dementia related to stroke. *Annals of Neurology, 33*, 568–575.

Taub, E., Miller, N. E., Novack, T. A., Cook, E. W., Fleming, W. C., Nepomuceno, C. S., et al. (1993). Technique to improve chronic motor deficit after stroke. *Archives of Physical Medicine and Rehabilitation, 74*(4), 347–354.

Taylor, D. C. (1969). Different rates of cerebral maturation between sexes and between hemispheres. *Lancet, 2*, 140–142.

Taylor, D. C. (1974). The influence of sexual differentiation on growth, development, and disease. In J. A. Davis & J. Dobbing (Eds.), *Scientific foundations of pediatrics.* Philadelphia: W. B. Sanders.

Taylor, E. S. (1976). *Beck's obstetric practice and fetal medicine* (10th ed.). Baltimore: Lippincott Williams & Wilkins.

Taylor, J. R., Tompkins, R., Demers, R., & Anderson, D. (1982). Electroconvulsive therapy and memory dysfunction: Is there evidence for prolonged defects? *Biological Psychiatry, 17*(10), 1169–1193.

Taylor, M. A., & Amir, N. (1995). Sinister psychotics: Left-handedness in schizophrenia and affective disorder. *Journal of Nervous and Mental Disease, 183*(1), 3–9.

Teeter, P. A., & Semrud-Clikeman, M. (1997). *Child neuropsychology: Assessment and interventions for neurodevelopmental disorders.* Boston: Allyn & Bacon.

Teng, E. L., & Chui, H. C. (1987). The Modified Mini-Mental State (3MS) examination. *Journal of Clinical Psychiatry, 48*(8), 314–318.

Terzian, H., & Dalle-Ore, P. C. (1955). Syndrome of Klüver-Bucy reproduced in man by bilateral removal of the temporal lobes. *Neurology, 5*, 373–380.

Tezner, D., Tzavaras, A., Gruner, J., & Hecaen, H. (1972). L'asymmetrie droite-gauche due planum temporale: A propos de l'etude anatomique de 100 cerveaux. *Revue Neurologique, 126,* 444–449.

Tolosa, E., Marti, M. J., Valldeoriola, F., & Molinuevo, J. L. (1998). History of levodopa and dopamine agonists in Parkinson's disease treatment. *Neurology, 50*(6, Suppl. 6), S2–S10.

Tonnessen, F. E., Lokken, A., Hoien, T., & Lundberg, I. (1993). Dyslexia, left-handedness, and immune disorders. *Archives of Neurology, 50*(4), 411–416.

Tooby, J., & Cosmides, L. (1990). On the universality of human nature and the uniqueness of the individual: The role of genetics and adaptation. *Journal of Personality, 58*(1), 17–67.

Tooby, J., & Cosmides, L. (1992). The psychological foundations of culture. In J. H. Barkow, L. Cosmides, & J. Tooby (Eds.). *The adapted mind: Evolutionary psychology and the generation of culture.* New York: Oxford University Press.

Tooby, J., & Cosmides, L. (2000). *Toward mapping the evolved functional organization of mind and brain: The new cognitive neurosciences* (pp. 1167–1178). Cambridge, MA: MIT Press.

Torgerson, J. (1950). Situs Inversus, asymmetry, and twinning. *American Journal of Human Genetics, 2,* 361–370.

Tovee, M. J., Rolls, E. T., & Azzopardi, P. (1994). Translation invariance in the responses to faces of single neurons in the temporal visual cortical areas of the alert macaque. *Journal of Neurophysiology, 72*(3), 1049–1060.

Town, C. H. (1913). Aphasia. *Psychological Bulletin, 10*(6), 237–244.

Trankell, A. (1955). Aspects of genetics in psychology. *American Journal of Human Genetics, 7,* 264–276.

Treatikoff, C. (1974). Thesis for doctorate in medicine, 1919. In J. Marks (Ed.), *The treatment of Parkinsonism with L-dopa.* Lancaster, England: MTP Medical and Technical Publishing.

Treisman, A. M., & Gelade, G. (1980). A feature-integration theory of attention. *Cognitive Psychology, 12*(1), 97–136.

Trimble, M. R. (1988). Body image and the temporal lobes. *British Journal of Psychiatry, 153*(Suppl. 2), 12–14.

Trinkaus, E., & Zimmerman, M. R. (1982). Trauma among the Shanidar Neandertals. *American Journal of Physical Anthropology, 57,* 61–76.

Troster, A. I., Jacobs, D., Butters, N., Cullum. M., & Salmon, D. P. (1989). Differentiating Alzheimer's disease with the Wechsler Memory Scale-Revised. In F. J. Pirozzolo (Ed.), *Clinics in geriatric medicine (Vol. 5, No. 3).* Philadelphia: W. B. Saunders.

Tsai, L. Y. (1982). Handedness in autistic children and their families. *Journal of Autism and Developmental Disorders, 12*(4), 421–423.

Tsal, Y., Shalev, L., Zakay, D., & Lubow, R. E. (1994). Attention reduces perceived brightness contrast. *Quarterly Journal of Experimental Psychology: Human Experimental Psychology, 47A*(4), 865–893.

Tucha, O., Steup, A., Smely, C., & Lange, K. W. (1997). Toe agnosia in Gerstmann syndrome. *Journal of Neurology, Neurosurgery and Psychiatry, 63*(3), 399–403.

Tucker, D. M., Watson, R. T., & Heilman, K. M. (1977). Discrimination and evocation of affectively intoned speech in patients with right parietal disease. *Neurology, 27*(10), 947–958.

Umilta, C. (2001). Mechanisms of attention. In B. Rapp (Ed.), *The handbook of cognitive neuropsychology: What deficits reveal about the human mind.* Philadelphia: Psychology Press/Taylor and Francis.

Umilta, C., Bagnara, S., & Simion, F. (1978). Laterality effects for simple and complex geometrical figures and nonsense patterns. *Neuropsychologia, 16,* 165–174.

Vakil, E., Grunhaus, L., Nagar, I., Ben-Chaim, E., Dolberg, O. T., Dannon, P. N., et al. (2000). The effect of electroconvulsive therapy (ECT) on implicit memory: Skill learning and perceptual priming in patients with major depression. *Neuropsychologia, 38*(10), 1405–1414.

Valenza, N., Ptak, R., Zimine, I., Badan, M., Lazeyras, F., & Schnider, A. (2001). Dissociated active and passive tactile shape recognition: A case study of pure tactile apraxia. *Brain, 124*(Pt. 11), 2287–2298.

van der Lely, H. K., & Stollwerck, L. (1996). A grammatical specific language impairment in children: An autosomal dominant inheritance? *Brain and Language, 52*(3), 484–504.

van der Linden, G. J. H., Stein, D. J., & van Balkom, A. J. L. M. (2000). The efficacy of the selective serotonin reuptake inhibitors for social anxiety disorder (social phobia): A meta-analysis of randomized controlled trials. *International Clinical Psychopharmacology, 15*(Suppl. 2), S15–S23.

van Gelder, R. S., & Borod, J. C. (1990). Neurobiological and cultural aspects of facial asymmetry. *Journal of Communication Disorders, 23*(4–5), 273–286.

van Strien, J. W., Bouma, A., & Bakker, D. J. (1987). Birth stress, autoimmune diseases, and handedness. *Journal of Clinical and Experimental Neuropsychology, 9*(6), 775–780.

Varma, T. R. (1979). Ultrasound evidence of early pregnancy failure in patients with multiple conceptions. *British Journal of Obstetrics and Gynaecology, 86*(4), 290–292.

Vecera, S. P., & Gilds, K. S. (1998). What processing is impaired in apperceptive agnosia? Evidence from normal subjects. *Journal of Cognitive Neuroscience, 10*(5), 568–580.

Velasco, M., Velasco, F., Velasco, A. L., Brito, F., Jimenez, F., Marque, L., et al. (1997). Electrocortical and behavioral responses produced by acute electrical stimulation of the human centromedian thalamic nucleus. *Electroencephalography and Clinical Neurophysiology, 102*(6), 461–471.

Vellutino, F. R. (1987). Dyslexia. *Scientific American. 256*(3), 34–41.

Vessie, P. R. (1932). On the transmission of Huntington's chorea for 300 years: The Bures family group. *Journal of Nervous and Mental Disorders, 76,* 533–565.

Vignolo, L. A. (1996). Auditory perceptual disorders. In J. G. Beaumont, P. M. Kenealy, & M. J. C. Rogers (Eds.), *The Blackwell dictionary of neuropsychology* (pp. 128–133). Cambridge, MA: Blackwell Publishers.

Vignolo, L. A., Boccardi, E., & Caverni, L. (1986). Unexpected CT-scan findings in global aphasia. *Cortex, 22*(1), 55–69.

Villarreal, G., Hamilton, D. A., Petropoulos, H., Driscoll, I., Rowland, L. M., Griego, J. A., et al. (2002). Reduced hippocampal volume and total white matter volume in posttraumatic stress disorder. *Biological Psychiatry, 52*(2), 119–125.

Villarreal, G., Petropoulos, H., Hamilton, D. A., Rowland, L. M., Horan, W. P., Griego, J. A., et al. (2002). Proton magnetic resonance spectroscopy of the hippocampus and occipital white matter in PTSD: Preliminary results. *Canadian Journal of Psychiatry, 47*(7), 666–670.

Vles, J. S., Grubben, C. P., & Hoogland, H. J. (1989). Handedness not related to foetal position. *Neuropsychologia, 27*(7), 1017–1018.

Volpe, B. T., Sidtis, J. J., Holtzman, J. D., Wilson, D. H., & Gazzaniga, M. S. (1982). Cortical mechanisms involved in praxis: Observations following partial and complete section of the corpus callosum in man. *Neurology, 32*(6), 645–650.

von Economo, C. V., & Horn, L. (1930). Uber Windungsrelief, Masse, and Rindernarchitektonik der Supratemporalflache, ihre individuellen und ihre Seitenunterschiede. *Zeitschrift fur Neurologie and Psychiatrie, 130,* 678–757.

Vroon, P. A., Timmers, H., & Tempelaars, S. (1977). On the hemispheric representation of time. In S. Dornic (Ed.), *Attention and performance VI: Procedings of the Sixth International Symposium on Attention and Performance.* Hillsdale, NJ: Erlbaum.

Vymazal, J., Righini, A., Brooks, R. A., Canesi, M., Mariani, C., Leonardi, M., et al. (1999). T1 and T2 in the brain of healthy subjects, patients with Parkinson disease, and patients with multiple system atrophy: Relation to iron content. *Radiology, 211*(2), 489–495.

Wada, J., & Rasmussen, T. (1960). Intracarotid injection of sodium amytal for the lateralization of speech dominance. *Journal of Neurosurgery, 17,* 266–282.

Wada, J. A., Clarke, R., & Hamm, A. (1975). Cerebral hemispheric asymmetry in humans: Cortical speech zones in 100 adults and 100 infant brains. *Archives of Neurology, 32*(4), 239–246.

Walsh, V. (2000). Hemispheric asymmetries: A brain in two minds. *Current Biology, 10*(12), R460–R462.

Warrington, E. K. (1982). Neuropsychological studies of object recognition. *Philosophical Transactions of the Royal Society of London, Series B, 295,* 411–423.

Warrington, E. K., & McCarthy, R. A. (1994). Multiple meaning systems in the brain: A case for visual semantics. *Neuropsychologia, 32*(12), 1465–1473.

Warrington, E. K., & Rudge, P. (1995). "Apperceptive visual agnosia: A case study": Comment. *Brain and Cognition, 28*(2), 173–177.

Warrington, E. K., & Shallice, T. (1984). Category specific semantic impairments. *Brain, 107*(Pt. 3), 829–854.

Warrington, E. K., & Taylor, A. M. (1973). The contribution of the right parietal lobe to object recognition. *Cortex, 9*(2), 152–164.

Watanabe, M. (1996). Reward expectancy in primate prefrontal neurons [see comments]. *Nature, 382*(6592), 629–632.

Watanabe, M. (1998). Cognitive and motivational operations in primate prefrontal neurons. *Review of Neuroscience, 9*(4), 225–241.

Watkins, K. E., Paus, T., Lerch, J. P., Zijdenbos, A., Collins, D. L., Neelin, P., et al. (2001). Structural asymmetries in the human brain: A voxel-based statistical analysis of 142 MRI scans. *Cerebral Cortex, 11*(9), 868–877.

Watson, J. B. (1924). *Behaviorism.* New York: Norton.

Webb, M., & Trzepacz, P. T. (1987). Huntington's disease: Correlations of mental status with chorea. *Biological Psychiatry, 22*(6), 751–761.

Webster, W. G., & Poulos, M. (1987). Handedness distributions among adults who stutter. *Cortex, 23*(4), 705–708.

Weintraub, S., Mesulam, M. M., & Kramer, L. (1981). Disturbances in prosody: A right-hemisphere contribution to language. *Archives of Neurology, 38*(12), 742–744.

Weiskrantz, L. (1995). Blindsight: Not an island unto itself. *Current Directions in Psychological Science, 4*(5), 146–151.

Wessinger, C. M., Buonocore, M. H., Kussmaul, C. L., & Mangun, G. R. (1997). Tonotopy in human auditory cortex examined with functional magnetic resonance imaging. *Human Brain Mapping, 5*(1), 18–25.

Westby, G. W., & Partridge, K. J. (1986). Human homing: Still no evidence despite geomagnetic controls. *Journal of Experimental Biology, 120,* 325–331.

Wild, B., Erb, M., & Bartels, M. (2001). Are emotions contagious? Evoked emotions while viewing emotionally expressive faces: Quality, quantity, time course and gender differences. *Psychiatry Research, 102*(2), 109–124.

Wilkins, W. K., & Wakefield, J. (1995). Brain evolution and neurolinguistic preconditions. *Behavioral and Brain Sciences, 18*(1) 161–226.

Wills, K. (1993). Neuropsychological characteristics of children with spina bifida/hydrocephalus. *Journal of Clinical Child Psychology, 22*(2), 247–265.

Wilson, C. M., Grace, G. M., Munoz, D. G., He, B. P., & Strong, M. J. (2001). Cognitive impairment in sporadic als: A pathologic continuum underlying a multisystem disorder. *Neurology, 57*(4), 651–657.

Wilson, D. (1872). Righthandedness. *The Canadian Journal, 75,* 193–203.

Winocur, G., Kinsbourne, M., & Moscovitch, M. (1981). The effect of cuing on release from proactive interference in korsakoff amnesic patients. *Journal of Experimental Psychology [Human Learning], 7*(1), 56–65.

Witelson, S. F., & Pallie, W. (1973). Left hemisphere specialization for language in the newborn. Neuroanatomical evidence of asymmetry. *Brain, 96*(3), 641–646.

Wolf, P. & Cobb, J. (1991). Left-handedness and life expectancy: Letter. *New England Journal of Medicine, 325,* 1042.

Wood, L. C., & Cooper, D. S. (1992). Autoimmune thyroid disease, left-handedness, and developmental dyslexia. *Psychoneuroendocrinology, 17*(1), 95–99.

Woolf, L. I. (1986). The heterozygote advantage in phenylketonuria. *American Journal of Human Genetics, 38*(5), 773–775.

Wright, L. (1995). Double mystery. *The New Yorker* (August 7), 45–62.

Wright, P., Williams, J., Currie, C., & Beattie, T. (1996). Left-handedness increases injury risk in adolescent girls. *Perceptual and Motor Skills, 82*(3, Pt. 1), 855–858.

Wright, R. (1995). The evolution of despair. *Time, 146*(9), 50–57.

Yarnell, P. R., & Lynch, S. (1970). Retrograde memory immediately after concussion. *Lancet, 1*(7652), 863–864.

Yeo, R. A., Gangestad, S. W., Thoma, R., Shaw, P., & Repa, K. (1997). Developmental instability and cerebral lateralization. *Neuropsychology, 11*(4), 552–561.

Young, A., & Willatts, S. (1998). Controversies in management of acute brain trauma. *Lancet, 352*(9123), 164–166.

Young, R. M. (1990). *Mind, brain and adaptation in the nineteenth century.* New York: Oxford University Press.

Yurgelun-Todd, D. A., Gruber, S. A., Kanayama, G., Killgore, W. D., Baird, A. A., & Young, A. D. (2000). fMRI during affect discrimination in bipolar affective disorder. *Bipolar Disorders, 2*(3, Pt. 2), 237–248.

Zaidel, D., & Sperry, R. W. (1977). Some long-term motor effects of cerebral commissurotomy in man. *Neuropsychologia, 15*(2), 193–204.

Zeki, S. (1983). The distribution of wavelength and orientation selective cells in different areas of monkey visual cortex. *Proceedings of the Royal Society of London: Series B, Biological Sciences, 217*(1209), 449–470.

Zhang, G., & Simon, H. A. (1985). STM capacity for Chinese words and idioms: Chunking and acoustical loop hypotheses. *Memory and Cognition, 13*(3), 193–201.

Zillmer, E. A., & Spiers, M. V. (2001). *Principles of human neuropsychology.* Toronto, Canada: Wadsworth.

Zimmerman, A. M., Abrams, M. T., Giuliano, J. D., Denckla, M. B., & Singer, H. S. (2000). Subcorticol volumes in girls with Tourette syndrome: Support for a gender effect. *Neurology, 54*(12), 2224–2229.

Zoccolotti, P., Passafiume, D., & Pizzamiglio, L. (1979). Hemispheric superiorities on a unilateral tactile test: Relationship to cognitive dimensions. *Perceptual and Motor Skills, 49*(3), 735–742.

Zola-Morgan, S., Squire, L. R., & Amaral, D. G. (1986). Human amnesia and the medial temporal region: Enduring memory impairment following a bilateral lesion limited to field CA1 of the hippocampus. *Journal of Neuroscience, 6*(10), 2950–2967.

Grow Your Own Phantom Hand!

Complete instructions for this experiment appear on page 165.

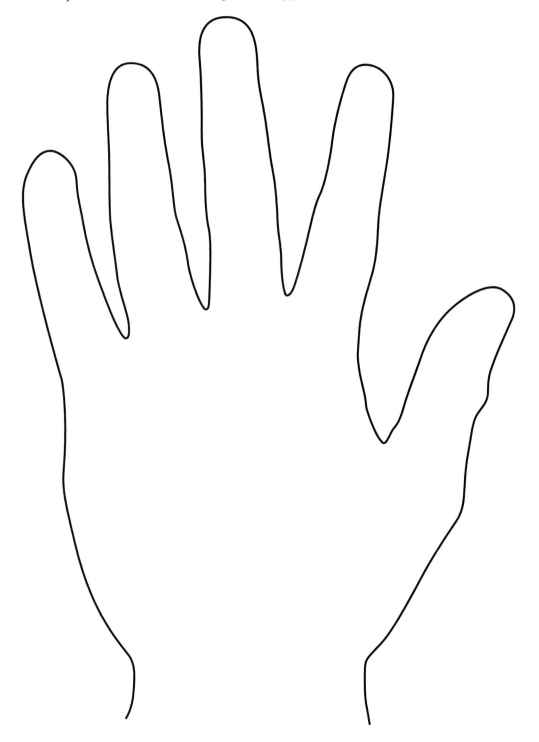

Index